National Key Book Publishing Planning Project of the 13th Five-Year Plan

“十 三 五” 国 家 重 点 图 书 出 版 规 划 项 目

International Clinical Medicine Series Based on the Belt and Road Initiative

“一 带 一 路” 背 景 下 国 际 化 临 床 医 学 丛 书

Surgery

外科学（下）

Chief Editors Ma Qingyong Liang Guiyou Bai Yuting Qiu Xinguang Wang Wenjun Wu Xuedong

主编 马清涌 梁贵友 白育庭 邱新光 王文军 吴学东

郑州大学出版社

ZHENGZHOU UNIVERSITY PRESS

图书在版编目(CIP)数据

外科学 = Surgery：英文 / 马清涌等主编. — 郑州：郑州大学出版社，2020. 12
(“一带一路”背景下国际化临床医学丛书)
ISBN 978-7-5645-7692-9

Ⅰ. ①外… Ⅱ. ①马… Ⅲ. ①外科学 - 英文 Ⅳ. ①R6

中国版本图书馆 CIP 数据核字(2020)第 272606 号

外科学 = Surgery：英文

项目负责人	孙保营　杨秦予	策划编辑	李龙传
责任编辑	陈文静	装帧设计	苏永生
责任校对	张彦勤	责任监制	凌　青　李瑞卿

出版发行	郑州大学出版社有限公司	地　　址	郑州市大学路 40 号(450052)
出 版 人	孙保营	网　　址	http://www.zzup.cn
经　　销	全国新华书店	发行电话	0371-66966070
印　　刷	河南文华印务有限公司		
开　　本	850 mm×1 168 mm　1 / 16		
总 印 张	77.25	总 字 数	2 976 千字
版　　次	2020 年 12 月第 1 版	印　　次	2020 年 12 月第 1 次印刷

书　　号	ISBN 978-7-5645-7692-9	总 定 价	389.00 元(上、下)

Staff of Expert Steering Committee

专家指导委员会

Staff of Editor Steering Committee

编审委员会

Editorial Staff

Honorary Chief Editor

Li Yuming Lanzhou University

Chief Editors

Ma Qingyong The First Affiliated Hospital of Xi' an Jiaotong University
Liang Guiyou Guizhou Medcial University
Bai Yuting Hubei University of Science and Technology
Qiu Xinguang The First Affiliated Hospital of Zhengzhou University
Wang Wenjun The First Affiliated Hospital of University of South China
Wu Xuedong The First Affiliated Hospital of Dali University

Vice Chief Editors

Ma Zhenhua The First Affiliated Hospital of Xi' an Jiaotong University
Wang Shufeng The First Affiliated Hospital of Xi' an Jiaotong University
Fan Jinhai The First Affiliated Hospital of Xi' an Jiaotong University
Cao Gang The Second Affiliated Hospital of Xi' an Jiaotong University
Wang Tuo The First Affiliated Hospital of Xi' an Jiaotong University
Wang Zheng The First Affiliated Hospital of Xi' an Jiaotong University
Wang Cheng The First Affiliated Hospital of University of South China

Editorial Board Member

Bai Hongliang The First Affiliated Hospital of Xi' an Jiaotong University
Cai Qingyong The Affiliated Hospital of Zunyi Medical University
Chen Chen The First Affiliated Hospital of Xi' an Jiaotong University
Chen Wei The First Affiliated Hospital of University of South China
Chen Zhiwei The First Affiliated Hospital of University of South China
Cui Feibo The First Affiliated Hospital of Xi' an Jiaotong University
Cui Juncheng The First Affiliated Hospital of University of South China
Dai Zhu The First Affiliated Hospital of University of South China
Deng Youwen The Third Xiangya Hospital of Central South University
Ding Chenguang The First Affiliated Hospital of Xi' an Jiaotong University
Ding Xiaoming The First Affiliated Hospital of Xi' an Jiaotong University
Fan Lin The First Affiliated Hospital of Xi' an Jiaotong University
Fan Weijie The First Affiliated Hospital of University of South China

Gao Hui	Hubei University of Science and Technology
Gao Jie	The First Affiliated Hospital of Xi'an Jiaotong University
Geng Zhimin	The First Affiliated Hospital of Xi'an Jiaotong University
Huang Jun	The Second Xiangya Hospital of Central South University
Huo Xiongwei	The First Affiliated Hospital of Xi'an Jiaotong University
Ke Xixian	The Affiliated Hospital of Zunyi Medical University
Li Jian	The Affiliated Hospital of Guizhou Medical University
Li Junhui	The Second Affiliated Hospital of Xi'an Jiaotong University
Li Ruichun	The First Affiliated Hospital of Xi'an Jiaotong University
Li Shaobo	The First Affiliated Hospital of Dali University
Liu Daxing	The Affiliated Hospital of Zunyi Medical University
Liu Qing	The Third Xiangya Hospital of Central South University
Liu Senyuan	The First Affiliated Hospital of Zhengzhou University
Liu Yang	The Second Affiliated Hospital of Xi'an Jiaotong University
Lu Le	The Second Affiliated Hospital of Xi'an Jiaotong University
Ma Xing	The First Affiliated Hospital of Xi'an Jiaotong University
Mao Ping	The First Affiliated Hospital of Xi'an Jiaotong University
Mao Xinzhan	The Second Xiangya Hospital of Central South University
Ouyang Zhihua	The First Affiliated Hospital of University of South China
Qi Lei	The First Affiliated Hospital of Xi'an Jiaotong University
Qiu Guanglin	The First Affiliated Hospital of Xi'an Jiaotong University
Qu Kai	The First Affiliated Hospital of Xi'an Jiaotong University
Shan Tao	The Second Affiliated Hospital of Xi'an Jiaotong University
Shen Xin	The First Affiliated Hospital of Xi'an Jiaotong University
Song Yongchun	The First Affiliated Hospital of Xi'an Jiaotong University
Wang Ning	The First Affiliated Hospital of Dali University
Wang Suoliang	The First Affiliated Hospital of Xi'an Jiaotong University
Wang Wei	The First Affiliated Hospital of Xi'an Jiaotong University
Wu Tao	The Second Affiliated Hospital of Xi'an Jiaotong University
Xu Gang	The Affiliated Hospital of Zunyi Medical University
Xu Kedong	The First Affiliated Hospital of Xi'an Jiaotong University
Xue Wujun	The First Affiliated Hospital of Xi'an Jiaotong University
Yan Yiguo	The First Affiliated Hospital of University of South China
Yao Nüzhao	The First Affiliated Hospital of University of South China
Yi Guoliang	The First Affiliated Hospital of University of South China
Yin Ke	The First Affiliated Hospital of University of South China
Zha Wenliang	Hubei University of Science and Technology
Zhang Dong	The First Affiliated Hospital of Xi'an Jiaotong University
Zhang Hanchong	Shenzhen People's Hospital
Zhang Yangchun	The First Affiliated Hospital of University of South China
Zheng Jianbao	The First Affiliated Hospital of Xi'an Jiaotong University
Zheng Xin	The First Affiliated Hospital of Xi'an Jiaotong University

Zhu Guodong The First Affiliated Hospital of Xi' an Jiaotong University
Zhu Yulin The First Affiliated Hospital of Xi' an Jiaotong University

Editor

Sun Wenjuan The First Affiliated Hospital of Xi' an Jiaotong University

作者名单

名誉主编

李玉民　　兰州大学

主　编

马清涌　　西安交通大学第一附属医院
梁贵友　　贵州医科大学
白育庭　　湖北科技学院
邱新光　　郑州大学第一附属医院
王文军　　南华大学附属第一医院
吴学东　　大理大学第一附属医院

副主编

马振华　　西安交通大学第一附属医院
王曙逢　　西安交通大学第一附属医院
范晋海　　西安交通大学第一附属医院
曹　罡　　西安交通大学第二附属医院
王　拓　　西安交通大学第一附属医院
王　铮　　西安交通大学第一附属医院
王　程　　南华大学附属第一医院

编　委　（以姓氏汉语拼音排序）

柏宏亮　　西安交通大学第一附属医院
蔡庆勇　　遵义医科大学附属医院
陈　晨　　西安交通大学第一附属医院
陈　魏　　南华大学附属第一医院
陈志伟　　南华大学附属第一医院
崔飞博　　西安交通大学第一附属医院
崔俊成　　南华大学附属第一医院
戴　祝　　南华大学附属第一医院
邓幼文　　中南大学湘雅三医院
丁晨光　　西安交通大学第一附属医院
丁小明　　西安交通大学第一附属医院
樊　林　　西安交通大学第一附属医院
范伟杰　　南华大学附属第一医院

高　卉　湖北科技学院
高　洁　西安交通大学第一附属医院
耿智敏　西安交通大学第一附属医院
黄　俊　中南大学湘雅二医院
霍雄伟　西安交通大学第一附属医院
柯希贤　遵义医科大学附属医院
李　剑　贵州医科大学附属医院
李军辉　西安交通大学第二附属医院
李瑞春　西安交通大学第一附属医院
李绍波　大理大学第一附属医院
刘达兴　遵义医科大学附属医院
刘　擎　中南大学湘雅三医院
刘森源　郑州大学第一附属医院
刘　阳　西安交通大学第二附属医院
卢　乐　西安交通大学第二附属医院
马　兴　西安交通大学第一附属医院
冒　平　西安交通大学第一附属医院
毛新展　中南大学湘雅二医院
欧阳智华　南华大学附属第一医院
祁　磊　西安交通大学第一附属医院
仇广林　西安交通大学第一附属医院
曲　凯　西安交通大学第一附属医院
单　涛　西安交通大学第二附属医院
申　新　西安交通大学第一附属医院
宋永春　西安交通大学第一附属医院
王　宁　大理大学第一附属医院
王锁良　西安交通大学第一附属医院
王　炜　西安交通大学第一附属医院
吴　涛　西安交通大学第二附属医院
徐　刚　遵义医科大学附属医院
许克东　西安交通大学第一附属医院
薛武军　西安交通大学第一附属医院
晏怡果　南华大学附属第一医院
姚女兆　南华大学附属第一医院
易国良　南华大学附属第一医院
尹　科　南华大学附属第一医院
查文良　湖北科技学院
张　东　西安交通大学第一附属医院
张晗翀　深圳市人民医院
张阳春　南华大学附属第一医院
郑见宝　西安交通大学第一附属医院
郑　鑫　西安交通大学第一附属医院

朱国栋　　西安交通大学第一附属医院
朱宇麟　　西安交通大学第一附属医院

编　辑

孙文娟　　西安交通大学第一附属医院

Preface

At the Second Belt and Road Summit Forum on International Cooperation in 2019 and the Seventy-third World Health Assembly in 2020, General Secretary Xi Jinping stated the importance for promoting the construction of the "Belt and Road" and jointly build a community for human health. Countries and regions along the "Belt and Road" have a large number of overseas Chinese communities, and shared close geographic proximity, similarities in culture, disease profiles and medical habits. They also shared a profound mass base with ample space for cooperation and exchange in Clinical Medicine. The publication of the International Clinical Medicine series for clinical researchers, medical teachers and students in countries along the "Belt and Road" is a concrete measure to promote the exchange of Chinese and foreign medical science and technology with mutual appreciation and reciprocity.

Zhengzhou University Press coordinated more than 600 medical experts from over 160 renowned medical research institutes, medical schools and clinical hospitals across China. It produced this set of medical tools in English to serve the needs for the construction of the "Belt and Road". It comprehensively coversaspects in the theoretical framework and clinical practicesin Clinical Medicine, including basic science, multiple clinical specialities and social medicine. It reflects the latest academic and technological developments, and the international frontiers of academic advancements in Clinical Medicine. It shared with the world China's latest diagnosis and therapeutic approaches, clinical techniques, and experiences in prescription and medication. It has an important role in disseminating contemporary Chinese medical science and technology innovations, demonstrating the achievements of modern China's economic and social development, and promoting the unique charm of Chinese culture to the world.

The series is the first set of medical tools written in English by Chinese medical experts to serve the needs of the "Belt and Road" construction. It systematically and comprehensively reflects the Chinese characteristics in Clinical Medicine. Also, it presents a landmark achievement in the implementation of the "Belt and Road" initiative in promoting exchanges in medical science and technology. This series is theoretical in nature, with each volume built on the mainlines in traditional disciplines but at the same time introducing contemporary theories that guide clinical practices, diagnosis and treatment methods, echoing the latest research findings in Clinical Medicine.

As the disciplines in Clinical Medicine rapidly advances, different views on knowledge, inclusiveness, and medical ethics may arise. We hope this work will facilitate the exchange of ideas, build common ground while allowing differences, and contribute to the building of a community for human health in a broad spectrum of disciplines and research focuses.

Nick Lemoine

Foreign Academician of the Chinese Academy of Engineering

Dean, Academy of Medical Sciences of Zhengzhou University

Director, Barts Cancer Institute, London, UK

6th August, 2020

Foreword

With the development of medical international communication and education in China, there is an urgent need for an English version of surgery textbooks to meet the domestic demand for clinical medical English teaching in the current Chinese education system. In view of this, we compiled this textbook, together with 9 medical colleges and universities in China. In the process of compiling, we use the syllabus of undergraduates in clinical medicine as the basis, draw on the contents of the Chinese version of the textbook of surgery, and refer to the presentation, typesetting and professional vocabulary of textbooks in overseas medical schools. On the basis of following the principles of surgical treatment, this book highlights the characteristics of disease spectrum, diagnosis and treatment in China. We wish this book could be used as a bridge and link between domestic and foreign surgeon training methods, and could be widely used in medical schools in China.

The content of the book is mainly for international students and undergraduates, while it can also be used for the continuing education of domestic undergraduates and graduate students. We believe this book can bring you professional improvement. At the same time, we hope everyone can improve their English level. Regarding the shortcomings in the book, we really appreciate if you can give us valuable advices.

Authors

Contents

Part 27 Stomach and Duodenum

Part 28 Ileus and Bowel Obstruction

Part 29 The Appendix

Part 30 Anorectal Disease

Part 31 Liver Diseases

Part 32 Portal Hypertension

Part 33 Biliary Tract Disease

Part 34 Pancreas Disease

Part 35 Upper Gastrointestinal Hemorrhage

Part 36 Spleen Diseases

Part 37 Arterial Aneurysms

Part 38 The Diseases of Veins and Lymphoduct

Part 39 Anatomy of the Genitourinary Tract

Part 40 Development Anomalies of the Urologic and Male Genital Tract

Part 41 Urinary Tract Trauma

Part 42 Urinary Tract and Male Genital Infections

Part 43 Genitourinary Tuberculosis

Part 44 Urinary Tract Obstruction

Part 45 Urolithiasis

Part 46 Urologic and Male Genital Tumors

Part 47 Other Diseases and Disorders of Genitourinary Tract

Part 48 General Principles of Fracture Treatment

Part 49 Fractures of Upper Limb

Part 50 Fracture of Lower Limb

Part 51 Fracture and Dislocations of the Pelvis

Part 52 Fracture of the Spine

Part 53 Arthrosis Dislocation

Part 54 Chronic Lacomotor System Damnification

Part 55 Purulent Infection of Bone and Joint

Part 56 Pain Syndrome of Low Back and Leg

Part 57 Bone and Joint Tuberculosis

Part 58 Tumors of the Bone

Part 59 Musculoskeletal Malformation

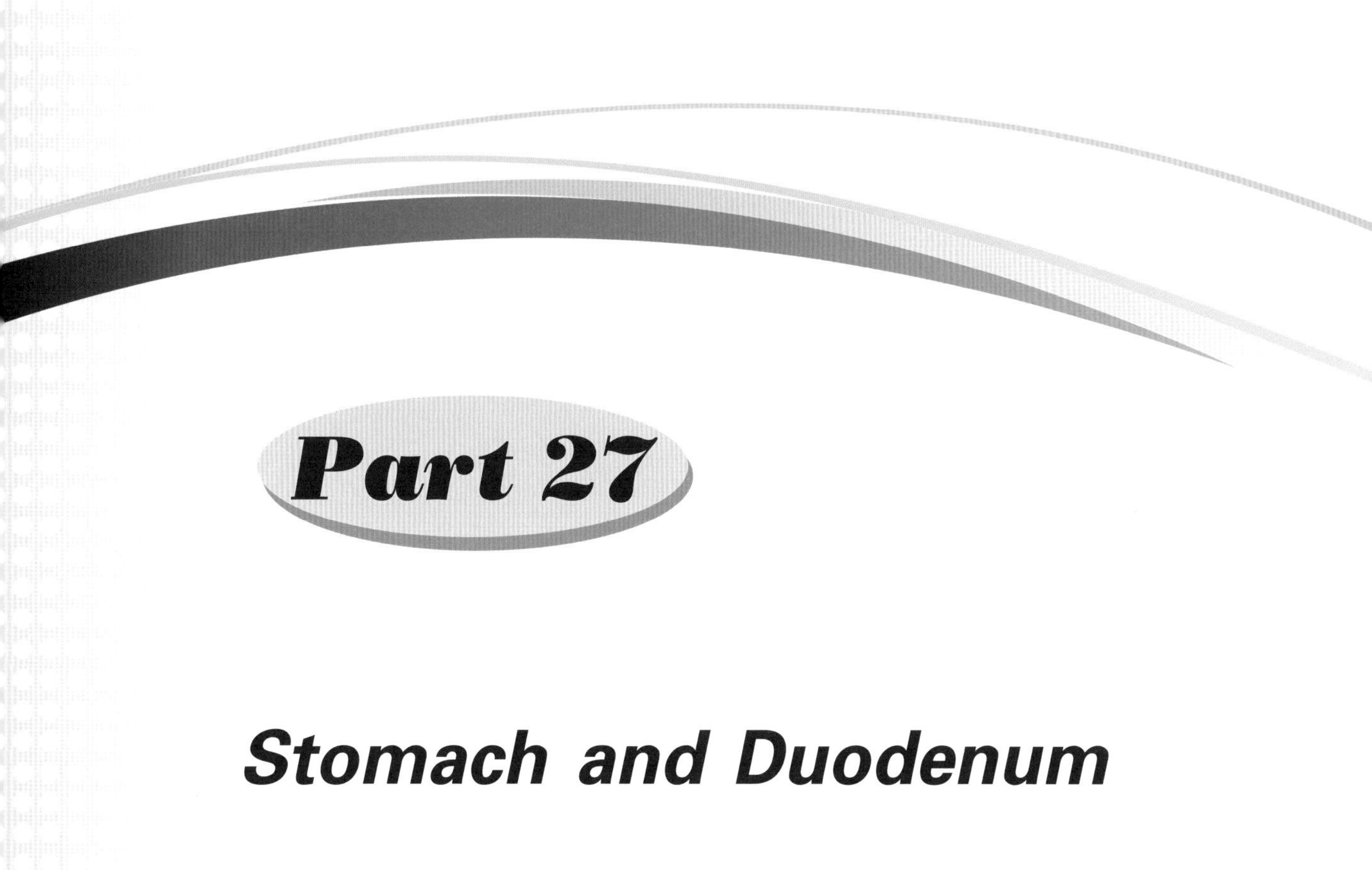

Stomach and Duodenum

Chapter 1

Duodenal Ulcer

1.1 Clinical Findings

1.1.1 Symptoms and signs

Pain, the presenting symptom in most patients, is usually located in the epigastrium and is variably described as aching, burning, or gnawing. Radiologic survey studies indicated, however, that some patients with active duodenal ulcer have no gastrointestinal complaints.

The daily cycle of the pain is often characteristic. The patient usually has no pain in the morning until an hour or more after breakfast. The pain is relived by the noon meal, only to recur in the later afternoon. Pain may appear again in the evening, and in about half of cases it arouses the patient during the night. Food, milk, or antacid preparations give temporary relief.

When the ulcer penetrates the head of the pancreas posteriorly, back pain is not relieved, concomitantly, the cyclic pattern of pain may change to a more steady discomfort, with less relief from food and antacids.

Varying degrees of nausea and vomiting are common. Vomiting may be a major feature even in the absence of obstruction.

The abdominal examination may reveal localized epigastric tenderness to the right of the midline, but in many instances no tenderness can be elicited.

1.1.2 Endoscopy

Gastroduodenoscopy is useful in evaluating patients withan uncertain diagnosis those with bleeding from the upper intestine, and those who have obstruction of the gastroduodenal segment and for assessing response to therapy.

1.1.3 Diagnosis test

(1) Gastric analysis: A gastric analysis may be indicated in certain cases. The standard gastric analysis consists of the following: ①Measurement of acid production by the unstimulated stomach under basal fasting

conditions; the result is expressed as H^+ secretion in mEq/h and is termed the basal acid output (BAO). ②Measurement of acid production during stimulation by histamine or pentagastrin given in a dose maximal for this effect. The result is expressed as H^+ secretion in mEq/h and is termed the maximal acid output (MAO).

(2) Serum gastrin: Depending on the laboratory, normal basal gastric levels average 50-100 pg/mL, and levels over 200 pg/mL can almost always be considered high.

Gastrin concentration may raise in hypo secretory and hypersecretory states. In the former conditions (e. g., atrophic gastritis, pernicious anemia), the cause is higher antral pH with loss of antral inhibition for gastrin release. More important clinically is elevated gastrin levels with concomitant hypersecretion, where the high gastrin level is responsible for the increased acid and resulting peptic ulceration. The best defined clinical condition in this category is Zollinger-Ellison syndrome (gastrinoma).

A fasting serum gastrin determination should be obtained in patients with peptic ulcer disease that is unusually severe or refractory to therapy.

1.1.4 Radiographic studies

On an upper gastrointestinal series, the changes induced by duodenal ulcer consist of duodenal deformities and an ulcer niche. Inflammatory swelling and scarring may lead to distortion of the duodenal bulb, eccentricity of the pyloric channel, or pseudodiverticulum formation. The ulcer itself may be seen either in profile or, more commonly, enface.

1.2 Treatment

Acute duodenal ulcer can be controlled by suppressing acid secretion in most patients, but the long term course of the disease (i. e., frequency of relapses and of complications) is unaffected unless H pylori infection is eradicated. Surgical therapy is recommended principally for the treatment of complications; bleeding, perforation, or obstruction.

1.2.1 Medical treatment

The goals of medical therapy are to heal the ulcer and to cure the disease. Treatment in the first category is aimed at decreasing acid secretion or neutralizing acid. The principal drugs consist of H_2 receptor antagonists (e. g., cimetidine, ranititdine) and proton pump blockers (e. g., omeprazole). One of the H_2 receptor antagonists is usually the first choice, and when given in therapeutic doses, it will bring about healing of the ulcer in 80% of patients within 6 weeks. Omeprazole is reserved for patients whose ulcers are refractory to H_2 antagonists or for those with Zollinger-Ellison syndrome. Antacids may be use alternatively as primary therapy or on an as needed basis to treat ulcer pain. Antacids are just as effective as H_2 receptor antagonists but slightly more difficult to administer.

After the ulcer has healed, discontinuation of therapy results in an 80% recurrence rate within 1 year, which may be avoided by chronic nighttime administration of a single dose of H_2 receptor antagonists. A better approach is to treat the H pylori infection along with the ulcer, since eradication of H pylori eliminates recurrent ulceration unless the infection recurs an uncommon event. At present, the optimal daily regimen consists of the following combination of drugs. ① An H_2 receptor antagonists (e. g., cimetidine, 1.2g). ② A bismuth compound (Pepto-Bismol, 8 tablets; De-Nol). ③ Tetracycline, 2 g. ④metronidazole, 750 mg. The

H_2 receptor antagonists is given until the ulcer has healed or for 16 weeks. The last three drugs are given for 3 weeks.

1.2.2 Surgical treatment

If medical treatment has been optimal, a persistent ulcer may be judged intractable, and surgical treatment is indicated. This is now uncommon.

The surgical procedures that can cure peptic ulcer are aimed at reduction of gastric acid secretion. Excision of the ulcer itself is not sufficient for either duodenal or gastric ulcer, recurrence is nearly inevitable with such procedures.

The surgical methods of treating duodenal ulcer are vagotomy (several varieties) and antrectomy plus vagotomy. All of these procedures can be performed laparoscopically. With rare exceptions, on of the vagotomy operations is sufficient.

1.2.2.1 Vagotomy

Truncal vagotomy consists of resection of a 1 or 2 cm segment of each vagal trunk as it enters the abdomen on the distal esophagus. The resulting vagal denervation of the stomach in many patients unless a drainage procedure is performed. The method of drainage most often selected is pyloroplasty (Heinek Mikulicz procedure), gastrojejunostomy is used less often. Both procedures give a superior functional result, and pyloroplasty is less time consuming.

Vagal denervation of just the parietal cell area of the stomach is called parietal cell vagotomy or proximal gastric vagotomy. The technique spares the main nerves of latarjet but divides all vagal branches that terminate on the proximal two thirds of the stomach. Since antral innervation is preserved, gastric emptying is relatively normal, and a drainage procedure is unnecessary. Nevertheless, parietal cell vagotomy plus pyloroplasty gives better results (i. e., fewer recurrent ulcers) than parietal cell vagotomy alone. Pariteal cell vagotomy appears to have about the same effectiveness as truncal or selective vagotomy for curing the ulcer disease, but dumping and diarrhea are much less frequent. It is probably the procedure of choice for intractable and perforated duodenal ulcers and is relatively less useful for obstructing and bleeding ulcers.

The vagotomy procedures have the advantages of technical simplicity and preservation of the entire gastric reservoir capacity. The principal disadvantage is recurrent ulceration in about 10% of patients. The recurrence ulceration rate after parietal cell vagotomy is about twice as high in patients with prepyloric ulcer, and most surgeons use different operation for an ulcer in this location.

1.2.2.2 Antrectomy and vagotomy

This operation entails a distal gastrectomy of 50% of the stomach with the line of gastric transection carried high on the lesser curvature to conform with the boundary of the gastrin producing mucosa.

The terms antrectomy and hemigastrectomy are loosely synonymous. The proximal remnant may be reanastomosed to the duodenum (Billroth Ⅰ resection) or to the side of the proximal jejunum (Billroth Ⅱ resection). The Billroth Ⅰ technique is most popular, but there is no conclusive evidence that the results are superior. When creating a Billroth Ⅱ (gastrojejunostomy) reconstruction, the surgeon may bring the jejunal loop up to the gastric remnant either anterior to the transverse colon or posterior through a hole in the transverse mesocolon. Since either method is satisfactory, an antecolic anastomosis is elected in most cases because it is simpler. Truncal vagotomy is performed as described in the preceding section; antrectomy by itself will not prevent a high recurrence rate. In most instances the surgeon will be able to remove the ulcerated portion of duodenum in the course of the resection of duodenum in the course of resection.

Vagotomy and antrectomy is associated with a low incidence of marginal ulceration (2%) and a generally good overall outcome, but the risk of complications is higher than after vagotomy without resection.

1.2.2.3 Subtotal gastrectomy

This operation consists of resection of 2/3–3/4 of the distal stomach. After subtotal gastrectomy for duodenal ulcer, a Billroth Ⅱ reconstruction is preferable. Subtotal gastrectomy is largely of historical interest.

1.2.3 Complication of surgery for peptic ulcer

1.2.3.1 Early complications

Duodenal stump leakage, gastric retention, and hemorrhage may develop in the immediate postoperative period.

1.2.3.2 Late complications

(1) Recurrent ulcer (marginal ulcer, stomal ulcer, anastomotic ulcer)

Recurrent ulcers form in about 10% of duodenal ulcer patients treated by vagotomy and pyloroplasty or parietal cell vagotomy and in 2%–3% after vagotomy and antrectomy or subtotal gastrectomy. Recurrent ulcers nearly always develop immediately adjacent to the anastomosis on the intestinal side.

The usual complaint is upper abdominal pain, which is often aggravated by eating and improved by antacids. In some patients, the pain is felt more to the left in the epigastrium, and left axillary or shoulder pain is occasionally reported. About 1/3 of patients with stomach ulcer will experience major gastrointestinal hemorrhage. Free perforation is less common (5%).

Diagnosis and treatment are essentially the same as for the original ulcer.

(2) Gastrojejunocolic and gastrocolic fistula

A deeply eroding ulcer may occasionally produce a fistula between the stomach and colon. Most examples have resulted from recurrent peptic ulcer after an operation that included a gastrojejunal anastomosis.

Severe diarrhea and weight loss are the presenting symptoms in over 90% of cases. Abdominal pain typical of recurrent peptic ulcer often precedes the onset of the diarrhea. Bowel movements number 8–12 or more a day they are water and often contain particles of undigested food.

The degree of malnutrition ranges from mild to very severe. Laboratory studies reveal low serum proteins and manifestations of fluid and electrolyte depletion. Appropriate tests may reflect deficiencies in both water soluble and fatsoluble vitamins.

An upper gastrointestinal series reveals the marginal ulcer in only 50% of patients and the fistula in only 15%. Barium enema demonstrates the fistulous tract.

Initial treatment should replenish fluid and electrolyte deficits. The involved colon and ulcerated gastrojejunal segment should be excised and colonic continuity reestablished. Vagotomy, partial gastrectomy, or both are required to treat the ulcer diathesis and prevent another recurrent ulcer. Results are excellent in benign disease. In general, the outlook for patients with a malignant fistula is poor.

(3) Dumping syndrome

Symptoms of the dumping syndrome are noted to some extent by most patients who have an operation that impairs the ability of the stomach to regulate its rate of emptying, within several months. However, dumping is a clinical problem in only 1%–2% of patients. Symptoms fall into two categories, cardiovascular and gastrointestinal. Shortly after eating, the patient may experience palpitation, sweating, weakness, dyspnea, flushing, nausea, abdominal cramps, belching, vomiting, diarrhea, and rarely, syncope. The degree of severity varies widely, and not all symptoms are reported by all patients. In severe cases, the patient must lie down for 30–40 minutes until the discomfort passes.

Diet therapy to reduce jejunal osmolality is not successful in all but in a few cases. The diet should be low in carbohydrate and high in fat and protein content. Sugars and carbohydrates are least well tolerated, some patients are especially sensitive to milk. Meals should be taken dry, with fluids restricted to between meals. This dietary regimen ordinarily suffices, but anticholinergic drugs may be of help in some patients; others have reported improvement with supplemental pectin in the diet, and the use of somatostatin analogues offers some promise.

(4) Alkaline gastritis

Reflux of duodenal juices into the stomach is an invariable and usually innocuous situation after operations that interfere with pyloric function, but in some patients it may cause marked gastritis. The principle symptom is prostpransial pain, and the diagnosis rests on endoscopic and biopsy demonstration of an edematous inflamed gastric mucosa. Since a minor degree of gastritis is found in most patients after Billroth Ⅱ gastrectomy, the endoscopic findings are to some degree nonspecific. Persistent severe pain is an indication for surgical reconstruction. Roux-en-Y gastrojejunostomy with a 40 cm efferent jejunal limb is the treatment of choice.

(5) Anemia

Iron deficiency anemia develops in about 30% of patients within 5 years after partial gastrectomy. It is caused by failure to absorb food iron bound in an organic molecule. Before this diagnosis is accepted, the patient should be checked for blood loss, marginal ulcer, or an unsuspected blood loss, marginal ulcer, or an unsuspected tumor. Inorganic iron ferrous sulfate or ferrous gluconate is indicated for treatment and is absorbed normally after gastrectomy. VitaminB_{12} deficiency and megaloblastic anemia appear in a few cases after gastrectomy.

(6) Postvagotomy diarrhea

5%-10% of patients who have had truncal vagotomy require treatment with antidiarrheal agents at some time, and perhaps 1% are seriously troubled by this complication. The diarrhea may be episodic, in which case the onset is unpredictable after symptom free intervals of weeks to months. An attack may consist of only one or two watery movements or, in severe cases, may last for a few days. Other patients may continually produce 3-5 loose stools per day.

Most cases of postvagotomy diarrhea can be treated satisfactorily with constipating agents.

(7) Chronic gastroparesis

Chronic delayed gastric emptying is seen occasionally after gastric surgery. Prokinetic agents (e. g., metoclopramide) are often helpful, but some cases are refractory to any therapy except a completion gastrectomy and Roux-en-Y esophagojejunostomy (i. e., total gastrectomy).

Chapter 2

Gastric Ulcer

2.1 Clinical Findings

2.1.1 Symptoms and signs

The principal symptom is epigastric pain relived by food or duodenal ulcer. Epigastric tenderness is a variable finding. Compared with duodenal ulcer, the pain in gastric ulcer tends to appear earlier after eating, often within 30 minutes. Vomiting, anorexia and aggravation of pain by eating are also more common with gastric ulcer.

Gastroscopy and biopsy: Gastroscopy should be performed as part of the initial workup to attempt to find malignant lesions. The rolled-up margins of the ulcer that produce the meniscus sign on X-ray can often be distinguished from the flat edges characteristic of a benign ulcer. Multiple biopsy specimens and brush biopsy should be obtained from the edge of the lesion. False positives are rare, false negatives occur in 5%-10% of malignant ulcers.

2.1.2 Imaging studies

Upper gastrointestinal X-rays will show an ulcer, usually on the lesser curvature in the pyloric area. In the absence of a tumor mass, the following suggest that the ulcer is malignant.

(1) The deepest penetration of the ulcer is not beyond the expected border of the gastric wall.

(2) The meniscus sign is present, i. e., a prominent rim of radiolucency surrounding the ulcer, caused by heaped up edges of tumor.

(3) Cancer is more common (10%) in ulcers greater than 2 cm in diameter. Coexistence of duodenal deformity or ulcer favors a diagnosis of benign ulcer in the stomach.

2.1.3 Differential diagnosis

The characteristic symptoms of gastric ulcer are often clouded by numerous nonspecific complaints. Uncomplicated hiatal hernia, atrophic gastritis, chronic choecystitis irritable colon syndrome, and undifferentiated functional problems are distinguishable from pepticulcer only after appropriate radiologic studies and sometimes not even then.

Gastroscopy and biopsy of the ulcer should be performed to rule out malignant gastric ulcer.

2.2 Treatment

2.2.1 Medical treatment

Medical management of gastric ulcer is the same as for duodenal ulcer. The patient should be questioned regarding the use of ulcerogenic agents, which should be eliminated as far as possible.

Repeated endoscopy should be obtained to document the rate of healing. After 4–16 weeks (depending on the initial size of the lesion and other factors), healing usually has reached a plateau. In order to cure the disease and avoid recurrent ulcers, H. pylori must be eradicated. Serologic testing for H. pylori antibodies in this regard can check the success of therapy.

2.2.2 Surgical treatment

Before the significance of H. pylori in the etiology of gastric ulcer was appreciated, the most effective surgical treatment was distal hemigastrectomy (including the ulcer), somewhat less effective but still useful in high risk patients was vagotomy and pyloroplasty. Parietal cell vagotomy for prepyloric ulcers was followed by a high (e. g., 30%) recurrence rate, but parietal cell vagotomy plus pyloroplasty worked well.

Intractability to medical therapy has now become a rare indication for surgery in gastric ulcer disease. since H_2 receptor antagonists or omeprazole can bring the condition under control, and treatment of H. pylori infection can almost eliminate the problem of recurrence. Consequently, surgery will be needled principally for complications of the disease, bleeding perforation, or obstruction.

2.2.3 Hemorrhage from peptic Ulcer

Approximately 20% of patients with peptic ulcer will experience a bleeding episode and this complication is responsible for about 40% of the deaths from peptic ulcer. Pepticulcer is the most common cause of massive upper gastrointestinal hemorrhage, accounting for over half of all cases. Chronic gastric and duodenal ulcers have about the same tendency to bleed, but the former produce more severe episodes. Bleeding ulcers are more common in persons with blood group O, though the reason for this association is not known.

Bleeding ulcers in the duodenum are usually located on the posterior surface of the duodental bulb. As the ulcer penetrates, the gastroduodenal artery is exposed and may become eroded. Since no major blood vessels lie on the anterior surface of the duodenal bulb, ulcerations at this point are not as prone to bleed. Patients with concomitant bleeding and perforation usually have two ulcers, a bleeding posterior ulcer and a perforated anterior one. Postubulbar ulcers (those in the second portion of the duodenum) bleed frequently, though ulcers are much less common in this site than near the pylorus.

In some patients, the bleeding is sudden and massive, manifested by hematemesis and shock. In others, chronic anemia and weakness due to slow blood loss are the only findings. The diagnosis is unreliable when based on clinical findings, also endoscopy should be performed early (i. e., within 24 hours) in most cases.

In the preceding section, the management of acute upper gastrointestinal hemorrhage, the selection of diagnostic tests, and the factors suggesting the need for operation were discussed. Most patients (75%) with bleeding peptic ulcer can be successfully managed by medical means alone. Initial therapeutic efforts usually halt the bleeding H_2 cimetidine decreases the risk of rebleeding, but blockers and omeprazole decrease the risk of rebleeding but have no effect on active bleeding.

After 12–24 hours have passed and the bleeding has clearly stopped, a patient who feels hungry should be fed. Twice daily hematocrit readings should be ordered as a check on slow continued blood loss. Stools should be tested daily for the presence of blood. They will usually remain guaiac positive for several days after bleeding stops.

Rebleeding in the hospital has been attendee by a death of about 30%. A policy of early surgery for those who rebleed would improve this figure. Patients who are over age 60, present with hematemesis, is actively bleeding at the time of endoscopy, or whose admission hemoglobin is below 8 g/dL having a higher risk of rebleeding. About three times as many patients with gastric ulcer(30%) rebleed compared with those duodenal ulcer. Most instances of rebleeding occur within 2 days from the time the first episode has stopped. In one study, only 3% of patients who stopped bleeding for this long bled again.

2.2.4 Endoscopic therapy

Treatments administered through the endoscope may stop active bleeding or prevent rebleeding. Effective methods include injection of epinephrine, epinephrine plus 1 % polidocanonl (a sclerosing agent), or ethanol, or cautery using the heater probe, monopolar electrocautery, or the YAG laser. At least two modalities should be available to the endoscopist in the event one is unsuitable for a specific case or fails to work. Except for the laser, all are inexpensive. The indication for treatment are active bleeding at the time of endoscopy and the presence of a visible vessel in the base of the ulcer. Endoscopic therapy decreases transfusion requirements(by about half) and the rate of rebleeding(by about half) and the rate of rebleeding(by about three quarters) compared with sham treated controls. When treatment fails the first time, it may often be repeated with a good chance of success. It is important, however, not to allow the patient to deteriorate during nonoperative attempts at halting the bleeding.

2.2.5 Emergency surgery

About 10% of patients bleeding form a peptic ulcer require emergency surgery. Selection of those most likely to survive with surgical compare with medical treatment rests on the rate of blood loss and the other factors associated with a poor prognosis.

The overall death rate is significantly less after vagotomy and pyloroplasty than after gastrectomy for bleeding ulcer, and rebleeding occurs with about equal frequeney afereither procedure.

During laparototmy, the first step is to make a pyloroplasty incision if the endoscopic diagnosis is a bleeding duodental ulcer, if a dodeal ulcer is found, the bleeding vessel should be sutureligated and the duodenal ulcer is found, the bleeding vessel should be sutureligated and the duodenum and antrum inspected for additional ulcers. The pyloroplasty incision should then be closed and a truncal vagotomy performed. If a giant duodenal ulcer has destroyed the posterior wall of the duodenal bulb a gastrectomy and Billroth Ⅱ gastrojejunostomy may be preferable, since this somewhat uncommon ulcer is especially with the stomach. Gashtric ulcers can be handled by either gastrectomy or vagotomy and pyloropasty. A thorough search should always be made for second ulcers or other causes of bleeding.

Chapter 3

Pyloric Obstruction due to Peptic Ulcer

3.1 Clinical Findings

3.1.1 Symptoms and signs

Most patients with obstruction have a long history of symptomatic peptic ulcer, and as many as 30% have been treated for perforation or obstruction in the past. The patient often notes gradually increasing ulcer pains over weeks or months, with the eventual development of anorexia, vomiting, and failure to gain relief from antacids. The vomitus often contains food ingested several hours previously, and absence of bile staining reflects the site of blockage. Weight loss may be marked if the patient has delayed seeking medical care.

Dehydration and malnutrition may be obvious on physical examination but are not always present. A succession, splash can often be elicited from the retained gastric contents. Peristalsis of the distended stomach may be visible on gross inspection of the abdomen but this sign is relatively rare. Most patients have upper abdominal tenderness. Tetany may appear with advanced alkalosis.

3.1.2 Laboratory findings

Anemia is found in about 25% of patients. Prolonged vomiting leads to unique form of metabolic alkalosis with dehydration. Measurement of serum electrolytes shows hypochloremia, hypokalemia, hyponatremia, and increased bicarbonate. Vomiting depleted the patient of Na^+, K^+, and Cl^-, the later is lost in excess of Na^+ and K^+ as HCl, gastric HCl loss causes excreted in the urine with the HCO_3^-. Increasing Na^+ deficit evoles aldosterone secretion, which in turn brings about renal Na^+ conservation at the expense of more renal loss of K^+ and H^+. GRF may drop and produce a prerenal azotemia. The eventual result of the process is a marked deficit of Na^+, Cl^-, K^+ and H_2O. Treatment involves replacement of water and NaCl until a satisfactory urine flow has been established. KCl replacement should then be started.

3.1.3 Saline load test

This is a simple means of assessing the degree of pyloric obstruction and is useful in following the patient' progress during the first few days of nasogastric suction.

Through the nasogastric tube of 700 mL of normal saline(at room temperature) is infused over 3–5 minutes and the tube is clamped. 30 minutes later, the stomach is aspirated and the residual volume of saline recorded. Recovery of more than 350 mL indicates obstruction. It must be recognized that the results of a saline load test do not predict how well the stomach will handle solid food. Solid emptying can be measured solid food. Solid emptying can be measured with technetium Tc^{99m} labeld chicken liver.

3.1.4 Imaging studies

Plain abdominal X–rays may show a large gastric fluid level. An upper gastrointestinal series should not be performed gastrointestinal series should not be performed until the stomach has been emptied because dilution of the barium in the retained secretions makes a worthwhile study impossible.

3.1.5 Endoscopy

Gastroscopy is usually indicated to rule out the presence of an obstructing neoplasm.

3.2 Treatment

(1) Medical treatment: A large (32F) Ewald tube should be passed and the stomach emptied of its contents and lavaged until clean. After the stomach has been completely decompressed, a smaller tube should be inserted and placed on suction for several days to allow pyloric edema and spasm to subside and to permit the gastric musculature to regain its tone. A saline load test may be performed at this point to provide a baseline for later comparison if chronic obstruction has produced severe malnutrition total parenteral nutrition should be instituted.

(2) After decompression of the stomach for 48–72 hours, the saline load test should be repeated if this indicates sufficient improvement, the tube should be withdrawn and a liquid diet may be stated. Gradual resumption of solid foods is permitted as tolerated.

(3) Surgical treatment: If 5–7 days of gastric aspiration do not result in relief of the obstruction, the patient should be effort beyond this point in the absence of progress rarely achieves the result hoped for. Failure of the obstruction to resolve completely(e. g. , if the patient can take only liquids) and recurrent obstruction of any degree are indications for surgery.

Surgery treatment may consist of a truncal or parietal cell vagotomy and drainage procedure. Truncal vagotomy and gastrojejunostomy is the easiest perform laparoscopically.

Chapter 4

Perforated Peptic Ulcer

4.1 Clinical Findings

4.1.1 Symptoms and signs

The perforation usually elicits a sudden severe upper abdominal pain whose onset can be recalled precisely. The patient may or may not have had preceding chronic symptoms of peptic ulcer disease. Perforation rarely is heralded by nausea or vomiting and if typically occurs several hours after the last meal. Shoulder pain, if present reflects diaphragmatic irritation. Back pain is uncommon.

The initial reaction consists of a chemical peritonitis caused by gastric acid or bile and pancreatic enzymes. The peritoneal reaction dilutes these irritants with a thin exudates and as a result the patient's symptoms may temporarily improve before bacterial peritonitis occurs. The physician who sees the patient for the first time during this symptomatic lull must not be misled into interpreting it as representing bona fide improvement.

The patient appears severely distressed lying quietly with the knees drawn up and breathing shallowly to minimize abdominal motion. Fever is absent at the start. The abdominal muscles are rigid owing to severe involuntary spasm. Epigastric tenderness may not be as marked as expected because the board like rigidity protects the abdominal viscera from the palpating hand, escaped air from the stomach may enter the space between the liver and abdominal wall, and upon percussion the normal dullness over the liver will be tympanitic. Peristaltic sounds are reduced or absent. If delay in treatment allows continued escape of air into the peritoneal cavity, abdominal distention and diffuse tympany may result.

The above description applies to the typical case of perforation with classic findings. In as many as 1/3 of patients, the presentation is not as dramatic, diagnosis is less obvious, and serious delays in treatment may result from failure to consider this condition and to obtain the appropriate abdominal X-rays. Many of these atypical perforations occur in patients already hospitalized for some unrelated illness and the significance of the new symptom of abdominal pain is not appreciated. The only way to improve this record is to routinely obtain abdominal films on patients with abdominal pain of recent onset.

Lesser degrees of shock with minimal abdominal findings occur if the leak is small or rapidly sealed. A small duodenal perforation may slowly leak fluid that runs down the lateral peritoneal gutter, producing pain and muscular rigidity in the right lower quadrant and thus raising a problem of confusion with acute appendicitis.

Perforations may be sealed by omentum or by the liver, with the later development of a subhepatic or subdiaphragmatic abscess.

4.1.2 Laboratory findings

A mild leukocytosis in the range of 12,000/μL is common in the early stages. After 12–24 hours, this may rise to 20,000/μL or more if treatment has been inadequate. The mild rise in the serum amylase value that occurs in many patients is probable caused by absorption of the enzyme from duodenal secretions within the peritoneal cavity. Direct measurement of fluid obtained by paracentesis may show very high levels of amylase.

4.1.3 Imaging studies

Plain X-ray of the abdomen reveal free subdiaphragmatic air in 85% of patients. Films should be taken with the patient in both supine and upright. A film in the left lateral decubitus position may be a more practical way to demonstrate free air in the uncomfortable patient. If the findings are questionable, 400 mL of air can be insufflated into the stomach through a nasogastric tube and the films repeated. Free air in the abdomen in a patient with sudden upper abdominal pain should clinch the diagnosis.

If no free air is demonstrated and the clinical picture suggests perforated ulcer, an emergency upper gastrointestinal series should be performed. If the perforation has not sealed, the diagnosis is established by noting escape of the contrast material from the lumen, barium is more reliable than water soluble contrast media, and, contrary to previous views, does not appear to aggravate infection or to be difficult to remove.

4.1.4 Differential diagnosis

The differential diagnosis includes acute pancreatitis and acute cholecystitis. The former does, not have as explosive an onset as perforated ulcer and is usual accompanied by a high serum amylase level. Acute cholecystitis with perforated gallbladder could mimic perforated ulcer closely but free air would not be present with ruptured gallbladder. Intestinal obstruction has a more gradual onset and is characterized by less severe pain that is crampy and accompanied by vomiting.

The simultaneous onset of pain and free air in the abdomen in the absence of trauma usually means perforated peptic ulcer. Free perforation of colonic diverticulitis and acute appendicitis are other rare causes.

4.2 Treatment

The diagnosis is often suspended before the patient is sent for confirmatory X-rays. Whenever a perforated ulcer is considered, the first step should be to pass a nasogastric tube and empty the stomach to reduce further contamination of the peritoneal cavity. Blood should be drawn for laboratory studies, and intravenous antibiotics (e. g. , cefazolin, cefoxitin) should be started. If the patients overall condition is precarious owing to delay in treatment, fluid resuscitation should precede diagnostic measures. X-rays should be obtained as soon as the clinical status will permit.

The simplest surgical treatment, laparoscopy (or laparotomy) and suture closure of the perforation solves the immediate problem. The closure most often consists of securely plugging the hole with omentum sutured into place rather than bringing together the two edges with sutures. All fluid should be aspirated from the peritoneal cavity, but drainage is not indicated. Reperforation is rare in the immediate postoperative period.

About 3/4 of patients whose perforation is the culmination of a history of chronic symptoms continue to have clinically severe ulcer disease after simple closure, this has gradually led to a more aggressive treatment policy involving a definitive ulcer operation for most patients with acute perforation, e. g. , parietal cell vagotomy plus closure of the perforation or truncal vagotomy and pyloroplasty. Now that eradicating H. pylori can cure ulcer disease, the value of anything more than simple closure will have to be reexamined.

Concomitant hemorrhage and perforation are most often due to two ulcers, an anterior perforated one and a posterior one that is bleeding. Perforated ulcers that also obstruct obvious can not be treated by suture closure of the perforation alone. Vagotomy plus gastroenterostomy or pyloroplasty should be performed. Perforated anastomotic ulcers require a vagotomy or gastrectomy, since in the long run, closure alone is nearly always inadequate.

Nonoperative treatment of perforated ulcer consists of continuous gastric suction and the administration of antibiotics in high doses. Although this has been shown to be effective therapy, with a low death rate, a peritoneal and subphrenic abscess occasionally accompanies if and side effects are greater than with laparoscopic closure.

Chapter 5

Upper Gastrointestinal Hemorrhage

5.1 Initial Management

In an apparently healthy patient, melena of a week or more suggests that the bleeding is slow. In this type of patient, admission to the hospital should be followed by a deliberate but nonemergency workup. However, patients who present with hematemesis or melena of less than 12 hours duration should be handled as if exsanguinations were imminent. The approach entails a simultaneous series of diagnostic and therapeutic steps with the following initial goals: Assess the status of the circulatory system and replace blood loss as necessary. Determine the amount and rate of bleeding. Slow or stop the bleeding by ice water lavage. Discover the lesion responsible for the episode. The last step may lead to more specific treatment appropriate to the underlying condition.

The patient should be admitted to the hospital and a history and physical examination performed. Experienced clinicians are to make a correct diagnosis of the cause of bleeding from clinical findings in only 60% of patients. Peptic ulcer, acute gastritis, esophageal varices, esophagitis, and Mallory Weiss tear account for over 90% of cases. Questions for factors should be asked. The patient should be questioned about salicyate intake and any history of a bleeding tendency.

Of the diseases commonly responsible for acute upper gastrointedtinal bleeding, only portal hypertension is associated with diagnostic clues on physical examination. However, gatrointestinal bleeding should not be automatically attributed to esophageal varices in a patient with jaundice, ascites, splenomegaly spider angiomas, or hepatomegaly, over half of cirrhotic patients who present with acute hemorrhage are bleeding from gastritis or peptic ulcer.

Blood should be drawn for cross matching, hematocrit, hemoglobin, creatinine, and tests of liver function. An intravenous infusion should be started and, in the massive bleeder, a large bore nasogastric tube inserted. In cases of melena, the gastric aspirate should be examined to verify the gastroduodenal source of the hemorrhage, but about 25% of patients with bleeding duodenal ulcers have gastric aspirates than the standard nasogastric tube(16F) so the stomach can be lavaged free of liquid blood and clots. After its contents have been removed, the stomach should be irrigated with copious amounts of ice water or saline solution until blood no longer returns. If the patient was bleeding at the time the nasogastric tube was inserted, iced saline irrigation usually stops it. The large tube can then be exchanged for a standard nasogastric tube attached to continuous suction so further blood loss can be measured.

It is common to give H_2 receptor antagonists or omeprazole, though controlled trials have shown no benefit. If bleeding continues or if tachycardia or hypotension is present, the patient should be monitored and treated as for hemorrhagic shock.

In acute rapid hemorrhage, the hematocrit may be normal or only slightly low. A very low hematocrit without obvious signs of shock indicates more gradual blood loss.

All of the above tests and procedures can be performed within 1 or 2 hours after admission. By this time, in most instances, bleeding is under control, blood volume has been restored to normal, and the patient is being adequately monitored so that recurrent bleeding can be detected promptly. When this stage is reached, additional diagnostic tests should be performed.

5.2 Diagnosis of Cause of Bleeding

Once the patient is stabilized, endoscopy should be the first study. In general, endoscopy should be performed within 24 hours, after admission, and under these circumstances the source of bleeding can be demonstrated in about 80% of cases. Longer delays will give a lower diagnostic yield. Two lesions are seen in about 15% of patients. An upper gastrointestinal series should be performed if endoscopy is equivocal or unavailable. Although the diagnostic information provided by endoscopy does not appear to have resulted in decreased blood loss or improved outcome, endoscopic therapy, in the form of sclerosis of varices or injection of a bleeding ulcer, may do so. Having the diagnosis will also help in planning subsequent treatment, including the surgical approach if surgery becomes necessary.

Rarely, selective angiography will i have diagnostic or therapeutic usefulness. For diagnosis, it is most helpful when other studies fail to demonstrate the cause of bleeding. Infusion through the angiographic catheter of vasoconstrictors (e. g., vasopressin) and embolization of the bleeding vessel with Gelfoam may be able to halt the bleeding in special cases.

5.3 Later Management

Although a precise diagnosis of the cause of the bleeding may be valuable in later management, the patient must not be allowed to slip out of clinical control during the search for definitive diagnostic information. The decision for emergency surgery depends more on the rate and duration of bleeding than on its specific cause.

The need for transfusion should be determined on a continuing basis, and blood volume must be maintained. Blood pressure, pulse, central venous pressure, hematocrit, hourly urinary volume, and amount of blood obtained from the gastric tube or from the rectum all enter into this assessment. Many studies have shown the tendency to underestimate blood loss and inadequately transfuse massively bleeding patients who truly need aggressive therapy. Continued slow bleeding is best monitored by serial determinations of the hematocrit.

The following criteria define patients with a very low risk of serious bleeding: age less than 75 years, no unstable comorbid illness, no ascites evident on physical examination, normal prothrombin time, and, within

1 hour after admission, a systolic blood pressure above 100 mmHg and nasogastric aspirate free of fresh blood. Patients with all six of these findings may be spared emergency endoscopy and discharged from the hospital early to undergo outpatient workup.

Several factors are associated with a worse prognosis with continued medical management of the bleeding episode. These are not absolute indications for laparotomy, but they should alert the clinician that emergency surgery might be required.

High rates of bleeding or amounts of blood loss predict high failure rates with medical treatment. Hematemesis is usually associated with more rapid bleeding and a greater blood volume deficit than melena. The presence of hypotension on admission to the hospital or the need for more than four units of blood to a worse prognosis, if bleeding continues and subsequent transfusion requirements exceed 1 unit every 8 hours, continued medical management is usually unwise. The level of serum fibrin degradation products, indicating endogenous fibrinolysis, correlates with the severity of hemorrhage and the death rate. This may be a useful prognostic test, and the results could be used as a guide for the administration of fibrinolytic inhibitors in therapy. Evidence for or against this view is not yet available.

Total transfusion requirements also correlate with death rates. Death is uncommon when fewer than seven units of blood have been used, and the death rate rises progressively thereafter.

In general, bleeding from a gastric ulcer is more dangerous than bleeding from gastritis or duodenal ulcer, and patients with gastric ulcer should always be considered for early surgery. Regardless of the cause, if bleeding recurs after it has once stopped, the chances of success without operation are low. Most patients who rebleed in the hospital should have surgery.

Patients over age 60 tolerate continued blood loss less well than younger patients, and their bleeding should be stopped before secondary cardiovascular, pulmonary, or renal complications arise.

In 85% of patients, bleeding stops within a few hours of admission. About 25% of patients rebleed once bleeding has stopped. Rebleeding episodes are concentrated within the first 2 days of hospitalization, and if the patient has had no further bleeding for a period of 5 days, the chance of rebleeding is only 2%. Rebleeding is most common in patents with varices, peptic ulcer, anemia, or shock. About 10% of patients require surgery to control bleeding, and most of these patients have bleeding ulcers or, less commonly, esophageal varices. The death rate is 30% among patients who rebleed and 3% among those who do not. The mortality rate is also high in the elderly and in patients who are already hospitalized at the onset of bleeding. Analyses of large series of patients suggest that a number of those who dies would not have done so if operation had been performed earlier and more often.

Chapter 6

Gastric Carcinoma

6.1 Clinical Findings

6.1.1 Symptoms and signs

The earliest symptom is usually vague postprandial abdominal heaviness that the patient does not identify as a pain. Sometimes the discomfort is no different from other vague dyspeptic symptoms that been intermittently resent for years but the frequency and persistence are new.

Anorexia develops early and may be most pronounced for meat. Weight loss is the most common symptom which averages about 6 kg. True postprandial pain suggesting a benign gastric ulcer is relatively uncommon but if it is present one may be misled if subsequent X-rays show an ulcer. Vomiting may be present and becomes a major feature of pyloric obstruction occurs. It may have a coffee ground appearance owing to bleeding by the tumor. Dysphagia may be the presenting symptom of lesions at the cardia.

An epigastric mass can be felt on examination in about one fourth of cases. Hepatomegaly is present in 10% of cases. The stool will be positive for occult blood in half of patients, and melena is seen in a few. Otherwise, abnormal physical findings are confined to sings of distant spread of the tumor. Metastases to the neck along the thoracic duct may reveal a Blumer shelf, a solid peritoneal deposit anterior to thel rectum. Enlarged ovaries (Krukenberg tumors) may be caused by intraperitoneal metastases; further dissemination may involve the liver, lungs, brain, or bone.

6.1.2 Laboratory findings

Anemia is present in 40% of patients. Carcinoembryonic antigen (CEA) levels are elevated in 65%, usually indicating extensive spread of the tumor.

6.1.3 Imaging studies

An upper gastrointestinal series is diagnostic for many tumors, but the overall false negative rate is about 20%. Major diagnostic problems are posed by ulcerating tumors, a few of which may not be distinguishable radiologically from benign peptic ulcers. The differential features are listed in the section on gastric a diagnosis of benign ulcer. All patients with a newly discovered gastric ulcer should undergo gastroscopy and gastric biopsy.

6.1.4 Gastroscopy and biopsy

Largegastric carcinomas can usually be identified as such by their gross appearance at endoscopy. All gastric lesions, whether polypoid or ulcerating, should be examined by taking multiple biopsy and brush cytology specimens during endoscopy. False results are seen occasionally as a result of sampling error, and a minimum of six biopsies is necessary for greatest accuracy.

6.2 Treatment

Surgical resection is the only curative treatment. About 85% of patients are operable, and in 50% the lesions amenable to resection of the respectable lesion, half are potentially curable(i. e. , no signs of spread beyond the limits of resection).

The surgical objective should be to remove the tumors, and duodenum, the regional lymph nodes, and, if necessary, portions margin should be a minimum of 6 cm from the gross tumor. If the tumor were located in the antrum, a curative resection would entail distal gastrectomy with enbloc removal of the omentum, a 3–4 cm cuff of duodenum and the subpyloric lymph nodes, and, in some instances, excision of the left gastric artery and nearby may be by either a Billrothe Ⅰ or Ⅱ procedure, but the latter is preferable because procedure growth of residual tumor near the pylorus may obstruct a gastroduodenal anastomosis early.

Total gastrectomy with splenectomy is required for tumors of the proximal half of the stomach and for extensive tumors(e. g. , linitis plastica). Whether or not the spleen should be removed such cases is a subject of debate. Alimentary continuity is most of the reestablished by a Roux-en-Y esophagojejunostomy. Construction of an intestinal pouch as a substitute food reservoir(e. g. , Hunt Lawrence pouch) of no nutritional value and if increases the risks of immediate complications.

Japanese surgeons have devised a more detailed staging system than the one used in most other countries and have also recommended more aggressive lymhadenectomy as a matter of routine in the resection of gastric. The results of resections as reported from Japan are better than those obtained by the standard operation described above so attempts are being made to determine whether the difference is due to the more radical operations.

The propensity for proximal submucosal spread must be appreciated at surgery. It is of ten advisable to perform a frozen section at the proximal margin before constructing the anastomosis. If tumor is found the gastrectomy should be extended.

Palliative resection is usually indicated if the stomach is still movable and life expectancy is estimated to be more than 1–2 months. Palliative gastrectomy is usually performed to remove an antral lesion and prevent obstruction but in selected cases, total gastrectomy is appropriate palliative treatment if the operation can be done safely and the amount of extragastric tumor is minimal. Whenever technically feasible, palliative gastrectomy is preferable to palliative gastrojejunostomy.

Adjuvant chemotherapy after curative surgery has not been of value with the regimens tested to date. For advanced disease doxorubicin or fluorouracil alone each of which results in 20% response rate is as good as a combination of chemotherapeutic agents.

Chapter 7

Duodenal Diverticula

Diverticula of the duodenum are found in 20% of autopsies and 5% -10% of upper gastrointestinal series. Symptoms are uncommon and only 1% of those found by X-rays warrant surgery.

Duodenal pulsion diverticula are acquired outpouchings of the mucosa and submucosa, 90% of which are on the medial aspect of the duodenum. They are rare before age 40. Most are solitary and within 2.5 cm of the ampulla of Vater. There is a high incidence of gallstone disease of the gallbladder in patients with juxtapapillary diverticula. Diverticula are not seen in the first portion of the duodenum where diverticular configurations are due to scarring by peptic configurations are due to sarring by peptic ulceration or cholecystitis.

A few patients have chronic postprandial abdominal pain or dyspepsia caused by a duodenal diverticulum. Treatment is with antacids and anticholinergics.

Serous complications are hemorrhage or perforation from inflammation, pancreatitis and biliary obstruction. Bile acid bilirubinate enteroliths are occasionally formed by bile stasis in a diverticulum. Enteroliths can precipitate diverticular inflammation of biliary obstruction and rarely have caused bowel obstruction after entering the intestinal lumen.

Surgical treatment is required for complications and rarely for persistent symptoms. Excision and a two layer closure are usually possible after mobilization of the duodenum and dissection of the diverticulum from the pancreas. Removal of the diverticulum and closure of the defect are superior to simple drainage in the case of perforation. If biliary obstruction appears in a patient whose bile duct empties into a diverticulum, excision might be more hazardous than a side to side choledochoduodenostomy.

The rare windsock type of intraluminal diverticulum usually presets with vague epigastric pain and postprandial fullness, though intestinal bleeding or pancreatitis is occasionally seen. The diagnosis can be made by barium X-ray studies. The diverticulum can be excised through a nearby duodenotomy. In some cases, the narrow diverticular outlet can be enlarged endoscopically.

Chapter 8

Duodenal Atresia

Duodenal atresia (DA) is more commonly proximal intestinal obstruction that causes bilious vomiting within the first 24–48 hours of life time following the first feeding. The first reported case of duodenal atresia was in the year 1733. DA is once the lethal disease in neonates. Over the past 30 years, the survival rate of effected neonates has gradually improved due to improved anesthetic and operation techniques.

8.1 Epidemiology

DA occurs about 1 in 6000 live births and represents up to 60% of intestinal atresia. There is a slight male preponderance (1.4 : 1).

Infants with DA often associated with other malformation, such as trisomy 21, Down syndrome, and congenital cardiac anomalies. Around 30% of patients with DA have Down syndrome.

8.2 Etiology

8.2.1 Embryology

Despite considerable efforts have been put into investigating the organogenesis of duodenum, but little has changed. In 1902, Tandler published his study of duodenal development and theorized the etiology of DA. During the 8th week of fetal life, there is exuberant growth of epithelial cells before the size of the gut increased sufficiently to accommodate it, obliterating the lumen. As the gut grows, vacuolization of the solid core of cells starts, and the lumen is recanalized by the end of the 10th week. The failure of lumen recanalization produces duodenal atresia.

8.2.2 Genome

Genetic tools are being applied to the investigation of duodenal atresia. Fibroblast growth factor-10 (FGF10) is not only active in duodenal developing but critical to normal development. A murine model by knock-out of the fibroblast growth factor receptor 2b produces multiple anomalies including DA. Aside from etiology study, works on FGF10 will provide a genetic model for DA studies.

8.3 Clinical Classification

Three types of DA are as follows. ① Type 1: two blind ends connected by intact muscularis with marked discrepancy in size between proximal and distal segment. ② Type 2: two blind ends connected by a short fibrous cord along the edge of the intact mesentery. ③ Type 3: separated blind ends without connected, and the absence of mesentery or V-shape defection.

8.4 Clinical Manifestations

(1) History

Neonates present with vomiting in the first 24–48 hours of life after the first feeding. The presence of bilious vomiting in 80% infants (post-ampullary). In the remaining 20% the vomit is not bilestained (pre-ampullary).

(2) Symptoms

Vomiting is usually delayed and progressive aggravation after the first feeding. Vomitus can be bilestained or not. Dehydration and weakness of infants are also common symptoms.

(3) Physical signs

There may be a fullness in the epigastrium because of the dilated stomach, but the rest of abdomen is quite scaphoid because of the absence of gas in the distal intestine. Excessive vomiting can cause hypokalemic hypochloremic metabolic alkalosis.

(4) Associated anomalies

About 30% of infants with DA have trisomy 21 and up to 25% with DA have structural cardiac defects. Around 10% of affected infants have midgut malrotation and another intestinal atresia.

8.5 Diagnosis

(1) Prenatal stage

Prenatal ultrasonography performed in any pregnant woman is an important method to rule out DA. Polyhydramnios is present in about 50% of effected women. Aside from the polyhydramnios, the presence of duodenal obstruction with a dilated, fluid-filled stomach and duodenum is also vital indications for DA.

(2) Postnatal stage

Infants with vomiting of the bilestained material within a few hours of births should be considered to the possibility of DA.

(3) Imaging study

The plain abdominal supine radiography is usually helpful to assist the diagnosis of DA. The classic radiographic finding is the double-bubble sign which the higher, larger bubble in the left side is the stomach and the another bubble is the dilated proximal duodenum. No air is seen in distal digestive tract. For unusual cases with lack of air in the obstructed segment, a small amount of air can be injected through a nasogastric tube to confirm the diagnosis. Generally speaking, further radiologic investigations and contrast barium swallow are not necessary which are potential hazards of vomiting with aspiration. Ultrasonography is also useful to show an associated annular pancreas.

8.6 Differential Diagnosis

It should to know the vomitus is bilious or not in differential diagnosis. Several considerations of infant with bilious vomiting are duodenal atresia, duodenal stenosis, annular pancreas, midgut volvulus, Ladd bands, or intraluminal diverticulum. Midgut volvulus often presents later in life than duodenal atresia. In cases with Down syndrome, it is essential to take other gastrointestinal malformations (such as anal atresia, Hirschsprung disease, and diaphragmatic hernia) into consideration.

8.7 Treatments

8.7.1 Preoperative managements

Correction of DA is not an emergency operation. Operative interruption should be postponed to ensure effected neonate is in optimal condition for operative procedures. The main preoperative managements are including the following: ① A nasogastric tube should be inserted into stomach and taped in place to aspirate gastric contents. ② Total parenteral nutrition should be started. ③ Vitamin K (1 mg) is given intramuscularly. ④ Infants are checked carefully to find other associated anomalies. ⑤ Possible metabolic or respiratory complications should be corrected before operation.

8.7.2 Operative repair

(1) Operation timing

Immediate operation is not necessary to correct DA. The infant is transferred to operation room for interruptive procedure when children's condition is stable after preoperative managements.

(2) Surgical method

An nasogastric tube is used to decompress the stomach and indicate the duodenal obstruction point. Laparotomy is performed through a transverse right upper quadrant supraumbilical incision. The choice of operation depends on the types of anomaly founded and the gape between two blinds of duodenum. The common methods of duodenal anastomosis are as follows: ① Direct incision: a simple duodenal web or diaphragm could be excised through a longitudinal incision across the obstruction point, but this method has the risk of Vater ampulla damage. ② Duodenoduodenostomy: side-to-side or diamond shaped duodenoduodenostomy can be performed to restore physiologic bypass of duodenum. ③ Retrocolic duodenojejunostomy: infants with difficult duodenoduodenostomy or a long distance between two blinds of duodenum can choice the retrocolic duodenojejunostomy.

(3) Operation principles

Removing duodenal obstruction, explorating multiple atresia, and reconstructing digestive tract are main objects of surgery to correct DA.

(4) Postoperative complications

Despite mortality rate of around 5% with DA is associated with other anomalies, postoperative complications can also increase the risks of death. The common complications are as follows: ① Pancreatic fistula: An annular pancreas has not been considered or cared during operation. Pancreatic tissue was divided but not bypassed. ② Ampulla of Vater injured: The damage of ampulla of Vater occurs when a simple duodenal web or diaphragm is excised through a longitudinal incision across the area of atresia. ③ Anastomotic leakage: Bacteria infection, higher anastomotic tension, and malnutrition will increase the possibility of anastomotic leakage. ④ Anastomotic stricture: Patients performed with side-to-side fashion in duodenoduodenostomy are more likely to be associated with anastomotic stricture than diamond shaped type.

8.8 Prognosis

The long-term outcome of successful treated duodenal atresia is excellent. The mortality rate of neonate associated with other anomalies is around 5%.

Chapter 9

Superior Mesenteric Artery Obstruction of the Duodenum

Rarely obstruction of the third portion of the duodenum is produced by compression between the superior mesenteric vessels and the aorta. It most commonly appears after rapid weight loss following injury, including burns. Patients in body casts are particularly susceptible.

The superior mesenteric artery normally leaves the aorta at an angle of 50–60 degrees and the distance between the two vessels there the duodenum passes between them is 10–20 mm. These measurements in patients with superior mesenteric artery syndrome average 18 degrees and 2. 5 mm. Acute loss of mesenteric fat is thought to permit the artery to drop posterior trapping the bowel like a scissors.

Skepticism exists regarding the frequency of this condition in adults who have not experienced acute loss of weight. Most of the patient in question is a thin nervous woman whose complaints of dyspepsia and occasional emesis are more properly explained on a functional basis. When a clear cut example is encountered it may actually represent form of intestinal malrotation with duodenal bands.

The patient complains of epigastric bloating and crampy pain relived by vomiting. The symptoms may remit in the prone position. Anorexia and postprandial pain lead to additional malnutrition and weight loss.

Upper gastrointestinal X–rays demonstrate a widened duodenum proximal to a sharp obstruction at the point where the artery crosses the third portion of the duodenum. When the patient moves to the knee chest position the passage of barium is suddenly unimpeded. Further verification can be provided if angiography shows an angle of 25 degrees or less between the superior mesenteric artery and the aorta. However, this procedure is not recommended for routine evaluation of obvious cases.

Many patients whose superior mesenteric artery makes a prominent impression on the duodenum are asymptomatic and in ambulatory patients one should hesitate to attribute vague chronic complaints to this finding.

In evolvement of the duodenum by scleroderma leads to duodenal dilation and hypomotility and an X–ray and clinical picture highly suggestive of superior mesenteric artery syndrome. In the latter increased duodenal peristalsis should be demonstrated proximal to the arterial blockage whereas diminished peristalsis characterizes scleroderma. Patients with duodenal scleroderma usually have dysphagia from concomitant esophageal involvement.

Malrotation with duodenal obstruction by congenital bands can mimic this syndrome. Postural therapy may suffice. The patient should be placed prone when symptomatic or in anticipation of postprandial dirriculties. Ambulator y patients should be instructed to assume the knee chest position, which allows the viscera and the artery to rotate forward off the duodenum. Chronic obstruction may require section of the suspensory ligament and mobilization of the duodenum or a duodenojejunostomy to bypass the obstruction. Mobilizing the duodenojejunal flexure which releases the duodenum form entrapment by congenital bands should treat patients with various forms of malrotation.

Part 28

Ileus and Bowel Obstruction

(1) Introduction

The purpose of this chapter is to provide an overview of the classification, pathophysiology, natural history, diagnosis, and management of mechanical obstruction and ileus of the small and large intestines. The development of the modern approach to intestinal obstruction and ileus paralleled the development of techniques for safe abdominal surgery. Chief among these accomplishments were the discovery of safe general anesthetics, the popularization of aseptic methods in the operating room and in the management of wounds, and the development of techniques for intestinal resection, intestinal anastomosis, and colostomy. The foundations of the recognition and management of intestinal obstruction and ileus are attributed to Frederick Treves.

(2) Classification

1) Mechanical obstruction and ileus: The term mechanical obstruction means that luminal contents cannot pass through the gut tube because the lumen is blocked. This obstruction is in contrast with neurogenic or functional obstruction in which luminal contents are prevented from passing because of disturbances in gut motility that prevent coordinated peristalsis from one region of the gut to the next. This latter form of obstruction is commonly referred to as ileus in the small intestine and pseudo-obstruction in the large intestine.

2) Simple obstruction and strangulation obstruction: In simple obstruction the intestinal lumen is partially or completely occluded without compromise of intestinal blood flow. Simple obstructions may be complete, meaning that the lumen is totally occluded, or incomplete, meaning that the lumen is narrowed but permitting distal passage of some fluid and air. In strangulation obstruction, blood flow to the obstructed segment is compromised and tissue necrosis and gangrene are imminent. Strangulation usually implies that the obstruction is complete, but some forms of partial obstruction can also be complicated by strangulation.

3) Classified according to etiology: The various forms of mechanical intestinal obstruction can be classified according to different but overlapping schemes. Most commonly, obstruction is classified according to etiology. Including intraluminal obturators such as foreign bodies or gallstones, intramural lesions such as tumors or intussusceptions, and extrinsic or extramural lesions such as adhesions.

4) Proximal or "high" obstructions and distant or "low" obstructions: In order to highlight the pathophysiology, presentation, and natural history, however, it is useful to classify obstruction according to the location of the obstructing lesion. Proximal or "high" obstructions involve the pylorus, duodenum, and proximal jejunum. Intermediate levels of obstruction involve the intestine from the midjejunum to the midileum. Distal levels of obstruction arise in the distal ileum, ileocecal valve, and proximal colon, whereas the most distant or "low" obstructions would arise in regions beyond the transverse colon. Clinical symptoms and signs of obstruction (pain, vomiting, abdominal distention, gas pattern on abdominal radiographs) vary with the level of obstruction.

5) Open-loop and closed-loop obstructions: It is also important to distinguish between open-loop and closed-loop obstructions. An open-loop obstruction occurs when intestinal flow is blocked but proximal decompression is possible through vomiting. A closed-loop obstruction occurs when inflow to the loop of bowel and outflow from the loop are both blocked. This obstruction permits gas and secretions to accumulate in the loop without a means of decompression, proximally or distally. Examples of closed-loop obstructions are torsion of a loop of small intestine around an adhesive band, incarceration of the bowel in a hernia, volvulus of the cecum or colon, and development of an obstructing carcinoma of the colon with a competent ileocecal valve. The primary symptoms of a closed-loop obstruction of the small intestine are sudden, severe abdominal pain and vomiting, whereas symptoms of the large intestine are pain and sudden abdominal distention.

This pain often occurs before associated findings of localized abdominal tenderness or involuntary guarding. When physical findings develop, there is a high level of suspicion that the viability of the bowel is compromised. When bowel obstruction is the most likely diagnosis, "abdominal pain out of proportion to physical findings" represents a surgical emergency.

Chapter 1

Mechanical Obstruction of the Intestines

1.1 Etiology

The causes of a small bowel obstruction can be divided into three categories:

(1) Obstruction arising from extraluminal causes (e. g., adhesions, hernias, carcinomas, abscesses).

(2) Obstruction intrinsic to the bowel wall (e. g., primary tumors).

(3) Intraluminal obturator obstruction (e. g., gallstones, enteroliths, foreign bodies, and bezoars).

The cause of small bowel obstruction has changed dramatically during the past century. At the turn of the 20th century, hernias accounted for more than half of mechanical intestinal obstructions. With the routine elective repair of hernias, this cause has dropped to the third most common cause of small bowel obstruction in industrialized countries. Adhesions secondary to previous surgery are by far the most common cause of small bowel obstruction today (Figure 28-1-1).

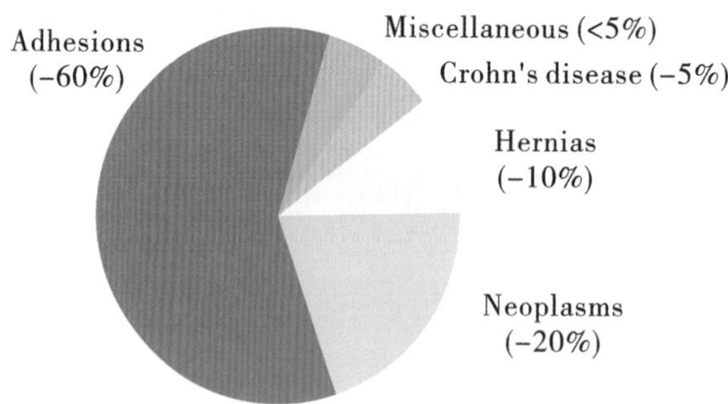

Figure 28-1-1 Common causes of small bowel obstruction in industrialized countries

1.1.1 Adhesions

Adhesions, particularly after pelvic operations (e. g., gynecologic procedures, appendectomy, and colorectal resection), are responsible for more than 60% of all causes of bowel obstruction. This preponderance of lower abdominal procedures to produce adhesions that result in obstruction is thought to be due to the fact that the bowel is more mobile in the pelvis and more tethered in the upper abdomen.

The causes of mechanical small intestinal obstruction in adults are as follows: lesions extrinsic to the intstinal wall, adhesions (usually postoperative), hernia includes external (e. g., inguinal, femoral, umbilical or ventral hernias) and internal (e. g., congenital defects such as paraduodenal, foramen of Winslow, and diaphragmatic hernias or postoperative secondary to mesenteric defects), neopiastic (includes carcinomatosis and extraintestinal neoplasms), intra-abdominal abscess, lesions intrinsic to the intstinal wall, congenital, malrotation, duplications, cysts, inflammatory, Crohn's disease, infections (includes tuberculosis, actinomycosis and diverticulitis), neoplastic (includes primary neoplasms and metastatic neoplasms), traumatic, hematoma, ischemic stricture, miscellaneous, intussusception, endometriosis, radiation enteropathy or stricture, intraluminal, obturator obstruction, gallstone and enterolith.

1.1.2 Malignant tumors

Malignant tumors account for about 20% of the cases of small bowel obstruction. Most of these tumors are metastatic lesions that obstruct the intestine secondary to peritoneal implants that have spread from an intra-abdominal primary tumor such as ovarian, pancreatic, gastric, or colonic. Less often, malignant cells from distant sites, such as breast, lung, and melanoma, may metastasize hematogenously and account for peritoneal implants and result in an obstruction. Large intra-abdominal tumors may also cause small bowel obstruction through extrinsic compression of the bowel lumen. Primary colonic cancers (particularly those arising from the cecum and ascending colon) may present as a small bowel obstruction. Primary small bowel tumors can cause obstruction but are exceedingly rare.

1.1.3 Hernias

Hernias are the third leading cause of intestinal obstruction and account for about 10% of all cases. Most commonly, these represent ventral or inguinal hernias. Internal hernias, usually related to prior abdominal surgery, can also result in small bowel obstruction. Less common hernias can also produce obstruction, such as femoral, obturator, lumbar, and sciatic hernias.

1.1.4 Crohn's disease

Crohn's disease is the fourth leading cause of small bowel obstruction and accounts for about 5% of all cases. Obstruction can result from acute inflammation and edema, which may resolve with conservative management. In patients with long-standing Crohn's disease, strictures can develop that may require resection and reanastomosis or strictureplasty.

1.1.5 Intra-abdominal abscess

An important cause of small bowel obstruction that is not routinely considered is obstruction associated with an intra-abdominal abscess, commonly from a ruptured appendix, diverticulum, or dehiscence of an intestinal anastomosis. The obstruction may occur as a result of a local ileus in the small bowel adjacent to the abscess. In addition, the small bowel can form a portion of the wall of the abscess cavity and become obstructed by kinking of the bowel at this point.

1.1.6 Miscellaneous causes

Miscellaneous causes of bowel obstruction account for 2%-3% of all cases but should be considered in the differential diagnosis. These include intussusception of the bowel, which in the adult is usually secondary to a pathologic lead point such as a polyp or tumor (Figure 28-1-2); gallstones, which can enter the intestinal lumen by a cholecystenteric fistula and cause obstruction; enteroliths originating from jejunal diverticula; foreign bodies; and phytobezoars.

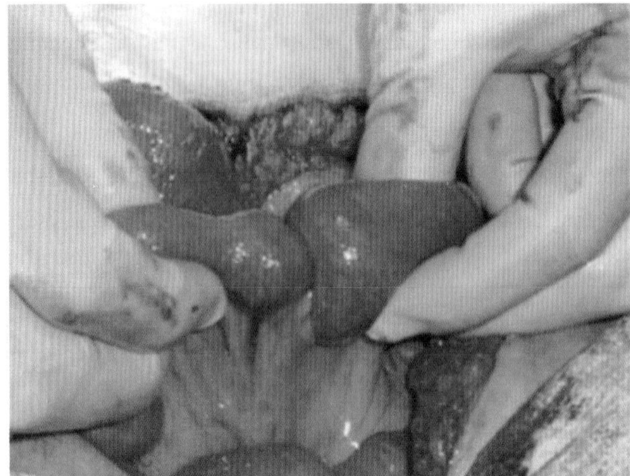

Figure 28-1-2 Jejunojenunal intussusception in an adult patient

1.2 Pathophysiology

1.2.1 Change in peristalsis

Early in the course of an obstruction, intestinal motility and contractile activity increase in an effort to propel luminal contents past the obstructing point. The increase in peristalsis that occurs early in the course of bowel obstruction is present both above and below the point of obstruction, thus accounting for the finding of diarrhea that may accompany partial or even complete small bowel obstruction in the early period. Later in the course of obstruction, the intestine becomes fatigued and dilates, with contractions becoming less frequent and less intense.

1.2.2 Dehydration and hypovolemia

As the bowel dilates, water and electrolytes accumulate both intraluminally and in the bowel wall itself. This massive third-space fluid loss accounts for the dehydration and hypovolemia. The metabolic effects of fluid loss depend on the site and duration of the obstruction. With a proximal obstruction, dehydration may be accompanied by hypochloremia, hypokalemia, and metabolic alkalosis associated with increased vomiting. Distal obstruction of the small bowel may result in large quantities of intestinal fluid into the bowel; however, abnormalities in serum electrolytes are usually less dramatic. Oliguria, azotemia, and hemoconcentration can accompany the dehydration. Hypotension and shock can ensue. Other consequences of bowel obstruction include increased intra-abdominal pressure, decreased venous return, and elevation of the diaphragm, compromising ventilation. These factors can serve to further potentiate the effects of hypovolemia.

1.2.3 Ischemia

As the intraluminal pressure increases in the bowel, a decrease in mucosal blood flow can occur. These alterations are particularly noted in patients with a closed-loop obstruction in which greater intraluminal pressures are attained. A closed-loop obstruction, produced commonly by a twist of the bowel, can progress to arterial occlusion and ischemia if left untreated and may potentially lead to bowel perforation and peritonitis.

1.2.4 Inflammation

In the absence of intestinal obstruction, the jejunum and proximal ileum of the human are virtually sterile. With obstruction, however, the flora of the small intestine changes dramatically, in both the type of organism (most commonly Escherichia coli, Streptococcus faecalis, and Klebsiella species) and the quantity, with organisms reaching concentrations of 10^9 to 10^{10}/mL. Studies have shown an increase in the number of indigenous bacteria translocating to mesenteric lymph nodes and even systemic organs. Bacterial translocation amplifes the local inflammatory response in the gut, leading to intestinal leakage and subsequent increase in systemic inflammation. This inflammatory cascade may result in systemic sepsis and multiorgan failure if it is unrecognized and untreated.

1.3 Clinical Manifestations

A thorough history and physical examination are critical to establishing the diagnosis and treatment of the patient with an intestinal obstruction. In most patients, a meticulous history and physical examination complemented by plain abdominal radiographs are all that is required to establish the diagnosis and to devise a treatment plan. More sophisticated radiographic studies may be necessary in certain patients in whom the diagnosis and cause are uncertain. However, a CT scan of the abdomen should not be the starting point in the workup of a patient with intestinal obstruction.

1.3.1 History (symptoms)

The cardinal symptoms of intestinal obstruction includecolicky abdominal pain, nausea, vomiting, abdominal distention, and a failure to pass flatus and feces (i. e., obstipation). These symptoms may vary with the site and duration of obstruction. The typical crampy abdominal pain associated with intestinal obstruction occurs in paroxysms at 4- to 5-minute intervals and occurs less frequently with distal obstruction. Nausea and vomiting are more common with a higher obstruction and may be the only symptoms in patients with gastric outlet or high intestinal obstruction. An obstruction located distally is associated with less emesis, and the initial and most prominent symptom is the cramping abdominal pain. Abdominal distention occurs as the obstruction progresses, and the proximal intestine becomes increasingly dilated. Obstipation is a later development, and it must be reiterated that patients, particularly in the early stages of bowel obstruction, may relate a history of diarrhea that is secondary to increased peristalsis. Therefore, the important point to remember is that a complete bowel obstruction can not be ruled out based on a history of loose bowel movements. The character of the vomitus is also important to obtain in the history. As the obstruction becomes more complete with bacterial overgrowth, the vomitus becomes more feculent, indicating a late and established intestinal obstruction.

1.3.2 Physical examination (signs)

The patient with intestinal obstruction may present with tachycardia and hypotension, demonstrating the severe dehydration that is present. Fever suggests the possibility of strangulation. Abdominal examination demonstrates a distended abdomen, with the amount of distention somewhat dependent on the level of obstruction. Previous surgical scars should be noted. Early in the course of bowel obstruction, peristaltic waves can be observed, particularly in thin patients, and auscultation of the abdomen may demonstrate hyperactive bowel sounds with audible rushes associated with vigorous peristalsis (i. e., borborygmi). Late in the obstructive course, minimal or no bowel sounds are noted. Mild abdominal tenderness may be present with or without a palpable mass; however, localized tenderness, rebound, and guarding suggest peritonitis and the likelihood of strangulation. A careful examination must be performed to rule out incarcerated hernias in the groin, the femoral triangle, and the obturator foramen. A rectal examination should be performed to assess for intraluminal masses and to examine the stool for occult blood, which may be an indication of malignancy, intussusception, or infarction.

1.3.3 Radiologic and laboratory examinations

1.3.3.1 Plain radiographs

The diagnosis of intestinal obstruction is often immediately evident after a thorough history and physical examination. Therefore, plain radiographs usually confirm the clinical suspicion and define more accurately the site of obstruction. The accuracy of diagnosis of the small intestinal obstruction on plain abdominal radiographs is estimated to be about 60%, with an equivocal or a nonspecific diagnosis obtained in the remainder of cases. Characteristic findings on supine radiographs are dilated loops of small intestine without evidence of colonic distention. Upright radiographs demonstrate multiple air-fluid levels, which often layer in a stepwise pattern (Figure 28-1-3). Plain abdominal films may also demonstrate the cause of the obstruction (e. g., foreign bodies or gallstones) (Figure 28-1-4). In uncertain cases or when one is unable to differentiate partial from complete obstruction, further diagnostic evaluations may be required.

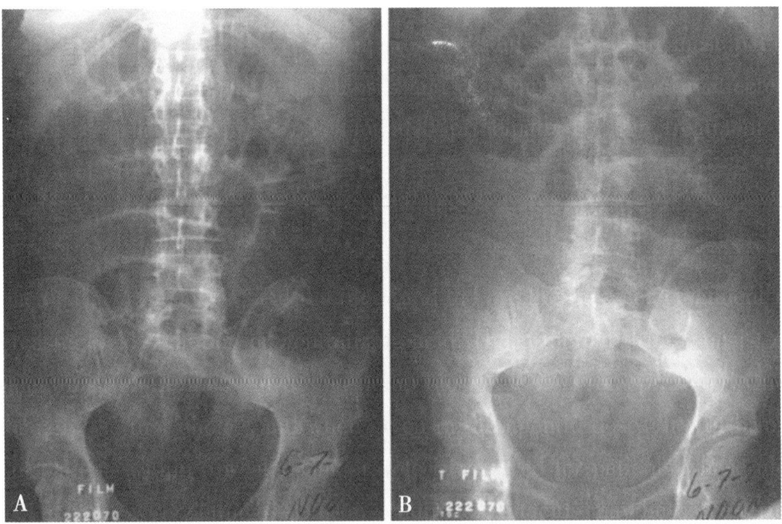

Figure 28-1-3 Plain abdominal radiographs of a patient with a complete small bowel obstruction

A. Supine film shows dilated loops of small bowel in an orderly arrangement, without evidence of colonic gas; B. Upright film shows multiple, short air-fluid levels arranged in a stepwise pattern.

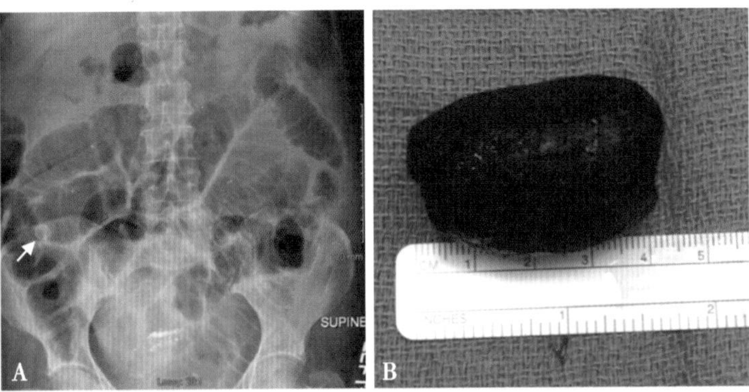

Figure 28-1-4 Plain radiograph of abdomen

A. Plain abdominal film shows complete bowel obstruction caused by a large radiopaque gallstone(arrow) obstructing the distal ileum; B. The large gallstone responsible for the obstruction seen in the corresponding plain abdominal film.

1.3.3.2 Computed tomography

In the more complex patient in whom the diagnosis is not readily apparent, CT has proved to be beneficial(Figure 28-1-5). CT is particularly sensitive for diagnosing complete or high-grade obstruction of the small bowel and for determining the location and cause of obstruction. The CT examination is less sensitive, however, in patients with partial small bowel obstruction. In addition, CT is helpful if an extrinsic cause of bowel obstruction(e. g. , abdominal tumors, inflammatory disease, or abscess) is suggested(Figure 28-1-6). CT has also been described as useful in determining bowel strangulation. Unfortunately, CT findings associated with strangulation are those of irreversible ischemia and necrosis. Importantly, the emergent surgical management of a toxic patient with a bowel obstruction identified by a thorough history and physical examination should not be delayed to perform further unnecessary and costly radiographic studies.

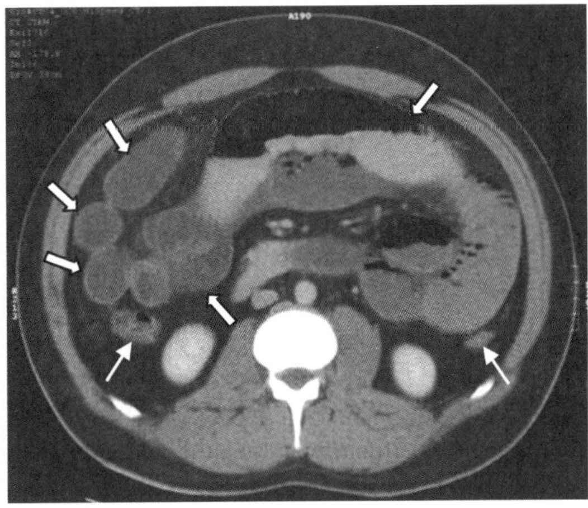

Figure 28-1-5 CT scans of small bowel obstruction

CT scan through the midabdomen shows dilated small bowel loops filled with fluid (thick arrows) and decompressed ascending and descending colon(thin arrows). These are typical CT findings in small bowel obstruction.

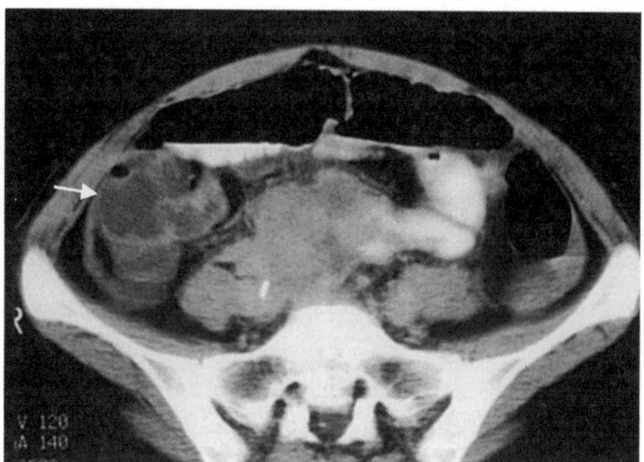

Figure 28-1-6 **CT scan of mechanical small bowel obstruction**

CT scan of the abdomen of a patient with a mechanical bowel obstruction secondary to an abscess in the right lower quadrant (arrow). Multiple dilated and fluid-filled loops of small bowel are noted.

1.3.3.3 Barium studies

Barium studies, namely, enteroclysis, have been a useful adjunct in certain patients with a presumed obstruction. This procedure involves the continued infusion of 500-1000 mL of thin barium sulfate and methylcellulose suspension into the intestine through a duodenal tube. The suspension is then viewed continuously with use of either fluoroscopy or standard radiographs taken at frequent intervals; therefore, this technique is a double-contrast procedure that allows detailed imaging of the entire small intestine. Enteroclysis has been advocated as the definitive study in patients in whom the diagnosis of low-grade, intermittent small bowel obstruction is clinically uncertain. In addition, barium studies can precisely demonstrate the level of the obstruction as well as the cause of the obstruction in certain instances (Figure 28-1-7). The main disadvantages of enteroclysis are the need for nasoenteric intubation, the slow transit of contrast material in patients with a fluid-filled hypotonic small bowel, and the enhanced expertise required by the radiologist to perform this procedure.

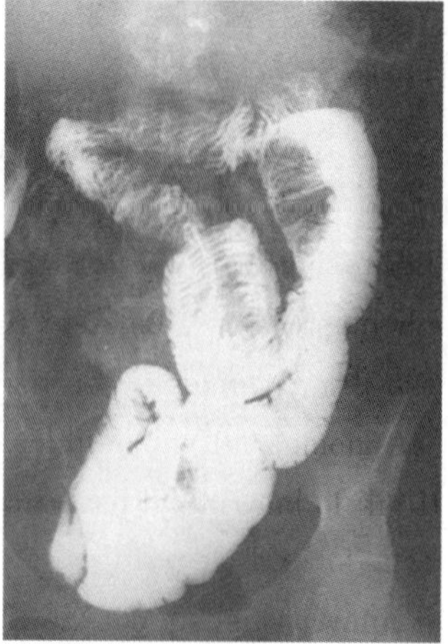

Figure 28-1-7 Barium study demonstrates jejunojejunal intussusception

1.3.3.4 Ultrasound

Ultrasound has been reported to be useful in pregnant patients because radiation exposure is a concern.

1.3.3.5 Magnetic resonance imaging

MRI has been described in patients with obstruction; however, it appears to be no better diagnostically than CT.

To summarize, plain abdominal radiographs are usually diagnostic of bowel obstruction in more than 60% of the cases, but further evaluation (possibly by CT or barium radiography) may be necessary in 20%–30% of cases. CT examination is particularly useful in patients with a history of abdominal malignancy, in postsurgical patients, and in patients who have no history of abdominal surgery and present with symptoms of bowel obstruction. Barium studies are recommended in patients with a history of recurring obstruction or low-grade mechanical obstruction to precisely define the obstructed segment and degree of obstruction.

Laboratory examinations: Laboratory examinations are not helpful in the actual diagnosis of patients with small bowel obstruction but are extremely important in assessing the degree of dehydration. Patients with a bowel obstruction should routinely have laboratory measurements of serum sodium, chloride, potassium, bicarbonate, and creatinine. The serial determination of serum electrolytes should be performed to assess the adequacy of fluid resuscitation. Dehydration may result in hemoconcentration, as noted by an elevated hematocrit. This value should be monitored because fluid resuscitation results in a decrease in the hematocrit, and some patients (e. g., those with intestinal malignancies) may require blood transfusions before surgery. In addition, the white blood cell count should be assessed. Leukocytosis may be found in patients with strangulation; however, an elevated white blood cell count does not necessarily denote strangulation. Conversely, the absence of leukocytosis does not eliminate strangulation as a possibility.

1.4 Diagnosis

The diagnostic evaluation should focus on the following goals:

(1) Distinguish mechanical obstruction from ileus.

(2) Determine the etiology of the obstruction.

(3) Discriminate partial from complete obstruction.

(4) Discriminate simple from strangulating obstruction.

Important elements to obtain on history include prior abdominal operations (suggesting the presence of adhesions) and the presence of abdominal disorders (e. g., intra-abdominal cancer or inflammatory bowel disease) that may provide insights into the etiology of obstruction. Upon examination, a meticulous search for hernias (particularly in the inguinal and femoral regions) should be conducted.

1.5 Differential Diagnosis

1.5.1 Paralytic ileus

Pain from paralytic ileus is usually not severe but is constant and diffuse, and the abdomen is distended and mildly tender. If ileus has resulted from an acute intraperitoneal inflammatory process(e. g. ,acute appendicitis),there should be symptoms and signs of the primary problem as well as the ileus. Plain films show gas mainly in the colon in uncomplicated postoperative ileus;gas in the small bowel suggests peritonitis. Small bowel X-rays may be required in order to distinguish ileus from mechanical obstruction in postoperative patients.

1.5.2 Obstruction of the large intestine

It is characterized by obstipation and abdominal distention;pain is less often colicky,and vomiting is an inconstant symptom. X-rays usually make the diagnosis by demonstrating colonic dilation proximal to the obstructing lesion. If the ileocecal valve is incompetent,the distal small bowel will be dilated,and a barium enema may be needed to determine the level of obstruction.

1.5.3 Acute gastroenteritis,acute appendicitis,acute pancreatitis,acute hemorrhagic pancreatitis and mesenteric vascular occlusion

Acute gastroenteritis,acute appendicitis,and acute pancreatitis can mimic simple intestinal obstruction. Strangulation obstruction may be confused with acute hemorrhagic pancreatitis or mesenteric vascular occlusion.

1.5.4 Intestinal pseudo-obstruction

It is a diverse group of disorders in which there are symptoms and signs of intestinal obstruction without evidence for an obstructing lesion. Acute pseudo-obstruction of the colon carries the risk of cecal perforation. Chronic or recurrent pseudo-obstruction affecting the small bowel with or without colonic involvement is often idiopathic. In other cases,pseudo-obstruction is associated with scleroderma,myxedema,lupus erythematosus,amyloidosis,drug abuse(e. g. ,phenothiazine ingestion),radiation injury,or progressive systemic sclerosis. Several variations of familial visceral myopathy have been identified with seemingly distinct patterns of intestinal pseudo-obstruction. Patients with familial visceral neuropathy have degeneration of axons and neurons of the myenteric plexus of the gastrointestinal tract,and pseudo-obstruction results.

Patients withchronic pseudo obstruction have recurrent attacks of vomiting,cramping abdominal pain, and abdominal distention. In some patients the esophagus,stomach,small bowel,colon,and urinary bladder all have abnormal motility,but in others one or more of these organs may be spared. Treatment is directed at the underlying disease if there is one. Management of idiopathic pseudo-obstruction is largely supportive, but cisapride may be effective in the neuropathic variety.

1.6 Simple Versus Strangulating Obstruction

Most patients with small bowel obstruction are classified as having simple obstructions that involve mechanical blockage of the flow of luminal contents without compromised viability of the intestinal wall. In contrast,strangulation obstruction,which usually involves a closed-loop obstruction in which the vascular supply to a segment of intestine is compromised,can lead to intestinal infarction. Strangulation obstruction is associated with an increased morbidity and mortality risk,and therefore recognition of early strangulation is important. In differentiating from simple intestinal obstruction,classic signs of strangulation have been described and include tachycardia,fever,leukocytosis,and a constant,noncramping abdominal pain. However, a number of studies have convincingly shown that no clinical parameters or laboratory measurements can accurately detect or exclude the presence of strangulation in all cases. This reinforces the dictum that a careful history and physical examination are key for an accurate and timely diagnosis.

CT examination is useful only in detecting the late stages of irreversible ischemia(e. g. ,pneumatosis intestinalis,portal venous gas). Various serum determinations,including lactate dehydrogenase,amylase,alkaline phosphatase,and ammonia levels,have been assessed with no real benefit. Initial reports have described some limited success in discriminating strangulation by measuring serum D-lactate,creatine phosphokinase isoenzyme(particularly the BB isoenzyme),or intestinal fatty acid-binding protein;however, these are only investigational and can not be widely applied to patients with obstruction. Finally,noninvasive determinations of mesenteric ischemia have been described using a superconducting quantum interference device(SQUID)magnetometer to noninvasively detect mesenteric ischemia. Intestinal ischemia is associated with changes in the basic electrical rhythm of the small intestine. This technique remains investigational and is not in widespread clinical use.

Thus,it is important to remember that bowel ischemia and strangulation can not be reliably diagnosed or excluded preoperatively in all cases by any known clinical parameter,combination of parameters,or current laboratory and radiographic examinations.

1.7 Treatment

1.7.1 Non-operative

1.7.1.1 Fluid resuscitation

Patients with intestinal obstruction are usually dehydrated and depleted of sodium,chloride,and potassium,requiring aggressive intravenous(IV) replacement with an isotonic saline solution such as lactated Ringer's. Urine output should be monitored by the placement of a Foley catheter. After the patient has formed adequate urine,potassium chloride should be added to the infusion if needed. Serial electrolyte measurements,as well as hematocrit and white blood cell count,are performed to assess the adequacy of fluid repletion. Because of large fluid requirements,patients,particularly the elderly,may require central venous assessment and,in some cases,the placement of a Swan-Ganz catheter.

1.7.1.2 Antibiotics

Broad-spectrum antibiotics are given prophylactically by some surgeons based on the reported findings of bacterial translocation occurring even in simple mechanical obstructions;however,there is no substantial evidence to support the use of antimicrobial therapy in nontoxic-appearing patients or those without suspected bacterial overgrowth of the small intestine. Antibiotics are administered preoperatively in the event that the patient requires surgery.

1.7.1.3 Tube decompression

In addition to IV fluid resuscitation,another important adjunct to the supportive care of patients with intestinal obstruction is nasogastric suction. Suction with a nasogastric tube empties the stomach,reducing the hazard of pulmonary aspiration of vomitus and minimizing further intestinal distention from preoperatively swallowed air. Nasogastric decompression in a patient with small bowel obstruction is still considered standard of care.

The use of long intestinal tubes(e. g. ,Cantor or Baker tube) has been advocated by some. However, prospective randomized trials have demonstrated no significant differences with regard to the decompression achieved, success of non-operative treatment, or morbidity rate after surgical intervention compared with the use of nasogastric tubes. Furthermore, the use of these long tubes has been associated with a significantly longer hospital stay, duration of postoperative ileus, and postoperative complications in some series. Therefore, it appears that long intestinal tubes also offer no benefit in the preoperative setting over nasogastric tubes.

Patients with a partial intestinal obstruction may be treated conservatively with resuscitation and tube decompression alone. Resolution of symptoms and discharge without the need for surgery have been reported in up to 85% of patients with a partial obstruction. Enteroclysis can assist in determining the degree of obstruction, with higher-grade partial obstructions requiring earlier operative intervention. Although an initial trial of non-operative management of most patients with partial small bowel obstruction is warranted, it should be emphasized that clinical deterioration of the patient or increasing small bowel distention on abdominal radiographs during tube decompression warrants prompt operative intervention. The decision to continue to treat a patient non-operatively with a presumed bowel obstruction is based on clinical judgment and requires constant vigilance to ensure that the clinical course has not changed.

1.7.2 Operative management

In general, the patient with acomplete small bowel obstruction requires operative intervention. A nonoperative approach to selected patients with complete small intestinal obstruction has been proposed by some, who argue that prolonged intubation is safe in these patients provided that no fever, tachycardia, tenderness, or leukocytosis is noted. Nevertheless, one must realize that nonoperative management of these patients is undertaken at a calculated risk of overlooking an underlying strangulation obstruction. This delay of definitive treatment often necessitates an urgent surgical intervention and can result in increased morbidity and mortality compared with patients who undergo a more prompt intervention. Retrospective studies have reported that a 12-24 hour delay of surgery in these patients is safe but that the incidence of strangulation and other complications increases significantly after this time period.

The nature of the problem dictates the approach to man agement of the obstructed patient. Patients with intestinal obstruction secondary to anadhesive band may be treated with lysis of adhesions. Great care should be used in the gentle handling of the bowel to reduce serosal trauma and avoid unnecessary dissection and inadvertent enterotomies. Incarcerated hernias can be managed by manual reduction of the herniated segment of bowel and closure of the defect.

The treatment of patients with an obstruction and a history of malignant tumors can be particularly challenging. In the terminal patient with widespread metastasis, non-operative management, if successful, is usually the best course; however, only a small percentage of cases of complete obstruction can be successfully managed nonoperatively. In this case, a simple bypass of the obstructing lesion, by whatever means, may offer the best option rather than a long and complicated operation that may entail bowel resection.

An obstruction secondary to Crohn's disease will often resolve with conservative management if the obstruction is acute. If a chronic fibrotic stricture is the cause of the obstruction, then a bowel resection or strictureplasty may be required.

Patients with anintra-abdominal abscess can present in a manner indistinguishable from those with mechanical bowel obstruction. CT is particularly useful in diagnosing the cause of the obstruction in these patients; percutaneous drainage of the abscess may be sufficient to relieve the obstruction, but laparotomy and abdominal washout may be required for large and established abscesses. Laparoscopic drainage is also an option in cases not amenable to image-guided percutaneous drainage for patients who would not otherwise tolerate a laparotomy; it has reduced wound morbidity and is also useful in multiloculated collections and allows a washout of the peritoneal cavity at the same time.

Radiation enteropathy, as a complication of radiation therapy for pelvic malignant neoplasms, may cause bowel obstruction. Most cases can be treated non-operatively with tube decompression and possibly corticosteroids, particularly during the acute setting. In the chronic setting, non-operative management is rarely effective and will require laparotomy with possible resection of the irradiated bowel or bypass of the affected area.

At the time of exploration, it can sometimes be difficult to evaluate bowel viability after the release of astrangulation. If intestinal viability is questionable, the bowel segment should be completely released and placed in a warm, saline-moistened sponge for 15-20 minutes and then reexamined. If normal color has returned and peristalsis is evident, it is safe to retain the bowel. A prospective controlled trial comparing clinical judgment with the use of a Doppler probe or the administration of fluorescein for the intraoperative discrimination of viability found that the Doppler flow probe added little to the conventional clinical judgment of the surgeon. In difficult borderline cases, fluorescein fluorescence may supplement clinical judgment. Intraoperative near-infrared angiography to determine the presence of ischemic bowel has shown promising results, but this technique is currently not in wide clinical use. Another approach to the assessment of bowel viability is the so-called second look laparotomy 18-24 hours after the initial procedure. This decision should be made at the time of the initial operation. A second-look laparotomy is clearly indicated in a patient whose condition deteriorates after the initial operation.

Some studies have evaluated the efficacy of laparoscopic management of acute small bowel obstruction. The laparoscopic treatment of small bowel obstruction appears to be effective and leads to a shorter hospital stay and reduced overall complications in a highly selected group of patients. Patients fitting the criteria for consideration of laparoscopic management include those with the following symptoms: ①Mild abdominal distention allowing adequate visualization. ②Proximal obstruction. ③Partial obstruction. ④Anticipated single-band obstruction.

In particular, laparoscopic treatment has been found to be of greatest benefit in patients who have undergone fewer than three previous operations, were seen early after the onset of symptoms, and were thought to have adhesive bands as the cause. Currently, patients who have advanced, complete, or distal small bowel obstructions are not candidates for laparoscopic treatment. Similarly, patients with matted adhesions or carcinomatosis or those who remain distended after nasogastric intubation should be managed with conventional laparotomy. Therefore, the future role of laparoscopic procedures in the treatment of these patients remains to be completely defined. A multicenter, prospective, randomized trial comparing laparoscopic adhesiolysis to open surgery in patients with adhesive small bowel obstruction, diagnosed by CT scan, that fails to resolve with nonoperative management is currently accruing patients for evaluation.

1.8 Outcomes

Prognosis is related to the etiology of obstruction. The majority of patients who are treated conservatively for adhesive small bowel obstruction do not require future readmissions; less than 20% of such patients will have a readmission over the subsequent 5 years with another episode of bowel obstruction.

The perioperative mortality rate associated with surgery for nonstrangulating small bowel obstruction is less than 5%, with most deaths occurring in elderly patients with significant comorbidities. Mortality rates associated with surgery for strangulating obstruction range from 8% to 25%.

Considering the frequency of small bowel obstruction and the varied degree of clinical severity and presentation, there is often no consistency as to whether the patient is admitted to the medical or surgical service, and further variability in whether and when surgery is consulted. Recent studies have shown that a standard hospital-wide policy can help improve care of patients with bowel obstruction, reducing their time to surgery and shortening their length of hospital stay.

1.9 Prevention

With adhesive small bowel obstruction representing a large therapeutic burden, prevention of postoperative adhesions has become an area of great interest. Good surgical technique, careful handling of tissue, and minimal use and exposure of peritoneum to foreign bodies form the cornerstone of adhesion prevention. These measures alone are often inadequate. In patients undergoing colorectal or pelvic surgery, hospital readmission rates of greater than 30% over the subsequent 10 years have been reported for adhesive small bowel obstruction.

Use of laparoscopic surgery, when possible, has been strongly promoted. A recent study using the Swedish inpatient register has shown that, compared to laparoscopy, open surgery is associated with a four-fold increase in risk of small bowel obstruction within 5 years of the index procedure even after accounting for other risk factors such as age, comorbidity, and previous abdominal surgery.

In those undergoing open surgery, several strategies for adhesion prevention have been tried; however, the only therapy that has shown some success has been the use of hyaluronanbased agents, such as Seprafilm. The use of this barrier has been clearly shown to reduce the incidence of postoperative bowel adhesions; however, its effect in actually reducing the incidence of small bowel obstruction remains less well defined. The use of these products is often left to the discretion of the surgeon and the clinical context. Wrapping of an intestinal anastomosis with the material may be associated with increased leak rates and is generally discouraged.

1.10 Specific Types of Bowel Obstruction

1.10.1 Chronic adhesions

Peritoneal adhesions account for more than half of small-bowel obstruction cases. Lower abdominal procedures such as appendectomy, hysterectomy, colectomy, and abdominoperineal resection are common precursor operations to adhesive obstruction. Adhesions form after any abdominal procedure, however, including cholecystectomy, gastrectomy, and abdominal vascular procedures. In long-term follow-up, about 5% of patients undergoing laparotomy will develop adhesive obstruction; of these, 10%-30% will suffer from additional episodes. Up to 80% episodes of small-bowel obstruction due to adhesions may resolve nonoperatively. However, an index episode and three recurrences indicate a likelihood of over 80% that there will be more recurrences. Surgical management of an acute episode appears to reduce subsequent recurrence rates from 15% ~6% ;but no studies have been able to establish whether the immediate benefit of laparotomy for any given episode of simple adhesive obstruction outweighs the overall benefit of expectant management and operation only for serial recurrences. Thus, a previous history of a laparotomy simply provides a reasonable basis for expectant management of patients in whom it is not yet possible to diagnose a complete obstruction. Ultimately, patients who present with signs and symptoms from bowel obstruction are managed according to the CT findings and clinical course.

The pathobiology of adhesion formation has been the subject of considerable investigation. Histologic examination of chronic adhesions reveals foreign body reaction, usually to talc, starch, lint, intestinal content, or suture. Talc and starch are found less commonly now than previously, because of improvements in techniques of manufacture and sterilization of surgical gloves. Mesothelial cells are the presumed origin of tissue plasminogen activator(TPA). TPA binds fibrin and plasminogen, thereby preventing adhesion formation. In early studies, inflammatory cells, including mast cells, were implicated in the process that produces adhesions. Recent studies have emphasized the role of various cytokines in exacerbating or inhibiting adhesion formation in different animal models. Biologically active substances that might prove useful in preventing postoperative adhesions include transforming growth factor-β(TGF-β) and vascular endothelial growth factor(VEGF), both of which may be targeted for inhibition with less fear of compromising the response to bacterial infection.

Current strategies to prevent adhesions after a first laparotomy include targeting the fibrinolytic system, which enhances rapid healing and appears to minimize formation of peritoneal adhesions. Attempts to minimize or prevent adhesion formation have resulted in development of a hyaluronic acid-carboxymethylcellulose membrane(Seprafilm, Genzyme, Cambridge, MA). This compound mechanically prevents adhesion formation by physically separating adjoining tissues. It is absorbed by the body in 7 days and thus is present only during the phase of fibrosis, and not as a persistent foreign body. Randomized trials have suggested that this compound prevents, minimizes severity, and decreases density and vascularity of adhesions. Other trials corroborate decreased severity, density, and vascularity of adhesions but not total prevention of adhesions or reduction of the incidence of subsequent bowel obstruction. Seprafilm and similar barriers have been advocated for use in patients in whom a second abdominal procedure is planned or significant adhesions anticipated(e. g., Hartmann procedure, ileal pouch anal anastomosis with protecting ileostomy, pelvic surgery, gynecologic procedures, and colon surgery), though it has been proposed for all surgeries by the manufacturers. Meta-analyses in gynecologic procedures support claims that numbers and density of adhesions are reduced, without necessarily improving the incidence of subsequent intestinal obstruction.

More important than pharmacologic approaches, however, are the efforts of the surgeon to pay meticulous attention to hemostasis and surgical technique, and to carefully inspect for and remove foreign material from the peritoneal cavity. It is also possible that the use of monofilament sutures for fascial closure and avoidance of closure of the peritoneum as a separate layer may lower the formation of adhesions between viscera and the abdominal wall.

1.10.2 Early postoperative adhesions

Obstruction in the immediate period following abdominal surgery is uncommon but may occur in up to 1 percent of patients in the 4 weeks following laparotomy. Adhesions are responsible for approximately 90% of such cases and hernias for approximately 7%. Intussusception, abscess, or technical errors may be responsible for the remainder of cases. Most cases occur after surgery of the colon, especially abdominoperineal resections, or operations in the lower abdomen. It is rare for upper abdominal surgery to cause such obstructions. A common scenario is that a patient will undergo colectomy uneventfully, pass flatus, and have bowel sounds by postoperative day 3. On the fourth postoperative day the patient suddenly becomes distended and uncomfortable, and stops passing flatus and stool. Patients with acutely evolving symptoms and signs represent complete obstruction and should be managed as such. In this latter setting, the mortality may be as high as 15%; due to delays in recognition and operative intervention. The loss of bowel sounds after a short period of normal or hyperactive activity is worrisome for ischemia of the obstructed segment. The vast majority of such cases may be treated as partial intestinal obstruction; nasogastric suction and intravenous fluids will help resolve symptoms within a few days. When the clinical course does not demand earlier intervention, a nonoperative approach may be tried for 10-14 days and will resolve the obstruction in over 75% of such cases.

1.10.3 Hernia

Hernias of all types are second only to adhesions as the most frequent causes of obstruction in western countries. External hernias such as inguinal (Figure 28-1-8) or femoral hernias may present with the symptoms of obstruction and will not be diagnosed unless sought. Femoral hernias are particularly prone to incarceration and bowel necrosis due to the small size of the hernia inlet. Other hernias such as umbilical, incisional, paracolostomy, or lumbar hernias are obvious. Still others such as internal hernias are usually diagnosed at laparotomy for obstruction. These include obturator hernias, paraduodenal hernias (Figure 28-1-9), and hernias through the foramen of Winslow or mesenteries. When hernia has been identified as the cause of the obstruction, the patient is quickly resuscitated, given antibiotics, and taken to the operating room. The hernia is then reduced and the viability of the bowel assessed. If viable, the bowel is left alone; if not, it is resected. The hernia defect is then repaired. One important consideration is the Richter hernia. In this variant, only a portion of the wall of the bowel is incarcerated and thus incarceration and strangulation may not be associated with complete obstruction. These most frequently occur in association with femoral or inguinal hernias. Complete obstruction can occur if more than half of the bowel circumference is incarcerated.

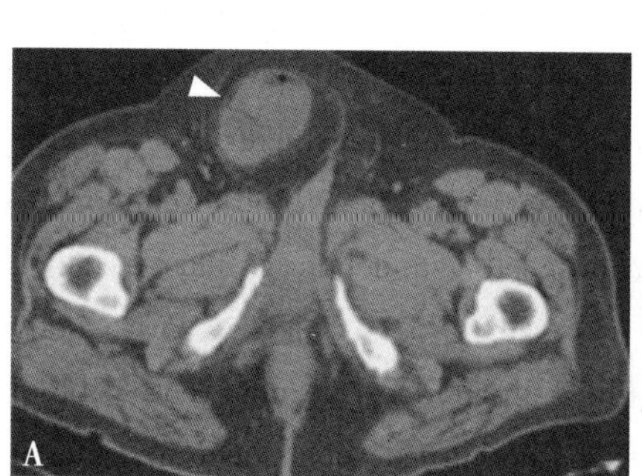

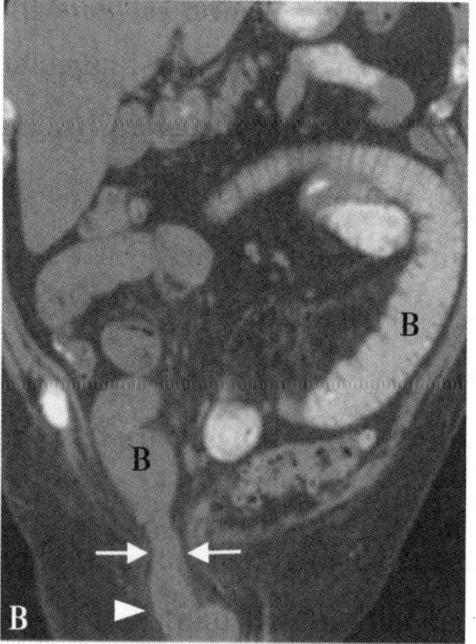

Figure 28-1-8 Computed tomography images of an inguinal hernia

Axial (A) and coronal CT scan (B) images showing incarcerated right inguinal hernia with air and fluid filled loop of small bowel (arrowhead) in the right inguinal canal (arrow) causing small bowel obstruction with dilated loops of proximal small bowel (B).

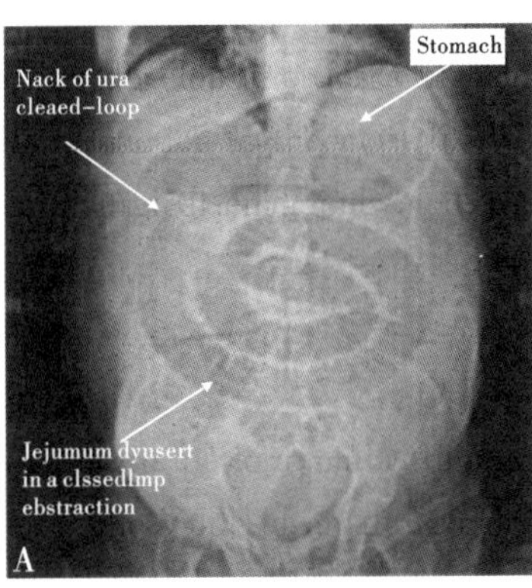

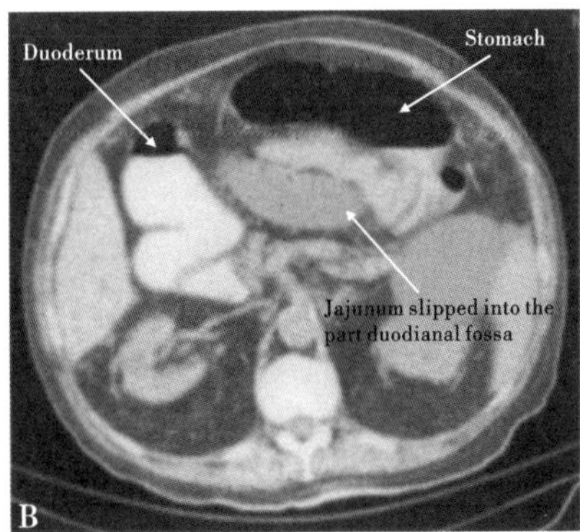

Figure 28-1-9 Paraduodenal hernia

A. Plain film of closed-loop obstruction with neck of the closed loop in the right upper abdomen; B. Computed tomography scan showing slippage of the jejunum behind the stomach, with dilatation and obstruction of the duodenum.

For external(abdominal wall)hernias, it may be possible to perform taxis, that is, the manual reduction of an incarcerated/irreducible hernia. Taxis is usually successful in reduction of an irreducible hernia. Occasionally, taxis results in reduction of the contents of the hernia sac en mass(still obstructed), reduction of strangulated bowel resulting in generalized peritonitis, or reduction of an obstructed Richter hernia. This is one reason for using circumspection in relying on taxis as a mode of treatment for incarcerated inguinal, femoral, and incisional hernias. In general, taxis should be followed expeditiously by operative repair.

1.10.4 Gallstone ileus

As a result of intense inflammation surrounding a gallstone, a fistula may develop between the biliary tree and the small or large intestine. Most fistulas develop between the gallbladder fundus and duodenum. If the stone is greater than 2.5 cm in diameter, it can lodge in the narrowest portion of the terminal ileum, which is just proximal to the ileocecal valve. This complication is rare, accounting for less than 6 in 1000 cases of cholelithiasis and no more than 3% of cases of intestinal obstruction. Typically, the patient is elderly and presents with intermittent symptoms over several days, as the stone tumbles distally toward the ileum. The classic findings on plain radiographs include those of intestinal obstruction, a stone lying outside the right upper quadrant, and air in the biliary tree(Figure 28-1-10). Treatment includes removal of the stone and resection of the obstructed segment only if there is evidence of tissue necrosis. The risk of a recurrent gallstone ileus is 5%-10%. Such recurrences usually occur within 30 days of the initial episode and are usually due to stones in the small intestine that were missed at the original operation.

The difficult decisions in management of gallstone ileus focus on the fistula. The arguments in favor of disconnecting the fistula and removing the gallbladder have been the possibility of recurrence of gallstone ileus and the risk of cholangitis due to reflux of intestinal content into the biliary tree. When the latter operation is included, the mortality may be doubled as compared to simple removal of the gallstone. It is used selectively in good-risk patients. The long-term incidence of biliary tract infections has not been common enough to warrant the more aggressive approach at the initial operation. Some authors have advocated cholecystectomy at a second operation, especially if the patient is young and fit. The consensus is that cholecystectomy should not be performed at the initial operation for gallstone ileus, except in highly selected patients. A careful search of the entire intestine should be performed to exclude the possibility of additional large stones.

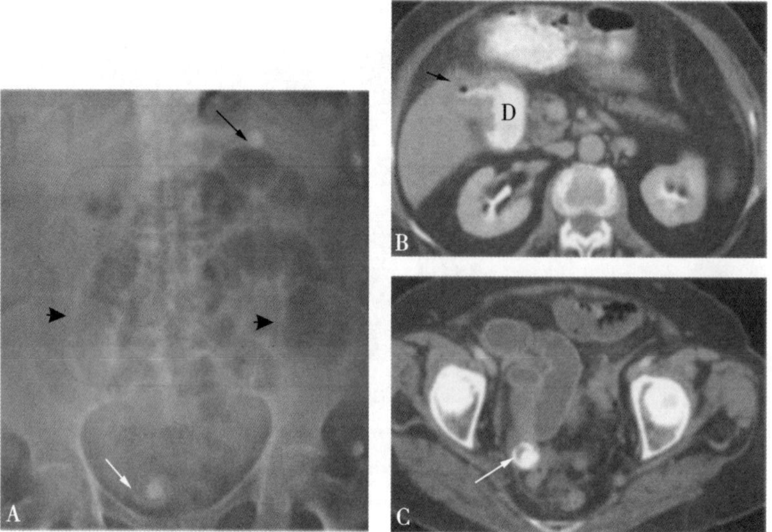

Figure 28-1-10 Plain radiograph and CT scans of a patient with gallstone ileus

A. Plain radiograph of a patient with gallstone ileus, showing obstructed loops of small intestine (black arrow) in the abdomen and a gallstone (white arrow) in the pelvis [gallstone was initially misinterpreted as an EKG lead (black arrow)]; B. Computed tomography (CT) scan showing a cholecystoduodenal fistula (black arrow) with air in the biliary tree (D, duodenum); C. CT scan showing gallstone (white arrow) in the distal ileum and fecalization of luminal content adjacent to the stone.

1.10.5 Intussusception

About 5% of intussusceptions occur in adults. An intussusception occurs when one segment of bowel telescopes into an adjacent segment, resulting in obstruction and ischemic injury to the intussuscepting segment (Figure 28-1-11), and the obstruction may become complete, particularly if tissue inflammation and necrosis occur. Of adult cases, 90% are associated with pathologic processes. Tumors, benign or malignant, act as the lead point of intussusception in more than 65% of adult cases. A significant proportion of cases have been reported to occur after abdominal surgery for lesions other than neoplasm. In cases not associated with neoplasm, Sarr et al. reported that approximately 20% were related to the suture line, approximately 30% to adhesions, and approximately 60% to intestinal tubes. Intussusception related to long tubes can occur when the tube is withdrawn, but most frequently occurs with the tube in place. Perioperative intussusception frequently subsides without intervention.

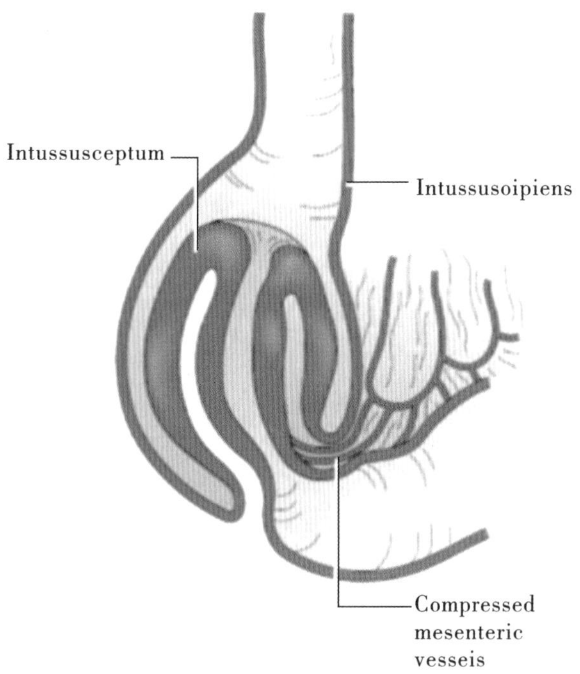

Figure 28-1-11 Anatomy of intussusception. The intussusceptum is the segment of bowel that invaginates into the intussuscipiens

Four types of intussusception are recognized: enteric (Figure 28-1-12), ileocolic, ileocecal, and colonic. In the ileocolic form, the ileum telescopes into the colon past a fixed ileocecal valve. In the ileocecal form, the valve itself may be the lead point of the intussusception. Radiographic features of intussusception are not specific. Plain films reveal evidence of partial or complete obstruction. Occasionally, a sausage-shaped soft tissue density will be seen, outlined by two strips of air. Recently, in both pediatric and adult cases, it has been suggested that sonography may be useful in diagnosis. Nevertheless, the mainstays of diagnosis are contrast studies or CT scan. Because of the high incidence of tumors, surgery has generally been recommended. Reduction by hydrostatic pressure, which is the standard of care in pediatric cases, is not usually attempted in adults. Clear indications for operation include long length and wide diameter of the intussusception, presence of a lead point, or evidence of bowel obstruction. Recent studies have called into question the need to operate in all cases detected on sensitive imaging studies such as CT scan, arguing that a number of these patients can be safely managed without operation. However, in the opinion of these authors, it is difficult to advise expectant management except in unusual circumstances.

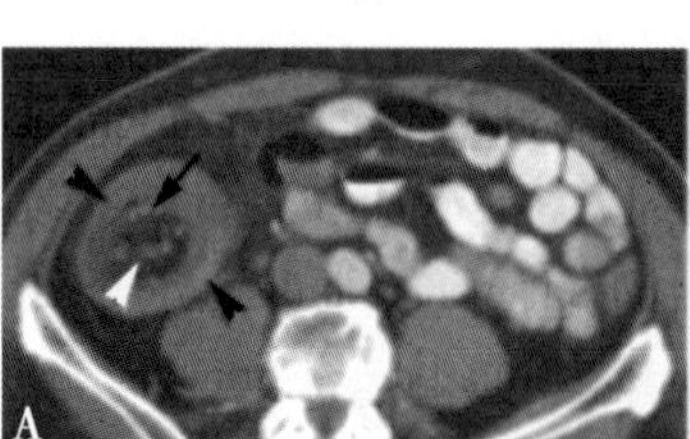

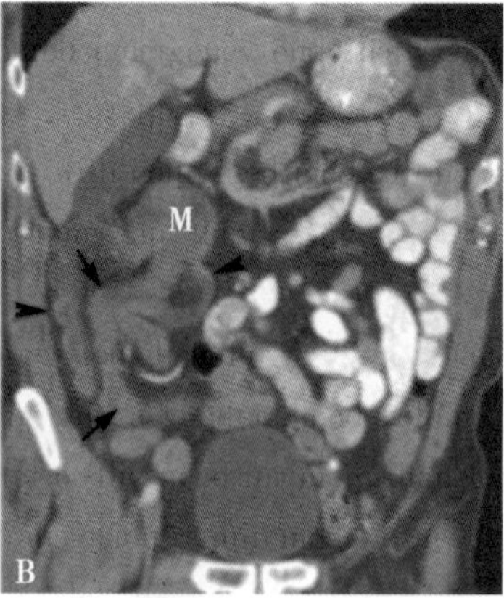

Figure 28-1-12 **CT scan images of an ileocolic intussusception**

Axial(A) and coronal CT scan(B) images of an ileocolic intussusception secondary to colon carcinoma(M) as a lead point. Intussusceptum(long arrows) and intussuscipiens(arrowhead). Mesenteric vessels and fat(white arrowhead) accompany the intussusceptum.

1.10.6 Crohn disease

Indications for surgery in Crohn disease are discussed elsewhere in this book. In this disease, obstruction occurs under two different sets of circumstances. When the disease has flared acutely, the lumen may be narrowed by a reversible inflammatory process. The result is an open-loop obstruction that may respond first to intravenous hydration and nasogastric decompression, and ultimately to therapy with corticosteroids or other anti-inflammatory regimens. Alternatively, obstruction may occur in the setting of a chronic stricture. Such strictures will not respond to conservative measures and, once diagnosed, operative therapy should not be delayed. One important clinical point is that about 7%, of strictures in the colon, and an uncertain proportion of those in the small intestine, are malignant. Extent of resection is thus based on intraoperative findings, that is, to margins beyond visibly diseased bowel and not necessarily including enlarged lymph nodes in the mesentery. If there is suspicion for malignancy, a lymphadenectomy is performed.

A second clinical point is that Crohn-affected bowel may not be dilated proximal to the obstruction but can be complicated by a small perforation. Such a microperforation may not be large enough to be associated with free air on plain films. The patient may thus present with significant abdominal pain and tenderness. A CT scan is likely to be the most sensitive imaging modality for obtaining evidence that differentiates conditions that require immediate surgery(closed-loop obstruction, microperforation) from simple obstruction that would otherwise be observed. In the absence of clinical progression of symptoms and signs, however, extended conservative management is warranted before the patient is committed to surgery.

1.10.7 Malignant obstruction

Obstruction can complicate malignancies of the small and large bowel in a number of settings. Studies have documented that 10%-28% of patients with colorectal cancer and 20%-50% of patients with ovarian cancer will present with a malignant bowel obstruction at some point during the course of their disease. Most commonly, a primary lesion such as an adenocarcinoma or lymphoma will enlarge until the lumen of the intestine is blocked. The lesion then presents with symptoms and signs associated with the level of obstruction and is managed accordingly.

A second setting involves a patient who previously has undergone surgery for malignancy and now returns with evidence of bowel obstruction. The likelihood that the obstruction is due to recurrent disease is based on several factors, including the origin of the primary malignancy, the stage of the primary malignancy, and the designation of the original surgery as curative or palliative. Gastric and pancreatic carcinomas often present with or are subsequently complicated by peritoneal carcinomatosis and thus the subsequent obstruction is most likely due to malignancy. With respect to colon and rectal carcinomas, as many as 50% of cases presenting with obstruction after resection of the primary malignancy may be due to adhesions and not recurrent malignancy. In addition, even if the obstruction is due to now unresectable disease, significant palliation can be obtained through bypass or enterostomy in up to 75% of patients (Figure 28-1-13). However, the underlying diagnosis of cancer in this patient population mandates careful attention be paid to patient selection prior to any surgical intervention and risk factors for poor outcome. In patients presenting with gastroduodenal and colorectal obstructing lesions who are not candidates for surgical bypass or enterostomy, endoscopic management options including percutaneous endoscopic gastrostomy tube (PEG) placement and self-expanding metallic stent (SEMS) placement are available. These options have been associated with symptomatic relief in more than 75% of patients.

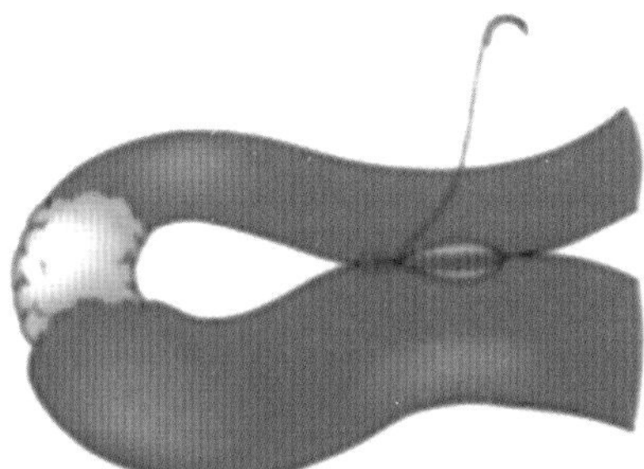

Figure 28-1-13 **Enteroenterostomy is performed to bypass the obstructing segment**

Significant palliation can be achieved in a patient with obstructing but unresectable malignancy.

Management of incurable malignant obstruction may require an approach that moves away from classical surgical teaching of nothing by mouth, nasogastric tube, intravenous fluids, and serial radiographs. Patients with advanced malignant obstruction in the absence of a solitary or correctable obstructing lesion are generally managed without surgery. Patients are managed without a nasogastric tube if possible. They are encouraged to eat as soon as obstructive symptoms resolve using a low-fiber diet. Antiemetics and opioids via continuous subcutaneous infusions are used to manage nausea and vomiting and colic, respectively. In addition, octreotide, a somatostatin analogue, is used in palliation of refractory malignant intestinal obstruction by improving intestinal mucosal absorption, improving motility, reducing gastrointestinal hormone levels and intestinal secretions, and having a direct antineoplastic effect on the obstructing tumor. This allows true palliative care outside a hospital setting saving patients the pain, discomfort, and complications of hospitalization and unproductive surgery.

1.10.8 Volvulus

The term volvulus indicates that a loop of bowel is twisted more than 180 degrees about the axis of its mesentery. Volvulus has been reported for the cecum, transverse colon, splenic flexure, and sigmoid colon. A special variant of volvulus, complicating a condition known as Chilaiditi syndrome, can occur when redundant loops of the transverse colon slip between the liver and diaphragm and then torse. Generally, the condition is asymptomatic, but when associated with volvulus it must be relieved surgically.

The most common site for volvulus is the sigmoid colon, accounting for 65% of cases. By definition, a volvulus is a form of closed-loop obstruction of the colon. Air is always present in the colon and rectum, and thus volvulus of any segment of the colon is associated with abdominal distention and, usually, severe abdominal pain. As shown in Figure 28-1-14, the most common radiographic feature is the "bent inner tube" appearance of the sigmoid, which is located in the upper abdomen. The preferred method of management involves endoscopic decompression. A rigid or flexible proctosigmoidoscope is advanced gently into the rectum until a rush of air and feces indicate that the loop has been untorsed. A rectal tube is then advanced well into the loop as a stent to prevent retorsion. Gangrene of the colon does not usually complicate the picture if the patient is seen and treated promptly. This conservative approach resolves the volvulus in 85%-90% of cases and elective resection or fixation of the redundant segment can then be planned. Following endoscopic decompression, recurrence of the volvulus is higher than 60%. Thus, an operation to remove the sigmoid should be performed if the patient is fit for surgery. However, a majority of these patients are elderly and infirm and approximately 15%; have a history of psychiatric disorder. As a result, the patient may present with peritoneal findings, sepsis, and shock. In this setting, rapid resuscitation followed by urgent resection and colostomy is warranted. Other forms of volvulus generally can not be detorsed without operation. Fixation of the torsed segment(e. g., via cecostomy or cecopexy) is generally a less satisfactory solution than resection of the involved segment and is not generally recommended.

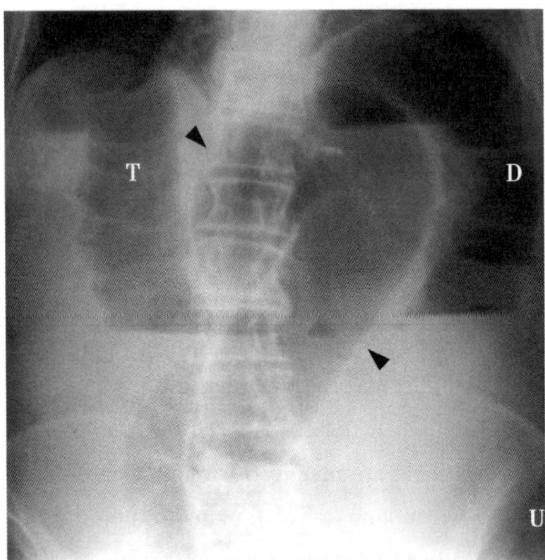

Figure 28-1-14 **Plain upright abdominal film of a patient with sigmoid volvulus**

The dilated centrally located sigmoid loop is seen(arrowheads). The proximal colon is dilated and gas filled.

1.10.9 Radiation enteritis

After asymptomatic periods lasting at least 10 years, chronic intestinal obstruction can result. Radiation injury elicits an underlying vasculitis and fibrosis that lead to chronic, recurring low-grade partial obstruction of the small intestine or stricturing and bleeding in the colon and rectum. Operation is indicated for incapacitating symptoms and obstruction not resolved by conservative management. Recurrence of the original tumor as a cause of obstruction should be considered and excluded. However, the diffuse nature of the injury and pathologic responses can lead to massive resections that leave the patient with short-bowel syndrome. Attempts to suture scarred loops can also result in chronic inflammation and formation of interloop abscesses and fistulas. The incidence of suture line leak is high.

Chapter 2

Ileus and other Disorders of Intestinal Motility

Ileus and intestinal pseudo-obstruction designate clinical syndromes caused by impaired intestinal motility and are characterized by symptoms and signs of intestinal obstruction in the absence of a lesion-causing mechanical obstruction. Ileus is a major cause of morbidity in hospitalized patients. Postoperative ileus is the most frequently implicated cause of delayed discharge following abdominal operations.

Ileus is a temporary motility disorder that is reversed with time as the inciting factor is corrected. In contrast, chronic intestinal pseudo-obstruction comprises a spectrum of specific disorders associated with irreversible intestinal dysmotility.

2.1 Etiologies and Pathophysiology

The most frequently encountered factors are abdominal operations, infection and inflammation, electrolyte abnormalities, and drugs. Common etiologies of ileus are as follows: abdominal surgery, infection, sepsis, intra-abdominal abscess, peritonitis, pneumonia, electrolyte abnormalities, hypokalemia, hypomagnesemia, hypermagnesemia, hyponatremia, medications, anticholinergics and opiates.

Following most abdominal operations or injuries, the motility of the GI tract is transiently impaired. Among the proposed mechanisms responsible for this dysmotility are surgical stress-induced sympathetic reflexes, inflammatory response mediator release, and anesthetic/analgesic side effects, each of which can inhibit intestinal motility. The return of normal motility generally follows a characteristic temporal sequence, with small-intestinal motility returning to normal within the first 24 hours after laparotomy and gastric and colonic motility returning to normal by 48 hours and 3-5 days, respectively. Because small bowel motility is returned before colonic and gastric motility, listening for bowel sounds is not a reliable indicator that ileus has fully resolved. Functional evidence of coordinated GI motility in the form of passing flatus or a bowel movement is a more useful indicator. Resolution of ileus may be delayed in the presence of other factors capable of inciting ileus such as the presence of intra-abdominal abscesses or electrolyte abnormalities.

Chronic intestinal pseudo-obstruction can be caused by a large number of specific abnormalities affecting intestinal smooth muscle, the myenteric plexus, or the extraintestinal nervous system (Table 28-2-1). Visceral myopathies constitute a group of diseases characterized by degeneration and fibrosis of the intestinal muscularis propria. Visceral neuropathies encompass a variety of degenerative disorders of the myenteric and submucosal plexuses. Both sporadic and familial forms of visceral myopathies and neuropathies exist. Systemic disorders involving the smooth muscle, such as progressive systemic sclerosis and progressive muscular dystrophy, and neurologic diseases, such as Parkinson's disease, can also be complicated by chronic intestinal pseudo-obstruction. In addition, viral infections, such as those associated with cytomegalovirus and Epstein-Barr virus, can cause intestinal pseudo-obstruction.

Table 28-2-1 Chronic intestinal pseudo-obstruction: etiologies

Primary Causes
Familial types
Familial visceral myopathies (types I, II, and III)
Familial visceral neuropathies (types I and II)
Childhood visceral myopathies (types I and II)
Sporadic types
Visceral myopathies
Visceral neuropathies
Secondary Causes
Smooth muscle disorders
Collagen vascular diseases (e. g., scleroderma)
Muscular dystrophies (e. g., myotonic dystrophy)
Amyloidosis
Neurologic disorders
Chagas disease, Parkinson's disease, spinal cord injury
Endocrine disorders
Diabetes, hypothyroidism, hypoparathyroidism
Miscellaneous disorders
Radiation enteritis
Pharmacologic causes, e. g., phenothiazines and tricyclic antidepressants
Viral infections

2.2 Clinical Presentation

The clinical presentation of ileus resembles that of small bowel obstruction. Inability to tolerate liquids and solids by mouth, nausea, and lack of flatus or bowel movements are the most common symptoms. Vomiting and abdominal distension may occur. Bowel sounds are characteristically diminished or absent, in contrast to the hyperactive bowel sounds that usually accompany mechanical small bowel obstruction. The clinical manifestations of chronic intestinal pseudo-obstruction include variable degrees of nausea and vomiting and abdominal pain and distention.

2.3 Diagnosis

Routine postoperative ileus should be expected and requires no diagnostic evaluation. If ileus persists beyond 3-5 days postoperatively or occurs in the absence of abdominal surgery, diagnostic evaluation to detect specific underlying factors capable of inciting ileus and to rule out the presence of mechanical obstruction is warranted.

Patient medication lists should be reviewed for the presence of drugs, especially opiates, known to be associated with impaired intestinal motility. Measurement of serum electrolytes may demonstrate electrolyte abnormalities commonly associated with ileus. Abdominal radiographs are often obtained, but the distinction between ileus and mechanical obstruction may be difficult based on this test alone. In the postoperative setting, CT scanning is the test of choice because it can demonstrate the presence of an intra-abdominal abscess or other evidence of peritoneal sepsis that may be causing ileus and can exclude the presence of complete mechanical obstruction. Distinction of postoperative ileus from early postoperative obstruction can be difficult but is helpful in developing the appropriate management plan.

The diagnosis of chronic pseudo-obstruction is suggested by clinical features and confirmed by radiographic and manometric studies. Diagnostic laparotomy or laparoscopy with full-thickness biopsy of the small intestine may be required to establish the specific underlying cause.

2.4 Therapy

The management of ileus consists of limiting oral intake and correcting the underlying inciting factor. If vomiting or abdominal distention is prominent, the stomach should be decompressed using a nasogastric tube. Fluid and electrolytes should be administered intravenously until ileus resolves. If the duration of ileus is prolonged, TPN may be required.

Given the frequency of postoperative ileus and its financial impact, a large number of investigations have been conducted to define strategies to reduce its duration. Although often recommended, the use of early ambulation and routine nasogastric intubation has not been demonstrated to be associated with earlier resolution of postoperative ileus. There is some evidence that early postoperative feeding protocols and are generally well tolerated, reduce postoperative ileus, and can result in a shorter hospital stay. The administration of nonsteroidal anti-inflammatory drugs such as ketorolac and concomitant reductions in opioid dosing have been shown to reduce the duration of ileus in most studies. Similarly, the use of perioperative thoracic epidural anesthesia/analgesia with regimens containing local anesthetics combined with limitation or elimination of systemically administered opioids has been shown to reduce duration of postoperative ileus, although they have not reduced the overall length of hospital stay. Interestingly, recent data have suggested that limiting intra-and postoperative fluid administration can also result in reduction of postoperative ileus and shortened hospital stay. Table 28-2-2 summarizes some of the measures used to minimize postoperative ileus.

Table 28-2-2 Measures to reduce postoperative ileus

Measures
Intraoperative measures
Minimize handling of the bowel
Laparoscopic approach, if possible
Avoid excessive intraoperative fluid administration
Postoperative measures
Early enteral feeding
Epidural anesthesia, if indicated
Avoid excessive intravenous fluid administration
Correct electrolyte abnormalities
Consider mu-opioid antagonists

Most other pharmacologic agents, including prokinetic agents, are associated with efficacy–toxicity profiles that are too unfavorable to warrant routine use. Recently, administration of alvimopan, a novel peripherally active mu–opioid receptor antagonist with limited oral absorption, has been shown to reduce duration of postoperative ileus, hospital stay, and rate of readmissions in several prospective, randomized, placebocontrolled trials and a subsequent meta–analysis. However, any cost savings associated with the use of this drug outside of a clinical trial have been debated.

Surgical interest in minimizing postoperative ileus has led to exploration of other potential avenues. Experiments in rodents have shown reduced postoperative ileus with enteral administration of lipid–rich nutrition, which is believed to work through a CCK–dependent vagovagal reflex.

Therapy of patients with chronic intestinal pseudo–obstruction focuses on palliation of symptoms as well as fluid, electrolyte, and nutritional management. Surgery should be avoided if at all possible. No standard therapies are curative or delay the natural history of any of the specific disorders causing intestinal pseudo–obstruction. Prokinetic agents, such as metoclopramide and erythromycin, are associated with poor efficacy. Cisapride has been associated with palliation of symptoms; however, because of cardiac toxicity and reported deaths, this agent is restricted to compassionate use.

Patients with refractory disease may require strict limitation of oral intake and long–term TPN administration. Despite these measures, some patients will continue to have severe abdominal pain or such copious intestinal secretions that vomiting and fluid and electrolyte losses remain substantial. These patients may require a decompressive gastrostomy or an extended small bowel resection to remove abnormal intestine. Small–intestinal transplantation has been applied in these patients with increasing frequency; the ultimate role of this modality remains to be defined.

Part 29

The Appendix

Chapter 1

Anatomy and Function

The appendix first becomes visible during embryologic development in the eighth week of life as a protubance of the terminal portion of the cecum. During both antenatal and postnatal development, the growth rate of the cecum exceeds that of the appendix, displacing the appendix medialy toward the ileocecal valve. The relationship of the base of the appendix to the cecum remains constant, whereas the tip can be found in a retrocecal, pelvic, subcecal, preileal, or right pericolic position. These anatomic considerations have significant clinical importance in the context of acute appendicitis. The three taenia coli converge at the junction of the cecum with the appendix and can be a useful landmark to identify the appendix. The appendix can vary in length from less than 1 cm to greater than 30 cm; most appendices are 6–9 cm in length. Appendiceal absence, duplication, and diverticula have all been described.

For many years, the appendix was erroneously viewed as a vestiglal organ with no known function. It is now well recognized that the appendix is an immunologic organ which actively participates in the secretion of immunoglobulins, particularly IgA. Though the appendix is an integral component of the gut associated l ymphoid tissue (GALT) system, its function is not essential and appendectomy has not been associated with any predisposition to sepsis or any other manifestation of immune compromise. Lymphoid tissue first appears in the appendix about 2 weeks after birth. The amount of lymphoid tissue increases throughout puberty, remains steady for the next decade, and then begins a steady decrease with age. After the age of 60, virtually no lymphoid tissue remains within the appendix and complete obliteration of the appendiceal lumen is common.

Chapter 2

Acute Appendicitis

2.1 Historical Background

There is evidence in the literature that alchemists and physicians in the 1500 s recognized the existence of a clinical entity associated with severe inflammation of the cecal region, known as "perityphlitis". Although the firstsuccessful appendectomy was reported in 1736. It was not until 1886 that Reginad Fitz helped establish the role of surgical removal of the inflamed appendix as curaive therapy for this disease, which was once though to be fatal. In 1889, Charles MeBumey presented his classic report before the New York Surgical Society on the importance of early operative intervention for acute appendicitis in which he described the point of maximal abdominal tenderness to be determined by the pressure of one finger placed one third of the distance between the anterior superior iliac spine and the umbilicus. 5 years later he devised the muscle spliting incision which today bears his name.

2.2 Incidence

Appendicitis remains one of the most common acute surgical diseases. The incidence of acute appendicitis rough parallels that of lymphoid development, with the peak incidence in early adulthood. Appendicitis occurs more frequently in males especially at the time of puberty. A review of over 2000 patients with appendicitis demonstrated an overall 1.3 : 1 male predominance.

A decline from 100 cases per 100,000 population to 52 cases per 100,000 population was demonstrated over a study period from 1975 to 1991. This degree of change does not seem to be explained by improved diagnosis, and the explanation for phenomenon remains elusive. Currently, 84% of all appendectomies are performed for acute pathology. The rate of normal appendectomy averages 16%, with females comprising 68% of those patients found to have a normal appendix at exploration.

2.3 Pathophysiology

The pathogenesis of acute appendicitis is dependent primarily on obstruction of the appendiceal lumen. The most common pathologic cause of obstruction is marked hyperplasia of the lymphoid follicles, which obstruct the lumen. This occurs in approximately 60% of patients, most of whom are in the younger age groups. The presence of a fecalith may also be a cause of obstruction and occurs in some 35% of patients. In the remainder, foreign bodies inflammatory strictures, and other rare causes are responsible. At times, no specific inciting cause can be found, and in some of these patients, it is probable that a fecalith initiated the inflammation and peristalsis propelled it into the lumen of the cecum.

Mucus continues to be secreted into the lumen following obstruction of the appendiceal lumen. Stasis is created by the obstruction, and bacteria multiply and secrete exotoxins and endotoxins, which damage the epithelium and ulcerate the mucosa. Bacteria can then penetrate through the ulcerated mucosa into the muscular layers of the appendix and establish an inflammatory process. The increased pressure within the lumen also elevat6s the interstitial pressure in the wall of the appendix, impeding arterial blood flow and creating a state of ischemia, with ultimate infarction and gangrene of the appendix. As the muscular layers become necro ti. , perforation of the appendix occurs. Depending on the duration of the inflammatory process, either a walled off abscess occurs at the site or, if the pathologic process has advanced rapidly, the perforation occurs free into the peritoneal cavity and causes generalized peritonitis. If the latter occurs, a very serious clinical situation ensues. , and mutiple intraperitoneal abscesses may follow at various sites in. pelvis and subhepatic and subdiaphragmatic spaces.

2.4 Clinical Manifestations

Symptoms: Abnominal pain is the prime symptom of acute appendicitis. Classically the pain is initially diffusely centered in the lower epigastrium or umblical area, is moderately severe, and is steady, sometimes with intermittent cramping superimposed. After a period varying from 1 to 12 h, but usually within 4 to 6 h, the pain localizes in the right lower quadrant. The classic pain sequencc, though usual, is not invariable. In some patients the pain of appendicitis begins in the right lower quadrant and remains there. Variations in the anatomic location of the appendix account for many of the variations in the principal locus of the somatic phase of the pain. For example, a long appendix with the inflamed tip in the left lower quadrant causes pain in that area; a rectrocecal appendix may cause principally flank or back pain; a pelvic appendix, a principally suprapubic pain; and a retroileal appendix may cause testicular pain, presumably from irritation of the spermatic artery and ureter. Malrotaon is also responsible for puzzling pain patterns. The visceral component is in the normal location, but the somatic component is felt in that part of the abdomen where the cecum has been arrested in rotation.

Anorexia nearly always accompanies appendicitis. It is so constant that the diagnosis should be questioned if the patient is not anorectic. Vomiting occurs in about 75% of patients, but is not prominent or prolonged, and most patients vomit only once or twice.

Most patients give a history of obstruction before the onset of abdominal pain, and many feel that defecation would relieve their abdominal pain. However, diarrhea occurs in some patients, particulary children so that the pattern of bowel function is of little differentinal diagnostic value. The sequence of symptom appearance has great differential diagnostic significance. In over 95% of patients with acute appendicitis, anorexia is the first symptom, followed by abdominal pain, which is followed in turn by vomitting (if vomiting occurs). If vomiting precedes the onset of pain, the diagnosis should be questioned.

2.5 Signs

Physical findings are determined principally by the anatomic position of the inflamed appendix as well as by whether the organ has already ruptured when the patient is first examined.

Vital signs are not changed very much by uncomplicated appendicitis. Temperature elevation is rarely more than 1℃, the pulse rate is normal or slightly elevated. Changes of greater magnitude usually mean that a complication has occurred or that another diagnosis should be considered.

Patients with appendicitis usually prefer to lie supine, with the thighs, particularly the right thighs, drawn up, because any motion increases pain. If asked to move, they do so slowly gingerly.

The classic right 1 ower quadrant physical signs are present when the inflamed appendix lies in the anterior position. Tenderness is often maximal at or near the point described by McBurmey as being "Located exactly between an inch and a half and two inches from the anterior spinous process of the ileum on a straight line drawn from that process to the umbilicus".

Direct rebound tenderness usually present, and referred or indirect rebound tenderness is frequently present, and the tenderness is felt maximally in the right lower quardrant, indicating peritoneal irritation. Rovsing's sign pain in the right lower quadrant when palpatory pressure is exerted in the left lower quadrant also indicates the site of peritoneal irritation. Cutaneous hyperesthesia in the area supplied by the spinal-nerves on the right at T_{10}, T_{11}, and T_{12} frequently but not always accompanies acute appendicitis. In patients with obvious appendicitis, this sign is superfluous, but in some early cases it may be the first positive sign. It is elicited I either by needle prick or, better, by gently picking up the skin between the forefinger and thumb. This ordinarily is not unpleasant but is painful areas of cutaneous hyperesthesia.

Muscular resistance to palpation of the abdominal wall roughly parallels the severity of the inflammatory process. Early in the disease, resistance, if present, consists mainly of voluntary guarding. As peritoneal irritation progresses, muscle spasm increases and becomes largely invol untary true reflex rigidity as opposed to voluntary guarding.

2.6 Laboratory Data

The clinical history and physical examination are most important in establishing a diagnosis of acute appendicitis, but laboratory findings may be helpful. The majority of patients with acute appendicitis have an elevated leukocyte count of 10,000 to 20,000. For those in whom the level is normal, there is generally a shift to the left in the differential leukocyte count, indicating acute inflammation. However, it should be emphasized that a number of patients have a normal leukocyte count, especially the elderly urinary analysis may show a few red cells, indicating some inflammatory contact with the ureter or urinary bladder la significant number of erythrocytes in the urine indicates a primary disorder of the urinary tract.

Radiographic studies are not indicated in classic cases of acute appendicitis but may be useful when the diagnosis is in doubt. Plain films of the abdomen may show a dilated cecum and fluid level and occasionally a calcified fecalith or foreign body Barium enema may show an absence of fling of the appendix, which is suggestive of acute appendicitis. If the lumen of the appendix fills with barium, acute appendicitis is quite unlikely. Ultrasonography examination is sometimes helpful and may show signs indicating an enlarged appendix or an abscess. Similarly, a computed tomography scan of the abdomen may be helpful, particularly in establishing the presence of an abscess. However, it should be emphasized that in the vast majority of patients, these special studies are unnecessary and delay surgical therapy. It should also be mentioned that laparoscopic examination may be used to establish the diagnosis and, in appropriate instances, for appendectomy.

2.7 Differential Diagnosis

The diagnosis of acute appendicitis is particularly difficult in the very young and in the elderly. Infants manifest only lethargy, irritability, and anorexia in the early stages, but vomiting, fever, and pain are apparent as the disease progresses. Classic symptoms are seldom elicited in aged patients, and the diagnosis is often not considered by the examining physician. The course of appendicitis is more virulent in the elderly, and perforation occur sat an earlier stage. Other types of patients presenting diagnostic problem include muscular males(in whom the only symptom may be the "gas stoppage sensation"), pregnant women, and patients recovering from recent abdominal operations. For this reasons, appendicitis should never be lower than second in the differential l diagnosis of any acute abdominal complaint.

The condition that is perhaps most commonly: confused with appendicitis is vague gastrointestinal upset; in man such cases, a specific diagnosis is never established.

2.8 Gastroenteritis

Gastroenteritis often simulates acute appendicitis. The differential diagnosis is especially challenging if gastroenteritis initiates inflammatory changes in appendiceal lymphoid follicles and evolves into true acute appendicitis. It is common to see a few cases of acute appendicitis in a college population in the midst of an epidemic of gastroenteritis. The history is important in differentiating these two conditions: in gastroenteritis, nausea, vomiting, or diarrhea precedes the onset of pain, whereas pain is virtually always the initial symptom in acute appendicitis. Diffuse myalgias, photophobia, headache, etc. , may suggest a viral illness. On physical examination, tenderness is less sharply localized than in acute appendicitis.

Mesenteric lymphadenitis in children and young adults is often a diagnostic problem.

Enterocolitis caused by Salmonella or Yersinia spp may simulate appendicitis. The history and physical signs provide the best guide to a correct diagnosis.

2.9 Female Pelvic Disorders

(1) A ruptured ovarian follicle in a young woman (mittelschmerz) may mimic acute appendicitis. A careful history usually indicates sudden onset of pain in the middle of the menstrual cycle. The pain is most

severe initially and gradually subsides thereafter a sequence not likely to occur in appendicitis. Gastroenteritis symptoms are less prominent than in appendicitis, but sharply localized right lower quadrant tenderness may be quite misleading. These patients seldom appear ill, but at times a differential diagnosis is impossible and operation becomes safer than risking delay.

(2) Pelvic inflammatory disease (specifically, acute salpingitis) often masquerades as appendicitis. Fever tends to be higher in salpingitis and abdominal tenderness is more diffuse, but the patient does not appear acutely ill. By the time high fever and diffuse tenderness complicate appendicitis, the disease is far advanced and the patient is in desperate straits, pelvic examination reveals a tender cervix, and demonstration of intracellular gram negative diplococci in cervical smears clinches the diagnosis of salpingitis.

(3) Twisted ovarian cyst is difficult to distinguish from acute pelvic appendicitis. Pain is severe, abdominal findings may be typical of appendicitis, and the ovarian mass may not be felt on pelvic examination because tenderness is exquisite. The cyst may be palpated by repeating the pelvic examination under anesthesia, and the appropriate incision can then be made for its removal.

(4) Ectopic pregnancy may be distinguished from appendicitis by the history of menstrual irregularity, sudden onset of pain, and diffuse pelvic tenderness. Pain may be referred to the shoulder because of free blood in the peritoneal cavity, and on occasion there are signs of hypovolemic shock. Bloody fluid is usually obtained by culdocentesis.

2.10 Genitourinary Diseases

(1) Ureteral or renal calculi can produce right lower quadrant pain, nausea, and vomiting suggestive of retrocecal or pelvic appendicitis. A history of colicky pain radiating into the groin, findings on urinalysis, and a plain film of the abdomen often clarity the diagnosis, but an intravenous urogram is frequently required.

(2) Pyelonephritis, with or without renal calculi, is also confused with appendicitis. High fever and chills are common with renal infection but infrequent in acute appendicitis. Costovertebral angle tenderness and pyuria establish the diagnosis.

2.11 Other Acute Surgical Emergencies

A variety of acute surgical emergencies such as perforated ulcer, acute cholecystitis, pancreatitis, diverticculitis, intestinal obstruction, Meckel's diverticulitis, and perforated carcinoma of the colon any simulate appendicitis. Differential diagnosis is discussed separately under each of these conditions. Acute regional enteritis, a nonsurgical condition, may be difficult to distinguish from appendicitis.

An additional word about Meckel's diverticulitisis appropriate at this point. Whenever right lower quadrant pain simulating appendicitis is associated with signs of mechanical small bowel obstruction, the possibility of Meckel's diverticulitis should be entertained. The point of maximal tenderness is more medial than in classic appendicitis, but the differential diagnosis may be impossible. If the appendix is found to be normal during an operation for appendicitis, the surgeon must search for Meckel's diverticulum.

2.12 Systemic Diseases

Any condition producing diaphragmatic irritation(e. g. ,pneumonia) may cause right sided abdominal pain. Connective tissue diseases that have vasculitis as a prominent feature may present with abdominal pain,and some of these patients require abdominal operation. Nonsurgical disorders associated with abdominal pain and peritoneal signs are discussed in the section on peritonitis.

2.13 Complications

The complications of acute appendicitis include perforation,peritonitis,abscess,and pylephlebitis.

(1) Perforation: It is unusual for the acutely inflamed appendix to perforate within the first 12 hours, although cathartics or enemas may cause perforation at an earlier stage. Perforation may relieve pain temporarily,but the signs of advancing peritonitis are soon apparent.

The consequences of perforation vary from generalized peritonitis to formation of a tiny abscess that may not appreciably alter the symptoms and signs of appendicitis.

(2) Peritonitis: Localized peritonitis results from microscope perforation of a gangrenous appendix, while spreading or generalized peritonitis usually implies gross perforation into the free peritoneal cavity. Increasing tenderness and rigidity,abdominal distention,and adynamic ileus are obvious in patients with peritonitis. High fever and severe toxicity mark progression of this catastrophic illness in untreated patients.

(3) Abscess: localized perforation of the appendix leads to formation of an appendiceal abscess,which is protected from the free peritoneal cavity by omentum or loops of small bowel. In retrocecal or retroileal appendicitis,an abscess is walled off by adjacent structures. If perforation is not contained,abscesses may form in any part of the peritoneal cavity.

Fever,pain,ileus,and sometimes a palpable mass are manifestations of intraperitoneal abscess. When plus collects in the pelvis,diarrhea is a common symptom,and rectal examination discloses tenderness and fullness in the pouch of Douglas. A pelvic abscess may resorb spontaneously,may perforate into the rectum or other neighboring viscus,or may enlarge and require surgical drainage per rectum or vaginam.

Subphrenic abscess is most often seen following generalized peritonitis,but retrocecal appendicitis in particular can cause subphrenic abscess in the absence of generalized peritoneal contamination.

Postoperative abscesses are a significant problem. Intraperitoneal abscesses may occur anywhere but most commonly are near the surgical incision. Wound abscesses develop in 5% of primarily closed incisions after removal of an acutely inflamed appendix. If the appendix has perforated,the incidence of wound infection is greater than 30%. When skin and subcutaneous tissues are left open and the wound allowed to close by secondary intention,the rate of wound infection can be reduced to 5%. Delayed primary closure has not been effective in preventing wound infection following perforated appendicitis.

(4) Pylephlebitis: Pylephlebitis is suppurative thrombophlebitis of the portal venous system. Chills, high fever,low grade jaundice,and,later,hepatic abscesses are the hallmarks of this grave condition. The appearance of shaking chills in a patient with acute appendicitis demands vigorous antibiotic therapy to prevent the development of pylephlebitis.

Gas in the hepatic veins may be seen on X-ray in cases of pylephlebitis,and this is an ominous sign requiring immediate operation if findings indicate appendicitis or peritonitis from any cause.

2.14 Treatment

For the vast majority of patients with a diagnosis of acute appendicitis, the appropriate management is appendectomy. For patients with simple acute appendicitis, intravenous fluids should be initiated as well as an antibiotic agent effective against both aerobic and anaerobic organisms. All patients are begun on antibiotics preoperatively and maintained postoperatively as needed. If the appendix is tmruptured and not gangrenous, antibiotics can be discontinued after 24 hours. Although many agents are effective, cefoxitin is often the agent of choice on the basis of a multicenter randomized trial of 1735 patients. Half received 2 g. of cefoxitin preoperatively. Three groups were evaluated, a patients with a normal appendix, those with an acutely inflamed appendix, and those with a gangrenous appendix. The incidence of wound infection was significantly lower in all three groups. However, the formation of intra abdominal abscess was not influenced by preoperative antibiotics. In a recent double blind controlled study, prophylactic cefotetan was compared with prophylactic cefoxitin in the development of postoperative wound infections in patients with acute nonperforated appendicitis. The results showed that single dose cefotetan and multiple dose cefoxitin are equally effective. However, because of the greater convenience and decreased cost, single dose cefotetan was considered the prophylaxis of choice in appendectomy for nonperforated appendicitis. Clindamycin with an aminoglycoside is indicated when Bacteroides fragilis is present metronidazole can also be used for this organism.

2.14.1 Surgical management

After appropriate preoperative preparation, a decision is made whether the appendix is to be removed by the open or the laparoscopic approach. If the open operation is done, anesthesia is administered, and a transverse incision is made in the skin lines in the right lower quadrant. The appendix is exposed through a gridiron, muscle splitting incision. If peritoneal fluidor exudate is present upon opening the peritoneum, the fluid should be cultured and the appendix exposed. Careful observation is made of the pathologic state and especially of the site of perforation or abscess formation. The appendix is then removed. If an abscess is present, it maybe drained, but if generalized peritonitis is present, this is usually unnecessary. If a normal appendix is found, additional exploration should follow to eliminate other possible causes, including inspection of the cecum and colon for inflammatory or neoplastic lesions, the terminal ileum for a Meckel's diverticulum, and the gallbladder and duodenum for primary disease. If further evidence of intra abdominal disease is present, it may be necessary to enlarge the incision or perform a midline incision for more adequate exposure.

The laparoscopic approach may be chosen for selected patients. When the diagnosis is uncertain, this approach is helpful in achieving a more thorough examination of the abdominal contents. In a prospective, randomized trial comparing open versus laparoscopic appendectomy, 37 patients were assigned to the open appendectomy group and 38 patients to the laparoscopic group. It was concluded that patients who underwent laparoscopic appendectomy had a shorter duration of pain and returned to full activities sooner postoperatively than those undergoing open appendectomy. It was concluded that laparoscopic appendectomy is the procedure of choice in patients with acute appendicitis.

2.14.2 Nonsurgical management of appendiceal abscess

At times, a patient with an appendiceal perforation is seen late in the course of the disease and has a walled off abscess in the right lower quadrant. At this point, the process may be subsiding, with minimal systemic findings. In this situation, it may be appropriate to treat the patient with antibiotics and intravenous fluids and careful observation. When the process resolves, usually requiring 6 weeks to 3 months, an interval appendectomy should be performed, because the likelihood of recurrent appendicitis is quite high. Under these circumstances, it is preferable to remove the appendix electively rather than as an emergency.

Incidental appendectomy during the course of other abdominal operations has been raised, and opinion is divided. Elective appendectomy is probably performed most often in conjunction with gynecologic procedures. Removal of the appendix in these circumstances eliminates the possibility of postoperative acute appendicitis in patients who may later develop problems in the right lower quadrant. However, most surgeons do not electively remove a normal apperidix during the course of general surgical procedures. There is also the likelihood that the rate of wound infection would be increased.

Chapter 3

Special Features of Acute Appendicitis

Appendicitis in infants and young children is difficult to diagnose preoperatively, since these patients can not provide a history. Therefore, it is unusual to make a firm diagnosis in a patient under the age of 1 year unless perforation has occurred.

Acute appendicitis during pregnancy also presents diagnostic problems, because during the third trimestef, the uterus is rapidly enlarging and causes displacement of the cecum and appendix into the right upper abdomen. Thus, acute appendicitis in these patients causes symptoms and signs higher and more lateral during the third trimester. Appendicitis in young women also introduces a number of specific differential diagnoses, particularly those involving tubo ovarian disorders. For these, culdoscopy or laparoscopy may be helpful in revealing the problem. In the elderly, appendicitis may present with different clinical manifestations than in younger patients. The general tendency is for the inflammatory components to be less pronounced. The temperature is usually lower, as is the leukocyte count, and there is frequently less pain and tenderness. At times, the appendix in this age group may perforate with an abscess without causing the patient a significant earlier problem.

Chapter 4

Carcinoma of Theappendix

In one series of 5000 appendices, 41 cases of adenocarcinoma were found. Therefore, carcinoma of the appendix is an unusual neoplasm. The most common lesion is a carcinoid and accounts for some 90% of all primary tumors of the appendix. Malignant mucoceles are regarded as being well differentiated adenocarcinomas. The clinical presentation of most patients with appendiceal carcinoma is typical of that for acute appendicitis. In many instances, the appendix is perforated, with a localized appendiceal abscess that requires drainage. In a study from the Mayo Clinic, 94 consecutive patients with adenocarcinoma of the appendix were evaluated (excluding patients with carcinoia) of the group, 52 patients (55%) had mucinous tumors, of which 22 had pseudomyxoma peritonei. The most common presentation was that of acute appendicitis. The 5 year cure rate was 55% and varied with the stage: 100%, 67%, 50%, and D, 6%. Right hemicolectomy produced a higher survival (68%) than appendectomy alone (20%). For this reason, it was concluded that right hemicolectomy is indicated in treating carcinoma of the appendix.

Part 30

Anorectal Disease

Chapter 1

Anatomy

1.1 Anus and Rectum

1.1.1 Anal canal structure, anus, and anal verge

The anal canal is anatomically peculiar and has a complex physiology, which accounts for its crucial role in continence and, in addition, its susceptibility to a variety of diseases. The anus or anal orifice is an anteroposterior cutaneous slit, that along with the anal canal remains virtually closed at rest, as a result of tonic circumferential contraction of the sphincters and the presence of anal cushions. The edge of the anal orifice, the anal verge or margin (anocutaneous line of Hilton), marks the lowermost edge of the anal canal and is sometimes the level of reference for measurements taken during sigmoidoscopy. Others favor the dentate line as a landmark because it is more precise. The difference between the anal verge and the dentate line is usually 1–2 cm. The epithelium distal to the anal verge acquires hair follicles, glands, including apocrine glands, and other features of normal skin, and is the source of perianal hidradenitis suppurativa, inflammation of the apocrine glands.

1.1.2 Anatomic versus surgical anal canal

Two definitions are found describing the anal canal (Figure 30-1-1). The "anatomic" or "embryologic" anal canal is only 2.0 cm long, extending from the anal verge to the dentate line, the level that corresponds to the proctodeal membrane. The "surgical" or "functional" anal canal is longer, extending for approximately 4.0 cm (in men) from the anal verge to the anorectal ring (levator ani). This "long anal canal" concept was first introduced by Milligan and Morgan10 and has been considered, despite not being proximally marked by any apparent epithelial or developmental boundary, useful both as a physiologic and surgical parameter. The anorectal ring is at the level of the distal end of the ampullary part of the rectum and forms the anorectal angle, and the beginning of a region of higher intraluminal pressure. Therefore, this definition correlates with digital, manometric, and sonographic examinations.

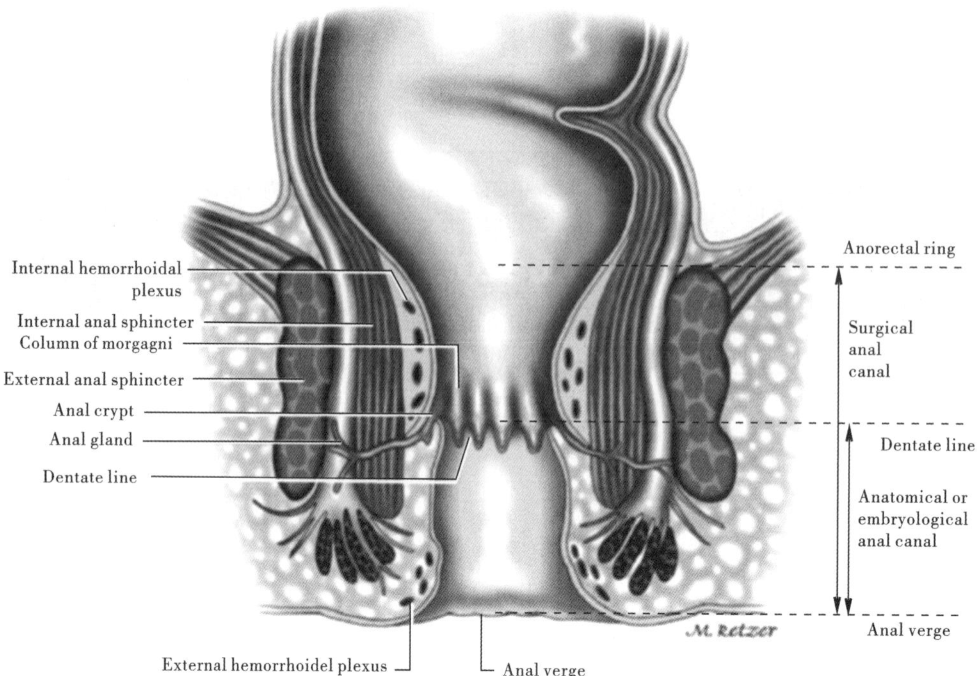

Figure 30-1-1 Anal canal

1.1.3 Anatomic relations of the anal canal

Posteriorly, the anal canal is related to the coccyx and anteriorly to the perineal body and the lowest part of the posterior vaginal wall in the female, and to the urethra in the male. The ischium and the ischio-rectal fossa are situated on either side. The fossa ischiorectal contains fat and the inferior rectal vessels and nerves, which cross it to enter the wall of the anal canal.

1.1.4 Muscles of the anal canal

The muscular component of the mechanism of continence can be stratified into three functional groups: lateral compression from the pubococcygeus, circumferential closure from the internal and external anal sphincter, and angulation from the puborectalis. The internal and external anal sphincters, and the conjoined longitudinal are intrinsically related to the anal canal, and will be addressed here.

1.1.5 Internal anal sphincter

The internal anal sphincter represents the distal 2.5–4.0 cm condensation of the circular muscle layer of the rectum. As a consequence of both intrinsic myogenic and extrinsic autonomic neurogenic properties, the internal anal sphincter is a smooth muscle in a state of continuous maximal contraction, and represents a natural barrier to the involuntary loss of stool and gas.

The lower rounded edge of the internal anal sphincter can be felt on physical examination, about 1.2 cmdistal to the dentate line. The groove between the internal and external anal sphincter, the inter-sphincteric sulcus, can be visualized or easily palpated. Endosonographically, the internal anal sphincter is a 2–3 mm thick circular band and shows a uniform hypoechogenicity.

1.1.6 External anal sphincter

The external anal sphincter is the elliptical cylinder of striated muscle that envelops the entire length of the inner tube of smooth muscle, but it ends slightly more distal than the internal anal sphincter. The deepest part of the external anal sphincter is intimately related to the puborectalis muscle, which can actually be considered a component of both the levator ani and the external anal sphincter muscle complexes. In the male, the upper half of the external anal sphincter is enveloped anteriorly by the conjoined longitudinal muscle, whereas the lower half is crossed by it. In the female, the entire external anal sphincter is encapsulated by a mixture of fibers derived from both longitudinal and internal anal sphincter muscles. The automatic continence mechanism is formed by the resting tone, maintained by the internal anal sphincter, and magnified by voluntary, reflex, and resting external anal sphincter contractile activities. In response to conditions of threatened incontinence, such as increased intra-abdominal pressure and rectal distension, the external anal sphincter and puborectalis reflexively and voluntarily contract further to prevent fecal leakage. The external anal sphincter and the pelvic floor muscles, unlike other skeletal muscles, which are usually inactive at rest, maintain unconscious resting electrical tone through a reflex arc at the cauda equina level.

1.1.7 Conjoined longitudinal muscle

Whereas the inner circular layer of the rectum gives rise to the internal anal sphincter, the outer longitudinal layer, at the level of the anorectal ring, mixes with fibers of the levator ani muscle to form the conjoined longitudinal muscle. This muscle descends between the internal and external anal sphincter, and ultimately some of its fibers, referred to as thecorrugator cutis ani muscle, traverse the lowermost part of the external anal sphincter to insert into the perianal skin.

Possible functions of the conjoined longitudinal muscle include attaching the anorectum to the pelvis and acting as a skeleton that supports and binds the internal and external sphincter complex together.

1.1.8 Epithelium of the anal canal

The lining of the anal canal consists of an upper mucosal (endoderm) and a lower cutaneous (ectoderm) segment. The dentate (pectinate) line is the "saw-toothed" junction between these two distinct origins of venous and lymphatic drainage, nerve supply, and epithelial lining. Above this level, the intestine is innervated by the sympathetic and parasympathetic systems, with venous, arterial, and lymphatic drainage to and from the hypogastric vessels. Distal to the dentate line, the anal canal is innervated by the somatic nervous system, with blood supply and drainage from the inferior hemorrhoidal system. These differences are important when the classification and treatment of hemorrhoids are considered.

The pectinate or dentate line corresponds to a line of anal valves that represent remnants of the proctodeal membrane. Above each valve, there is a little pocket known as an anal sinus or crypt. These crypts are connected to a variable number of glands, in average 6 (range, 3-12). More than one gland may open into the same crypt, whereas half the crypts have no communication. The anal gland ducts, in an outward and downward route, enter the submucosa; two-thirds enter the internal anal sphincter, and half of them terminate in the intersphincteric plane. Obstruction of these ducts, presumably by accumulation of foreign material in the crypts, may lead to perianal abscesses and fistulas. Cephalad to the dentate line, 8-14 longitudinal folds, known as the rectal columns (columns of Morgagni), have their bases connected in pairs to each valve at the dentate line. At the lower end of the columns are the anal papillae. The mucosa in the area of the columns consists of several layers of cuboidal cells and has a deep purple color because of the underlying internal hemorrhoidal plexus. This 0.5–1.0 cm strip of mucosa above the dentate line is known as the anal transition or cloacogenic zone. Cephalad to this area, the epithelium changes to a single layer of columnar cells and macroscopically acquires the characteristic pink color of the rectal mucosa.

The cutaneous part of the anal canal consists of modified squamous epithelium that is thin, smooth, pale, stretched, and devoid of hair and glands.

1.1.9 Rectum

Both proximal and distal limits of the rectum are controversial: the rectosigmoid junction is considered to be at the level of the third sacral vertebra by anatomists but at the sacral promontory by surgeons, and likewise the distal limit is regarded to be the muscular anorectal ring by surgeons and the dentate line by anato mists. The rectum measures 12–15 cm in length and has three lateral curves: the upper and lower are convex to the right and the middle is convex to the left. These curves correspond intraluminally to the folds or valves of Houston. The two left-sided folds are usually noted at 7–8 cm and at 12–13 cm, respectively, and the one on the right is generally at 9–11 cm. The middle valve (Kohlrausch's plica) is the most consistent in presence and location and corresponds to the level of the anterior peritoneal reflection. Although the rectal valves do not contain all muscle wall layers from a clinical point of view, they are a good location for performing rectal biopsies, because they are readily accessible with minimal risk for perforation.

The rectum is characterized by its wide, easily distensible lumen and the absence of taeniae, epiploic appendices, haustra, or a well-defined mesentery. The word "mesorectum" has gained widespread popularity among surgeons to address the perirectal areolar tissue, which is thicker posteriorly, containing terminal branches of the inferior mesenteric artery and enclosed by the fascia propria. The "mesorectum" may be a metastatic site for a rectal cancer and is removed during surgery for rectal cancer without neurologic sequelae ecause no functionally significant nerves pass through it.

The upper third of the rectum is anteriorly and laterally invested by peritoneum; the middle third is covered by peritoneum on its anterior aspect only. Finally, the lower third of the rectum is entirely extraperitoneal, because the anterior peritoneal reflection occurs at 9.0–7.0 cm from the anal verge in men and at 7.5–5.0 cm from the anal verge in women.

1.1.10 Anatomic relations of the rectum

The rectum occupies the sacral concavity and ends 2–3 cm anteroinferiorly from the tip of the coccyx. At this point, it angulates backward sharply to pass through the levators and becomes the anal canal. Anteriorly, in women, the rectum is closely related to the uterine cervix and posterior vaginal wall; in men, it lies behind the bladder, vas deferens, seminal vesicles, and prostate. Posterior to the rectum lie the median sacral vessels and the roots of the sacral nerve plexus.

1.1.11 Fascial relationships of the rectum

The parietal endopelvic fascia lines the walls and floor of the pelvis and continues on the internal organs as a visceral pelvic fascia. Thus, the fascia propria of the rectum is an extension of the pelvic fascia, enclosing the rectum, fat, nerves, and the blood and lymphatic vessels. It is more evident in the posterior and lateral extraperitoneal aspects of the rectum.

The lateral stalks are comprised essentially of connective tissue and nerves, and the middle rectal artery does not traverse them. Branches, however, course through in approximately 25% of cases. Consequently, division of the lateral stalks during rectal mobilization is associated with a 25% risk for bleeding. One theoretical concern in ligation of the stalks is leaving behind the lateral mesorectal tissue, which may limit adequate lateral or mesorectal margins during cancer surgery.

The presacral fascia is a thickened part of the parietal endopelvic fascia that covers the concavity of the sacrum and coccyx, nerves, the middle sacral artery, and presacral veins. Operative dissection deep to the presacral fascia may cause troublesome bleeding from the underlying presacral veins. Presacral hemorrhage occurs as frequently as 4.6%–7.0% of resections for rectal neoplasms, and despite its venous nature, can be life threatening. This is a consequence of two factors: the difficulty in securing control because of retraction of the vascular stump into the sacral foramen and the high hydrostatic pressure of the presacral venous system.

The rectosacral fascia is an anteroinferiorly directed thick fascial reflection from the presacral fascia at the S4 level to the fascia propria of the rectum just above the anorectal ring. The rectosacral fascia, classically known as the fascia of Waldeyer, is an important landmark during posterior rectal dissection.

The visceral pelvic fascia of Denonvilliers is a tough fascial investment that separates the extraperitoneal rectum anteriorly from the prostate and seminal vesicles or vagina.

1.1.12 Urogenital considerations

Identification of the ureters is advisable to avoid injury to their abdominal or pelvic portions during colorectal operations. On both sides, the ureters rest on the psoas muscle in their inferomedial course; they are crossed obliquely by the spermatic vessels anteriorly and the genitofemoral nerve posteriorly. In its pelvic portion, the ureter crosses the pelvic brim in front of or a little lateral to the bifurcation of the common iliac artery, and descends abruptly between the peritoneum and the internal iliac artery. Before entering the bladder in the male, the vas deferens crosses lateromedially on its superior aspect. In the female, as the ureter traverses the posterior layer of the broad ligament and the parametrium close to the side of the neck of the uterus and upper part of the vagina, it is enveloped by the vesical and vaginal venous plexuses and is crossed above and lateromedially by the uterine artery.

1.1.13 Arterial supply of the rectum and anal canal

The superior hemorrhoidal artery is the continuation of the inferior mesenteric artery, once it crosses the left iliac vessels. The artery descends in the sigmoid mesocolon to the level of S3 and then to the posterior aspect of the rectum. In 80% of cases, it bifurcates into right, usually wider, and left terminal branches; multiple branches are present in 17%. These divisions, once within the submucosa of the rectum, run straight downward to supply the lower rectum and the anal canal.

The superior and inferior hemorrhoidal arteries represent the major blood supply to the anorectum. In addition, it is also supplied by the internal iliac arteries.

The contribution of the middle hemorrhoidal artery varies with the size of the superior hemorrhoidal artery; this may explain its controversial anatomy. Some authors report absence of the middle hemorrhoidal artery in 40%–88%, whereas others identify it in 94%–100% of specimens. The middle hemorrhoidal artery is more prone to be injured during low anterior resection, when anterolateral dissection of the rectum is performed close to the pelvic floor and the prostate and seminal vesicles or upper part of the vagina are being separated. The anorectum has a profuse intramural anastomotic network, which probably accounts for the fact that division of both superior and middle hemorrhoidal arteries does not result in necrosis of the rectum.

The paired inferior hemorrhoidal arteries are branches of the internal pudendal artery, which in turn is a branch of the internal iliac artery.

1.1.14 Venous drainage and lymphatic drainage of the rectum and anal canal

The anorectum also drains, via middle and inferior hemorrhoidal veins, to the internal iliac vein and then to the inferior vena cava. The external hemorrhoidal plexus, situated subcutaneously around the anal canal below the dentate line, constitutes when dilated the external hemorrhoids. The internal hemorrhoidal plexus is situated submucosally, around the upper anal canal and above the dentate line. The internal hemorrhoids originate from this plexus.

Lymph from the upper two-thirds of the rectum drains exclusively upward to the inferior mesenteric nodes and then to the para-aortic nodes. Lymphatic drainage from the lower third of the rectum occurs not only cephalad, along the superior hemorrhoidal and inferior mesentery arteries, but also laterally, along the middle hemorrhoidal vessels to the internal iliac nodes. In the anal canal, the dentate line is the landmark for two different systems of lymphatic drainage: above, to the inferior mesenteric and internal iliac nodes, and below, along the inferior rectal lymphatics to the superficial inguinal nodes, or less frequently along the inferior hemorrhoidal artery. In the female, drainage at 5 cm above the anal verge in the lymphatic may also spread to the posterior vaginal wall, uterus, cervix, broad ligament, fallopian tubes, ovaries, and cul-de-sac, and at 10 cm above the anal verge, spread seems to occur only to the broad ligament and cul-de-sac.

1.2 Innervation of the Rectum and Anal Canal

1.2.1 Innervation of the rectum

The sympathetic supply of the rectum and the left colon arises from L-1, L-2, and L-3. Preganglionic fibers, via lumbar sympathetic nerves, synapse in the preaortic plexus, and the postganglionic fibers follow the branches of the inferior mesenteric artery and superior rectal artery to the left colon and upper rectum. The lower rectum is innervated by the presacral nerves, which are formed by fusion of the aortic plexus and lumbar splanchnic nerves. Just below the sacral promontory, the presacral nerves form the hypogastric plexus (or superior hypogastric plexus). Two main hypogastric nerves, on either side of the rectum, carry sympathetic innervation from the hypogastric plexus to the pelvic plexus. The pelvic plexus lies on the lateral side of the pelvis at the level of the lower third of the rectum, adjacent to the lateral stalks.

The parasympathetic fibers to the rectum and anal canal emerge through the sacral foramen and are called the nervi erigentes (S2, S3, and S4). The periprostatic plexus, a subdivision of the pelvic plexus situated on Denonvilliers' fascia, supplies the prostate, seminal vesicles, corpora cavernosa, vas deferens, urethra, ejaculatory ducts, and bulbourethral glands. Sexual function is regulated by cerebrospinal, sympathetic, and parasympathetic components. Erection of the penis is mediated by both parasympathetic (arteriolar vasodilatation) and sympathetic inflow (inhibition of vasoconstriction).

All pelvic nerves lie in the plane between the peritoneum and the endopelvic fascia and are in danger of injury during rectal dissection. Permanent bladder paresis occurs in 7%-59% of patients after abdominoperineal resection of the rectum; the incidence of impotence is reported to range from 15% to 45% and that of ejaculatory dysfunction from 32% to 42%. The overall incidence of sexual dysfunction after proctectomy has been reported to reach 100% when wide dissection is performed for malignant disease. Dissections performed for benign conditions are undertaken closer to the bowel wall, thus reducing the possibility of nerve injury.

Trauma to the autonomic nerves may occur at several points. During high ligation of the inferior mesenteric artery, close to the aorta, the sympathetic preaortic nerves may be injured. Division of both superior hypogastric plexus and hypogastric nerves may occur also during dissection at the level of the sacral promontory or in the presacral region. In such circumstances, sympathetic denervation with intact nervi erigentes results in retrograde ejaculation and bladder dysfunction. The nervi erigentes are located in the posterolateral aspect of the pelvis and at the point of fusion with the sympathetic nerves are closely related to the middle hemorrhoidal artery. Injury to these nerves will completely abolish erectile function. The pelvic plexus may be damaged either by excessive traction on the rectum, particularly laterally, or during division of the lateral stalks when this is performed close to the lateral pelvic wall. Finally, dissection near the seminal vesicles and prostate may damage the periprostatic plexus, leading to a mixed parasympathetic and sympathetic injury. This can result in erectile impotence as well as a flaccid, neurogenic bladder. Sexual complications after rectal surgery are readily evident in men but are probably underdiagnosed in women.

1.2.2 Anal canal

The internal anal sphincter is supplied by sympathetic (L5) and parasympathetic nerves (S2, S3, and S4) following the same route as the nerves to the rectum. The external anal sphincter is innervated on each side by the inferior rectal branch of the pudendal nerve (S2 and S3) and by the perineal branch of S4. Despite the fact that the puborectalis and external anal sphincter have somewhat different innervations, these muscles seem to act as an indivisible unit. After unilateral transection of a pudendal nerve, external anal sphincter function is still preserved because of the crossover of the fibers at the spinal cord level.

Anal sensation is carried in the inferior rectal branch of the pudendal nerve and is thought to have a role in maintenance of anal continence.

1.2.3 Anorectal spaces

The potential spaces of clinical significance in close relation to the anal canal and rectum include ischiorectal, perianal, intersphincteric, submucosal, superficial postanal, deep postanal, supralevator, and retrorectal spaces.

The ischiorectal fossa is subdivided by a thin horizontal fascia into two spaces: the perianal and ischiorectal.

The perianal space surrounds the lower part of the anal canal and contains the external hemorrhoidal plexus, the subcutaneous part of the external anal sphincter, the lowest part of the internal anal sphincter, and fibers of the longitudinal muscle. This space is the typical site of anal hematomas, perianal abscesses, and anal fistula tracts. The intersphincteric space is a potential space between the internal and external anal sphincters. It is important in the genesis of perianal abscess, because most of the anal glands end in this space. The submucous space is situated between the internal anal sphincter and the mucocutaneous lining of the anal canal. This space contains the internal hemorrhoidal plexus and the muscularis submucosae ani. It is continuous with the submucous layer of the rectum, and, inferiorly, it ends at the level of the dentate line.

The superficial postanal space is interposed between the anococcygeal ligament and the skin. The deep postanal space, also known as the retrosphincteric space of Courtney, is situated between the anococcygeal ligament and the anococcygeal raphe. Both postanal spaces communicate posteriorly with the ischiorectal fossa and are the sites of horseshoe abscesses. The supralevator spaces are situated between the peritoneum superiorly and the levator ani inferiorly. Supralevator abscesses may occur as a result of upward extension of a cryptoglandular infection or develop from a pelvic origin. The retrorectal space is located between the fascia propria of the rectum anteriorly and the presacral fascia posteriorly. The retrorectal space is a site for embryologic remnants and rare presacral tumors.

1.2.4 Pelvic floor musculature

The muscles within the pelvis can be divided into three categories: the anal sphincter complex, pelvic floor muscles, and muscles that line the sidewalls of the osseous pelvis.

1.2.5 Levator ani

The levator ani muscle, or pelvic diaphragm, is the major component of the pelvic floor. It is a pair of broad, symmetric sheets composed of three striated muscles: ileococcygeus, pubococcygeus, and puborectalis. A variable fourth component, the ischiococcygeus or coccygeus, is rudimentary in humans and represented by only a few muscle fibers on the surface of the sacrospinous ligament. The levator ani is supplied by sacral roots on its pelvic surface (S-2, S-3, and S-4) and by the perineal branch of the pudendal nerve on its inferior surface. The puborectalis muscle receives additional innervation from the inferior rectal nerves.

The pelvic floor is "incomplete" in the midline where the lower rectum, urethra, and either the dorsal vein of the penis in men or the vagina in women passes through it. This defect is called the levator hiatus and consists of an elliptic space situated between the two pubococcygeus muscles.

The puborectalis muscle is a strong, U-shaped loop of striated muscle that slings the anorectal junction to the posterior aspect of the pubis.

1.2.6 The anorectal ring and the anorectal angle

Two anatomic structures of the junction of the rectum and anal canal are related to the puborectalis muscle: the anorectal ring and the anorectal angle. The anorectal ring, a term coined by Milligan and Morgan, is a strong muscular ring that represents the upper end of the sphincter, more precisely the puborectalis, and the upper border of the internal anal sphincter, around the anorectal junction. It is of clinical relevance because division of this structure during surgery for abscesses or fistula inevitably results in fecal incontinence.

The anorectal angle is thought to be the result of the anatomic configuration of the U-shaped sling of the puborectalis muscle around the anorectal junction. Whereas the anal sphincters are responsible for closure of the anal canal to retain gas and liquid stool, the puborectalis muscle and the anorectal angle are designed to maintain gross fecal continence.

Chapter 2

Anorectal Physiology

2.1 Introduction

Normal bowel continence and evacuation are complex processes that involve the coordinated interaction between multiple different neuronal pathways and the pelvic and perineal musculature. Understanding of anorectal anatomy and physiology is challenging due to the complex series of neural and behavioral-mediated interactions and the lack of ideal studies to evaluate the anatomy and physiology. Complicating this understanding are other factors such as systemic disease, sphincter integrity, bowel motility, stool consistency, evacuation efficiency, pelvic floor stability, and cognitive and emotional affects.

Conventional anorectal physiology testing using techniques such as manometry, endoanal ultrasound, electrophysiologic studies, and defecography help to elucidate anorectal structures and function. However, diagnostic dilemmas occur when patients report normal function with grossly abnormal test results or abnormal function with a normal test profile.

2.2 Muscles of the Pelvic Floor and Sphincter Complex

Control of stool can be thought of as a pressure vector diagram, with continence represented as a balance of propulsive and resistive forces. Contraction of the muscles of the pelvic floor and sphincter complex provides resistance, and tone is noted during periods of rest or deep sleep.

Voluntary contraction of the puborectalis and external sphincter increases resistance and defers defecation. The anal sphincter is not a paired muscle structure, like the biceps and triceps in the arm; there is no extensor ani muscle. Evacuation occurs when propulsive forces (increased intra-abdominal pressure and peristalsis of the colon and rectum) overcome the resistance of the pelvic floor and sphincter muscles. The pelvic floor consists of a striated muscular sheet through which viscera pass. This striated muscle, the paired levator ani muscles, is actually subdivided into four muscles defined by the area of attachment on the pubic bone. The attachments span from the pubic bone, along the arcus tendineus (a condensation of the obturator fascia), to the ischial spine. The components of the levator ani are therefore named the pubococcygeus, ileococcygeus, and ischiococcygeus. The pubococcygeus is further subdivided to include the puborectalis. Between the urogenital viscera and the anal canal lies the perineal body. The perineal body consists of the superficial and deep transverse perinei muscles and the ventral extension of the external sphincter muscle to a tendinous intersection with the bulbocavernosus muscle. The fourth sacral nerve innervates the levator ani muscles. Controversy continues regarding the innervation and origin of the puborectalis muscle. Cadaver studies differ from in vivo stimulation studies as to whether the puborectalis muscle receives innervation only from the sacral nerve or also from the pudendal nerve. Comparative anatomy and histological studies of fiber typing also support the inclusion of the puborectalis muscle with the sphincter complex and not as a pelvic floor muscle. In addition, electromyography(EMG) studies of the external anal sphincter(EAS) and puborectalis muscle indicate that the muscles function together with cough and strain. The rectal smooth muscle consists of an outer muscularis mucosa, inner circular muscle, and the outer longitudinal layer. The inner circular muscle forms the valves of Houston proximally and distally extends down into the anal canal becoming the internal anal sphincter(IAS). This is not a simple extension of muscle as there are histologic differences between the upper circular muscle and the IAS. For instance, the IAS is thicker than the circular muscle due to an increased number of smaller muscle cells. The outer longitudinal layer surrounds the sigmoid colon coalescing proximally into thicker bands called taenia coli. This same layer continues down to the anorectal junction where it forms the conjoined longitudinal muscle along with fibers from the pubococcygeus muscle.

Distally, this muscle lies in the intersphincteric plane, and fibers may fan out and cross both the internal and EAS muscles. In an ultrasound view of the anal canal, the longitudinal muscle is seen as a narrow hyperechoic line in the intersphincteric space. The puborectalis muscle, EAS, and IAS muscles are easily viewed with endoanal ultrasound. In the hands of an experienced ultrasonographer, the technique is highly sensitive and specific in identifying internal and external sphincter defects.

2.2.1 External anal sphincter(EAS)

Anatomical and sonographic studies indicate that the EAS begins development, along with the puborectalis muscle, at 9–10 weeks gestation. At 28–30 weeks it is mature, and the anal sphincter then consists of three components, the striated puborectalis muscle, the smooth IAS muscle, and the smooth and striated EAS muscle. Further differentiation of the EAS into two or three components is highly debated. In 1715, Cowper described it as a single muscle. Later, Milligan and Morgan promoted the naming of the components as subcutaneous, superficial, and deep. Recently, Dalley makes a convincing point that the three components can only be seen in the exceptionally dissected specimen, and, in most cases, the muscle is one continuous mass and should be considered as such. The EAS is innervated bilaterally by the pudendal nerve arising from S2 to S4. Motor neurons arise in the dorsomedial and ventromedial divisions of Onuf's nucleus in the ventral horn of the spinal cord. Crossover of the pudendal innervation was first suggested in studies by Swash and Henry on rhesus monkeys. Hamdy and associates evaluated corticoanal stimulation of humans and found variable crossover which was symmetric in some and either right or left-sided dominant in others. This has been offered as one possible explanation for the inconsistent relationship between unilateral pudendal neuropathy and fecal incontinence. The EAS maintains tonic activity at rest due to monosynaptic spinal reflex. The tone can be abolished with spinal anesthesia and in conditions such as tabes dorsalis, where large-diameter afferent sensory fibers are destroyed, and over distension of the rectum, due to the inflation response. Maximum tone, due to phasic activity in the EAS, can be maintained for only about 1 min, before fatigue is encountered. Of interest, the only other striated muscles that maintain continuous low level resting activity are the abductor of the larynx, the cricopharyngeus, and the external urinary sphincter.

2.2.2 Internal anal sphincter(IAS)

The IAS is an involuntary smooth muscle. It is the major source of anal resting pressure and is relatively hypoganglionic. There are nerve fibers expected in an autonomic muscle-cholinergic, adrenergic, and nonadrenergic noncholinergic fibers. It receives sympathetic innervation via the hypogastric and pelvic plexus. Parasympathetic innervation is from S1, S2, and S3 via the pelvic plexus. There is considerable evidence that the sympathetic innervation is excitatory but conflicting information regarding the parasympathetic effect. The IAS contributes 55% to the anal resting pressure. The myogenic activity that contributes 10% and 45% is due to the sympathetic innervation. The remainder of the resting tone is from the hemorrhoidal plexus(15%) and the EAS(30%). Spinal anesthesia decreases rectal tone by 50%, and the decreased resting tone seen in diabetic patients may be due to an autonomic neuropathy. The IAS has slow waves occurring 6-20 times each minute increasing in frequency toward the distal anal canal. Ultraslow waves occur less than 2 times a minute and are not present in all individuals occurring in 5%-10% of normal individuals. Ultraslow waves are associated with higher resting pressures, hemorrhoids, and anal fissures. The occurrence of anal slow-wave activity with rectal pressure waves exceeding anal resting pressure suggests a role for anal slow waves in preserving continence. Ultrasound examination of the anal canal shows the hypoechoic IAS ending approximately 10 mm proximal to the most distal portion of the hyperechoic EAS.

2.3 Sensory Factors

Conventional concepts of the sensory innervation of the rectum have been challenged by data from continent patients following sphincter-saving surgery and ileal pouch-anal anastomosis (IPAA). Anal canal sensation to touch, pinprick, heat, and cold are present from the anal verge to 2.5-15 mm above the anal valves. This sensitive area is thought to help discriminate between flatus and stool, but local anesthesia does not obliterate that ability. The rectum is only sensitive to distention. Rectal sensation may be due to receptors in the rectal wall but also in the pelvic fascia or surrounding muscle. The sensory pathway for rectal distention is the parasympathetic system via the pelvic plexus to S2, S3, and S4.

Below 15-cm rectal distention is perceived as flatus, but above 15-cm air distention causes a sensation of abdominal discomfort. Anal canal sensation is via the inferior rectal branch of the pudendal nerve that arises from S2, S3, and S4. This is the first branch of the pudendal nerve, and along with the second branch, the perineal nerve arises from the pudendal nerve in the pudendal canal(Alcock's canal). The remainder of the pudendal nerve continues as the dorsal nerve of the penis or clitoris.

Many articles report daytime continence following low rectal resections with coloanal or IPAA. The reports of nighttime soiling following these procedures suggest that the ability to interpret sensory input from the neo rectum requires conscious thought and not simple reflex contraction and relaxation. It is not clear if the decreased continence rate at night is solely due to impaired sensation(and subsequent defective discrimination of solid stool and gas) or if other factors limit fine control.

2.4 Reflexes

There are a great number of reflexes that end with the name "… anal reflex". The reason for this is, in part, that the EAS is readily accessible and represents a convenient end point for recording during electrophysiological study. Consequently, there are a number of ways that one can assess the integrity of neurological connection through or around the spinal cord.

2.4.1 Cutaneous-anal reflex

The cutaneous-anal reflex was first described by Rossolimo in 1891, as a brief contraction of the anal sphincter in response to pricking or scratching the perianal skin. This is a spinal reflex that requires intact S4 sensory and motor nerve roots. Both afferent and efferent pathways travel within the pudendal nerve. If a cauda equina lesion is present, this reflex will usually be absent. Henry et al. recorded the latency of the anal reflex in 22 incontinent patients as compared to 33 control subjects. The mean latency was 13.0 ms vs. 8.3 ms, respectively. The mean latency was within normal range in only three (14%) of the incontinent patients. However, Bartolo et al. have suggested that latency measurement of the cutaneous-anal reflex may be an inadequate means of demonstrating nerve damage in patients with fecal incontinence.

From a practical standpoint, this is a sacral reflex that can be interrogated during physical examination by simply scratching the perianal skin with visualization of contraction of the subcutaneous anal sphincter. The response to perianal scratch fatigues rapidly so it is important to test this as the first part of the sphincter examination.

2.4.2 Cough reflex

Chan et al. using intercostal, rectus abdominis, and EAS electrodes, studied the latencies in response to voluntary cough and sniff stimulation. When compared to latencies from transcranial magnetic stimulation, it appeared that the EAS response was consistent with a polysynaptic reflex pathway. Visible contraction of the subcutaneous EAS as a consequence to cough and sniff stimulation is a simple nonintrusive validation of the pathways involved in the anal reflex. This response can also be displayed during anal sphincter manometry. Amarenco et al. demonstrated that the greater the intensity of the cough, the greater was the electromyographic response within the anal sphincter. The reflex is preserved in paraplegic patients with lesions above the lumbar spine, but it is lost if the trauma involves the lumbar spine or with cauda equina lesions. The mechanism of the cough-anal reflex contributes to the maintenance of urinary and fecal continence during sudden increases in intra-abdominal pressure as might also be seen with laughing, shouting, or heavy lifting.

2.4.3 Bulbocavernosus reflex

The bulbocavernosus reflex (BCR) is pelvic floor contraction elicited by squeezing the glans penis or clitoris.

The EAS is used as the end point, because it is easily accessed either for visual assessment or by concentric needle electromyography (EMG) recording. The BCR latency will be prolonged by various disorders affecting the S2-S4 segments of the spinal cord.

2.4.4 Rectal anal inhibitory reflex

The rectoanal inhibitory reflex(RAIR) represents the relaxation of the IAS in response to distension of the rectum. It is felt that this permits fecal material or flatus to come into contact with specialized sensory receptors in the upper anal canal. This sampling process, the sampling reflex, creates an awareness of the presence of stool and a sense of the nature of the material present.

The process of IAS relaxation with content sampling is instrumental in the discrimination of gas from stool and the ability to pass them independently. The degree to which IAS relaxation occurs appears to be related to the volume of rectal distension more so in incontinent patients than in constipated or healthy control patients. Lower thresholds for the RAIR have been found to be associated with favorable response to biofeedback therapy in patients with fecal incontinence for formed stool. The amplitude of sphincter inhibition is roughly proportional to the volume extent of rectal distension. The RAIR is primarily dependent upon intrinsic nerve innervation in that it is preserved even after the rectum has been isolated from extrinsic influences, following transaction of hypogastric nerves and the presence of spinal cord lesions. The inhibition response is in part controlled by nonadrenergic, noncholinergic (NANC) mediators. The reflex matures quite early in that it is generally present at birth and has been detected in 81% of premature infants older than 26 weeks postmenstrual age. The reflex is destroyed in Hirschsprung's disease when myenteric ganglia are absent. In addition, the reflex is lost after circumferential myotomy and after generous lateral internal sphincterotomy. Saigusa et al. found that at an average of 23 months following closure of ileostomy after IPAA, only 53% of patients maintained a positive RAIR as compared to 96% preoperatively. The incidence of nocturnal soiling was significantly greater, 72% in those who did not have preserved or recovered RAIR as compared to those 40% who had postoperative preserved RAIR.

The RAIR appears to be nearly abolished in the early postoperative period following LAR resection for cancer. It often reappears with time. Loss of the RAIR is often a consequence of restorative proctocolectomy. Preservation of the RAIR correlated with less nocturnal soiling. The RAIR in children can be elicited even when general anesthetic agents or neuromuscular blockers are used. Glycopyrrolate, an anticholinergic, appears to inhibit RAIR. Disturbances in the RAIR appear to be involved in the incontinence that is associated with systemic sclerosis.

2.4.5 Rectal anal excitatory reflex

The rectal anal excitatory reflex(RAER) or inflation reflex is the contraction of the EAS in response to rectal distension. Rectal distension sensation is most likely transmitted along the S2, S3, and S4 parasympathetic fibers through the pelvic splanchnic nerves. However, on the motor side, a pudendal nerve block abolishes the excitatory reflex suggesting that pudendal neuropathy may interfere with the RAIR.

Common methodologies for assessing the integrity of the pudendal nerve involve both single fiber density(SFD) of the EAS and pudendal nerve terminal motor latency (PNTML). However, derangement of the distal RAER was shown by Sangwan et al. to compare favorably with these more traditional and discomforting methodologies as an indicator of neuropathic injury to the EAS. It would appear that patients that have both an abnormal PNTML and an abnormal distal RAER do not require further study with SFD.

2.5 Mechanical Factors of Continence and Defecation

2.5.1 Anorectal angle and flap valve

As a part of the pelvic floor musculature, the puborectalis arises from the pubic bone and passes horizontally and posteriorly around the rectum as the most medial portion of the levator ani muscle. This forms a U-shaped sling around the rectum near its anatomic junction with the anus, pulling the rectum anteriorly, and giving rise to the socalled anorectal angle. There are differences of opinion as to whether the puborectalis and anorectal angle are truly important in maintaining continence. Unlike the fine control of the external and internal sphincter muscles, the puborectalis sling is felt to be more involved with gross fecal continence. Parks postulated a mechanism by which this takes place. As intra-abdominal pressure is increased, such as with sneezing, coughing, or straining, the force is transmitted across the anterior wall of the rectum at the anorectal angle. The underlying mucosa is opposed against the upper anal canal, creating a flap-valve mechanism that prevents stool from passing to the lower anal canal and preserving continence. Yet other authors have disputed this flap-valve mechanism and downplayed the role and reliability of measuring the anorectal angle. Bannister et al., in a study of 29 patients including 14 patients with incontinence, found no evidence of a flap-valve in the normal subjects by using manometric measurements during rising intra-abdominal pressures. However, in the incontinent patients, the manometric pressures were consistent with a flap-valve. Yet subjects still had leakage of stool, questioning the contribution to overall continence.

Bartolo and colleagues also used manometric and EMG measurements in 13 subjects both at rest and during Valsalva, demonstrating a similar rise in rectal and sphincter pressures and puborectalis EMG recordings.

Yet, with concomitant barium studies the anterior rectal wall separated from the mucosa, allowing contrast to fill the rectum. The authors proposed that the puborectalis functions more like a sphincter rather than contributing to the flap-valve mechanism. Furthermore, quantifying the anorectal angle and relating that to patient symptoms have resulted in mixed views. One study noted significant interobserver variation in anorectal angle measurements between three interpreters but good intraobserver consistency, suggesting that variation in anorectal angle measurements may be due to subjective interpretation of the rectal axis along the curved rectal wall. In another study assessing the reproducibility of anorectal angle measurement in 43 defecating proctograms, the authors found significant intraand interobserver variations and concluded that the anorectal angle is an inaccurate measurement. Jorge and associates measured the anorectal angle during rest, squeeze, and push in 104 consecutive patients and also found highly significant differences in each measurement category.

2.5.2 Reservoir

As an additional part of the continence mechanism, the rectum must be able to function as a temporary storage site for liquid and solid stool. With passage of the fecal stream into the rectum, the pliable rectal walls are able to distend and delay the defecation sequence until an appropriate time. This process relies both on rectal innervation to sense and tolerate the rising volume of stool (capacity), as well as maintain a relatively low and constant pressure with increases in volume (compliance). Extremes of either of these components can lead to fecal incontinence through decreased accommodation or overflow states. Although decreased compliance has been demonstrated more often in patients with fecal incontinence, it has also been shown to occur as a normal consequence of aging. In addition, Bharucha and associates in a study of 52 women with fecal incontinence demonstrated that the rectal capacity was reduced in 25% of women, and these lower volume and pressure thresholds were significantly associated with rectal hypersensitivity and urge fecal incontinence. Furthermore, following low anterior resection for cancer, those patients with resultant lower rectal compliance and lower rectal volume tolerability (capacity) have been associated with higher rates of fecal incontinence.

2.5.3 Normal defecation

The awareness of the need to defecate occurs in the superior frontal gyrus and anterior cingulate gyrus. The process begins with movement of gas, liquid, or solid contents into the rectum. Distention of the rectum leads to stimulation of pressure receptors located on the puborectalis muscle and in the pelvic floor muscles, which in turn stimulates the RAIR.

The IAS relaxes allowing sampling of contents. If defecation is to be deferred, voluntary contraction of the EAS and levator ani muscles occurs, and the rectum accommodates with relaxation after an initial increase in pressure. When the anal canal is deemed to have solid contents and a decision to defecate is made, the glottis closes, pelvic floor muscles contract, and diaphragm and abdominal wall muscles contract, all increasing abdominal pressure. The puborectalis muscle relaxes, resulting in straightening of the anorectal angle, and the pelvic floor descends slightly. The EAS relaxes and anal canal contents are evacuated. Upon normal complete evacuation, the pelvic floor rises, and sphincters contract once more in a "closing reflex".

2.6 Continence

The interplay of all the aforementioned anatomy and physiology ensures continence, but a deficit in any one area does not lead to incontinence. An intact and functional puborectalis muscle can provide continence in the pediatric imperforate anus patient, but incontinence can ensue during adulthood. R. E. Karulf 61 Even profound deficits do not necessarily lead to incontinence if stool consistency is solid, while minor deficits can easily lead to incontinence to gas. Diagnosis and management of abnormal fecal incontinence requires a systematic approach focusing on identifying the specific deficits present, applying appropriate testing to elucidate anal physiology and anatomy, and then directing therapy accordingly.

2.7 Summary

Understanding the anatomy, innervation, and reflexes of the pelvic floor and anal sphincters is the key to assessing disorders of continence. Further work in this area remains promising.

Chapter 3

Anorectal Malformation

3.1 Introduction

Anorectal malformations are common in human being and consist of a series of congenital defects that represent a wide spectrum. There are different ways to classify because of different malformations and different combinations of anomalies. There are different prognoses because of different categories even though a good outcome can be obtained in almost of them after surgical repair.

3.2 Incidence

The cause of anorectal malformation is unknown. The average incidence worldwide is 1 in 5000 live births, although the condition is more common in some areas. A male preponderance (55% –65% of cases) is seen in larger series and in collected cases. Low lesions also occur in a majority of cases. 2/3 of the males with high abnormalities and 2/3 of females with low anomalies have been reported.

Most babies with imperforate anus have one or more abnormalities that affect other systems. The incidence of such defects depends on the zeal with which they are sought and varies from 50% –60% . In addition, the higher malformations are associated with more associated deformities. Some of them are incidental findings but others such as cardiovascular defects may be life–threatening. The incidence of such abnormalities might therefore be expected to increase.

Of all the anorectal malformations, there are 12% –22% with cardiovascular anomalies, 10% with tracheoesophageal abnormalities, 1% –2% with duodenal obstruction, 10% of low and 25% of high anomalies with vertebral abnormalities, 9% of low and 30% of high anomalies with genitourinary system abnormalities.

3.3 Embryology

The cloaca in the embryo is a cavity into which open hind gut, tail gut, allantois, and, later, the mesonephric ducts. The cloaca is first formed at around 21 days gestation. It is U-shaped, with the allantois lying anteriorly and the hind gut posteriorly. Standard teaching implies that the septum in the middle (urorectal septum) grows downward, fusing with folds until it joins the cloaca. By this process, two cavities would be created: a urogenital cavity anteriorly and an anorectal cavity posteriorly. This process is said to be complete at 6th weeks' gestation. A conflicting theory holds that the septum does not grow distally and does not fuse with the cloacal membrane. A cloacal canal persists between the two cavities. Rapid growth of the genital tubercle changes the shape of the cloaca and the orientation of the cloacal membrane, which is displaced posteriorly. The cloacal membrane breaks down at 7 weeks' gestation, thereby creating two openings: the urogenital and the anal ones.

The muscles that surround the rectum develop at the same time. The earliest promyoblasts of the levator ani are seen 6th week of gestation and of the external anal sphincter in the 7th week of gestation. The internal anal sphincter is first seen in the 8th week of gestation; by the 9th week, all relevant structures are in place. At this stage, differentiation into male or female external genitalia has not occurred.

It is apparent that none of the embryologic description can adequately explain all the abnormalities encountered in practice. In standard teaching, defective formation of the urorectal septum accounts for a wide variety of defects in both males and females. By contrast, the newer theory suggests that defects in the shape of the dorsal (posterior) cloaca and an absence of the dorsal cloacal membrane result in anorectal malformations. This has been shown in pigs and mice bred for the abnormality. By inference, the same processes may apply in humans. Because the Mullerian ducts appear when most of the other structures are already formed, the incorporation of these ducts into the range of anorectal malformations is difficult to explain under either theory. It is fortunate that satisfactory results may be achieved in the absence of clear embryologic guidelines.

3.4 Classification

There are different ways to classify, it can be clarified to "high" and "low" or "high" "intermediate" and "low" categories according to the position of rectal distal end, and also clarified to "male" and "female" categories according to sexuality. To date, no single classification system has achieved worldwide acceptance or been adopted into universal use. Classification in Table 30-3-1 is purely descriptive and related more to surgical imperatives than to embryologic concepts.

Table 30-3-1 Classifications of anorectal anomalies

category	males	females
1	Perineal fistula	
2	Rectourethral fistula (prostatic or bulbar)	Rectovestibular fistula
3	Rectovesical fistula (bladder or neck)	Persistent cloaca with a common channel (<3 cm or >3 cm)
4	Imperforate anus without fistula	
5	Rectal atresia	
6	Complex defects	

On the good side of the spectrum of anorectal anomalies, there are a very good functional post-operative prognosis, meaning that the majority of patients have normal bowel, urinary control, and sexual function. Unfortunately, on the bad side of the spectrum, the patient will not have bowel control, sometimes he or she will not have urinary control, and sometimes they will also suffer from a significant degree of sexual dysfunction after repair anatomically.

It is extremely important, therefore, to be sure that the patients born with what we call "benign defects", receive a technically correct operation to take advantage of their potential for bowel and urinary control.

3.5 Clinical Features

The clinical presentations are varied.

Some of the malformations can be found after birth at once, such as imperforate anus, perineal fistula and cloacal deformity can be diagnosed after birth immediately, but some of them are not so easy to be detected and less of them are so difficult to be diagnosed.

Digital examination should be done to detect rectum when acute or chronic intestine obstruction takes on in baby. Anorectal anomalies should be suspected such as rectal atresia, rectal or anus stenosis and Hirschsprung disease, even though the baby has a normal anus.

But the diagnosis of urethral fistula is so difficult to do and confirm where the fistula is. Sometimes even the colography, retrograde urethrography or cystoscopy has been done, the confirm diagnosis can't be established. Nevertheless, these investigations should be performed and that may give some evidence for diagnosis even not all.

Further investigation should be done to access if the patients suffer from complex malformations.

3.6 Diagnosis

The diagnosis of anorectal malformation is easy mostly, such as the imperforate anus, perineal fistula and cloacal deformity, according to the perineal inspection and other clinical findings. Beside the systematic examination, further investigations especially imaging should be done to confirm the diagnosis of fistula and how about it is and then any other associated anomalies. Finally, that is very important, define the type of malformation especially the distance of bowel-skin, different strategies should be carry out for the management of low, intermediate or high level anomalies.

3.6.1 Neonate

There are two important questions that must be answered when a newborn with anorectal malformation admitted: ①Does the baby have a serious associated life threatening defect? ②Does the baby need a colostomy or should we perform a primary repair of the malformation?

Based on the frequency of other associated defects, newborns with anorectal malformations must have the following diagnostic tests during the first 24 h of life: ①Clinical evaluation to rule out the other possibility of alimentary tract atresia and cardiovascular disease. ②Ultrasound detection to rule out the presence of hydronephrosis, megaureter, tethered cord and hydrocolpos in females. ③X-ray film at AP and lateral positions to evaluate for hemivertebrae and sacrum development. Babies with anorectal malformation should never be taken to the operating room without having ruled out the most important associated defects.

3.6.2 Male

For the "benign type of defect" (perineal fistula, imperforate anus with no fistula, a rectourethral bulbar fistula), Usually, the meconium will come out through the orifice after 12 or 24 h of life, because it is a very narrow track and it takes a significant intrarectal pressure to force the meconium out. The orifice of the perineal fistula is always located anterior to the center of the anal dimple, which represents the external sphincter mechanism. Sometimes the orifice is located in the midline raphe of the scrotum or at the base of the penis following a subepithelial tract that can be filled with meconium or mucus. If imperforate anus with no perineal orifice, there is a possibility that the baby has a rectourethral bulbar fistula and the baby will pass meconium into the urine during the first 24 h of life, so urinalysis should be done. Otherwise, there is a strong possibility that the baby has an imperforate anus with no fistula.

If none of these findings are detected after 24h, a crosstable lateral film or Ultrasound should be done and to measure the distance from the rectum to the skin, it may predict the type of malformations.

The "bad side" of the spectrum, includes malformations with poor functional prognosis. A flat-bottom baby connotes a very high defect, either a rectourethral prostatic or a rectobladder neck fistula. In addition, the sacrum is frequently hypodeveloped. An absent sacrum or a very abnormal short sacrum, hemisacrum or bifid scrotum is associated with higher defects.

3.6.3 Female

In female babies, the presence of a single perineal orifice makes the diagnosis of cloaca. The length of the common channel can be evaluated endoscopically. If the baby has a prominent midline groove and an obvious anal dimple, most likely she has a cloaca with a common channel shorter than 3 cm, particularly if the sacrum is normal. On the other hand, if the baby has a flat bottom and an abnormal sacrum, most likely she has a cloaca with a common channel longer than 3 cm.

If the baby has an absent anus but one can see rather normal-looking female genitalia, including the presence of a urethra and vagina, most likely the baby has a rectovestibular fistula which is the most common defect seen in females, and the orifice just in the vestibule of the genitalia outside the hymen.

Meconium may not pass in the first few hours of life, but most likely will start passing very soon after that. The diagnosis of a vestibular fistula requires a meticulous examination of the perineum of a female baby. A perineal fistula is a very obvious malformation and the diagnosis is made just by inspection of the perineum. These babies have an orifice located somewhere between the center of the anal dimple(sphincter) and the female genitalia. Usually, the orifice is abnormally narrow and is not surrounded by sphincter.

3.7 Management

A crosstable lateral X-ray film is indicated if the female baby has not a single Derineal orifice, no vestibular fistula, no eviderce of a perineal orifice, and no pass meconium after 24 h of birth, a crosstable lateral film is inaicated. The analysis of the diagnostic tests already described, as well as the result of the examination of the baby's perineum, that allow us to make an accurate diagnosis of the type of malformation and give us enough information to make a wise decision concerning the question of colostomy or primary repair.

In general, cases of imperforate anus with no fistula should be treated primarily, without a colostomy. A colostomy performed first is adaptable for the imperforate newborns with rectobladder neck fistula, rectal prostatic fistula or rectourethral bulbar fistula and a secondary repair at several months of life. Females born with a cloaca receive a diverting colostomy.

The patients with cloaca require a cystoscopy and vaginoscopy to measure the length of the common channel to do a future plan for the definitive repair. During the definitive reconstruction, the rectum is separated meticulously from the vagina, trying to respect both structures. The next step is a maneuver called "total urogenital mobilization", the vagina and urethra together, are dissected and mobilized, dividing the suspensory ligaments of urethra and vagina, which gains between 2 and 4 cm of length, enough to have a nice repair of the urethra and vagina with a good cosmetic and functional result. The limits of the sphincter are electrically determined and the perineum is repaired. The rectum is then placed within the limits of the sphincter and an anoplasty is performed.

3.8 Results

Functional results also represent a spectrum. Males with rectobladder neck fistula have poor functional results. Most of those babies have urinary control, but, constipation is the most common postoperative sequela in anorectal malformations. Patients operated on for a cloaca, frequently suffer from an incapacity to empty their bladder; consequently, intermittent catheterization is indicated in 80% of those patients born with a common channel longer than 3 cm and in 20% of those with a common channel shorter than 3 cm. Depending on the quality of the sacrum, approximately 70% of the patients born with a cloaca will have voluntary bowel movements.

Patients with vestibular fistula with normal sacrum have a 95% chance of having voluntary bowel movements; All patients with perineal fistula have voluntary bowel movements with minimal soiling very occasionally, depending on the efficiency in the treatment for constipation.

Chapter 4

Anal Fissure

4.1 Introduction

An anal fissure is a linear or oval tear distal to the dentate line that can be extremely painful with bowel movements and may lead to bright red blood per rectum. The estimated prevalence is inaccurate as many people with an anal fissure never seek medical treatment. Anal fissures occur equally in men and women and tend to occur in younger patients(mean age 40 years). 75% are located in the posterior midline, but anal fissures can be seen anteriorly in 25% of women and 8% of men. 7% can have both anterior and posterior fissures. If the fissure is in an atypical location or there are multiple fissures, other complicated diseases such as Crohn's disease, trauma, tuberculosis, syphilis, HIV/AIDS, or anal carcinoma should be investigated. Acute fissures appear as a simple tear. Symptoms lasting longer than 8–12 weeks are considered chronic and the fissure may demonstrate evidence of chronic inflammation such as sentinel piles/skin tags at the distal fissure margin and a hypertrophied anal papilla proximal to the fissure in the anal canal. Also in chronic fissures, fibers of the internal anal sphincter may be visible.

4.2 Etiology

The etiology of an anal fissure is debatable, but typically anal trauma after either a hard or loose stool is reported prior to symptoms. Sustained anal resting hypertonia is found in patients with anal fissures. Since many patients may experience constipation or diarrhea and never develop a fissure, other contributing factors were investigated. The concept of ischemia of the area is supported by cadaver studies, which showed a paucity of blood vessels in the posterior midline in 85% studied. Also by Doppler laser flowmetry, the posterior midline had the lowest perfusion compared to other quadrants of the anal canal.

4.3 Symptoms

Patients with symptomatic fissures report pain during and after defecation. With chronic fissures, this can last hours to all day. Due to this severe pain, patients can have fear of defecation. Many patients report limited bright red rectal bleeding seen on the toilet tissue. Anal fissure is the most common cause of painful bright red rectal bleeding.

4.4 Diagnosis

The diagnosis of a symptomatic anal fissure is suggested by the characteristic pain description. With gentle spreading of the buttocks, the fissure can usually be seen. Anal exam with a finger or scope should be avoided due to the exquisite tenderness of the fissure and the limited additional information obtained from the digital exam. The differential diagnosis includes perianal abscess, anal fistula, inflammatory bowel disease, a sexually transmitted disease, and anal carcinoma. Atypical fissures (off the midline, multiple, painless, and nonhealing fissures) warrant further evaluation with an exam under anesthesia, possible biopsy, and culture. Figure 30-4-1 illustrates the location of the anal fissure correlated with possible etiologies of the fissure.

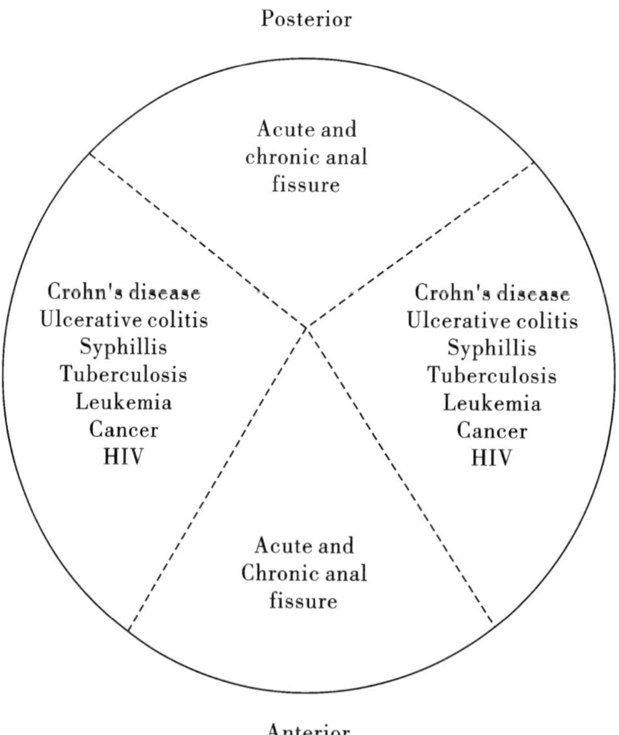

Figure 30-4-1 The location of anal fissure suggests etiology

4.5 Management

50% of acute fissures heal with sitz baths, psyllium, and topical anesthetics or anti-inflammatory ointments. 18% -27% recur within 5 years.

(1) Sphincter relaxants

Many agents to reduce mean and maximum anal resting pressure have been tested. Many of the topical preparations are only available through compounding pharmacies. Clinicians should be familiar with their available pharmaceutical resources before recommending a medical treatment that requires compounding.

(2) Topical nitrates

The internal sphincter is a smooth muscle and topical nitrates relax smooth muscle to theoretically improve blood flow to the fissure and promote healing. Initial healing rates were encouraging with the use of topical 0.2% nitrates (nitroglycerin cream). Headaches and problems with patient compliance following the planned treatment regiment were a problem with this therapy. Sustained healing of anal fissures has not been optimal, and combined with adverse reactions such as headaches (and some reports of orthostatic hypotension) has limited the use of topical nitrates.

(3) Calcium channel blockers

Calcium channel blockers can be administered in an oral form (as 20 mg oral or sublingual nifedipine) or topically (2% diltiazem gel) to treat anal fissures. There have not been sufficient studies with large enough numbers comparing oral versus topical therapy to give a definitive conclusion as to superiority of one delivery method over the other. From several randomized studies, it appears that topical calcium channel blockers have at least similar healing potential compared to topical nitroglycerin with fewer side effects. This has led some authors to conclude that calcium channel blockers should be the first line of treatment. Topical calcium channel blockers compared to lateral internal sphincterotomy showed fewer relapses with surgery. Studies comparing these two types of treatment for initial fissure healing, pain relief, and compliance show conflicting results. There are few long-term studies looking at sustained healing rates for calcium channel blockers. Therefore, definitive assessment of long-term healing is not possible.

(4) Adrenergic antagonists

Despite reduction of anal sphincter resting pressures, (limited) studies have failed to demonstrate that oral administration of alpha-1 adrenergic blockers will heal fissures.

(5) Cholinergic agonists

0.1% bethanechol gel reduces maximal anal resting pressures and has been shown to heal anal fissures in one limited study.

(6) Phosphodiesterase inhibitors

Topical administration of a phosphodiesterase-5 inhibitor (sildenafil) was shown to significantly reduce anal sphincter pressures in one study. Whether this effect will lead to sustained healing of anal fissures has yet to be demonstrated.

(7) Botulinum toxin

Botulinum toxin is an exotoxin that, when locally injected, binds to presynaptic nerve terminals of the neuromuscular junction preventing release of acetylcholine and temporarily paralyzing the muscle. Studies have shown that the predominant effect on the internal sphincter is through sympathetic blockade. Authors report that this treatment can be easily injected/administered in the outpatient setting and is well tolerated.

After evaluation of multiple studies focusing on the optimal dose and injection site of botulinum toxin, it appears that 20 units injected on either side of the anterior midline in the intersphincteric groove provides the best results. Comparative studies of botulinum toxin versus topical nitroglycerin showed conflicting results as to healing. Studies comparing lateral internal sphincterotomy with botulinum toxin injection showed superior long-term healing in the surgical group. One study showed that flatal incontinence was a side effect in 16% of patients that underwent surgery versus no side effects in the botulinum group. Late recurrences may be seen in up to 40% of patients who initially healed after injection of botulinum toxin. A higher risk of recurrences was associated with fissures that had an anterior location, disease longer than 12 months, and those requiring multiple injections of botulinum toxin. Some authors advocate repeat injection(s) if a patient experiences a recurrent fissure. They also cite improvement of symptoms and possibility of healing with repeated injections. The Food and Drug Administration (FDA) has issued a warning based on a small number of patients who had adverse reactions after injection of botulinum toxin including respiratory failure and death. It is speculated that this may be related to overdosing.

4.6 Operative Treatment

The goal of anal fissure treatment is to decrease elevated anal resting tone. Operative procedures produce permanent reduction in maximum resting anal pressures.

(1) Anal dilatation

Anal dilatation can reduce anal resting pressures. This treatment was standardized to mean dilatation by means of opening a Parks' anal retractor to 4.8 cm or a pneumatic balloon inflated to 40 mm. Performing dilatation with one of these measures found fissure healing in 94%. Widespread criticism toward the use of this technique focuses on fecal incontinence due to diffuse sphincter damage. Comparison of sphincterotomy with dilatation showed conflicting results as far as which surgical treatment is superior for healing of fissures and which leads to fewer problems with fecal incontinence. While dilatation is still performed in some centers, this procedure is not commonly used across North America as a primary treatment for anal fissures.

(2) Fissurectomy

While excision of the anal fissure has been proposed as a therapeutic option, given the accepted etiology of a fissure being secondary to inadequate blood flow and spasm, the benefit of fissurectomy is questioned.

(3) Lateral internal sphincterotomy

Lateral internal sphincterotomy is recommended in the American Society of Colon and Rectal Surgeons practice parameters as the surgical procedure of choice for refractory anal fissures. Division of the internal anal sphincter is done on the lateral sides of the anus.

Persistent incontinence to gas and stool is a major concern after sphincterotomy and this rate varies greatly between studies, mostly due to differences in definition and intensity of follow-up. Etiology of incontinence is related to type and extent of sphincter division. Care is needed when dividing the internal sphincter in women due to an inherent shorter anal canal versus men. Additionally, external anal sphincter defects in women should be recognized before the sphincterotomy procedure.

Chapter 5

Anorectal Abscess

Ducts from anal glands empty into the anal crypts at the level of the dentate line. Anal glands penetrate into deeper tissue: 80% submucosal, 8% internal sphincter, 8% conjoined longitudinal muscle, 2% intersphincteric space, and 1% penetrate the internal sphincter.

5.1 Pathophysiology

5.1.1 Etiology

Etiologies of anorectal abscesses. 90% are from nonspecific cryptoglandular suppuration. Abscesses result from obstruction of the anal glands (Park's cryptoglandular theory published in 1961). Persistence of anal gland epithelium in the tract between the crypt and the blocked duct results in fistula formation.

Predisposing factors for abscess formation are diarrhea and trauma from hard stool. Associated factors may be anal fissures, infection of a hematoma, or Crohn's disease.

5.1.2 Classification

Abscesses are classified by their location within the potential anorectal spaces (Figure 30-5-1 and Figure 30-5-2).

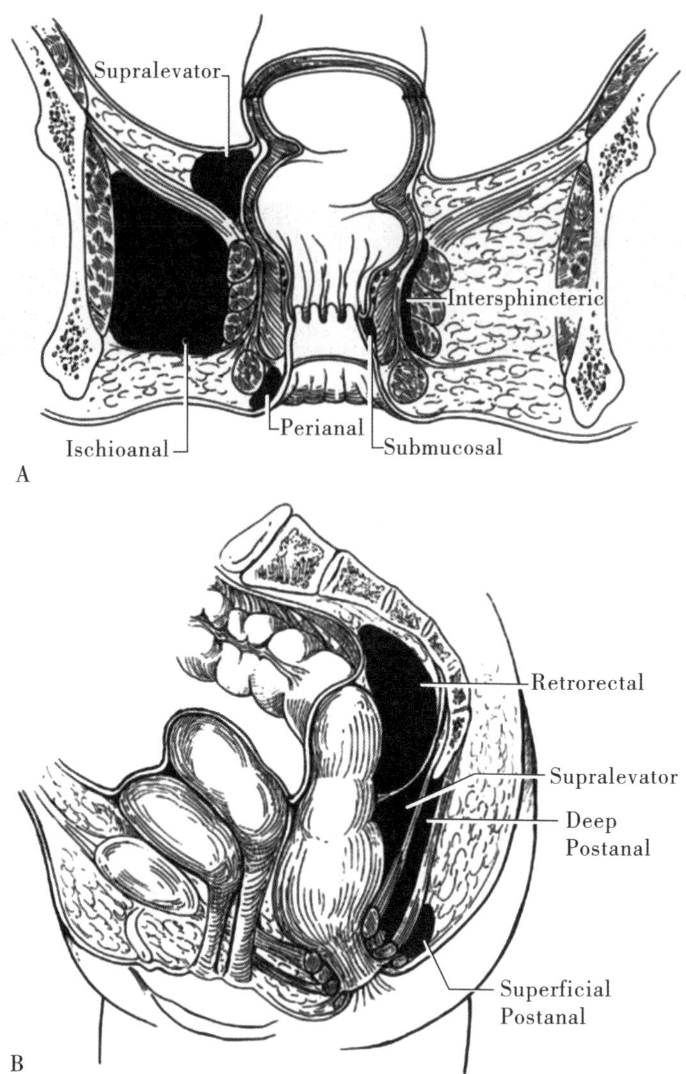

Figure 30-5-1 Anorectal spaces

A. Coronal section; B. Sagittal section.

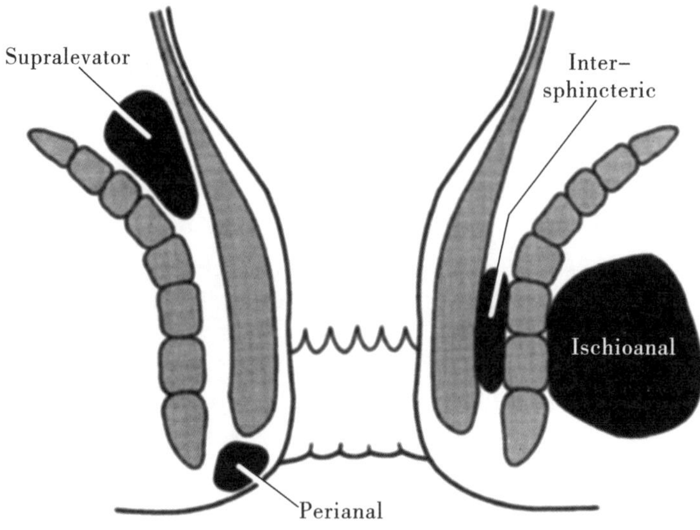

Figure 30-5-2 Classification of anorectal abscess

5.2 Evaluation

(1) Symptoms

Pain, swelling, and fever are the hallmarks associated with an abscess. The patient with a supralevator abscess may complain of gluteal pain. Rectal bleeding has been reported.

Severe rectal pain accompanied by urinary symptoms such as dysuria, retention, or inability to void may be suggestive of an intersphincteric or supralevator abscess.

(2) Physical examination

Inspection will reveal erythema, swelling, and possible fluctuation. It is crucial to recognize that no visible external manifestations will be present with the intersphincteric or supralevator abscesses despite the patient's complaint of excruciating pain. Although digital examination may not be possible because of extreme tenderness, palpation, if possible, will demonstrate tenderness and a mass. With a supralevator abscess, a tender mass may be palpated on rectal or vaginal examination. Anoscopy and sigmoidoscopy are inappropriate in the acute setting.

5.3 Treatment

5.3.1 General principles

The treatment of an anorectal abscess is prompt incision and drainage. Watchful waiting with antibiotics is ineffective and may lead to a more complicated abscess with sphincter mechanism damage. Delay in treatment may lead to a life-threatening necrotizing infection and death.

5.3.2 Operative management

5.3.2.1 Incision and drainage

Aperianal abscess may be drained with local anesthesia. A cruciate or elliptical incision is made over the point of maximal tenderness and the edges trimmed to prevent premature closing (which could lead to recurrence). No packing is required.

For pain out of proportion to physical findings, an exam under anesthesia is mandatory. An intersphincteric abscess may be established by palpation of a mass or aspiration of pus in the operating room. The treatment is division of the internal anal sphincter along the length of the abscess. The wound may be marsupialized for adequate drainage.

If the abscess is of pelvic origin, it can be drained via the area it is pointing: through the rectum, ischioanal fossa, or percutaneously via the abdominal wall.

5.3.2.2 Catheter drainage

An alternative method of treatment for selected patients is catheter drainage. Patients suitable for this technique should not have severe sepsis or any serious systemic illness. Several portions of this technique deserve further comment. First, the stab incision should be placed as close as possible to the anus, minimizing the amount of tissue that must be opened if a fistula is found after resolution of inflammation. Second, the size and length of the catheter should correspond to the size of the abscess cavity. A catheter that is too small or too short may fall into the wound. Third, the length of time that the catheter should be left in place requires clinical judgment. Factors involved in this decision should include the size of the original abscess cavity, the amount of granulation tissue around the catheter, and the character and amount of drainage. If there is doubt, it is better to leave the catheter in place for a longer period of time.

5.3.2.3 Primary fistulotomy

Primary fistulotomy at the time of abscess drainage is controversial. A meta-analysis showed that when the fistula is identified, drainage plus primary fistulotomy decreased the rate of subsequent fistula formation (by 83%) with no increase in incontinence.

Those younger than 40 years old have a significantly higher risk of developing a fistula or recurrent abscess after initial drainage of a perianal abscess. Abscess recurrence is more often observed after drainage of an ischioanal abscess. If the internal opening of a low transsphincteric fistula is readily apparent at the time of abscess drainage, primary fistulotomy is feasible except in patients with Crohn's disease, acquired immune deficiency syndrome (AIDS), advanced age, high transsphincteric fistula, and an anterior fistula (in women).

5.3.2.4 Antibiotics

Antibiotics are only used as an adjunct for patients with valvular heart disease, prosthetic heart valves, extensive soft tissue cellulitis, prosthetic devices, diabetes, immunosuppression, or systemic sepsis.

5.3.3 Postoperative care

Postoperatively, patients are instructed to take a regular diet, bulk-forming agents, the prescribed analgesia, and sitz baths. Follow-up for patients is generally 2-4 weeks after the procedure, but those with an intersphincteric or supralevator abscess may be seen sooner at about 2 weeks.

If catheter drainage has been done, these patients are seen 7-10 days after catheter placement. If the cavity has closed around the catheter and the drainage ceased, the catheter is removed. Otherwise, the catheter is left in place or a smaller catheter placed. In all cases, patients are observed until complete healing occurs.

5.4 Complications

(1) Recurrence

Up to 89% of patients after drainage of an ischioanal or intersphincteric abscess will develop a recurrent abscess or fistula. Recurrence is higher in those who had a previous abscess drained. Recurrence of anorectal infections may be due to missed infections in adjacent anatomic spaces, presence of an undiagnosed fistula or abscess at the initial drainage, or failure to completely drain the initial abscess.

(2) Extra-anal causes

Extra-anal etiologies that can lead to abscess recurrence include hidradenitis suppurativa, pilonidal abscess (with downward extension), Crohn's disease, tuberculosis, human immunodeficiency virus (HIV) infection, perianal actinomycosis, rectal duplication, lymphogranuloma venereum, trauma, foreign bodies, and perforated rectal carcinoma.

(3) Incontinence

Iatrogenic injury can lead to incontinence, which occurs with division of external sphincter muscle during drainage of a perianal or deep postanal space abscess(in a patient with borderline continence) or division of puborectalis muscle in a patient with a supralevator abscess. Prolonged packing of an abscess cavity may impair continence by leading to excessive scar formation. Primary fistulotomy at the time of initial abscess drainage may lead to continence disturbances while unnecessarily dividing sphincter muscle.

Chapter 6

Fistula in Ano

6.1 Pathophysiology

6.1.1 Etiology

A fistula is defined as an abnormal communication between any two epithelium-lined surfaces. A fistula-in-ano is an abnormal tract or cavity communicating with the rectum or anal canal by an identifiable internal opening. Most fistulas are thought to arise as a result of cryptoglandular infection.

6.1.2 Classification

The classification of anal fistula is divided into several categories according to the relationship between fistula and sphincter: intersphincteric, transsphincteric, suprasphincteric and extrasphincteric. Intersphincteric type includes simple low tract, high blind tract, high tract with rectal opening, rectal opening without perineal opening, extrarectal extension and secondary to pelvic diseasc. Transsphincteric type includes uncomplicated and high blind tract. Suprasphincteric type is also divided into two categories: uncomplicated and high blind tract. And extrasphincteric type includes secondary to anal fistula, secondary to trauma, secondary to anorectal disease and secondary to pelvic inflammation.

6.1.2.1 Intersphincteric fistula-in-ano

This fistula is the result of a perianal abscess. The tract passes within the intersphincteric space (Figure 30-6-1A). This is the most common type of fistula and accounts for approximately 70% of fistulas. A high blind tract passing from the fistula tract to the rectal wall may occur; in addition, the tract may also pass into the lower rectum. The infectious process may pass into the intersphincteric plane and terminate as a blind tract. There is no downward extension to the anal margin, and thus no external opening is present. Infection may also spread in the intersphincteric plane to reach the pelvic cavity to lie above the levator ani muscles. Lastly, an intersphincteric fistula may originate in the pelvis as a pelvic abscess but manifest itself in the perianal area.

6.1.2.2 Transsphincteric fistula-in-ano

In its usual variety, this fistula results from an ischioanal abscess and constitutes approximately 23% of fistulas seen. The tract passes from the internal opening through the internal and external sphincters to the ischioanal fossa(Figure 30-6-1B). A high blind tract may also occur in this situation in which the upper arm of the tract may pass toward the apex of the ischioanal fossa or may extend through the levator ani muscles and thereby into the pelvis. One form of transsphincteric fistula is the rectovaginal fistula.

6.1.2.3 Suprasphincteric fistula-in-ano

This fistula results from a supralevator abscess and accounts for approximately 5% of fistulas in some series. The tract passes above the puborectalis after arising as an intersphincteric abscess. The tract curves downward lateral to the external sphincter in the ischioanal space to the perianal skin(Figure 30-6-1C). A high blind tract may also occur in this variety and result in a horseshoe extension.

6.1.2.4 Extrasphincteric fistula-in-ano

This constitutes the rarest type of fistula and accounts for 2% of fistulas. The tract passes from the rectum above the levators and through them to the perianal skin via the ischioanal space(Figure 30-6-1D). This fistula may result from foreign body penetration of the rectum with drainage through the levators, from penetrating injury to the perineum, or from Crohn's disease or carcinoma or its treatment. However, the most common cause may be iatrogenic secondary to vigorous probing during fistula surgery.

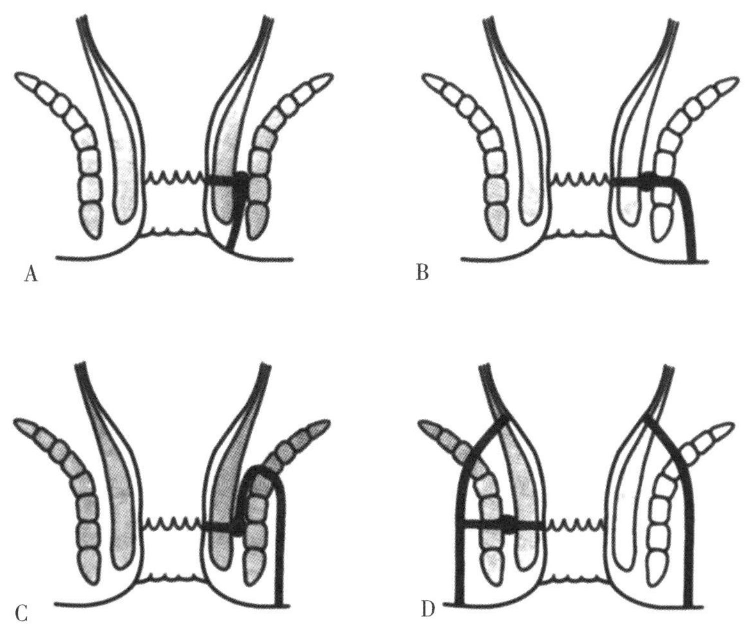

Figure 30-6-1 Classification of fistula-in-ano

A. Intersphincteric; B. Transsphincteric; C. Suprasphincteric; D. Extrasphincteric.

6.2 Evaluation

(1) Symptoms

Most patients with a fistula-in-ano recall an abscess(that was incised or drained spontaneously). They may also have continual drainage, pain with defecation, bleeding(if there is granulation tissue at the internal opening), or a decrease in their swelling/pain when spontaneous drainage occurs. Bowel symptoms may be present if the fistula results from Crohn's disease, actinomycosis, or anorectal carcinoma. Systemic diseases like HIV, carcinoma, or lymphoma should also be considered.

(2) Physical examination

The number and location of external openings may be helpful to locate the primary opening on digital exam, the internal opening may feel like a nodule or pit. An indurated cord-like structure may be palpable beneath the skin oriented toward the direction of the internal opening. Posterior or lateral induration may reflect a deep postanal space or horseshoe fistula. Digital exam also should note any relation of the tract to the sphincter muscle, along with the bulk, tone, and voluntary squeeze of the anal sphincter muscle.

(3) Investigations

Prior to operative intervention, anoscopy may identify an internal opening. Proctoscopy can exclude underlying proctitis or neoplasia.

Colonoscopy (or barium enema) and small bowel evaluation (as a small bowel series, CT enterography, or MRI enterography) are indicated if there are multiple fistulas, recurrent fistula, or bowel symptoms suggestive of inflammatory bowel disease.

Anal manometry may be useful in planning the operative approach in a patient with a history of obstetrical trauma (in women), advanced age, Crohn's disease, AIDS, or recurrent fistula.

Preoperative imaging is strategically used to decrease recurrence rates after fistula surgery by demonstrating clinically undetected sepsis, guide surgery, and determine the relationship of the fistula to the sphincters.

(4) Fistulography

Cannulation of the external opening and injection of a water-soluble contrast into the fistula tract are considered when the anatomy may be altered such as in recurrent fistulas or in Crohn's disease. Accuracy is variable and reported to be between 16% and 96%. This test may not demonstrate secondary tracts, distinguish an abscess located in the high ischioanal fossa versus supralevator space, or fail to precisely show the internal opening. One study found that fistulography altered surgical management or revealed other pathology 48% of the time.

(5) Computed tomography scan

A CT scan performed with IV and rectal contrast may distinguish an abscess from cellulitis. It may assess the degree of rectal inflammation in inflammatory bowel disease. It may not visualize fistula tracts in relation to the levators.

(6) Endoanal Ultrasound

Establishes the relation of the primary tract to the anal sphincters, determines simple from complex fistula, determines the primary internal opening, and assesses the adequacy of drainage. An enhancing agent such as hydrogen peroxide injected into the tract at the time of endosonography improves accuracy. This study is operator dependant and scars or defects from previous sepsis or surgery impede ultrasonographic interpretation.

(7) Magnetic resonance imaging

MRI is valued to assess complex fistulas particularly in patients with anatomic distortion from previous surgery. An MRI is felt by some to be the most accurate technique to delineate the internal opening along with showing the course of primary and secondary extensions.

6.3 Treatment

6.3.1 General principles

The surgical principles are to eliminate the fistula, prevent recurrence, and preserve sphincter function. This is done by finding the internal opening and dividing the least amount of sphincter muscle.

Steps to identify the internal opening are as follows:

(1) Passage of a probe from the external to the internal opening (or vice versa).

(2) Injection of dye (dilute methylene blue, milk, or hydrogen peroxide) in the external opening and noting its presence at the dentate line.

(3) Following the granulation tissue in the fistula tract while incising over the extrasphincteric component of the tract.

(4) Placing traction on the tract and noting puckering in the anal crypt associated with its internal opening. This maneuver is less successful for complicated fistula.

6.3.2 Operative management

(1) Lay-open technique

For a simple intersphincteric or low transsphincteric fistula (while typically in the prone position), gently passing a probe from the external opening through the internal opening and incising the overlying tissue can be done. No packing is required if adequate unroofing is accomplished.

(2) Seton

When the tract transverses a high and significant amount of sphincter muscle, a combination of the lay-open technique with a seton insertion may be chosen in an effort to preserve anal incontinence. The seton may be from silk or other nonabsorbable sutures, a Penrose drain, rubber bands, vessel loops, or Silastic catheters. The distal internal sphincter along with the skin leading up to the external opening is incised.

For a cutting seton, the seton is threaded through the tract and tied with multiple knots to create a handle. At regular intervals, the seton is tightened. The seton slowly cuts through the muscle and the proximal sphincter that it cuts through heals with fibrosis. This, in theory, prevents separation and retraction of the sphincter muscle. If it does not totally cut through the external sphincter, the seton allows delineation of the remaining external sphincter muscle, so at a second procedure 8 weeks later, the remaining external sphincter muscle may be divided. A cutting seton is preferred for treatment of low transsphincteric fistula, but its use in higher transsphincteric fistula risks fecal incontinence. The seton may also be tied loosely and left as a draining seton.

(3) Fistulectomy

Not recommended as it creates large wounds and has a greater risk of injuring the anal sphincter muscle.

6.3.3 Postoperative care

Following the lay-open technique, patients eat a regular diet, use bulk agents, and are given analgesic medication. Frequent sitz baths ensure perianal hygiene. Patients are seen at 2-week intervals to ensure healing is from the bottom up.

Chapter 7

Hemorrhoids

7.1 Anatomy

Hemorrhoids are normal components of anorectal anatomy. Hemorrhoids are vascular cushions in the submucosal space of the anal canal. Hemorrhoids are classically described as occurring in the left lateral, right anterior, and right posterior position. However, this finding was identified in less 20% of cadavers. They are composed of blood vessels, connective tissue, and smooth muscles. The smooth muscle is known as Treitz's muscle and originates from conjoined longitudinal muscle and internal sphincter.

Histologically, hemorrhoids lack a muscular wall and are therefore sinusoids (not veins or arteries). Blood inflow to hemorrhoids is from the superior hemorrhoidal artery with some contribution from middle hemorrhoidal artery, and most distally from inferior hemorrhoidal artery. pH analysis of hemorrhoidal bleeding confirms that it is arterial blood. Venous drainage distal to dentate line (external hemorrhoids) is to the inferior hemorrhoidal veins which flow into the pudendal and ultimately the internal iliac veins. Internal hemorrhoids (proximal to the dentate line) drain into the middle hemorrhoidal veins which also drain into the iliac veins. Innervation proximal to dentate line is from sympathetic and parasympathetic nerves (non-cholinergic/nonadrenergic mediators).

Distal to dentate line is from somatic nerves (sensitivity to touch, pain, temperature, and stretch). Exact function of hemorrhoids is unknown. Theories include maintaining closure of anal canal which could contribute to continence and protecting the sphincters from trauma related to passing stool. Internal hemorrhoids are covered by columnar epithelium. Near the dentate line, there is transitional epithelium which is viscerally innervated. External hemorrhoids are covered by anoderm which is a specialized squamous epithelium devoid of hair follicles or sweat glands. The most distal aspect is covered by normal skin. Anoderm and perianal skin are somatically innervated.

7.2 Etiology

The etiology of hemorrhoidal symptoms is poorly understood but most likely multifactorial. Contributors include the following:

(1) Venous congestion with hypertrophy of internal hemorrhoids due to straining, constipation, pregnancy, chronic cough, pelvic mass, pelvic floor dysfunction, and ascites.

(2) Conditions that promote prolapse of vascular cushions with secondary attenuation of fibers in Treitz's muscle and the elastic tissue in the submucosa.

(3) Dietary patterns such as low fiber which leads to hard stool and excessive straining. Hard stools may cause local tissue trauma.

(4) Behavior features such as prolonged time sitting on the commode.

(5) Diarrhea and frequent bowel movements have the same effect as constipation.

(6) Advanced age which leads to less supportive tissue (Treitz's muscle).

(7) Elevated sphincter pressures which may impair venous drainage.

7.3 Epidemiology

The true incidence is difficult to assess as patients may not seek medical attention, self-medicate themselves, seek care from a diverse group of specialists, or self-diagnose other anal problems as hemorrhoids. Prevalence in the USA is estimated to be 4.4% (8.5 million patients) with 1.9-3.5 million doctor visits and 168 000 hospitalizations annually. 2 million prescriptions are written annually for hemorrhoid therapies (over $43 000 000 which does not include over-the-counter, herbal, or homeopathic treatments).

7.4 Classification

Internal hemorrhoids originate proximal to dentate line and are lined by columnar epithelium.

External hemorrhoids are located distal to the dentate line and are lined by anoderm and most distally by skin.

Mixed hemorrhoids have both internal and external components.

Internal hemorrhoids are classified based on prolapse:

(1) Grade Ⅰ——internal bulge into the anus without prolapse.

(2) Grade Ⅱ——internal hemorrhoids that prolapse during defecation and spontaneously reduce.

(3) Grade Ⅲ——internal hemorrhoids that prolapse and require manual reduction.

(4) Grade Ⅳ——hemorrhoids that prolapse and are irreducible.

7.5 Clinical Presentation

(1) Internal hemorrhoid symptoms

1) Bleeding is typically bright red blood with bowel movements, or seen on the toilet paper, dripping in the toilet, or squirting into the toilet at the completion of a bowel movement. Anemia due to hemorrhoids is rare and patients with anemia should be considered for a full GI tract assessment.

2) Itching and burning which may be caused from mucous related to prolapse.

3) Sensation of fullness, urge to defecate, or feeling of incomplete evacuation can be from internal pro-

lapse.

4) Difficulty with perineal hygiene.

5) Sense of anal wetness or soiling of undergarments or sense of a lump if internal hemorrhoid prolapses through the anal canal.

6) Even though not somatically innervated, patients still may report pain. Severe pain may be from thrombosis or strangulation.

7) Internal hemorrhoids may spontaneously reduce, or may require manual reduction.

(2) External hemorrhoid symptoms

Pain (mild to excruciating) can result from acute thrombosis. This is often associated with a firm anal lump. As the thrombus erodes through the skin, patients may see bleeding. After the external hemorrhoid resolves, a skin tag (redundant skin) may remain. This could lead to difficulty maintaining hygiene or itching.

7.6 Differential Diagnosis Based on Anal Symptoms

The differential diagnosis based on anal symptoms are as shown in Table 30-7-1.

Table 30-7-1 Differential diagnosis based on anal symptoms

Symptom	Differential diagnoses
Pain	Thrombosed hemorrhoids, fissure, abscess, fistula, pruritus, anorectal Crohn's disease, anismus, abscess
Bleeding	Internal or external hemorrhoids, fissure, fistula, hypertophic papilla, polyps, anal or colorectal cancer, ulcerative colitis, Crohn's disease, infectious colitis, draining thrombosed hemorrhoids, rectal prolapse
Pruritis	Prolapsing hemorrhoids, fistula, incontinence, anal condylomata, rectal prolapse, reuritus ani, anal papilla, dermatitis, dietary causes
Mass	Thrombosed or prolapsed hemorrhoids, abscess, anal cancer, prolapsing polyp or papilla, skin tags, prolapsing tumor, rectal prolapse, condylomata

7.7 Evaluation

7.7.1 History

Document the patient's bowel habits, including constipation, diarrhea, urgency, frequency, and changes in bowel habits. A prospectively maintained bowel diary may be helpful. History can help differentiate hemorrhoids from other anal pathology. It can also elicit "red flag" symptoms such as bleeding or change in bowel habits that may be indicative of malignancy. Dietary history is included particularly focusing on fiber and fluid intake with attention to foods that cause diarrhea or constipation. Changes in bowel and diet habits due to an acute illness or travel should be noted.

7.7.2 Physical examination

Includes a general exam that focuses on liver disease, COPD, or coagulopathy. The abdominal exam will focus on signs of constipation. An anal exam may be embarrassing and same gender chaperone should be offered to be in the room to help relax the patient. Also reassure your patient and communicate what you will be doing. The prone jackknife position allows for maximal anal exposure. If impractical(too obese, pregnant, or orthopedic issues), then left lateral or lithotomy position is chosen. Describe anatomy and pathology in anatomical terms(left, right, anterior, posterior), and avoid using the position of the clock(patient's position may change). Inspect the anoderm and sacrococcygeal region. Identify external hemorrhoids, skin tags, prolapsing internal hemorrhoids, rectal prolapse, excoriated skin, fissures, fistulas, abscesses, anal cancer, thrombosed external hemorrhoids, rashes, or dermatitis. Palpate the area to assess induration, tenderness, masses, or thrombus in external hemorrhoids.

Use the digital exam to assess sphincter tone(both rest and squeeze), and identify masses, abscesses, and localized pain. The degree of prolapse is examined by asking the patient to strain. If there is any concern, an evaluation with the patient on a commode(which is a more physiologic situation) may be required. Anoscopy is performed using one of the several types of anoscopes available. Rigid or flexible proctoscopy evaluates the rectum for inflammation.

Colonoscopy or barium enema is ordered if red flag symptoms are present. These are considered in the context of the patient's age, personal and family history of colorectal pathology, duration of symptoms, and nature of bleeding. Due to concerns of inflaming hemorrhoids with a bowel preparation, treatment of the hemorrhoids for several weeks to months may be reasonable prior to a more in-depth colonic evaluation.

7.8 Treatment

Control of symptoms is the primary treatment goal. Reassure patient that hemorrhoids are normal components of human anatomy and removal of all hemorrhoid tissue is not necessary.

Treatment is categorized into three groups.

7.8.1 Medical management(dietary and behavioral therapies)

Modify stool through increased dietary fiber(25 g/day for women and 38 g/day for men) and increased water intake(64 oz daily).

Encourage regular sleep/wake cycle and exercise to maintain regular bowel habits.

Add bulk-forming agents such as psyllium to modify quality of stool. Taken with oral fluid, the goal is to add moisture and soften stools. Optimally, patients should ingest supplements in the morning so fluid can be consumed throughout the day to hydrate the supplements. If needed(inadequate stool mixing), divide doses throughout the day. Longterm compliance may be difficult due to poor palatability, bloating, excessive flatus, or crampy abdominal pain. Start at a low dose and titrate up for the desired effect to minimize side effects.

Stool softeners (docusate), lubricants (mineral oil), and laxatives [hyperosmolar (polyethylene glycol), saline (magnesium citrate), or stimulant (senna or bisacodyl)] are used to treat constipation. Transition to fiber and stool softeners as quickly as feasible. Goal is a bulky but soft stool that is easy to pass.

Diarrhea may require additional evaluation including diet recommendations to increase fiber and reduce fat consumption, along with assessment of caffeine intake, alcohol intake, and irregular sleep/wake cycle which can all contribute to diarrhea. Profound or bloody diarrhea needs further evaluation with stool cultures, fecal fat analysis, and endoscopy. Loose stools can be treated with fiber supplementation that is titrated according to the patient's symptoms.

The trial of increased fiber should be from 4 to 6 weeks followed by reevaluation of symptoms. The goal of medical management is symptom control. The appearance of the hemorrhoids may not change.

7.8.2 Toileting behavior

Patients should spend only 3–5 min on toilet. Do not read on toilet.

Patients that can not avoid excessive straining or require >30 min on the commode to evacuate stool should be evaluated for a pelvic floor disorder.

Avoid compulsive wiping which can lead to local trauma, contribute to inflammation from internal hemorrhoids, increase bleeding from external skin, and worsen pruritus. Use premoistened wipes, i. e. , witch hazel, but avoid those with alcohol.

7.8.3 Sitz baths

Use warm, approximately 40 ℃ water (without additives such as salt or oils), in a bathtub or portable device.

Limit duration to 15 min.

This treatment can provide relief of pain, itching, and burning and may aid hygiene (particularly after bowel movements).

May alleviate sphincter and pelvic floor muscle spasms.

Limited objective evidence regarding the use of sitz baths, but low cost and low risk, makes this an attractive treatment.

7.8.4 Medications

(1) Topical medications have little objective evidence to support firm recommendations, but since they are so commonly used by patients to selfmedicate themselves, surgeons need to be familiar with them. Many employ a combination of agents.

(2) Local anesthetics may provide temporary relief of pain, itching, and burning. The medication delivery mechanism may cause local irritation. Some contain vasoconstricting agents in an effort to reduce swelling.

(3) Barrier protectants prevent skin irritation by eliminating contact of mucous and stool with the skin.

(4) Astringents clean and dry skin.

(5) Analgesics sooth the skin.

(6) Corticosteroids relieve perianal inflammation. Prolonged use may thin the skin.

(7) Suppositories do not typically remain localized in the anal canal. However, they may provide indirect relief by delivering the medication to the rectum and anal skin. Suppositories frequently contain a combination of medicating agents.

7.8.5 Phlebotonics

These are a heterogeneous collection of substances used to treat many vascular conditions including hemorrhoids purportedly by improving venous flow, improving venous tone, stabilizing capillary permeability, and increasing lymphatic drainage. Safety concerns with some phlebotonics include flavonoids that can cause GI side effects and calcium dobesilate which can cause agranulocytosis. Citrus bioflavonoids are used in Europe. Commercially available nutritional supplements can contain diosmin and patients can obtain these. Calcium dobesilate is a synthetic product which can stabilize capillary permeability, decrease platelet aggregation, and improve lymphatic transport. In a randomized trial comparing this to fiber, patients significantly improved after 2 weeks using calcium dobesilate. Meta-analysis of 14 trials showed that flavonoids appear to give a beneficial effect.

7.9 Rubber Band Ligation

Most common office procedure to treat internal hemorrhoids due to its efficiency, safety, and cost-effectiveness. A small rubber band is applied at the apex and fixes the pedicle into its normal anatomical position. Ischemia causes hemorrhoids to shrink which corrects prolapse and improves venous drainage. No bowel prep is needed, but an enema may improve visualization. Ideally, the patient is positioned in prone jackknife position, but can be in left lateral position. Rarely, if the patient can not tolerate a full anoscopic exam, sedation in a monitored setting may be needed. Additionally, a bright light for viewing the anal canal and an assistant are usually required.

7.10 Operative Procedures

Only 5%-10% of patients will require operative hemorrhoidectomy. An operative approach is considered for patients that fail lesser techniques, have advanced disease, or have significant external hemorrhoids that require excision. Some patients with other anal pathology (fissures or fistula disease) may elect for an operative hemorrhoidectomy to address all anal pathology at the same setting. Patients intolerable of an office procedure or if coagulopathic may require operative hemorrhoidectomy for definitive treatment. Surgical treatment is divided into two categories: excisional hemorrhoid ectomy, stapled hemorrhoidopexy.

7.10.1 Complications of hemorrhoidectomy

Postoperative bleeding, most likely as a result of technical factors, is a more common complication. Massive postoperative bleeding can be controlled with anal canal packing or inflation of a balloon-tipped catheter into the rectum and then pulled back against the anorectal junction. If these maneuvers are unsuccessful, an exam under anesthesia is appropriate. Other complications include urinary retention, infection, fecal incontinence, fecal impaction, and anal stenosis.

7.10.2 Stapled hemorrhoidopexy

· Using a modified circular end-to-end stapler, transanally, circumferential sections of mucosa and submucosa are excised well proximal to the dentate line. This will pexy the hemorrhoid pedicles and secures the internal hemorrhoids into a normal anatomical position. This will improve venous outflow.

· The staple line may divide arterial inflow in the submucosal space, thus devascularizing the hemorrhoid.

· This treatment is advantageous as a single setting procedure without painful incisions.

· Multiple synonyms exist for this procedure: stapled anopexy, stapled prolapsectomy, stapled mucosectomy, and procedure for prolapse and hemorrhoids (PPH).

· Specific complications that are important to note include rectal obstruction, rectal perforation, retroperitoneal sepsis, pelvic sepsis, the potential for sphincter injury (if muscle is incorporated into stapler), and rectovaginal fistula.

Chapter 8

Colon Cancer

8.1 Anatomy

The colon is the tubular structure that extends from the end of the ileum to the junction between the sigmoid colon and rectum, including the ileocecal valve and appendix, and wraps the small intestines like an arch. Together with the rectum and anus, it forms the whole large intestine. Classical divisions of the colon are the cecum, ascending colon, transverse colon, descending colon, and sigmoid colon. The colon is approximately one fourth the length of the small intestines, with a length of 150 cm(120–200 cm). It is widest at the cecum(7.5 cm) and narrowest at the rectosigmoid junction(2.5 cm).

Three structures are helpful in making the macroscopic differentiation of the colon from the small intestine: the tenia coli, haustra coli, and appendix epiploica. The tenia coli is formed by the concentration of longitudinal muscular layer of large intestines in the form of three bands and continues from the appendix root to the rectosigmoid junction. As these tenias are shorter than the intestine length, they form the haustras that give the colon its saccular appearance. Except for the appendix and the cecum, most parts of the colon are surrounded by the appendix epiploica formed by the adipose tissue, which is mostly covered by peritoneum.

8.1.1 Cecum

The cecum is the widest part of the colon, situated on the right iliac fossa and starting at the termination of the terminal ileum. It is 6–8 cm diameter. As the cecum and ascending colon are close to the psoas major muscle posteriorly, the lateral femoral cutanous nerve, the femoral nerve, the genitofemoral nerves, the gonadal arteries and veins, and the ureter, caution must be exercised to preserve these structures while the right colon is liberalized. The cecum is adjacent to the anterior abdominal wall anteriorly.

In many people, more than 90% of the cecum's surface is covered by peritoneum. A peritoneal fold separated from terminal ileum mesentery may cross over the ileum to attach to the bottom part of the colon and cecum. This is called the superior ileocecal fold, and the anterior cecal artery passes through it. On the anterior part of the terminal ileum and anterior to the appendix mesentery, the inferior ileocecal fold is present, and no anatomic structure passes through it.

The ileum opens by a conical papillary eminence, called the ileocecal valve in humans, extending toward the cecum. Kumar and Philips noted that the superior and inferior ileocecal ligaments were responsible for the ileocecal valve's competence. This valve not only prevents the cecum's contents from refluxing into the ileum, but also prevents ileal content from passing too quickly to the cecum. Bogers and Van Mark stated that this valve has a sphincter function. However, barium enema studies have shown that ileocecal valve function is often not sufficient, even in people without any disease.

The appendix vermiformis is a blind-ended tubular structure situated approximately 3 cm from the ileocecal junction. Its length is 2–20 cm (average of 8–10 cm) and its diameter is 5 mm. Because of its high mobility, the appendix may be in many positions. While it is in the posteromedial position in 85% of humans, it may be in the retrocecal, pelvic, subcecal, preileal, or retroileal position. The point where three tenias conjoin on the cecum may assist in locating the appendix root.

The wall of the cecum is thin compared with the walls of other colonic segments.

For this reason, tenias are the most appropriate parts for such surgical procedures as anastomoses and cecopexy. Cecum volvulus is rarely seen because of posterior fixations.

8.1.2 Ascending colon

The ascending colon extends at the right side of the cavity in front of the quadratus lumborum and transverses the abdominis muscle. The ascending colon, which is the division between the cecum and the hepatic flexure, is 12–20 cm long on average. It is in relation with the m. iliacus, ileolumbar ligament, quadratus lumborum, transversus abdominis, perirenal fat tissue, right kidney, lateral cutaneous nerve, and ilioinguinal and iliohypogastric nerves posteriorly. It resides near the ureter, which extends over the psoas muscle and gonadal veins. Anteriorly, it neighbors the small intestines, omentum, and anterior abdominal wall. The ascending colon is covered with peritoneum, except at its posterior surface, but it is not rare that it is fully covered and has a short mesocolon. Reduced mobility of the colon may be because of abnormal connective tissue bands that crosscut the ascending colon under the peritoneum. If the band is wide enough to cover a large part of the colon, it is called Jackson's membrane. Treves determined that there was mesocolon in 12% of the ascending colon and 22% of the descending colon of the cadavers.

The ascending colon forms the hepatic flexure by turning to the left below the inferior part of the liver, lateral to the gallbladder. Sometimes, it extends over the second part of the duodenum by attaching to it via a peritoneal fold called a duodenocolic ligament. The hepatic flexure may move between 2. 5 and 7. 5 cm vertically during respiration.

8.1.3 Transverse colon

The transverse colon starts at the point where the colon sharply turns to left (hepatic flexure), just below the right lobe inferior face of the liver. Its approximate length is 45 cm, and it is the longest segment of the colon. Almost all of the transverse colon is covered with peritoneum, and it is attached to the posterior abdominal wall with a long mesentery, which gives it mobility.

The root of the transverse mesocolon begins at the inferior pole of the right kidney and crosses over the second part of duodenum, continues past the pancreas head, body, and tail, and ends at the hilus of the left kidney. This is generally accepted as an anatomic landmark separating the supramesocolic and inframesocolic compartments. This region is like a barrier separating both compartments in infectious situations.

Different from the ascending and descending colon, the transverse colon has a mesentery that is formed by the subsequent junction with the omental bursa's posterior face. Because of the splenic flexure's proximity to the inferior face of the spleen and its relation with the diaphragm through the phrenocolic ligament, caution must be exercised during mobilization. Dissection should be performed from the transverse colon toward the splenic flexure. The transverse mesocolon includes the middle colic artery and vein along with the lymph nodes and nerves. Sometimes, the transverse mesocolon's superior fold attaches to the stomach's posterior wall. Gastric ulcers and benign or malignant tumors may tightly attach to the mesocolon, and the middle colic artery may be damaged during the separation of the stomach wall from the mesocolon.

8.1.4 Descending colon

The descending colon, approximately 25 cm length, is the colonic segment extending from the splenic flexure to the pelvic unit. It arrives at the iliac crest by descending vertically from the lateral border of the left kidney between the psoas and quadratus and ends at the sigmoid colon, turning medially on the anterior of the psoas muscle and iliac bone. Like the ascending colon, the descending colon is surrounded by peritoneum on the anterior, medial, and lateral surfaces and has a short mesocolon. Existence of the fascia of Toldt, which provides posterior fixation of the colon in many people, enables dissection with little bleeding during an operation.

At its posterior face, the descending colon neighbors the lower pole of the left kidney, the origin of the transversus abdominis muscle, the quadratus lumborum, the iliac and psoas major muscles, the subcostal vein and nerves, the iliohypogastric and ilioinguinal nerves, the 4th lumbar artery, the lateral femoral, femoral, and genitofemoral nerves, the gonadal veins, and the external iliac artery. Anteriorly, however, it neighbors the small intestines and anterior abdominal wall anteroinferiorly. Having a deeper settlement compared with the ascending colon, the descending colon is more posterolaterally settled, especially in young females.

8.1.5 Sigmoid colon

When the descending colon comes to the iliac crest level, it becomes the sigmoid colon and has a mesentery. Sigmoid colon, with an average length of 35-40 cm, may show variations in terms of length, position, and fixation. The sigmoid colon has two parts; the iliac part is settled and fixed in the left iliac fossa while the pelvic part is mobile. The sigmoid colon starts at the level of iliac crest and ends at the level of the 3rd sacral vertebra.

The sigmoid colon, which is fully covered with peritoneum, generally has a V-shaped and sometimes U-shaped mesocolon, extending from the left iliac fossa to the pelvic unit. The apex of the "V" points at the bifurcation point of the common iliac veins extending over the sacroiliac junction. The left ureter passes at this point between the peritoneum and the common iliac artery and is an important landmark in the detection of the ureter. The sigmoid mesocolon is longer at the center, whereas it is shorter in the rectum and descending colon junctions, and this causes a relative fixation at the tips of the sigmoid.

In the 1800s, because it was observed that the sigmoid colon was generally empty and contracted, this part of the colon was thought to have a role in continence as a fecal reservoir. Later, as the thickening of the circular muscular layer between the rectum and sigmoid was noted, the terms "sphincter ani" "tertius rectosigmoid sphincter" and "piloris sigmoido rectalis" came into use.

The rectosigmoid junction may be described by surgeons as a zone between the last 5-8 cm of the sigmoid and the upper 5 cm of the rectum. By endoscopists, however, it is seen as a narrow and sharp-angled segment, in spite of knowledge that it is a well-identified segment that is the narrowest part of the large intestine.

In a study on cadavers, the rectosigmoid junction was identified as the zone where the tenia libera and the tenia omentalis form a single anterior tenia below 6-7 cm of the promontorium and the haustra and mesocolon disappear. Although it does not fit the definition of an anatomic sphincter formed by thickened circular muscle layers closing the lumen by rectosigmoid contraction, this segment may be accepted as a functional sphincter because of its active dilatation and passive closing mechanisms.

8.1.6 Arterial supply

The superior mesenteric artery (SMA) is a large–diameter artery that originates from a narrow opening on the aorta. This situation makes it the mesenteric vessel that is most prone to embolic events. It is the second largest intra–abdominal branch of the aorta and supplies the whole embryologic midgut. Generally, the AMS has many more branches supplying the distal intestine. This creates a higher potential for distal anastomoses. The AMS originates 1 cm below the a. coeliacus, at the L1 vertebra level, travels down and rightward, and ends as the a. ileocolica. Its main branches are the a. pancreaticoduodenale inferior, the a. colica media, the a. colica dextra, and 4–6 jejunal and 9–13 ileal branches. The a. colica media typically originates from the AMS's proximal part, supplies the transverse colon, and forms anastomoses with the branches of the a. mesenterica inferior. The splenic flexure is a border zone between these two mesenteric veins. Therefore, ischemic colitis is seen more commonly here.

The inferior mesenteric artery (IMA) is the smallest of the mesenteric arteries and originates 6–7 cm below the AMS at the L3 level and supplies the distal transverse colon, splenic flexure, descending colon, and rectosigmoid. The IMA is a small diameter artery and its branching angle to the aorta protects it against embolic events. Its main branches are the a. colica sinistra, the sigmoid, and the hemorrhoidal arteries. The branches of the a. colica sinistra reach the splenic flexure in 80% –85% and extend to middle transverse colon in 15% –20% of population. At this point, they anastomose with the branches of the a. colica media, coming from the AMS. Its sigmoid branches anastomose with the a. colica sinistra and a. hemorrhoidalis superior. The a. hemorrhodialis superior supplies the upper two–thirds wall of rectum and the mucosa of the lower one–third. The a. hemorrhoidalis media originates from the anterior face of the a. iliaca or its vesical branch. It crosses over the infraperitoneal pelvis at the lateral ligaments and supplies the middle one–third of the rectum. The a. hemorrhoidalis inferior is a branch of the a. iliaca internas' anterior face. After traveling for a short distance at the hip, it turns toward the pelvis by passing the ischiarectal fossa. This may lead to significant bleeding during abdominoperitonial rectum resection. This artery supplies the m. levator ani and sphincters as well as the lower rectum and anal canal.

8.1.6.1 Venous drainage

The colon's veins escort the arteries. On the right (cecum, descending, and right transverse colon), veins join and form the V. mesenterica. The hepatic flexure veins and rightside veins of the transverse colon pour into V. gastroepiploica and V. pancreaticoduodenale anterior superior. Voiglio was the first to identify V. gastrocolica and reported two avulsion cases that were secondary to abdominal trauma. It is a short (< 25 mm) (3–10 mm) vein that is present in 70% of population. It is situated in front of the pancreatic head, under the transverse mesocolon's root and at the intersection point of the V. gastroepiploica dextra and the right upper colic vein. The importance of this vein in abdominal trauma, pancreas surgeries, and portal hypertension has been reported. The left side of the transverse colon drains into the V. mesenterica inferior. The V. rectalis superior drains the ascending and sigmoid colon, ascends, and forms the V. mesenteric inferior.

Rectal veins drain into the V. rectalis, which drains into the V. mesenterica inferior. This part drains into the portal system. The V. rectalis inferior and V. rectalis media drain into the iliac vein and thereby into the systemic venous circulation.

8.1.6.2 Lymphatic drainage

Gastrointestinal system lymphatics show reverse flow along the arteries toward the lymphatic nodes. Colonic lymphatics are studied in four groups. The lymphatics on the colon walls primarily drain into epiploic appendix and subserosal epiploic nodes. The epiploic nodes drain into the paracolic nodes, which are on the posterior part of the peritoneum, located at the upper level of the transverse colon and the mesentery of the colon segments. Intermediate nodes are the third lymphatic stations and are related to the main colonic arteries such as the ileocolic artery(ICA), right colic artery(RCA), middle colic artery(MCA), left colic artery (LCA), and sigmoid branches. The intermediate lymph nodes become involved in the two main colonic flows(SMA and IMA) and lymphatic drainage occurs through these two main ways into the paraaortic lymph nodes, cisterna chyli, and ductus thoracicus. The lymphatic vessels of the left colon drain into the lymph nodes in the inferior mesenteric truncus and into the SMA lymph nodes, into which most of the right colon and small intestinal lymphatics drain. The lymphatics of the appendix drain into the lymph nodes of the mesoappendix and into paracolic nodes that are around the ileocolic artery.

The lymphatics of the cecum and ascending colon drain into the epicolic nodes that pass at the left side of the intestines and into the ileocolic nodes situated behind the peritoneum and into the paracolic nodes situated along the right colic artery. The transverse colon drains into the epicolic nodes and paracolic nodes situated along the middle colic artery, located at the transverse mesocolon. Drainage of the left part of the colon from splenic flexure to the beginning of the rectum drains into the epicolic nodes located at the right side of left kidney. From there, they drain into the paracolic nodes that extend along the branches of the IMA located behind the peritoneum and into the inferior mesenteric nodes in order. The upper two-thirds of the rectum drains into the inferior mesenteric nodes and the paraaortic nodes, in order. The lower third drains not only upward through the superior hemorrhoidal and inferior mesenteric vessels but also to the iliac nodes through the middle hemorrhoidal veins. The dentate line is a landmark for these two different lymphatic drainages in the anal canal. They drain into the inferior mesenteric and internal iliac nodes above and into the inguinal nodes with the inferior rectal lymphatics below. In females, drainage at 5 cm above the anal verge may spread to the posterior vaginal wall, uterus, cervix, broad ligament, fallopian tubes, ovaries, and cul-de-sac at the same time. At 10 cm, it is only to the broad ligament and cul-de-sac.

Yada et al. analyzed vascular anatomy in colon cancer and lymph node metastasis as follows. As the ileocecal artery always originates from the superior mesenteric artery and lymph node metastasis in cecum cancers is limited to nodes along the ileocolic artery, ileocecal resection is curative in surgical treatment of cecum cancer. When the origin of the right colic artery shows variations, lymph node metastasis in colon cancers may follow different paths. For this reason, right hemicolectomy should be performed in colon cancers. The right colic artery is divided into right and left branches and every branch shows a different branching pattern; if the right colic and middle colic arteries have a common stem, a right hemicolectomy can be performed in cancers of the right side of the transverse colon. If the left branch of the middle colic artery shows independent relocation, lymph node dissection should be changed according to the variation. If the left colic artery and first sigmoidal artery have a common stem, lymph nodes extending along this common stem have to be resected in descending colon and sigmoid colon cancers.

8.1.6.3 Innervation

The colon is innerved by both sympathetic(11th and 12th thoracic, 1st and 2nd lumbar) and parasympathetic(vagus and 2nd, 3rd, and 4th sacral nerves) systems. While sympathetic nerves show an inhibitor effect on colon peristaltism and secretion, parasympathetic stimuli increases the colon peristaltism and secretion. Sympathetic preganglionic nerves are organized in branches that will form the origin of splanchnic nerves by advancing toward paravertebral chains of the ganglion. Splanchnic nerves form such network-like structures as the celiac superior and inferior mesenteric that form synapses with the paravertebral ganglions. The proximal part of the colon is innervated by the celiac plexus via the superior mesenteric plexus; however, the descending colon takes its sympathetic fibers from the superior hypogastric plexus that provides nerve fibers via the lumbar part of the sympathetic tract and parallel to branches of IMA.

The parasympathetic innervation of the proximal colon is provided by the celiac branch of the right vagus. The branches coming to the preaortic and superior mesenteric plexuses reach the intestinal wall by following the route of the SMA. The distal colon and rectum receive their parasympathetic stimuli from pelvic splanchnic nerves, originating from S2 and S4. The nerve fibers extending to the superior hypogastric plexus (nerves going to the rectum and anus continue to the inferior hypoastric plexus) innerve the distal transverse, descending colon, and sigmoid colon in the neighborhood of the IMA.

8.2 Physiology

The colon has functions of digestion, absorption, storage, secretion, and excretion. The colon does not produce digestive enzymes, but it contains a large amount of bacteria, and its digestion is accomplished by bacterial fermentation. The absorption function of the colon is mainly semi-colonic and mainly absorbs water, electrolytes, glucose, urea and bile acids. Colonic mucosa, containing goblet cells, secrete alkaline mucus, can protect the mucous membrane, lubricate the stool, in order to promote the stool. Colonic movement advances the feces stored in the colon to the distal end, and the colonic movement is regulated by various factors such as eating, activity, age, and sleep.

8.3 Diagnostic Studies

A number of different diagnostic interventions have been used to detect colorectal cancer, often guided by local expertise and preference. These interventions are colonoscopy, barium enema/flexible sigmoidoscopy and CT colonography. However the optimum diagnostic strategy for colorectal cancer has not yet been defined.

All initial diagnostic investigations require rigorous bowel cleansing preparation.

Colonoscopy has for many years been regarded as the reference standard for diagnosing colonic pathology. Colonoscopy is known to have high sensitivity and specificity for detection of cancer, pre-malignant adenomas and other symptomatic colonic diseases. Colonoscopy also has the facility to take a biopsy from any suspected lesion (thereby increasing diagnostic accuracy and also permits complete removal of most benign lesions during the same procedure). However, it may not be possible to perform complete colonoscopy in a proportion of patients due to inadequate bowel preparation, poor tolerance of the procedure, inter-operator variation in terms of completion rate or the presence of an obstructing lesion in the distal colon. Patients with serious cardiorespiratory or neurological co-morbidity may beat high risk from potential complications of colonoscopy (for example colonic perforation, effects of sedation). Such patients might be better served by alternative investigations.

Barium enema is a long-established radiological investigation of the colon and rectum offering completion rates higher than those historically recorded for colonoscopy, without the need for patient sedation and with a lower incidence of serious complications. However, there is limited published evidence of the diagnostic accuracy of barium enema and there is concern that it is less sensitive than colonoscopy. This has led many centres to offer patients a combined investigative pathway of flexible sigmoidoscopy (endoscopic examination of the distal large bowel) followed by barium enema. There is a perception that this combination has comparable sensitivity to colonoscopy for detection of cancer. This investigative route also allows biopsy of lesions detected during flexible sigmoidoscopy.

Computerised tomography colonography is a more recent radiological investigation in which cross-sectional images of the abdomen and pelvis are obtained following laxative preparation and insufflation of the large bowel with air or carbon dioxide. The images are then analysed using 2-D and 3-D image reconstruction techniques. Colonoscopy can be performed at a later date to obtain biopsy confirmation of suspected tumours. It is thought that CT colonography may approach the sensitivity of colonoscopy for detection of larger polyps (>1 cm). By inference, CT colonography may therefore have high sensitivity for cancer detection, but no study of sufficient statistical power has been published that supports this inference. Some studies of CT colonography suggest large variations in performance between individual operators and different centres. Reported complication and completion rates for CT colonography compare favourably with those for colonoscopy. The technique is substantially less invasive than colonoscopy and does not require patient sedation. In addition to allowing interrogation of the large bowel, CT colonography produces images of all the abdominal and pelvic organs, and this can result in clinically important chance findings of abnormalities at other sites.

When a patient is referred for investigation of symptoms suspicious of colorectal cancer, to maximise the benefit of the diagnostic intervention it is essential that the initial clinical consultation includes the following:

(1) Accurate recording of the nature and duration of symptoms.

(2) With the patient's consent, thorough digital examination of the rectum and palpation of the abdomen.

(3) Accurate recording of significant comorbidities which may increase the risks arising from investigative procedures.

(4) Explanation of the investigations which may be offered, including the morbidity, risks and benefits.

(5) Discussion of the patient's preferences.

Clinical question: What is the most effective diagnostic intervention(s) for patients with suspected colorectal cancer to establish a diagnosis?

The quality of evidence available varied according to the intervention with high quality evidence available for CT colonography and very low quality evidence available for flexible sigmoidoscopy plus barium enema. No evidence was available for flexible sigmoidoscopy plus colonoscopy.

Staging of colorectal cancer

TNM staging system for colorectal cancer and comparison with Dukes' stage.

Tumour

T1: the tumour is confined to the submucosa.

T2: the tumour has grown into (but not through) the muscularis propria.

T3: the tumour has grown into (but not through) the serosa.

T4: the tumour has penetrated through the serosa and the peritoneal surface. If extending directly into other nearby structures (such as other parts of the bowel or other organs/body structures) it is classified as T4a. If there is perforation of the bowel, it is classified as T4b.

Nodes

N0: no lymph nodes contain tumour cells.

N1: there are tumour cells in up to 3 regional lymph nodes.

N2: there are tumour cells in 4 or more regional lymph nodes.

Metastases

M0: no metastasis to distant organs.

M1: metastasis to distant organs.

Dukes' stage

Dukes stage A = T1N0M0 or T2N0M0.

Dukes stage B = T3N0M0 or T4N0M0.

Dukes stage C = any T, N1, M0 or any T, N2, M0.

Dukes stage D = any T, any N, M1.

8.4 Management of Colon Cancer

8.4.1 Stage I colorectal cancer

Stage I colorectal cancer encompasses tumours which have extended either into the submucosa (T_1) or into, but not beyond, the muscularis propria (T_2) and in which there is no evidence of spread into the lymph nodes (N_0). In patients found to have stage I colorectal cancer a 5 year cancer specific survival of >95% can be expected following segmental resection with clear surgical margins (where there is removal of a segment of large bowel including its associated mesentery) and in these cases, surgery is essentially a curative procedure. Stage I colorectal cancer may be identified following histopathological assessment of an endoscopically resected polyp (malignant polyp), usually unsuspected at the time of polypectomy. Alternatively, and less commonly, it may be suspected in a polypoid lesion (usually laterally spreading) that appears amenable to local resection. In these cases, specialised techniques such as endoscopic submucosal dissection (ESD) or transanal endoscopic micro surgery (TEMS) may be used to perform complete "en bloc" resection of the lesion, particularly if it is situated in the left colon or rectum.

Following the introduction of the NHS bowel cancer screening programme in England and Wales, malignant colonic polyps are being detected with increasing frequency. Almost all locally removed malignant polyps are stage I cancers and would therefore be expected to have a very good prognosis. Endoscopic resection of malignant polyps may be sufficient as the only management but there is a risk of local recurrence or metastatic spread, particularly to local lymph nodes, since the mesentery, which contains the local lymph nodes, is not resected. It is uncertain, therefore, whether the same prognostic outcome can be expected as that seen in stage I tumours following segmental resection. These risks may be reduced by subsequent surgery, but the associated potential complications such as bleeding, infection or peri-operative death, and the effects on quality of life, need to be balanced against the potential benefits.

A number of retrospective studies have attempted to identify risk factors associated with recurrent malignancy in local resections, although none of these data have proven conclusive. The completeness of the endoscopic excision appears to be the most reliable predictor of tumour recurrence and, although publications vary, it can be assumed that a distance of less than 1 mm from the tumour to the margin of excision is associated with a high risk of cancer recurrence. Studies have tried to refine further the prognostic features in polyp cancers that have clear margins and arc thus deemed to have been completely excised. The risk of recurrence appears to correlate with degree of local advancement. Thus, in the Haggitt classification (applicable only to polyp cancers with long stalks), it is only the most advanced lesions, where there is extension of the tumour beyond the polyp stalk (Haggitt level 4), which is suggested to be associated with a poor outcome. The Kikuchi classification (for sessile polyps) suggests that lesions extending into the lower third of the submucosa are of the highest risk (Kikuchi level SM 3). The Ueno classification suggests that the tumour volume is directly correlated with risk of recurrence. These systems are, however, not easy to apply due to the nature of the polypectomy specimens, making assessment and subsequent decision-making problematic. Furthermore, the depth of invasion, or proximity of the tumour to the resection margin, may not be possible to assess when the lesion has been resected piecemeal and thus these lesion are best regarded as high risk. Other factors that have been suggested to predict poor outcome include tumour differentiation, (with poorly differentiated tumours conferring the highest risk), the presence of venous or lymphatic invasion and tumour budding. Uncertainty exists about the benefit to patient outcome of using these prognostic factors to guide subsequent management.

8.4.1.1 Laparoscopic surgery

(1) Laparoscopic (including laparoscopically assisted) resection is recommended as an alternative to open resection for individuals with colorectal cancer in whom both laparoscopic and open surgery are considered suitable.

(2) Laparoscopic colorectal surgery should be performed only by surgeons who have completed appropriate training in the technique and who perform this procedure often enough to maintain competence. The exact criteria to be used should be determined by the relevant national professional bodies. Cancer networks and constituent trusts should ensure that any local laparoscopic colorectal surgical practice meets these criteria as part of their clinical governance arrangements.

(3) The decision about which of the procedures (open or laparoscopic) is undertaken should be made after informed discussion between the patient and the surgeon. In particular, they should consider the suitability of the lesion for laparoscopic resection, the risks and benefits of the two procedures, and the experience of the surgeon in both procedures.

8.4.1.2 Adjuvant chemotherapy in rectal cancer

Colonic and rectal tumours occur anatomically in continuity, and have similar histopathological features. They might therefore be expected to respond similarly to chemotherapy.

Although it is established that patients with stage III (and possibly high-risk stage II) colon cancer will benefit from adjuvant chemotherapy, uncertainty remains around the benefits of such chemotherapy for patients with stage II and III rectal cancer.

8.4.2 Adjuvant chemotherapy for high-risk stage II colon cancer

A benefit from adjuvant chemotherapy in colorectal cancer was first demonstrated in 1990 in patients with stage III disease. The benefit for stage III patients has been confirmed and treatment schedules refined in the intervening years. Some of these studies of stage III disease included a proportion of patients with stage II disease. As the risk of recurrence is less with stage II disease the absolute benefit of adjuvant chemotherapy will be less than for stage III disease (assuming the relative risk reduction is the same for adjuvant chemotherapy in both stage II and stage III disease).

It is recognised that overall patients with stage II disease have a better prognosis than those with stage III disease, but that outcomes for patients within stage II vary and that there is a spectrum of risk for recurrence.

There are several pathological features which have been shown to be associated with poor prognosis in stage II disease such as extramural vascular invasion, pT4 disease (serosal breach or perforation), poorly differentiated tumours, obstructed tumours, perineural invasion and low lymph node recovery from the resection specimen. These features have been used to identify "high-risk" patients and have become, de-facto, criteria for adjuvant chemotherapy in stage II disease but their value to predict for treatment outcome has not been established.

Other tumour features, such as microsatellite instability may have both prognostic and predictive characteristics, but their exact role in the selection for adjuvant chemotherapy in patients with colon cancer is not clear.

8.4.3 Adjuvant chemotherapy for stage III colon cancer

The recommendations in this section are from Capecitabine and oxaliplatin in the adjuvant treatment of stage III (Dukes' C) colon cancer', NICE technology appraisal guidance 100 (NICE 2006).

Recommendations

(1) The following are recommended as options for the adjuvant treatment of patients with stage III (Dukes' C) colon cancer following surgery for the condition: capecitabine10 as monotherapy oxaliplatin in combination with 5-fluorouracil and folinic acid.

(2) The choice of adjuvant treatment should be made jointly by the individual and the clinicians responsible for treatment. The decision should be made after an informed discussion between the clinicians and the patient; this discussion should take into account contraindications and the side-effect profile of the agent(s) and the method of administration as well as the clinical condition and preferences of the individual.

8.4.4 Management of patients presenting in stage IV

Approximately 25% of patients with colorectal cancer have metastatic disease at the time of initial presentation and it is thought that their outcome is often worse than for those patients who develop metachronous metastatic disease following apparently curative resection of their primary tumour.

The first question in managing this group of patients is whether the primary tumour needs immediate treatment because of established or impending obstructive symptoms, even in the presence of unresectable metastatic disease.

The second question is whether or not both the primary tumour and the metastases are surgically resectable with curative intent. If the disease sites are considered resectable then the next questions are whether there should be preoperative or post-operative adjuvant treatments (or a combination of both) and whether the surgery should be a staged or combined procedure? Current practice varies widely including synchronous resections, staged resections with or without initial systemic treatment.

Where metastases are unresectable, currently patients fall into two groups:

(1) The extent of metastatic disease is such that although inoperable at presentation, patients might become resectable with curative intent if they have a good response to chemotherapy.

(2) The extent of metastatic disease is such that patients are highly unlikely to be suitable for potentially curative surgery, even with a good response to chemotherapy. Advances in systemic therapy over the last 10 years have increased the potential for long-term survival and possible cure. However there remains uncertainty as to the best sequence of treatments to achieve optimal outcome.

Chapter 9

Rectal Cancer

Colorectal cancer is the second most common malignancy with the rectum being the most frequent site involved. The prognosis for rectal cancer is relatively good compared with that for other solid tumors such as lung cancer and stomach cancer. Improvement in outcome has come from meticulous surgical techniques and more sophisticated medical management.

9.1 Origin

It is now accepted that rectal cancer arises from adenomas in a stepwise progression in which increasing dysplasia in the adenoma is due to an accumulation of genetic abnormalities (the adenoma–carcinoma sequence). In approximately 5% of cases, there is more than one carcinoma present.

9.2 Risk Factors

☆Dietary factors. A diet rich in fat and meat, and low in fibre, is commonly associated with colorectal cancers.

☆Adenomatous polyps. Most if not all cancers originate within an adenoma. However, most adenomas do not become malignant.

☆Genetic factors. Familial adenomatous polyposis syndromes (FAP); Peutz–Jegher's syndrome and juvenile polyposis.

☆Family history. Individuals with a family history of colorectal cancer or large (>1 cm) adenoma have an increased risk of developing colorectal cancer.

☆Inflammatory bowel disease. Ulcerative colitis, Crohn's colitis when the disease is longstanding and extensive.

☆Irradiation. The risk of rectal cancer is increased following radiation therapy for cancer of the cervix. These cancers may appear 10–20 years later.

9.3 Pathology

The outcome of rectal cancer depends on its biological behaviour. The clinicopathological stage together with the histopathological features provide the most accurate prognostic index at the moment.

(1) Dukes' staging

Dukes classified carcinoma of the rectum into three stages.

☆A. The growth is limited to the rectal wall(15%): prognosis excellent(90% year survival).

☆B. The growth is extended to the extrarectal tissues, but no metastasis to the regional lymph nodes (35%): prognosis reasonable(70% year survival).

☆C. There are secondary deposits in the regional lymph nodes(50%).

C1, in which the local pararectal lymph nodes alone are involved.

C2, in which the nodes accompanying the supplying blood vessels are implicated up to the point of division.

This does not take into account cases that have metastasised beyond the regional lymph nodes or by way of the venous system: prognosis is poor(40 percent year survival).

A stage D is often included, which was not described by Dukes. This stage signifies the presence of widespread metastases, usually hepatic.

(2) TNM staging

Tumor-node-metastasis(TNM) classification is now recognised internationally as the optimum classification for staging.

T represents the extent of local spread and there are four grades:

☆T_1: tumor invasion through the muscularis mucosa, but not into the muscularis propria.

☆T_2: tumor invasion into, but not through the muscularis propria.

☆T_3: tumor invasion through the muscularis propria, but not through the serosa(on surfaces covered by peritoneum) or mesorectal fascia.

☆T_4: tumor invasion through the serosa or mesorectal fascia.

N describes nodal involvement:

☆N_0: no lymph node involvement.

☆N_1: between 1 and 3 involved lymph nodes.

☆N_2: 4 or more involved lymph nodes.

M indicates the presence of distant metastases:

☆M_0: no distant metastases.

☆M_1: distant metastases.

The prefix "p" indicates that the staging is based on histopathological analysis, and "y" that it is the stage after neoadjuvant treatment, which may have resulted in downstaging.

(3) Histological grading

In the great majority of cases, rectal cancer is a columnar-celled adenocarcinoma. The more nearly the tumor cells approach normal shape and arrangement, the less aggressive the tumor is. Conversely, the greater the percentage of cells of an undifferentiated type, the more aggressive the tumor is:

☆Low grade, well-differentiated 11% prognosis good.

☆Average grade, 64% prognosis fair.

☆High grade, undifferentiated tumors 25% prognosis poor.

Vascular and perineural invasion are poor prognostic features, as is the presence of an infiltrating margin and tumor budding. In a small number of cases, the tumor is a primary mucoid carcinoma. The mucus lies within the cells, displacing the nucleus to the periphery, like the seal of a signet ring. Primary mucoid carcinoma gives rise to a rapidly growing bulky growth that metastasises very early and the prognosis of which is very poor.

9.4 Spreading Types

9.4.1 Local spread

Local spread occurs circumferentially rather than in a longitudinal direction. Anteriorly, the prostate, seminal vesicles or bladder become involved in the male; in the female, the vagina or the uterus is invaded. In either sex, a ureter may become involved, while posterior penetration may reach the sacrum and the sacral plexus. Downward spread for more than a few centimetres is rare.

9.4.2 Lymphatic spread

Above the peritoneal reflection, lymphatic spread occurs almost exclusively in an upward direction; below that level, the lymphatic spread is still upwards, but when the neoplasm lies within the field of the middle rectal artery, primary lateral spread along the lymphatics that accompany it is not infrequent.

Downward spread is exceptional, with drainage along the subcutaneous lymphatics to the groins being confined to the lymph nodes draining the perianal rosette and the epithelium lining the distal 1–2 cm of the anal canal.

Metastasis at a higher level than the main trunk of the superior rectal artery occurs only late in the disease. Atypical and widespread lymphatic permeation can occur in highly undifferentiated neoplasms.

9.4.3 Venous spread

The principal sites for blood–borne metastases are liver (34%), lungs (22%) and adrenals (11%). The remaining 33% are divided among the many other locations where secondary carcinomatous deposits tend to lodge, including the brain.

9.4.4 Peritoneal dissemination

This may follow penetration of the peritoneal coat by a high–lying rectal carcinoma.

9.5 Clinical Features

Carcinoma of the rectum can occur early in life, but the age of presentation is usually above 55 years, when the incidence rises rapidly. Often, the early symptoms are so insignificant that the patient does not seek advice for 6 months or more, and the diagnosis is often delayed in younger patients as these symptoms are attributed to benign causes. Initial rectal examination and a low threshold for investigating persistent symptoms are essential to prevent this.

9.5.1 Bleeding

Bleeding is the earliest and most common symptom. There is nothing characteristic about the time at which it occurs, nor is the colour or the amount of blood distinctive; often, the bleeding is slight in amount and occurs at the end of defaecation, or is noticed because it has stained underclothing. And often the bleeding simulates that of internal haemorrhoids (haemorrhoids and carcinoma sometimes coexist).

9.5.2 Sense of incomplete defaecation

The patient's bowels open, but there is the sensation that there are more faeces to be passed (tenesmus). This is a very important early symptom and is almost invariably present in tumors of the lower half of the rectum. The patient may endeavour to empty the rectum several times a day (spurious diarrhea), often with the passage of flatus and a little bloodstained mucus ("bloody slime").

9.5.3 Alteration in bowel habit

This is the next most frequent symptom. The patient may find it necessary to start taking an aperient or to supplement the usual dose. A patient who has to get up early in order to defaecate, or one who passes blood and mucus in addition to faeces ("early-morning bloody diarrhea"), is usually found to be suffering from carcinoma of the rectum.

9.5.4 Pain

Pain is a late symptom, but pain of a colicky character may accompany advanced tumors of the rectosigmoid, and is caused by some degree of intestinal obstruction. When a deep carcinomatous ulcer of the rectum erodes the prostate or bladder, there may be severe pain. Pain in the back, or sciatica, occurs when the cancer invades the sacral plexus.

9.6 Investigations

9.6.1 Abdominal examination

Abdominal examination is normal in early cases. Occasionally, when an advanced annular tumor is situated at the rectosigmoid junction, signs of obstruction of the large intestine are present. By the time the patient seeks advice, metastases in the liver may be palpable. When the peritoneum has become studded with secondary deposits, ascites usually results.

9.6.2 Rectal examination

In many cases, the neoplasm can be felt as a nodule with an indurated base. When the centre ulcerates, a shallow depression will be found, the edges of which are raised and everted. After the finger has been withdrawn, if it has been in direct contact with a carcinoma, it is smeared with blood or mucopurulent material tinged with blood. In females, a vaginal examination should be performed and, when the neoplasm is situated on the anterior wall of the rectum, with one finger in the vagina and another in the rectum, very accurate palpation can be carried out.

9.6.3 Faecal occult blood

Faecal occult blood testing is generally used for screening asymptomatic individuals and not for investigating symptoms. A positive faecal occult blood test must be followed by further investigation of the entire colon and rectum.

9.6.4 Proctosigmoidoscopy

Proctosigmoidoscopy will always show a carcinoma, if present, provided that the rectum is emptied of faeces beforehand.

9.6.5 Biopsy

Using biopsy forceps via a sigmoidoscope, a portion of the edge of the tumor can be removed. If possible, another specimen from the more central part of the growth should also be obtained.

9.6.6 Colonoscopy

A colonoscopy is required if possible in all patients to exclude a synchronous tumor, be it an adenoma or a carcinoma. If a proximal adenoma is found, it can be conveniently snared and removed via the colonoscope. If a synchronous carcinoma is present, the operative strategy will need changing. If a full colonoscopy is not possible, a CT colonography or barium enema can be performed. When a stenosing carcinoma is present and a colonoscopy is impossible to use, it is imperative that a colonoscopy is always performed within a few months of surgical resection.

9.6.7 Computed tomography or magnetic resonance imaging

Computed tomography is used to screen for intra-abdominal metastases. Magnetic resonance imaging is helpful in defining the extent of loco-regional invasion of rectal cancer.

9.6.8 Endorectal ultrasound

A rigid endorectal ultrasound probe is a new but established method of assessing the depth of penetration of a rectal tumor through the bowel wall. Enlarged mesorectal lymph nodes can be identified. The test is helpful in planning the operative strategy.

9.7 Differential Diagnosis

When an adenoma shows evidence of induration or unusual friability, it is almost certain that malignancy has occurred, even in spite of biopsy findings to the contrary. On the other hand, biopsy is invaluable in distinguishing carcinoma from an inflammatory stricture or an amoebic granuloma. The possibility of a neoplasm being an endometrioma should always be considered in patients with dysmenorrhoea. The possibility of a carcinoid tumor in atypical cases must be remembered. In the last four instances, biopsy should establish the correct diagnosis.

9.8 Treatment

The principle of potential surgical cure demands that the cancer be excised with an adequate margin of surrounding tissue and lymphovascular clearance. For rectal tumors, a 5 cm margin of clearance is usually preferred, although as little as 2 cm may be taken for a small mid-rectal tumor. Spread is equally likely into surrounding tissues such as the mesorectum. Thus, a wide lateral resection including all of the mesorectum is important for a rectal cancer.

Now laparoscopy-assisted technique is being developed. When performed expertly, patients undergoing laparoscopic resection have significant benefits with smaller and more cosmetic scars, a shorter hospital stay and much earlier return to normal activity. The oncologic outcome is similar to conventional open surgery.

(1) Pre-operative preparation

1) Bowel preparation

Mechanical preparation with Golytely, Fleet phospho-soda or picolax on the pre-operative day are currently the most widely used methods. Reduction of faecal load reduces both the wound and anastomotic sepsis. In patients with partial bowel obstruction, a more gentle and prolonged bowel preparation over 2-3 days is necessary.

2) Antibiotic prophylaxis

Prophylactic broad-spectrum antibiotics against aerobic and anaerobic bowel pathogens have greatly reduced incidence of wound infection and intra-abdominal sepsis. While one good dose may be adequate, most clinicians would continue the prophylactic antibiotics for 24 hours post-operatively. An unnecessarily prolonged course of antibiotics is expensive, predisposes to pseudomembranous colitis and may encourage growth of antibiotic-resistant organisms.

3) Thromboembolism prophylaxis

Patients undergoing surgery for rectal carcinoma have many risk factors for deep vein thrombosis. Increasing age, malignancy, immobilisation and operations of the abdomen and pelvis are all well recognised risk factors.

(2) Operation

Management of rectal cancer is challenging because of the technical expertise and clinical judgement required to select patients for restorative anterior resection, transanal local excision, abdominoperineal resection (APR) or a palliative procedure. About 30 years ago, nearly all patients with a rectal cancer were treated by an APR of the rectum and anus with a permanent colostomy. In more recent times, APR is used in less than 10% of rectal cancers.

9.8.1 Factors influencing choice of operation

(1) Level of lesion

The distance of the lower edge of the tumor from the dentate line is the most important factor in the choice of operation. As a rule, a tumor that is less than 5 cm from the dentate line requires APR. A 2 cm distal margin is acceptable and may permit restorative resection in most cases without damaging the anal sphincter complex.

(2) Nature of carcinoma

A high-grade, poorly differentiated tumor tends to be more widely infiltrative. This is best treated by rectal resection with a greater margin. Evidence of tumor invasion into the anal sphincters or fixation in the pelvis will contraindicate sphincter preservation procedures.

(3) Patient factors

The age and medical fitness of the patient and the presence of metastases are important factors in deciding the magnitude of the operation.

(4) Mesorectal lymph node status

Endorectal ultrasound examination will give some guidance as to the presence of lymph node metastases. Resection should be performed in the presence of lymph node metastases.

9.8.2 Anterior resection

Anterior resection is the standard radical operation for cancers of the upper and mid-rectum. It is also used for the smaller tumors of the distal rectum when a 2 cm distal margin of resection is possible without damaging the anal sphincters. The level of rectal anastomosis may be as low as the dentate line.

The sigmoid colon and the rectum are resected. The inferior mesenteric artery and left colic artery are divided at the highest possible level to enable a tension free anastomosis between a well-vascularised left colon and the rectum, while ensuring an adequate resection of the lymphovascular pedicle. The mesorectum is removed as completely as possible beyond the distal line of rectal transection.

The functional results after anterior resection are usually good but vary with the level of anastomosis. Bowel function continues to improve spontaneously for 12-18 months post-operatively. With a very distal anastomosis, there is a loss of rectal reservoir and impairment of the internal anal sphincter function. There may be stool frequency of 3-6 times in 24 hours, urgency and impaired continence.

With improved techniques, anastomotic leakage has become less common. Although neither a protective defunctioning colostomy nor a pelvic drain prevents anastomotic leaks, it may abrogate generalised sepsis should anastomotic leakage occur.

9.8.3 Abdominoperineal resection of the rectum

Abdominoperineal resection of the rectum is now largely reserved for larger T_2, T_3 or poorly differentiated tumors of the distal rectum. The rectum is mobilised down to the pelvic floor through an abdominal incision. The large bowel is divided and the sigmoid colon brought out as a left iliac fossa end colostomy. A separate perianal elliptical incision is made to mobilise and deliver the anus and distal rectum. The surgery may be expedited by having the abdominal and perineal surgeons operating simultaneously.

9.8.4 Hartmann's operation

Hartmann's operation is an anterior resection of the rectum without an anastomosis. The operation is usually reserved for palliation or as a preliminary procedure for acute malignant obstruction or perforation.

9.8.5 Transanal local excision

Transanal local excision is considered in early-stage rectal cancers that are too distal to allow restorative resection, or when age or infirmity of the patient or presence of metastases precludes major resection. Appropriate guidelines for a curative local excision are as follows:

(1) Mobile tumor located in the lower third of the rectum.

(2) Tumor size <3 cm.

(3) T_1 (submucosal invasion) or T_2 (muscularis propria) tumor on endorectal ultrasound.

(4) Well or moderately differentiated histology on biopsy no detectable mesorectal lymph nodes clinically or by endorectal ultrasound.

Long-term surveillance is essential.

9.8.6 Palliative procedures

Palliative procedures include a diverting stoma, radiotherapy and chemotherapy. Local therapy includes laser therapy, electrocoagulation and cryosurgery. Severe pelvic and perineal pain may be improved by a variety of nerve block procedures.

9.8.7 Locally advanced rectal carcinoma

En bloc resection of the cancer with adherent viscera and portions of the abdominal wall is performed. This reduces the risk of seeding viable tumor cells. The increased morbidity of such radical en bloc resection should be weighed against the likelihood of cure and the effect on the patient. If vital structures such as the inferior vena cava or pancreas are involved, a palliative operation (e. g., bypass with ileocolic anastomosis) is preferred. A diverting stoma is considered if an internal bypass is not possible.

9.8.7.1 Adjuvant therapy

Patients with more bulky disease (T_3, N_1, N_2) are at greatest risk of having microscopic residual disease. Chemotherapy, radiotherapy and immunotherapy have all been tried alone and in various combinations as adjuvant treatments before and after surgery with variable success. Currently most countries would recommend 6 months of post-operative adjuvant therapy with 5-fluorouracil and pelvic radiotherapy for Dukes'C and some B2 rectal cancer. Combined chemotherapy and radiotherapy may be administered pre-operatively to "downstage" or shrink a large T_3 or T_4 rectal cancer fixed to the pelvis. This is followed by a resection 6-8 weeks later.

9.8.7.2 Treatment of metastases

The magnitude of treatment should be weighed against any potential gain, in the relief of symptoms and the quality of remaining life. The prospect of cure to some extent justifies radical therapy of isolated metastases. The treatment options include surgery, radiotherapy, chemotherapy and drug management of symptoms:

(1) Liver

☆ Resection.

☆ Hepatic artery embolisation or ligation.

☆ Chemotherapy.

☆ Cryosurgery or radiofrequency ablation.

(2) Small bowel

☆ Resection.

☆ Bypass.

(3) Pelvis

☆ Radiotherapy: 35-55 cGy.

☆ Systemic chemotherapy: 5-fluorouracil and folinic acid, immunotherapy (e. g., monoclonal antibody).

9.9 Follow-up

Follow-up review provides reassurance for patients and allows a surgical audit of outcome. Occasionally, a structured and directed review protocol (CT scan, chest X-ray, CEA, liver function test) may detect minimal recurrent disease, which enables earlier treatment. This may improve survival and give better palliation. As there is an increased risk of metachronous colorectal neoplasm, routine colonoscopy surveillance every 3-5 years is recommended.

Part 31

Liver Diseases

Chapter 1

Anatomy and Functions

1.1 Historical Perspective

The surface anatomy of the liver was described as early as 2000 years BC by the ancient Babylonians. Even Hippocrates understood and described the seriousness of liver injury. In 1654, Francis Glisson was the first physician to describe the essential anatomy of the blood vessels of the liver accurately. The beginnings of liver surgery are described as rudimentary excisions of eviscerated liver from penetrating trauma. The first documented case of a partial hepatectomy is credited to Berta, who amputated a portion of protruding liver in a patient with a selfinflicted stab wound in 1716.

In the late 1800s, the first gastrectomies and cholecystectomies were being performed in Europe. At that time, surgery on the liver was regarded as dangerous, if not impossible. In 1897, Elliot, in his report on liver surgery for trauma, said that the liver was so "friable, so full of gaping vessels and so evidently incapable of being sutured that it had always seemed impossible to successfully manage large wounds of its substance". European surgeons began to experiment with techniques of elective liver surgery on animals in the late 1800s. The credit for the first elective liver resection is a matter of debate and many surgeons have been given credit, but it certainly occurred during this time period.

The early 1900s saw some small but significant advances in liver surgery. Techniques for suturing major hepatic vessels and the use of cautery for small vessels were applied and reported. The most significant advance of that time was probably that of J. Hogarth Pringle. In 1908, he described digital compression of the hilar vessels to control hepatic bleeding from traumatic injuries. The modern era of hepatic surgery was ushered in by the development of a better understanding of liver anatomy and formal anatomic liver resection. Credit for the first anatomic liver resection is usually given to Lortat-Jacob, who performed a right hepatectomy in 1952 in France. Pack from New York and Quattelbaum from Georgia performed similar operations within the next year and were unlikely to have had any knowledge of Lortat-Jacob's report. Descriptions of the segmental nature of liver anatomy by Couinaud, Woodsmith, and Goldburne in 1957 opened the door even wider and introduced the modern era of liver surgery.

Despite these improvements, hepatic surgery was plagued by tremendous operative morbidity and mortality from the 1950s into the 1980s. Operative mortality rates in excess of 20% were common and usually related to massive hemorrhage. Many surgeons were reluctant to perform hepatic surgery because of these results and, understandably, many physicians were reluctant to refer patients for hepatectomy. With the courage of patients and their families, as well as the persistence of surgeons, safe hepatic surgery has now been realized. A complete list is not possible here, but courageous hepatic surgeons such as Blumgart, Bismuth, Longmire, Fortner, Schwartz, Starzl, and Ton deserve mention.

Advances in anesthesia, intensive care, antibiotics, and interventional radiologic techniques have also contributed tremendously to the safety of major hepatic surgery. Total hepatectomy with liver transplantation and live donor partial hepatectomy for transplantation are now performed routinely in specialized transplantation centers. Partial hepatectomy for a large number of indications is now performed throughout the world in specialized centers, with mortality rates of 5% or less. Partial hepatectomy performed on normal livers is now consistently performed, with mortality rates of 1%–2%.

Safely performed open hepatic surgery and its liberal use in the management of a wide variety of diseases is now a reality. Moreover, minimally invasive approaches to liver surgery have been developed and are now being used in significant numbers. However, the learning curve remains steep and the indications for this technique are still being carefully defined. Thermal ablative techniques to treat hepatic tumors, including radiofrequency and microwave ablation, have exploded in popularity. Finally, techniques to improve the safety of liver resection further, such as portal vein embolization to induce preoperative hypertrophy of the future liver remnant(FLR), have been developed and are now being used.

1.2 Anatomy

The liver, an organ only found in vertebrates, detoxifies various metabolites, synthesizes proteins, and produces biochemicals necessary for digestion. In humans, it is located in the right upper quadrant of the abdomen, below the diaphragm. Its other roles in metabolism include the regulation of glycogen storage, decomposition of red blood cells and the production of hormones.

The liver is a solid gastrointestinal organ whose mass(1.2–1.6 kg) largely occupies the upper right quadrant of the abdomen, below the diaphragm. Major part of the liver hides below the right diaphragm and covered deeply in the right hypochondrial region, minor crosses over the Ventral midline andextends to the left side of the abdomen. The large majority of the right liver and most of the left liver is covered by the thoracic cage. It extends superiorly to the height of the fifth rib on the right and the sixth rib on the left. The lower right margin is on the right costal margin level, and the lower left margin can be felted below the Processus xiphoideus during inspiration(Figure 31-1-1).

The peritoneal duplications on the liver surface are referred to as ligaments. On the superior and anterior of the liver, left and right trigonum ligaments, coronary ligaments, falciform ligaments and ligamentum teres help to connect the liver surface to the diaphragm, abdominal wall, and umbilicus. On the inferior and posterior, run the hepatoduodenal ligament and the ligamentum hepatogastricum. The hepatoduodenal ligament contains portal vein, hepatic artery, lymph-vessel, lymph-nodes and nerves.

Hepatic arterial and portal venous blood enter the liver at the hilum (orhepatic portal) and branch throughout the liver as a single portal pedicle unit, which also includes a bile ducts. The vessels(arteries, veins and bile ducts) and nerves are held together by a fine dense irregular fibroelastic connective tissue layer which extends into the structure of the liver, as a fibrous capsule called Glisson's capsule. Majority of the blood runs away from liver through hepatic veins, left, right and middle hepatic vein come together at the

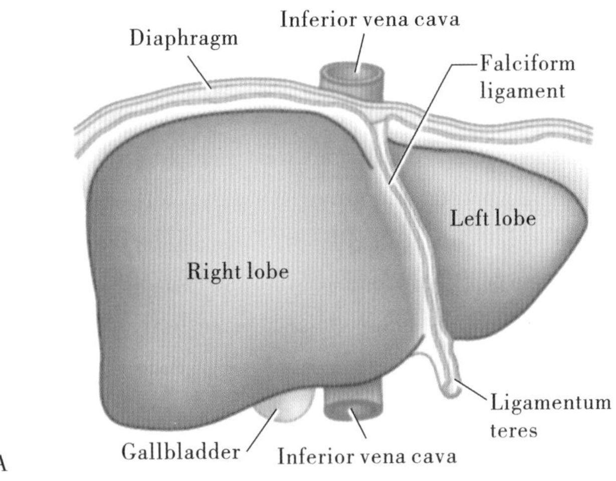

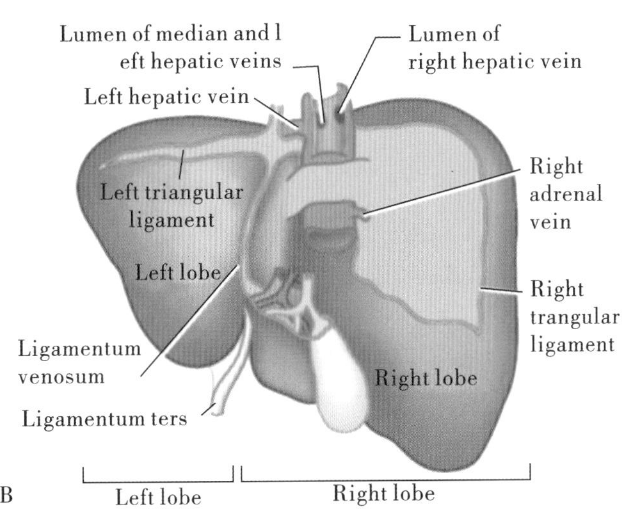

Figure 31-1-1 Anatomy of liver

A. Liver diaphragmatic view; B. View of liver viscera.

second hepatic portal. Other blood ties into the flow of the inferior vena cava through veins on the posterior of liver, called the third hepatic portal.

Historically, the liver was divided into two parts when viewed from above (a right and a left lobe) by the obvious external landmark of the falciform ligament, and four parts when viewed from below (left lobe, right lobe, caudate and quadrate lobes). Not only was this description oversimplified, but it was anatomically incorrect in relation to the blood supply to the liver. Later, a more accurate understanding of the lobar anatomy of the liver was developed. The liver now is divided into right and left lobes determined by portal and hepatic vein branches.

Our understanding of functional liver anatomy has become more sophisticated. Briefly, the liver is composed of eight segments, each supplied by a single portal triad (or pedicle) composed of a portal vein, hepatic artery, and bile duct. These segments are further organized into four sectors separated by scissurae containing the three main hepatic veins. The four sectors are even further organized into the right and left liver. The terms right liver and left liver are preferable to the terms right lobe and left lobe because there is no external mark that allows the identification of the right and left liver. This system was originally described in 1957 by Woodsmith and Goldburne, and by Couinaud. It defines hepatic anatomy because it is most relevant to surgery of the liver.

The organization of hepatic parenchyma into microscopic functional units has been described in a number of ways, referred to as an acinus or a lobule. A lobule is made up of a central terminal hepatic venule surrounded by four to six terminal portal triads that form a polygonal unit. This unit is lined on its periphery between each terminal portal triad by terminal portal triad branches. In between the terminal portal triads and the central hepatic venule, hepatocytes are arranged in one cell-thick plates, surrounded on each side by endothelial-lined and blood-filled sinusoids. Blood flows from the terminal portal triad through the sinusoids into the terminal hepatic venule. Bile is formed within the hepatocytes and empties into terminal canaliculi, which form on the lateral walls of the intercellular hepatocyte. These ultimately coalesce into bile ducts and flow toward the portal triads. This functional hepatic unit provides a structural basis for the many metabolic and secretory functions of the liver(Figure 31-1-2).

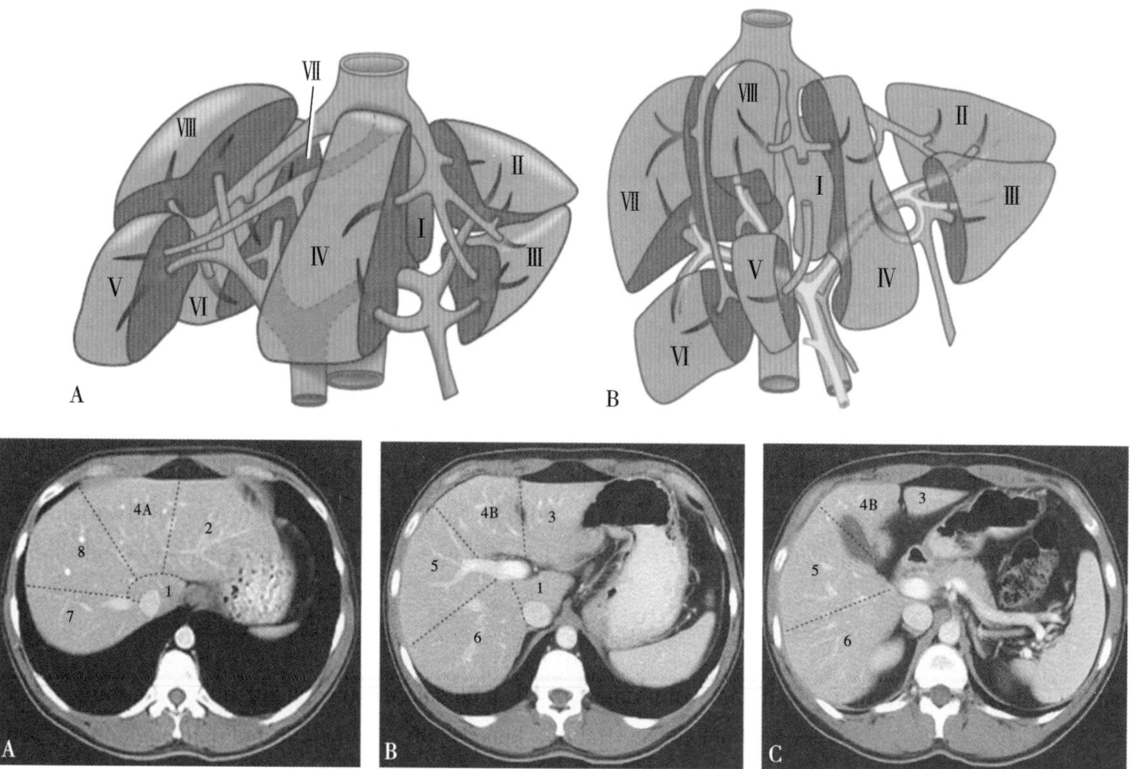

Figure 31-1-2 Couinaud segmental anatomy

A. Anatomy of the Couinaud segment of the diaphragmatic surface of the liver; B. Anatomy of the Couinaud segment of the visceral surface of the liver; C. Couinaud segments in different slice CT scanning.

The hepatic artery, representing high-volume oxygenated systemic arterial flow, provides 25%-30% of the hepatic blood flow and 40%-60% of its oxygenation. The portal vein provides 70%-75% of the hepatic blood inflow. Despite being postcapillary and largely deoxygenated, its high flow rate provides other 40% to 60% of the liver's oxygen. Moreover, it gathers the nutrition from intestine and supplies to liver. The blood flow of liver can reach 1500 mL/min normally, occupies 1/4 of cardiac output.

1.3 Functions

The unique anatomic arrangement of the liver described provides a remarkable landscape on which the multiple central and critical functions of this organ can be carried out. The following sections will summarize this broad range of functions.

1.3.1 Bile Formation

Bile production and secretion is one of the major functions of the liver, 600–1000 mL of bile are secreted daily. The physiologic role of bile is twofold. The first is to dispose of substances secreted into bile and the second is to provide enteric bile salts to aid in the digestion of fats as well as helping absorb lipid-soluble vitamin.

1.3.2 Metabolism

(1) Carbohydrate metabolism. The liver is the center of carbohydrate metabolism because it is the major regulator of storage and distribution of glucose to the peripheral tissues and, in particular, to glucose-dependent tissues such as the brain and erythrocytes.

(2) Lipid metabolism. Fatty acids are synthesized in the liver during states of glucose excess, when the liver's ability to store glycogen has been exceeded. Adipocytes have a limited ability to synthesize fatty acids. Therefore, the liver is the predominant source of synthesized fatty acids, although they are largely stored in adipose tissue.

(3) Protein metabolism. The liver is also a central site for the metabolism of proteins and is involved in protein synthesis, catabolism of proteins into energy or storage forms, and managing excess amino acids and nitrogen waste.

(4) Vitamin metabolism. Along with the intestine, the liver is responsible for the metabolism of the fat-soluble vitamins A, D, E, and K.

(5) Hormonc mctabolism. Estrogen and antidiuretic hormone are deactivated in liver; adrenal cortex hormone and aldosterone intermediary metabolisms occur in liver.

1.3.3 Coagulation

The liver is responsible for synthesizing almost all the identified coagulation factors, as well as many of the fibrinolytic system components and several plasma regulatory proteins of coagulation and fibrinolysis. As noted, the liver is critical for the absorption of vitamin K, synthesizes the vitamin K-dependent coagulation factors, and contains the enzyme that activates these factors. Also, the reticuloendothelial system of the liver clears activated clotting factors, activated complexes of the coagulation and fibrinolytic systems, and the end products of fibrin degradation.

1.3.4 Metabolism of drugs and toxins (xenobiotics)

The liver plays a central role in handling drugs and toxins through an enormously complex and numerous set of enzymes and reaction pathways, which are increasingly recognized as new chemicals are discovered.

1.3.5 Phagocytose and immune

Through Kupffer cells from the mononuclear phagocyte system, bacterial, immune complex and other chemical components can be cleared out from blood.

1.3.6 Regeneration

The liver possesses the unique quality of adjusting its volume to the needs of the body. This is observed clinically in its regeneration after partial hepatectomy or after toxic liver injury. It is also seen in liver transplantation, in that donor liver size mismatches adjust to the new host. Animal experiments confirmed that after 70% –80% volume lose, liver can maintain basic functions. Moreover, it can grow to normal volume in 6 weeks. However, this process can cost 1 year in human bodies. This quality is highly conserved evolutionarily because of the critical functions of the liver and the fact that the liver is the first line of exposure to ingested toxic agents.

1.3.7 Energy

The liver is the critical intermediary between dietary sources of energy and the extrahepatic tissues that require this energy. The critical and central nature of the liver in regulating the body's energy metabolism is evidenced by the fact that despite accounting for only 4% of the total body weight, the liver consumes about 28% of the total body blood flow and 20% of the total oxygen consumed. The liver also uses about 20% of the total body caloric intake.

Chapter 2

Hepatic Abscess

The liver abscess is a space-occupying suppurative cavity in the liver resulting from the invasion and multiplication of microorganisms, and infectious way included entering directly from an injury, through the blood vessels or by the way of the bile ducts. The most common forms of liver abscesses are amebic, or pyogenic, also there are some other pathogenesis special like tuberculous liver abscess, fungal liver abscess and parasitic liver abscess. Approximately 60% are solitary and mainly located in the right lobe of liver, as a result of the streaming pattern of portal blood flow, and because most of the hepatic volume is in the right lobe. When multiple abscesses are present, pyogenic or mixed abscesses are the most probable types. Clinically, because of low immunity of diabetic patients, it can lead to systemic suppurative disease. Including complications of the primary disease, the patient may have endophthalmitis or uveitis, pulmonary abscess, brain abscess or purulent meningitis. A detailed clinical history is useful in identifying the risk factors that suggest a possible etiology. Emerging new risk factors include the use of immunosuppressive drugs for neoplastic disease or for organ transplantation, sexual lifestyles, human immunodeficiency virus (HIV) infection, history of traveling to endemic areas, and the population migration phenomena. Here we mainly discuss pyogenic liver abscess, which is equivalent to the term called bacterial liver abscess.

2.1 Pyogenic Liver Abscess

2.1.1 Epidemiology

In America, there are 27-41 patients per 1 million in general population. And in China, the morbidity is about 5.7/100 thousands. PLA varies among different geographic regions influenced by the local prevalence of bacterial, parasitic, and helminthic infections, age of the population, and the presence of chronic debilitating diseases. Benign or malignant biliary tract disease, diverticulitis, and Crohn's disease are the most common predisposing factors. The frequency of PLA has increased as a complication of more aggressive treatment of liver or pancreatic malignancies—stent placement, sphincterotomy, embolization, ethanol injection, or radiofrequency ablation. In the past, PLA was primarily a complication of ruptured appendix. Accordingly, the age of presentation has moved forward from the second and third decades of life to the sixth and seventh. Advances in imaging techniques and new antibiotics, have decreased the morbidity and mortality of PLA.

2.1.2 Pathogenesis

Systemic bacterial infection, especially in the abdominal cavity infection, bacterial invasion of the liver, such as patient resistance, can develop bacterial liver abscess. Bile duct: when biliary ascariasis, bile duct stone and other concurrent suppurative cholangitis, bacteria along the bile duct up, which will becomes the most common pathogenesis. Hepatic artery: A suppurative lesion in any part of the body, such as pyogenic osteomyelitis, otitis media, carbuncle, while give a chance to bacteria to reach the liver along with hepatic artery. Portal vein: In the sanitation of gangrenous appendicitis, hemorrhoid infection, bacillary dysentery, bacteria can infect liver along the portal vein. In addition, lymphatic systems and surgical wounds are also the way bacteria invade the liver.

2.1.3 Clinical manifestations

An early clinical diagnosis relies on a high index of suspicion: Fever company with shiver, right upper quadrant abdominal pain and hepatomegaly, sometimes company with malaise, nausea anorexia and vomit, are the most common presentations. Sometimes we could differamebic liver abscess(ALA) with PLA by the clinical manifestations preliminarily. Abdominal pain in patients with PLA is similar to that found in patients with ALA. Other symptoms, anorexia, jaundice, and painful hepatomegaly are less prevalent in PLA as compared to ALA. Jaundice predicts a complicated clinical course but has no impact on mortality. Approximately 60% have an underlying debilitating condition or have had a recent interventional procedure(e. g. , biliary stent placement, ethanol injection). PLA should be suspected in elderly patients, in those taking steroids, or in patients with right-sided pulmonary abnormalities of unknown origin.

2.1.4 Diagnosis

For diagnosis of PLA, according to the medical history, clinical manifestations, and the reporters of x-ray examination and abdominal ultrasound, the doctor can diagnose the PLA easily. If necessary, ultrasound-guided diagnostic puncture is another choice to confirm the diagnosis.

When PLA is diagnosed, prognostic factors associated with increased mortality include low albumin, anemia, high blood urea nitrogen (BUN) and creatinine, prolonged prothrombin time, polymicrobial infection, pleural effusion, high acute physiological assessment and chronic health evaluation (APACHE) II score, disseminated intravascular coagulation, and septic shock. Multiple abscesses carry a high mortality risk independent of other risk factors. Regarding PLA in patients with cancer, morphology and topography are not different from noncancer patients.

2.1.5 Therapy

Antibiotic therapy choices involve combining broad-spectrum antibiotics: Third-generation cephalosporin plus clindamycin or metronidazole; broad-spectrum penicillin plus aminoglycosides; and second-generation cephalosporin plus aminoglycosides. Treatment should be started immediately after specimens have been obtained for culture without waiting for definitive results. Imipenem, aztreonam, piperacillin, tazobactam, ticarcillin, clavulanate, and quinolones are active against almost all aerobic gram-negative bacilli. Antibiotics should be given before, during, and after drainage and surgical procedures. Parenteral therapy for 2-3 weeks followed by oral antibiotics for 4-6 weeks is recommended. For a solitary abscess less than 5 cm in diameter, confirmed by aspirate and with available antimicrobial sensitivity, resolution can be achieved with antibiotics alone. For PLA greater than 5 cm with thick and viscous pus, or for those large multiloculate abscesses, surgical drainage may be necessary. Under imaging guidance, PLA can be aspirated and drained. Drainage is most effective when well-liguefied pus is completely evacuated. If the abscess is not well liquefied or has a thick wall, it is impossible to remove the pus completely. In such cases, most of the drainable pus is removed by needle aspiration, after which, antibiotic therapy is necessary to treat the residual abscess. Needle aspiration should be performed with an 18-gauge fine-walled needle. In multiloculate abscess, the needle tip should be inserted into the various loculi to evacuate pus as completely as possible. Percutaneous needle aspiration is considered unsuccessful when patients fail to improve clinically or radiologically after the second aspiration. Factors affecting drainage include accessibility, number, and size of the abscesses as well as the patient's general condition. Abscesses most accessible to percutaneous drainage are the posterior right lobe deep-seated lesions, those that adhere to the abdominal wall, and peripheral abscesses of the right lobe.

Surgical therapy is necessary for multiple macroscopic or multiloculate abscesses, or for those in the left lobe, after percutaneous drainage failure. Surgical drainage may be required in the presence of ascites or renal failure, evidence of clinical deterioration, persistent jaundice, or concomitant steroid therapy; or when abscesses are not accessible to radiologic manipulation; and in the case of a ruptured abscess.

In patients with stones or strictures of the bile duct and abscess formation in continuity with the biliary system, endoscopic therapy provides biliary drainage, promoting abscess drainage.

2.2 Amebic Liver Abscess

2.2.1 Epidemiology

Entamoeba histolytica infection is the common cause of liver abscess in the world, especially in tropical and subtropical regions. It is more prevalent in developing countries; it can be spread from person to person via food and water with Entamoeba histolytica in them. Landmark advances in epidemiology of amebiasis include the recognition that there are two distinct species, E. histolytica which is the cause of different kinds of diseases like dysentery, colitis, and liver abscess, unlike Entamoeba dispar which is a nonpathogenic form of ameba and recent technologic advances exploring the genome of the different strains of E. histolytica that ultimately may lead to the development of vaccines.

Specific probes derived from the analysis of repetitive deoxyribonucleic acid (DNA) sequence in the Entamoeba genome analysis have demonstrated possible candidates to distinguish between E. histolytica and E. dispar, such as transposable elements common in primitive eukaryotes that harbor non-long terminal-repeat (non-LTR) retrotransposons [also called long interspersed repetitive elements (LINEs)] or short interspersed repetitive elements known as EhSINE1.

Genotyping of E. histolytica has revealed an extensive genetic diversity among E. histolytica isolates preventing at present an association of a single genotype with hepatic disease. The HM-1 strain of E. histolytica, which was isolated from a dysenteric patient in Mexico more than 30 years ago, and those isolated in India and Bangladesh still cause disease in experimental animals and have been used for nearly all immunologic, biochemical, and molecular biologic studies of amebae.

2.2.2 Pathogenesis

Occurrence of an amebic liver abscess can be several months or years after the infection of pathogens.

The amoeba can penetrate intestinal wall and reach the liver via portal, lymph vessel or indirect. The immune system can remove the pathogens if the human is healthy, or else a few surviving protozoa continue to breed, which may cause trichodophlebitis and periphlebitis. In the branches of the portal vein, embolism caused by protozoa leads to the ischemia and hypoxia of the liver tissue. And large trophozoite release out form the blood vessels, which cause the focal necrosis of liver tissue which fuse and form the liver abscess finally. The center of the abscess is a large number of chocolate-like necrotic substances. It typically takes about 1 month from the invasion of the amebic to the formation of the abscess. Chronic abscess can be secondary to bacterial infection, in which situation the pus is yellow or yellowish green and loss the typical characteristic.

The invasive process is driven importantly by the parasite's motility. The parasite relies on a dynamic actomyosin cytoskeleton and on surface adhesion molecules for dissemination in the tissues. Myosin II is essential for E. histolytica intercellular motility through intestinal cell monolayers and for its motility in the liver, while galactose-binding lectins, mainly galactose/N-acetylglucosamine (Gal/GalNAc), modulate the distribution of trophozoites in the liver and their capacity to migrate in the hepatic tissue. Gal/GalNAc acts as a major cell surface antigen that activates target epithelial cells and triggers subsequent disease pathology and parasite survival. Lectin-stimulated cells show an immediate rise in Ca^{+}, which in turn activates cyclic nucleotides and other protein kinases, leading to activation of mitogen activated protein kinase (MAPK) cascade. Activation of MAPK pathway is implicated in events such as apoptosis, proliferation, cytoskeleton rearrangements, and permeability changes.

Initial steps in tissue invasion include the release of proteases by trophozoites, which are capable of degrading extracellular matrix components. E. histolytica is a cytotoxic effector cell with an extraordinary capacity to lyse the surrounding cells. The inflammatory response (mainly neutrophils and macrophages) initiated by amebic invasion may further contribute to tissue damage by added lysis of parenchymatous cells. When ameba is inoculated in the liver significant areas of apoptosis develop within the amebic liver abscess (ALA). The sequencing of the genome of E. histolytica has allowed a reconstruction of its metabolic pathways, many of which are unusual for a eukaryote. On the basis of the genome sequence, it appears that amino acids may play a larger role than previously thought in energy metabolism, with roles in both adenosine triphosphate (ATP) synthesis and nicotinamide adenine dinucleotide (NAD) regeneration. E. histolytica uses a complex mix of signal transduction systems to sense and interact with the different environments and encounters. The analysis of its genome has revealed almost 270 putative E. histolytica protein kinases.

2.2.3 Clinical manifestations

The severity of the clinical manifestation is mainly related to the location and size of the abscess and whether company with a secondary bacterial infection. ALA is found more frequently in men at age around 20-40 but can occur at any age. Gender differences in abscess formation in adults have been related to alcohol intake. Identification of risk factors including a history of travel to or residency in endemic areas several weeks or even months before, which is important to diagnosis and must be identified. The constant, dull, and intense right upper quadrant abdominal pain that exacerbates with movement and frequently radiates to the scapular region and right shoulder is the most common symptom. Patients have fever between 38 ℃ and 40 ℃, chills, and sweating, and the fever type remittene fever in majority. Very frequently they give a history of malaise and nausea in the previous 2 weeks and moderate weight loss. Some patients have cough and chest pain. Most of them do not have coexistent dysentery, although a past history of diarrhea or dysentery is present in approximately 50% of cases. At physical examination, the patient appears pale and wasted, with painful hepatomegaly, point tenderness over the liver, below the ribs, or in the intercostal spaces. When the abscess is located in the left lobe, the patient may have epigastric tenderness. Ventilation in the right lung is frequently restricted, respiratory sounds are reduced, but jaundice is infrequent. Alarm signs include abdominal rebound tenderness, guarding, absence of bowel sounds, and pleural or pericardial rub. The abscess may extend to the peritoneum, abdominal organs, great vessels, pericardium, pleura, bronchial tree, and lungs.

2.2.4 Diagnosis

Leukocytosis($>15\times10^9$ cells/L), with neutrophilia, increased erythrocyte sedimentation rate, slight anemia, and elevated alkaline phosphatase levels are common. But if there happened a secondary bacterial infection, the leukocytosis can be high to the level of 80×10^9 cells/L. Also, the trophozoite and cyst can be examined in the stool of patients. And the trophozoite is commonly found in liquid or semi-liquid stool and bloody purulent stool. An indirect hemagglutination(IHA) with a cutoff value of 1 : 512 is considered diagnostic. The enzyme immunoassay(EIA) with a sensitivity of 99% and specificity greater than 90% is also commonly used. In those patients in whom an aspirate is obtained, either for diagnostic or therapeutic purposes, the material should also be sent for Gram's staining and culture. Imaging studies are very important in the workup of patients with suspected ALA and have reduced the delay in diagnosis. Ultrasonography is the initial screening choice. The abscess appears as a hypoechoic round or oval lesion with well-defined margins. More advanced imaging techniques such as tomography or magnetic resonance are indicated for differential diagnosis. Chest X-ray may reveal elevation of the right diaphragm, atelectasis, and pleural effusion.

2.2.5 Therapy

The drug of choice is metronidazole at an oral dose of 1g twice daily for 10-15 days in adults and 30-50 mg/kg daily for 10 days divided in three doses in children; when given intravenously the dosage is 500 mg every 6 hours for adults and 7.5 mg/kg every 6 hours for children for 10 days. Other nitroimidazoles include tinidazole or ornidazole at a dose of 2 g orally daily for 10 days. Secondary drugs include chloroquine 1 g/day for 2 days orally followed by 500 mg/day for 2-3 weeks. In children the dose is 15 mg/kg Porally daily for 2-5 days followed by 5 mg/kg daily for 2 weeks. Percutaneous drainage may be necessary in non-responses to ant ameba therapy to rule out a pyogenic abscess or when less than 1 cm of rim liver tissue remains around a liquefied abscess.

Chapter 3

Echinococcosis of the Liver

Echinococcosis of the liver, which is also called hydatid disease of the liver or hepatic hydatid disease, is a kind of zoonosis caused by the infection of echinococcosis.

3.1 Epidemiology

Echinococcosis of the liver is mainly prevalent in animal husbandry area. There are four species that cause hydatid disease including Echinococcus granulosus, Echinococus multilocularis, Echinococcus vogeli and Echinococcus oligarthrus. The liver disease caused by the infection of Echinococcus granulosus is cystic echinococcosis(CE). The liver disease caused by the infection of Echinococus multilocularis is alveolar echinococcosis(AE). Their form, host and distribution area are slightly different.

In the world, the incidence and prevalence of echinococcosis of the liver have fallen dramatically over the past several decades. Nonetheless, echinococcosis of the liver remains a major public health issue in several countries and regions as a result of a reduction of control programmes due to economic problems. The annual incidence ranges from less than 1 case to as many as 42 cases/100 000 persons in some regions. Geographic distribution differs by country and region depending on the presence of large numbers of nomadic or semi-nomadic sheep and goat flocks that represent the intermediate host of the parasite, and their close contact with the final host, the dog, which mostly provides the transmission of infection to humans. The incidence rate of hepatic hydatid disease increases with the increase of regional population mobility.

Alveolar echinococcosis is high in local area. Rarely, alveolar echinococcosis can occur due to Echinococcus multilocularis. Cystic echinococcosis is the most common forms. It is endemic in parts of North America, central Europe, and northern and central Eurasia. Incidence is generally less than 1/100 000. The greatest prevalence of echinococcosis in human and animal hosts is found in countries of the temperate zone, including Mediterranean regions, southern and central parts of Russia, central Asia, China, Australia, South America and north and east Africa. At least 270 million people(58% of the total population) are at risk of cystic echinococcosis in Central Asia including areas of Mongolia, Kazakhstan, Kyrgyzstan, Tajikistan, Turkmenistan, Uzbekistan, Afghanistan, Iran, Pakistan and western China. The annual morbidity in some Tibetan communities in western China has been estimated to reaching 10% (range from 0.8% to 11.9%). Echinococcus transmission in the region is largely associated with social factors including limited community knowledge of echinococcosis, small-scale household animal production, home killing of livestock, and the feeding of dogs with uncooked offal. Alveolar echinococcosis is also endemic in Central Asia and is recognized as a major problem in some Tibetan communities with up to 6% of villagers infected in some villages. In western China, 5% - 30% of the population are seropositive against E. granulosus antigens, indicating that a large number of individuals have been exposed to the parasite.

3.2 Etiology and Pathology

Dogs are the common definitive host of E. granulosus. Foxes and wolves are also regarded as host definitive host of E. granulosus. The intermediate host of E. granulosus include sheep which is the most common, pig, horse, cow and human. Sheep are the usual intermediate host, but humans are the accidental intermediate host. Normally, it will not transmit in the people group. Up to thousands of ova are passed daily and deposited in the dog's feces. Humans are an end stage to the parasite. The parasitic embryo releases an oncosphere containing hooklets that penetrate the mucosa in the human duodenum. Oncosphere allowing access to the bloodstream. In the blood, the oncosphere reaches the liver (most commonly) or lungs, where the parasite develops its larval stage—the hydatid cyst. Hepatic hydatid disease is the most common type of echinococcosis in clinic, accounting for about 75%, followed by pulmonary echinococcosis, which accounts for about15%.

Three weeks after infection, echinococcus of the liver first developed into small capsules in human liver. Capsules grow and squeeze the parenchyma in the liver to form a multi-wall structure and a variety of contents of the cystic mass (hepatic hydatid cyst). Hepatic hydatid cyst wall is divided into two layers of the inner capsule and the outer capsule. The inner capsule is the structure of parasites which like the white powdery. The wall of the inner capsule is divided into the stratum corneum and germinal layer. The stratum corneum is located outside the germinal layer and is a translucent membrane of white powdery skin-like elastic formed by the secretions of the germinal layer. It can protect the germinal layer cells and provide nutrients to the germinal layer cells. The germinal layer is the true echinococcus granulosus, which consists of a row of reproductive cells that produce the fertility sacs (hair follicles), the head nodes, and the ascus. The outer capsule is a dense fibrous layer structure characterized by macrophage granulomatous lesions and fibrosis as a result of host immune rejection responses to parasites. With the expansion of cyst growth, the surrounding liver parenchymal pressure, hepatocellular degeneration, atrophy, disappearance of cystic fibrosis surrounding the system, a fibrous membrane structure is formed between the outer capsule and liver parenchyma. There is a potential separable gap between the fibrous membrane and the outer capsule along which the outer capsule can be substantially separated from the liver.

Hydatid cyst growth is the result of the interaction between the body and the parasite. Most hydatid cysts grow slowly, the pathological changes showed diversity. The size of hydatid cysts are different. The inner capsule can be single capsule, multiple ascicles, the collapse of the inner capsule or even necrosis. Cyst fluid can become cool and turbid. Cyst contents can become solid caused by moisture absorption and dry. The outer wall thickening, calcification; part of the rupture of the abdominal cavity or chest and bile duct, the formation of fistula. Hydatid cysts can die with degeneration of the membranes, development of cystic vacuoles, and calcification of the wall. Calcification of a hydatid cyst, however, does not always imply that the cyst is dead.

3.3 Clinical Manifestations

Due to the slow growth of cysts, there are no obvious symptoms in the early stage of infection of echinococcosis. The disease can be accidentally found because of physical examination after several years. The clinical presentation of a hydatid cyst is largely asymptomatic until excessive abdominal mass or oppression symptoms or complications occur. The most common presenting symptoms are abdominal pain, dyspepsia and vomiting. The most frequent sign is hepatomegaly. In consideration of the parasitic sites, the volume and number of cysts, the body's reactivity and complications, the symptoms of hepatic hydatid cyst are different.

(1) Bacterial superinfection of a hydatid cyst can occur in approximately 8% of patients. It present like a pyogenic abscess which clinical manifestations include jaundice and fever.

(2) Hydatid cyst rupture can cause a variety of diseases. Hydatid cyst contents can overflow into the abdominal cavity. It leads to multiple cysts, bloating or intestinal obstruction. Hydatid cyst rupturing into the biliary tract can cause obstructive jaundice or recurrent cholangitis. Hydatid cyst rupturing into the colon can be rectal discharge. Hydatid cyst rupturing into the lung through the transverse septum can result in recurrent lung infections and may cough up ascus. Hydatid cyst compression or rupture into the human hepatic vein, can cause Bad-Kyary Syndrome.

(3) Because the cystic fluid contains heterogeneous proteins and antigens. When hepatic hydatid cyst rupture, the cystic fluid goes into the biliary tree, bronchial tree, or free rupture into the peritoneal, pleural, pericardial cavities or out into the bloodstream. It can result in disseminated echinococcosis and/or occur repeated hives even cause the potentially fatal anaphylactic reaction. Membranous glomerulonephritis occurs when cyst fluid antigen is deposited in the glomerulus.

3.4 Diagnosis

The diagnosis of hepatic hydatid cyst is based on a high index of clinical suspicion and findings on imaging with ultrasonography, CT or MRI. The initial symptoms are usually caused by complications of the cysts or physical compression of adjacent organs by the cysts. The common clinical symptoms epigastric or right upper quadrant pain, fatigue, fever, nausea, and dyspepsia.

Ultrasound is most commonly used worldwide for the diagnosis of echinococcosis because of its availability, affordability, and accuracy. Calcifications in the wall of the cyst are highly suggestive of hydatid disease and can be helpful to the diagnosis. Ultrasound can help determine the stages of the cyst. A simple hydatid cyst is well circumscribed with budding signs on the cyst membrane and may contain free-floating hyperechogenic hydatid sand. A rosette appearance is seen when daughter cysts are present. The cyst can be filled with an amorphous mass, which can be diagnostically misleading.

CT or MRI are also used to diagnose echinococcosis. These cross-sectional imaging of CT or MRI is superior in identifying the location of the cysts and type of cyst. Besides, it can render detailed hepatic anatomic relationships to the cyst. Approximately 75% of hydatid cysts are located in the right liver and are solitary. If the cyst ruptures into the biliary tract, the endoscopic retrograde cholangiopancreatography (ERCP) or percutaneous transhepatic cholangiography (PTC) is needed for diagnosis.

In cases of diagnostic uncertainty, Serologic tests, including an indirect hemagglutination test and enzyme-linked immunosorbent assay for antibodies to Echinococcus antigens are available. The sensitivity of the test is approximately 90%. However, because of cross-reaction with other parasites, the teats may not distinguish cystic from alveolar disease.

3.5 Treatment

3.5.1 Surgical intervention

The treatment of hepatic hydatid cysts is optimally and primarily surgical. There is controversy about the surgical indication for cystic echinococcosis. In general, most cysts should be treated, but in elder patients with small, asymptomatic, densely calcified cysts, conservative management is appropriate. However, some advocate treatment even in asymptomatic patients to prevent complications such as rupture, infection, or anaphylaxis. The contraindications to surgery include complex or widespread injury, advanced patient age, pregnancy, comorbidities, multiple cysts that are difficult to access, partially inactive or calcified liver cysts, or patient refusal of surgery.

Radical surgery for hepatic hydatid cysts refers to pericystectomy and liver resection, whereas conservative surgery involves the removal of the cyst content and sterilization of the residual cavity, together with partial cyst resection which also called endocystectomy. Surgery can be curative if the parasites are removed completely. Frequently, surgical procedures are inconsistent and comprise liver resection or the opening of the parasitic cysts and subsequent removal of the parasite. Conservative procedures are safe and less complex than radical surgery, even though the risk of associated morbidity may be higher due to the presence of the residual cavity.

Endocystectomy is classic surgery for hepatic hydatid cysts. The core of endocystectomy is avoiding the overflow of cystic fluid and inactivation of the first head. A number of operations have been used but, in general, the abdomen is completely explored, the liver mobilized, and the cyst exposed. Packing off the abdomen is important because rupture can result in anaphylaxis and diffuse seeding. Usually, the cyst is then aspirated through a closed suction system and flushed with a scolicidal agent such as hypertonic saline. Then open the top of the cyst, which can be followed by a number of possibilities. including excision (or pericystectomy), marsupialization procedures, leaving the cyst open, drainage of the cyst, omentoplasty, or partial hepatectomy to encompass the cyst. Total pericystectomy or formal partial hepatectomy can also be performed without entering the cyst.

When bile duct communication is diagnosed preoperatively or at operation, biliary ducts leading to the lumen should be ligatured. Simple suture repair is often sufficient, but major biliary repairs, approaches through the common bile duct, or postoperative ERCP may be necessary. When the contents of the capsule rupture into the biliary tract, the choledochotomy is required. ERCP defines the cystobiliary relationship to guide management decisions during the pre-and postoperative periods. Pre-operative endoscopic sphincterotomy may decrease the incidence of postoperative external fistula from 11.1% to 7.6%. During the postoperative period, ERCP may provide an opportunity to manage postoperative external biliary fistulae.

3.5.2 Medical therapy

Medical therapy for early cysts small, thin outer wall, a wide spread and the risk of surgery patients. Recent 7 RCTs suggests that benzimidazole compound derivatives, albendazole (ALB) and mebendazole

(MBZ) may have a therapeutic effect on hepatic hydatid disease. From 1984 to 1986, the World Health Organization (WHO) carried out two multicenter trials in Europe to compare ALB and MBZ. Both drugs had similar efficacy, but MBZ required higher doses and a different treatment duration. The treatment duration of ALB course is more than half a year. Compared with a shorter treatment course, 3 months of oral ALB treatment appears to have better outcomes in terms of cyst degeneration (based on imaging) and cure rates. However, the cure rate for HC treated with ALB alone was below 60%. Only trials that included 3 months of ALB treatment and surgery had cure rates > 90%.

3.5.3 Puncture, aspiration, injection and re-aspiration (PAIR)

PAIR is a percutaneous treatment which present high success cure rates for hepatic hydatid cysts. It performs percutaneous aspiration and injection of scolicidal agents. PAIR may be a promising treatment for liver HC, but there is not sufficient evidence to support its use as a standard procedure for patients with uncomplicated cysts. The connection of the cyst to the biliary tree is an absolute contraindication for this procedure. Because the intracapsular pressure will affect the closure of bile duct fistula closure.

3.5.4 Liver transplantation

Due to the biological behavior of alveolar echinococcosis resembles cancer. It often involves the bile duct, hepatic vein, inferior vena cava and diaphragm, and lymphoid or hematogenous dissemination can occur. Liver transplantation can achieve better therapeutic effect.

3.6 Outcomes

The morbidity rate after surgery for hepatic hydatidosis has been reported to range from 6% to 47%. The main complications are wound infection and respiratory tract infection. Recurrence of hydatid disease in the liver constitutes a main concern in patients. It usually results from spillage of hydatid fluid containing daughter cysts during the operation or incomplete evacuation of the cyst following conservative procedures, leaving residual vesicles in place. Reported recurrence rates range from 6% to 25% when omentoplasty is used. Recommended practice is to follow up patients with ultrasonography every 6 months or an annual CT scan for at least 3 years, as most recurrences of hydatid disease are observed in this time period. Recurrent cysts should be managed by percutaneous drainage or radical surgery combined with albendazole therapy.

3.7 Prevention

Although echinococcosis control programs have been initiated in some countries in Central Asia, control efforts are generally fragmented and uncoordinated. Monthly deworming of dogs with praziquantel (PZQ), as a key measure to control the Echinococcus parasites, has been used in western China. However, the approach has proven difficult in local semi-nomadic communities. Additional control measures including health education, domestic livestock animal treatment/vaccination and dog vaccination are needed in CE-endemic areas to accelerate progress.

Chapter 4

Primary Liver Cancer

Hepatocellular carcinoma(HCC) is a neoplasm that mainly caused by chronic viral infection, alcohol excessive consumption and non-alcoholic fatty liver disease. These risks induce chronic liver disease, that is, cirrhosis, and induce genetic damage, leading to cancer occurrence and development.

HCC is the first cause of death in patients with cirrhosis. The sole approach to reduce cancer-related mortality is to detect cancer at an early stage and apply effective therapy. Patients with cirrhosis who would be treated if diagnosed with liver cancer should enter screening protocols. In cirrhotic patients, the annual incidence of HCC justifies periodic 6-monthly hepatic ultrasound screening. The aim of screening program is to diagnose the tumor as early as possible, so it can be treated with a curative intent.

Also, the early detection of HCC should be dependent on hepatic ultrasonography. Delete this sentence. So far, for patients diagnosed at early stages, curative treatments includes surgical resection, percutaneous ablation and transplantation provide the chance of long-term remission with 5-year survival rate of up to 75%. Among palliative approaches, transarterial chemoembolization is the sole approach with positive impact on survival of HCC.

Prevention of HCC should mainly derive from vaccination for the prevention of hepatitis B and maintenance of health and adequate lifestyle, meaning avoidance of risk factors. Antiviral therapy may cure viral infection and hence prevent progression to cirrhosis and cancer.

4.1 Epidemiology

Primary liver cancer is now is the second most lethal cancer worldwide and the third cause of cancer-related mortality. The number of new cases is estimated to be 564,000 per year, including 398,000 in men and 166,000 in women. In high-risk countries, liver cancer can arise before the age of 20 years, whereas, in countries at low risk, liver cancer is rare before the age of 50 years. Morbidity of liver cancer in men are typically 2-4 times higher than in women. Morbidity of primary liver cancer is increasing in several developed countries, including the United States, and the increase will likely continue to some decades. The trend is a result of a cohort effect related to infection with hepatitis B and C viruses, the incidence of which peaked in the 1950s to 1980s. In selected areas of some developing countries, the incidence of primary liver cancer has decreased, possibly as a result of the introduction of hepatitis B virus(HBV) vaccine. The geographic variability in incidence of primary liver cancer is largely explained by the distribution and the natural history of the hepatitis B and C viruses(HCV). The attributable risk estimates for the combined effects of these infections account for well over 80% of liver cancer cases worldwide. Studies suggest that the geographic heterogeneity is related to differences in the exposure rate to risk factors and time of acquisition rather than to genetic predisposition. In this regard, studies in migrant populations have demonstrated that first-generation immigrants carry with them the high incidence of HCC that is present in their native countries, but in the subsequent generations the incidence decreases. The age at which HCC appears varies according to gender, geographic area, and risk factors associated with cancer development.

4.2 Risk Factors for Hepatocellular Carcinoma

HCC affected by cirrhosis accounts for more than 80% individuals. Therefore, any drugs that cause chronic liver damage and ultimately cirrhosis should be considered as a risk factor for HCC. Obviously, the main cause of cirrhosis and HCC is HBV, HCV and alcohol, while less common diseases such as primary biliary cirrhosis, hemochromatosis, non-alcoholic steatohepatitis and Wilson's disease are also associated with the development of HCC. Patients with cirrhosis have an increased risk of developing liver dysfunction, and are at greater risk for males, patients older than 50 years, and those with elevated levels of alpha-fetoprotein(AFP). Pathological features such as increased cellular proliferation, the presence of atypical proliferative cells or irregular regeneration have also been suggested as useful risk markers but have not been fully validated.

4.2.1 Hepatitis B Virus

HBV is still a major health problem worldwide, unquestionable linking with HCC. An estimated 257 million people are currently chronically infected with HBV. About 887,000 die every year due to HBV complications. Active viral replication implies a higher risk and sustained reduction of HBV replication lowers the risk of HCC in HBV-related cirrhosis. The incidence of HCC in inactive HBV carriers without liver cirrhosis is less than 0.3%. The role of specific genotypes or mutations is not well established. HBV DNA can be incorporated into the genome of host cells during DNA recombination by means of host cell-associated enzymes, and can even occur early in HBV infection, resulting in antiviral treatment that is unlikely to completely eliminate the risk of HCC in patients after HBV infection. In 70%-90% of cases, HBV-associated cirrhosis leads to HCC. However, in the absence of cirrhosis, HBV is still a substantial risk factor. In addition, some of the HBV proteins, HBx, is often expressed at high levels in HBV-associated HCC and is modulated by the trans-action cell survival and proliferation related genes interact with intracellular proteins and tune a variety of signaling pathways, epigenetic changes induced by abnormal mechanisms such as promoting HCC happened. Interestingly, occult HBV infection may become apparent if properly investigated by molecular techniques even in the absence of serologic markers of HBV. Identification of the HBV genome has been reported in liver tumors of patients who are HCV positive and HBsAg negative in the serum. The rate of occult infection in these patients can be as high as 63%. Finally, the implementation of vaccination and drugs against HBV has resulted in a significant decrease in the incidence of HCC, which is the ultimate proof of the importance of the virus in the development of HCC.

4.2.2 Hepatitis C Virus

Hepatitis C virus plays a significant role in the development of hepatocellular carcinoma(HCC) globally. According to WHO, HCV infects 3-4 million people each year and the incubation period ranges from 2 to 24 weeks. Approximately 150 million individuals are infected with HCV and over 350,000 people die every year globally due to HCV-related liver diseases. A series of studies have revealed that certain ethnic groups are more susceptible to viral infection and the onset of HCC. In particular, Far-East Asian and Sub-Sharan African populations have a high rate of HCV-induced HCC. The pathogenic mechanisms of hepatocellular carcinoma with HCV infection are generally linked with inflammation, cytokines, fibrosis, cellular signaling pathways, and liver cell proliferation modulating pathways. HCV encoded proteins interact with a broad range of hepatocytes derived factors to modulate an array of activities such as cell signaling, DNA repair, transcription and translational regulation, cell propagation, apoptosis, membrane topology. Several cohort studies indicate that the incidence in patients with chronic hepatitis is low (below 1%) and that the risk increases sharply when cirrhosis is established. At this time, the annual incidence ranges between 2% and 8%. The transition from acute infection to cirrhosis may take decades, while some suggested the development of HCC even after a sustained response to interferon for the treatment of chronic hepatitis C. Patients infected with human immunodeficiency virus are now effectively treated with combined regimes and, if coinfected with HCV, they present a faster evolution to cirrhosis, meaning a higher risk for the development of HCC. In fact, liver disease and/or HCC are the major causes of death in these patients.

4.2.3 Alcohol, tobacco, and coffee

Alcohol excessive consumption is common cause ofcirrhosis in the Americas and Western Europe. In a recent meta-analysis, including 19 prospective studies, a positive association between the amount of alcohol intake and the risk of HCC was found. In particular, patients who drank three alcoholic units per day had a 16% increased risk of HCC, those who drank six units per day had a 22% increased risk. Smoking can slightly increase the oncogenic risk, whereas coffee consumption reduces the risk.

4.3 Pathogenesis

The development of HCC is a multistep process and determined with progressive and morphologically distinct preneoplastic lesions/alterations. These lesions are associated with chronic liver injury, inflammation, hepatocellular degeneration/regeneration, necrosis, and small-cell dysplasia which can be followed by low- and high-grade dysplastic nodules. Viral infections can cause chronic hepatitis B by causing the host's immune response, prolonged and repeated inflammation, injury, regeneration and fibrotic scar response, with local hypoxia, angiogenesis and tissue reconstruction, eventually leading to irreversible structural changes in cirrhosis. In addition, viral genomes can be integrated into host cell genomes by DNA-recombination-related enzymes of host cells, increasing cell genome instability. Long-term repeated liver inflammation and oxidative stress can also cause genetic damage and accumulation of hepatocytes, leading to the malignant transformation of hepatocytes to tumor cells.

4.4 Pathology

The appearance of HCC involves its transition from early to advanced stages. Gross appearance may be described as expansive, infiltrative, and diffuse. The first type shows distinct margins and a surrounding reticulin pseudocapsule. No distinct margins are seen in the infiltrative type, and the diffuse type corresponds to a multinodular tumor that mimics a cirrhotic liver. Usually, HCC appears as a distinct nodule of varying size that increases together with the development of additional tumor sites first in the vicinity or in separate segments. Some tumors may have envelopes, and tumors that are smaller than 3 cm are called small liver cancers. Tumors often invade the portal system to form portal thrombi. Under light microscope, cancer cells can be well differentiated (highly differentiated) or poorly differentiated (low differentiation). When highly differentiated, cells are often arranged in small trabeculae and often have pseudo-adenoid or alveolar structures, often with fatty changes. There are abundant sinusoid-like lacunae between tumor cells. Unlike normal hepatic sinusoids, endothelial cells in this sinusoid-like space are positive for CD34 and the 8th related antigenic factor and more like capillaries, so they are called capillaries. Some sinusoids are lined by tumor cells. When poorly differentiated, the type of solid growth was the main type, with few sinusoid-like lacunae and only fissure-like blood vessels. The proportion of cancerous cells in the nucleus pulposus was significantly increased, with obvious heteromorphism, including malformed tumor giant cells. In general, the tumor stroma is sparse and occasionally there are abundant interstitial, called sclerosing liver cancer. Well-differentiated HCC without such an invasive profile and without minute satellite nodules has been named very early HCC or carcinoma in situ. This initial lesion still does not have increased vascularization and, currently, is only confidently diagnosed after resection.

4.5 Clinical Manifestations

Because most HCC cases come from cirrhosis, the clinical picture observed in patients with HCC will be indistinguishable from patients with advanced cirrhosis. Generally, small HCC(s) seldom causes clinical symptoms, therefore it is often very difficult to diagnose small HCC(s) in patients without a prior history of liver disease. When clinical symptoms develop, HCC patients are usually presented with large tumor burden and poor general condition. Patients may present with jaundice, ascites, encephalopathy, or bleeding due to ruptured esophageal varices. Acute hemoperitoneum due to ruptured HCC is the first symptom in a minority of cases, whereas abdominal pain is the first symptom in a majority of cases. Advanced HCC is usually associated with increased bilirubin, alkaline phosphatase, and γ-glutamyl transpeptidase levels. The common indexes that can inflect hepatic function, such as alanine transaminase (ALT)/aspartate transaminase (AST) concentration has no diagnostic value. Paraneoplastic manifestations include polycythemia and severe hypoglycemia, which in some cases are the most relevant concern. Other manifestations include hypercalcemia, sexual changes, diarrhea, thrombophlebitis, and carcinoid syndrome.

4.6 Diagnosis and Staging

The preferred imaging method for surveillance is ultrasonography; it is well tolerated and widely available, and it has sensitivity of 60%-80% and specificity beyond 90%. The most used serological test is AFP. Unfortunately, even with the most efficient cutoff (10-20 μg/L), diagnostic sensitivity is around 60%. Surveillance should be initiated on development of cirrhosis and be restricted to patients who would be treated if diagnosed with HCC. Therefore, screening should be limited to Child-Pugh A and B patients, while Child-Pugh C patients should be evaluated for liver transplantation and HCC in them could become a contraindication for the procedure. Combined use of AFP and ultrasonography not only does not increase detection rates but also raises false-positive suspicions and cost. Other tumour markers, such as des-γ-carboxiprothrombin or AFP fractions, do not have better accuracy. On the basis of tumour-doubling times and data from the one available trial, screening of patients every 6 months is recommended. A 3-month interval increases detection of small nodules but has no effect on survival, and twice-yearly screening has better results than annual. Since tumour growth rate is not dictated by risk, increased risk should not prompt a shorter interval.

Nodules 1 cm or smaller are diagnosed infrequently as hepatocellular carcinoma and are almost impossible to diagnose confidently by available techniques (biopsy could miss the target and the diagnostic hypervascular profile is not in place at this stage). Furthermore, for these small lesions, pursuing a diagnosis of hepatocellular carcinoma would probably lead to more harm than benefit. When the nodule exceeds 1 cm, diagnosis can be established by biopsy or by imaging in the setting of liver cirrhosis. The specific imaging pattern is defined by intense contrast uptake during the arterial phase followed by contrast washout during venous or delayed phases in a contrast-enhanced study such as CT or MRI (magnetic resonance is being validated extensively). The value of these non-invasive criteria for hepatocellular carcinoma in cirrhosis has been confirmed prospectively. In nodules of 1-2 cm, typical imaging features have specificities and predictive positive values of near 100% and sensitivity that can reach 71%. Contrast-enhanced ultrasonography is not recommended as the sole diagnostic imaging technique because it can not distinguish intrahepatic cholangiocarcinoma from hepatocellular carcinoma and MRI or CT is still needed for staging. Non-invasive diagnostic criteria are valid only for investigation of screen-detected lesions in the liver in patients with either cirrhosis or long-lasting chronic HBV infection who might not have fully developed cirrhosis. In other clinical scenarios, a diagnostic biopsy should be requested. However, a negative finding after biopsy does not rule out hepatocellular carcinoma since the false-negative rate can reach 30% because of sampling error or absence of specific histological hallmarks for diagnosis of this cancer.

The classification that stratifies patients according to outcome and simultaneously links it with treatment indication is the Barcelona Clinic Liver Cancer (BCLC) strategy. The BCLC staging system is now the most widely used for incorporating tumor burden, liver function and patient general condition and it has been validated in different settings and establishes treatment recommendations for all stages of hepatocellular carcinoma. Patients with early-stage cancer are treated by resection, liver transplantation, or ablation, and prognosis can be refined for all these procedures according to different variables. The very early stage (BCLC 0) corresponds to patients with well-preserved liver function (Child-Pugh A) diagnosed with one asymptomatic nodule of less than 2 cm without vascular invasion or satellites. This stage corresponds to the carcinoma-in-situ entity that, if resected or ablated, would have excellent outcome with almost zero risk of recurrence. Currently, confident diagnosis is not feasible by imaging techniques or biopsy and it is classified as such at explant. End-stage patients are identified easily by any clinical method. They have a very poor prognosis and no intervention will be of benefit. Patients with end-stage liver disease (Child-Pugh C or advanced Child-Pugh B) should be considered for transplantation, but recognition of hepatocellular carcinoma could become a contraindication because of excessive tumour burden. Between these two extreme situations, the clinical profile is very heterogeneous; liver function includes Child-Pugh classes A and B, and tumour burden encompasses liver-only disease without vascular invasion or extensive disease with metastatic spread. Patients can be asymptomatic (performance status 0) or already have cancer-related symptoms such as pain or malaise (performance status 1-2). As a result, the term non-surgical hepatocellular carcinoma does not indicate any specific clinical profile or prognosis. The BCLC classification divides this heterogeneous group into two categories: the intermediate stage (BCLC B), defined by absence of any adverse predictor, and the advanced stage (BCLC C), which includes patients with symptoms, vascular invasion, extrahepatic spread, or a combination. The BCLC strategy has been validated externally in prospective studies and has been endorsed by several scientific associations, but further refinement is still needed. Liver function is assessed by the Child-Pugh classification, but class B includes a wide range of patients. Similarly, presence of ascites within Child-Pugh class A indicates impaired prognosis, which should be factored into individual assessment of patients and treatment proposals.

4.7 Prognostic Prediction

Assessment of prognosis is a crucial step in management of patients with hepatocellular carcinoma. Years ago, most affected individuals were diagnosed at an advanced symptomatic stage, when treatment was not feasible and short-term prognosis was dismal. Diagnosis has now advanced, and effective early treatment of patients is associated with median survival beyond 5 years. Any attempt to assess prognosis should account for tumour stage, degree of liver function impairment, and presence of cancer-related symptoms. Several proposals have been raised to stratify patients according to expected outcome. Some approaches do not take into account the presence of cancer-related symptoms that are major prognostic predictors. Others assess tumour burden roughly or investigate liver function according to the presence or absence of cirrhosis. This approach limits clinical usefulness.

Biomarkers should enable better stratification. High AFP concentration is associated with a poor prognosis, but no cutoff that would imply a modification in treatment decision has been defined. Other tumour markers do not refine prognosis or justify their use for staging or treatment selection. The same applies for biomarkers such as VEGF, angiopoietin 2, or the proto-oncogene c-Kit. They can refine prognostic prediction within statistical modelling but can not yet be incorporated into assessment of an individual patient.

4.8 Treatment

As far as we know, no large robust studies have been done to compare treatments regarded as potentially curative for early-stage disease (surgical resection, transplantation, percutaneous ablation), which represent only less than 40% of the patients, and no studies have compared these methods with no treatment. Surgical resection, transplantation, and ablation are treatments that offer a high rate of complete responses and, thus, potential for cure. The only non-curative treatments that improve survival are transarterial chemoembolisation and sorafenib. Arterial embolisation without chemotherapy, external radiotherapy, and radioembolisation have shown antitumour activity, but survival benefit has not been proven. Systemic chemotherapy has marginal activity with frequent toxic effects, without survival benefit, and agents such as tamoxifen, octreotide, or antiandrogens are completely ineffective. Treatment indication requires a careful evaluation of tumor stage, degree of liver failure, and general health. For treatment to be most effective, patients should be selected carefully and the treatment applied skilfully. In view of the complexity of hepatocellular carcinoma and the many potentially useful treatments, patients diagnosed with this malignant disease should be referred to multidisciplinary teams that include hepatologists, radiologists, surgeons, pathologists, and oncologists. Moreover, detection of vascular invasion or extrahepatic spread implies advanced disease stage and no any effective therapy. Although there is no functional impairment in patients with a normal underlying liver, in those with chronic liver disease, this aspect is of paramount relevance. Surgical resection is feasible only in patients with well-preserved liver function, and decompensated cirrhosis almost has not any forms of effective therapy methods, except liver transplantation.

4.8.1 Surgical treatment

HCC is a complex tumor with extremely heterogeneous biological behavior and multiple variables affecting treatment decision and outcome prediction. Liver function and patient general condition. According to BCLC staging system, surgical treatment should be reserved for patients with single lesion and normal bilirubin, but with no portal hypertension, while TACE and other palliative treatments are recommended as the first-line treatments to patients within BCLC stages B and C. It should not be overlooked that patients receiving surgery were often highly selected with younger age, better preoperative liver function, and lesser, smaller and more confined lesions. Some studies have suggested that surgical resection provides better long-term outcomes than other non-surgical treatments, even for patients with multiple lesions and major vascular invasion. Therefore, in carefully selected patients with low surgical risk and preserved liver function, surgical resection is safe, and it is effective for patients with resectable multiple and vascular invaded HCCs.

4.8.1.1 Resection

Hepatic resection is the treatment of choice for hepatocellular carcinoma in individuals without cirrhosis (5% of patients in the USA and Europe, 40% in Asia). These patients tolerate major resections with low rates of life-threatening complications. In individuals with cirrhosis, cirrhosis considerably limits surgical resection. Selection of candidates with cirrhosis should aim at a perioperative mortality of less than 3%, a transfusion rate less than 10%, and a 5-year survival rate higher than 50%, and careful selection of candidates is vital to avoid treatment-related complications, e. g., liver failure with increased risk of death.

For years, selection of candidates for resection has been based on the Child-Pugh classification, but this strategy has inconsistent predictive value. Some Child-Pugh A patients already have liver functional impairment with raised bilirubin concentrations, clinically significant portal hypertension, or even minor fluid retention necessitating diuretic treatment. In Japan, the indocyanine green retention rate is used to identify the best candidates for resection, whereas portal pressure and bilirubin are the variables used in Europe and the USA. Clinically relevant portal hypertension is defined as a hepatic vein pressure gradient greater than 10 mmHg, but it can also be confirmed by oesophageal varices or splenomegaly associated with a platelet count lower than 100×10^9/L. In patients without relevant portal hypertension and normal concentrations of bilirubin, survival at 5 years is 70%, whereas it is 50% for individuals with portal hypertension and is even lower when both adverse factors are present. With respect to the best candidates for resection, blood transfusion will be needed in fewer than 10% of cases, and treatment-related mortality should be less than 1%. Therefore, assessment of portal pressure is crucial for prediction of long-term survival.

Most groups restrict the indication for resection to patients with one tumour, because multifocality is associated with high recurrence and impaired survival. Although multifocality need not be viewed as a contraindication to resection, careful assessment to estimate survival (and associated risks) that might be offered by other options, such as transplantation, ablation, or chemoembolization, is mandatory. Tumour size is not a clear-cut limiting factor, but risk of vascular invasion and dissemination increases with diameter. Malignant vascular invasion should be viewed as a contraindication for resection. By application of these restrictive criteria, the proportion of patients in whom resection can be offered is 5% –10%.

Tumour recurrence complicates 70% of cases at 5 years, combining true recurrence, which usually arises within the first 2 years after resection, and de novo tumours. Microvascular invasion, poor histological differentiation, satellites, and multifocal disease predict early recurrence. Late recurrence depends mainly on the carcinogenic effect of underlying chronic liver disease. This risk can be estimated by liver function variables related to inflammatory activity, evolutionary stage, or both. No effective neoadjuvant or adjuvant treatment options to reduce risk of recurrence are available. Systemic chemotherapy and chemoembolisation have no effect, whereas immunotherapy, retinoids, and interferon have shown some potential efficacy, but evidence is not strong enough for them to be used in clinical practice. Findings of meta-analyses have reinforced the benefits of interferon but heterogeneity of the interferon used, the duration of the regimen, the patients recruited, and trial endpoints prevent valid assessment. The most effective option to prevent intrahepatic recurrence is liver transplantation. Although post-resection recurrence affects more than 70% of patients at 5 years in those with a risky profile, it affects fewer than 25% of individuals treated by transplantation. Transplantation can, therefore, be offered to patients initially treated by resection but with a high risk of recurrence according to pathological analysis. This policy not only allows some individuals to be treated effectively by resection with avoidance of transplantation but also permits best use of the few organs that are available by offering transplantation to patients whose cancer would recur after resection.

4.8.1.2 Transplantation

Hepatocellular carcinoma is the only solid cancer that can be treated by liver transplantation, especially for patients with small multi-nodular HCC (≤ 3 nodules ≤ 3 cm) or those with single tumours ≤5 cm without vascular invasion or extrahepatic spread (known as the Milano criteria) offered 4-year survival of 75%, with recurrence rates below 15%, and advanced liver dysfunction, which has completely changed the treatment strategy for this malignant disease. In theory, transplantation could simultaneously cure the tumour and underlying cirrhosis, and effectiveness of the procedure is not affected by the degree of liver function impairment. These results have been validated and are accepted as the benchmark for selection of patients in the USA and Europe.

These excellent results were achieved in an era with prompt availability of organs. The shortage of donors has imposed a delay before transplantation, and during this period the tumour can progress and impede transplantation. This delay impairs the effectiveness of liver transplantation when considered according to intention to treat. When waiting time exceeds 6 months, treatments aimed at delaying tumour progression (e.g., ablation, transarterial chemoembolisation) are done, even though effectiveness is unproven. Policies for transplantation are implemented that aim to prioritise the sickest patients. Moreover, several researchers have proposed expansion of current limits. Most suggestions are based on analysis of tumour stage in the explanted liver and not on imaging findings at the time of the patient's assessment. Furthermore, transplantation to patients who do not meet the Milano criteria is associated with increased prevalence of variables associated with risk of recurrence (microscopic vascular invasion or satellites). If the number of livers available exceeded the number of candidates for transplantation, a slight expansion would be feasible because it would not negatively affect patients with the best transplant profiles.

4.8.2 Percutaneous treatments

Percutaneous treatment of hepatocellular carcinoma (HCC) encompasses a vast range of techniques, including monopolar radiofrequency ablation (RFA), multibipolar RFA, microwave ablation, cryoablation and irreversible electroporation. Destruction or ablation of tumor cells can be achieved by the injection of chemical substances(e. g. ,ethanol,acetic acid,and boiling saline)or by the insertion of a probe that modifies local tumor temperature(e. g. , radiofrequency ablation, microwave, laser, and cryotherapy). This procedure can be done percutaneously with minimal invasiveness or during laparoscopy RFA is considered one of the main curative treatments for HCC of less than 5 cm developing on cirrhotic liver. And the imperfect sensitivity of imaging for detecting residual viable tumour, while obtaining a complete radiological response is the primary goal of ablative techniques, since complete ablation has been associated with prolonged overall survival. In line with the therapeutic algorithm of early HCC, percutaneous ablation could also be used as a bridge to liver transplantation or in a sequence of upfront percutaneous treatment, followed by transplantation if the patient relapses. Moreover, several innovations in ablation methods may help to efficiently treat early HCC, initially considered as "non-ablatable", and might, in some cases, extend ablation criteria beyond early HCC, enabling treatment of more patients with a curative approach. Besides, the combination of systemic therapy with percutaneous ablation aimed to reduce the incidence of distant tumour recurrence related both to intrahepatic metastasis from the initial tumour and de novo carcinogenesis in cirrhotic liver.

4.8.3 Palliative therapy

There are many options that have been proposed for patients with HCC, but unfortunately only chemoembolization has been recognized to have a beneficial impact on survival. Because the blood supply to HCC comes mostly through the hepatic artery, any intervention that blocks this vessel will result in tumor ischemia and necrosis of variable extent. Trans-arterial chemoembolisation(TACE) is a most effective technique of treatment that can be useful in cases of non-resectable liver tumors. This method involves intravascular administration of the chemotherapeutic agent to the tumor, and then embolisation of vessels supplying the tumor. The effectiveness of this method is based on a high concentration of chemotherapeutic agent in the tumor and embolisation of vessels supplying the lesion. TACE can reduce the toxicity of systemic chemotherapy. Hepatic artery obstruction requires an angiographic procedure with advancement of a catheter into the hepatic artery to interrupt blood flow to the tumor as selectively as possible and, therefore, to limit the injury of surrounding nontumor liver. There are several agents that can be used for arterial obstruction. The most common is Gelfoam prepared as 1 mm cubes, but active research aims to develop more effective obstructing agents. The method is save and less invasive. Side effects range from the postembolization syndrome with nausea, vomiting, fever and abdominal pain up to hepatic insufficiency, which is very rare. Stereotactic radiosurgery(stereotactic body radiation therapy-SBRT) is used for the treatment of liver lesions. High-precision treatment of lesions is possible with few side effects thanks to stereotaxy. This method is applicable for tumour sizes of 6-7 cm as well as in the case of numerous coexisting changes.

4.8.4 Future agents

Treatment of hepatocellular carcinoma has changed greatly within the past decade and has become a major area for research. Patients diagnosed with this malignant disease can benefit from effective options that will improve their survival, whatever the evolutionary stage at which they have been diagnosed. Obviously, improvement in several areas is still needed. Recurrence after ablation or resection is a major drawback, and effective preventive agents are needed. Also, progression after effective chemoembolisation is an area in which any positive strategy should result in relevant benefit. Finally, identification of novel targets and predictors through molecular cell biology will identify new therapeutic strategies for advanced stage hepatocellular carcinoma and provide better methods for outcome prediction. For that reason, collection of tissue samples should be considered in research studies. Molecular biology data might offer the insight to abrogate malignant transformation within cirrhotic livers. For these advances to take place, continuing active clinical and experimental research is essential. Only by combination of all areas of expertise will these hopes be realised.

Chapter 5

Secondary Liver Cancer

5.1 Epidemiology

Secondary liver disease mainly refers to secondary liver cancer(SLC), also known as metastatic liver cancer(MLC). The most common malignant tumors of the liver are metastatic lesions. The liver is a common site of metastases from gastrointestinal tumors, presumably because of dissemination via the portal venous system. The most relevant metastatic tumor of the liver to the surgeon is colorectal cancer because of the well-documented potential for long-term survival after complete resection. However, a large number of other tumors commonly metastasize to the liver, including cancers of the upper gastrointestinal system(stomach, pancreas, biliary), genitourinary system(renal, prostate), neuroendocrine system, breast, eye(melanoma), skin(melanoma), soft tissue(retroperitoneal sarcoma), and gynecologic system(ovarian, endometrial, cervix). The large majority of metastatic liver tumors that present with concomitant extrahepatic disease will have unresectable liver disease or are not curable with resection, limiting the role of the surgeon to highly select cases. It is worth reemphasizing that metastatic adenocarcinoma to the liver of unknown primary is often a primary intrahepatic cholangiocarcinoma, and this diagnosis must always be kept in mind.

5.2 Pathogenesis

There are six steps in the metastasis process. Not all cancers follow this process, but most do: ①Local invasion: Cancer cells move from the primary site into nearby normal tissue. ②Intravasation: Cancer cells move through the walls of nearby lymph vessels or blood vessels. ③Circulation: Cancer cells migrate through the lymphatic system or the bloodstream to other parts of the body. ④Arrest and extravasation: Cancer cells stop moving when they reach a distant location. They then move through the capillary(small blood vessel) walls and invade nearby tissue. ⑤Proliferation: Cancer cells grow at the distant location and create small tumors called micrometastases. ⑥Angiogenesis: Micrometastases stimulate the creation of new blood vessels, which supply the nutrients and oxygen needed for tumor growth.

Traditionally, cancer spread to a distant site was considered a systemic disease in which locoregional therapies(i. e. ,surgery) were not effective. Some metastatic tumors to the liver and, in particular, metastatic colorectal cancer have been shown to be an exception to this rule. Over 35 years of clinical research has documented that metastatic colorectal cancer isolated in the liver can be resected, with the potential for long-term survival and cure. Advances in systemic and regional chemotherapy have also broadened the number of patients eligible for surgical therapy and probably have improved long-term survival after resection. Patient selection is the most important aspect of surgical therapy for metastatic disease in the liver and clinical follow-up of resected patients has identified those most and least likely to benefit. Although long-term survival is common and occurs in up to 50%-60% of patients in current series, recurrence and chronic multimodal therapy are common, occurring in approximately 75% of patients. Therefore, realistic expectations and systemic patient education is an important aspect of treatment. Tumors other than colorectal cancer presenting as isolated or limited hepatic metastases can also be resected for potential long-term survival, but data on these other tumors are sparse and less compelling than for colorectal cancer.

5.3 Clinical Manifestation

The symptoms of MLC are mainly due to the primary cancer. Usually when the metastatic nodule is small, no symptoms can be realized until occasional lab or imaging tests. A small proportion of MLC patients even can't identify the primary extrahepatic cancerous focus. As the hepatic metastatic nodule grows bigger, you may feel loss of appetite, weight loss, abdominal swelling or bloating, a yellowing of the skin or the sclera, pain in the right shoulder or upper right abdomen, nausea, vomiting, confusion, sweats and fever. A lump can also be felt on the right side of the abdomen below the ribcage by physical examinations when the liver is obviously enlarged. Anemia, ascites and severe jaundice can occur in the late stage patients. Liver function tests are blood tests that indicate how well the liver is functioning. Liver enzyme levels are often elevated when there is a problem. Imaging tests including B-ultrasound, CT scan or enhancement CT, MRI and PET scan are essential tools for diagnosing MLC. A CT scan is a special kind of X-ray that takes visual images of soft-tissue organs in detail. Cancerous tissue will have a moth-eaten appearance. Ultrasound of the liver transmits high-frequency sound waves through the body. These sound waves produce echoes. The echoes are then used to create map-like computerized images of the liver's soft-tissue structures. MRI creates extremely clear images of internal organs and soft-tissue structures. In an angiogram, dye is injected into an artery. When images are taken of the body along that artery's pathway, it can produce high-contrast images of internal structures. The laparoscopy is a narrow tube with a light and a biopsy(tissue sample) tool. The laparoscope is inserted through a small incision, and biopsies are taken for study under a microscope. Laparoscopy is the most reliable minimally invasive method of diagnosing cancer. Tumor markers such as CEA, CA19-9 and CA125 are of great value particularly in the diagnosis of gastric cancer, colorectal cancer, carcinoma of gallbladder, pancreatic cancer, lung cancer, ovarian cancer and other primary cancer liver metastasis. However, AFP is rarely upregulated in MLC. When primary liver cancer is present, there may be higher levels of AFP detected in the blood which can help distinguish between primary liver cancer and liver metastasis. AFP markers can also be used to monitor treatment effects of primary liver cancer.

5.4 Treatment

MLC requires systemic multidisciplinary therapies according to the complex conditions of primary cancer. Generally, the choice of treatments will depend on the person's age and overall health; the size, location, and number of metastatic tumors; location and type of the primary cancer; the types of cancer treatment the patient had in the past. Systemic cancer therapies treat the whole body through the bloodstream. The therapeutic strategies for liver metastasis are similar to HCC. If it is solitary, or multiple though they are, they are limited to a lobe or a segment of liver, lobular or segmental section is a prior choice when the patient already free of the primary cancer is in good condition and there is no other metastasis. If the primary and metastatic cancer are detected simultaneously, evaluated resectable and meet the criterion of liver resection, staged or simultaneous hepatectomy can be performed to help patients get rid of both tumors after assessment of patients' conditions. Operation strategies should be adjusted if new cancerous focuses are found during the operation with the help of B-ultrasound. As for those unresectable tumors evaluated or found during the operation, regional therapies like TACE, PEI, radiofrequency ablation (RFA), etc., can be adopted as adjuvant approaches. These regional therapies can be conducted before the operation to shrink the tumor to make the tumor resectable. Surgical methods and RFA can also be combined to expand the applicable range of surgery. Recent studies showed that postoperative TACE can reduce recurrence rate and increase overall survival in patients who have undergone hepatectomy.

In most cases, treatment will be palliative because it has reached stage Ⅳ (TNM stage). These therapies include chemotherapy, biological response modifier (BRM) therapy, targeted therapy, hormonal therapy, localized therapies like RFA and TACE, radiation therapy, etc. Chemotherapy is a form of treatment that uses drugs to kill cancer cells. It targets cells that grow and multiply quickly, including some healthy cells. BRM therapy is a treatment that uses antibodies, growth factors, and vaccines to boost or restore the immune system. This helps your immune system's ability to fight cancer. BRM therapy does not have the usual side effects of other cancer therapies and, in most cases, is well tolerated. Targeted therapy also kills cancer cells, but it's more precise. Unlike chemotherapy drugs, targeted treatments can differentiate between cancer and healthy cells. These drugs can kill cancer cells and leave healthy cells intact. Targeted therapies have different side effects than some other cancer treatments. Side effects, which can be severe, include fatigue and diarrhea. Hormonal therapy can slow or stop the growth of certain types of tumors that rely on hormones to grow, such as breast and prostate cancer. Radiation therapy uses high-energy radiation to kill cancer cells and shrink tumors. It may come from radiation machines, such as external beam radiation; radioactive materials placed in the body near cancer cells, known as internal radiation; radioactive substances that travel through the bloodstream. RFA is commonly used to treat primary liver cancer and can be used to treat liver metastasis. RFA is a procedure that uses high-frequency electrical currents to create heat that destroys the cancer cells.

Intra-arterial therapy options for MLC include chemoinfusion via a hepatic arterial pump or port, irinotecan-loaded drug-eluting beads, and radioembolization using 90Y microspheres. Intra-arterial therapy allows the delivery of a high dose of chemotherapy or radiation into liver tumors while minimizing the impact on liver parenchyma and avoiding systemic effects. Specificity in intra-arterial therapy can be achieved both through preferential arterial flow to the tumor and through selective catheter positioning. There are two types of 90Y microspheres: resin and glass. Because glass microspheres have a higher activity per particle, they can deliver a particular radiation dose with fewer particles, likely reducing embolic effects. Glass microspheres thus may be more suitable when early stasis or reflux is a concern, in the setting of hepatocellular carcinoma with portal vein invasion, and for radiation segmentectomy. Because resin microspheres have a lower activity per particle, more particles are needed to deliver a particular radiation dose. Resin microspheres thus may be preferable for larger tumors and those with high arterial flow. In addition, resin microspheres have been approved by the U. S.

5.5 Outcome

The prognosis of MLC is closely associated with the characteristics and severity of both the primary and secondary tumors, responses to treatment and so on. Generally speaking, the outcome of MLC patients after hepatectomy remains unsatisfactory even though surgical techniques have been largely improved these years. CRC liver metastases in a small fraction (10% –20%) of patients are potentially resectable. Surgical resection of liver metastases results in long–term (>10–year) cure in 16% of patients. The principle for surgery is as follows: try to retain healthy liver tissue and remove cancerous tissue (marginal distance to the tumor > 1 cm). For patients with small–volume hepatic disease, thermal ablation is a less invasive alternative to surgery, and it has a comparable 5–year overall survival rate of about 50%. Ablation has been used extensively for patients with liver metastases smaller than 3–4 cm, especially patients who are not candidates for surgery, as well as for recurrences after hepatectomy that can be ablated with margins larger than 5 mm. In addition, ablation of resectable liver metastases allows for a "test–of–time" approach: surgery can be avoided in 76% of patients, either because they were disease–free after ablation or because they developed new metastases that could not be resected. Importantly, no tumors became unresectable after ablation because of the growth of existing metastases. About 50% recurrence cases of CRCLM remain limited to the liver. Serum CEA and liver ultrasound are necessary postoperative tests to monitor progression conditions.

Part 32

Portal Hypertension

32.1 Definition

Since pressure in the portal venous system is determined by the relationship P=Fx R, portal hypertension could result either from increased volume of portal blood flow or increased resistance to flow. Portal hypertension occurs whenever the flow of blood within the portal vein is impeded or obstructed and causes symptoms and signs including splenomegaly, hypersplenism, and then esophagogastric varices with hemorrhage (hematemesis, melena) and ascites. Portal venous pressure normally ranges from 13 to 24 cmH_2O (1.27–2.35 kPa), averaging 18 cmH_2O (1.76 kPa). In portal hypertension, portal pressure exceeds 24 cmH_2O and reaches–30–50 cmH_2O. If it is less than 25 cmH_2O, rupture and bleeding of esophogeal varices is a rare condition.

32.2 Etiology

There are two causes of portal hypertension. One cause is increased resistance to portal vein flow. There are also three types of increasing resistance to portal vein flow. The first type is prehepatic portal hypertension with portal vein obstruction. The reason of portal vein obstruction are congentialatresis or stenosis, thrombosis of portal vein, thrombosis of splenic vein, or extrinsic compression (such as tumor). The second type is hepatic portal hypertension. The main reason is cirrhosis, such as portal cirrhosis (nutritional or alcoholic), post necrotic cirrhosis, biliary cirrhosis or others (Wilson's disease or hemochromatosis). There are also some relative rare reasons, such as acute alcoholic liver disease, congenital hepatic fibrosis, idiopathic portal hypertension (hepatoportal sclerosis) and schistosomiasis. The last type is posthepatic portal hypertension, included Budd–Chiari syndrome and constrictive pericarditis. The other cause is increased portal blood flow. One type is Arterial–portal venous fistula. The other type is increased splenic flow, included Banti's syndrome and splenomegaly (such as tropical splenomegaly and myeloid metaplasia). Cirrhosis accounts for about 85% of cases of portal hypertension in the USA, and the most common form is due to alcoholism. Postnecrotic cirrhosis is next in frequency, followed by biliary cirrhosis.

32.3 Anatomy

32.3.1 The portal vein

It is formed by the confluence of the splenic (which collects blood from inferior mesenteric vein) and superior mesenteric veins at the level of the second lumbar vertebra behind the head of the pancreas. The blood of splenic vein accounts for 20% of portal flow. Portal vein is located between two capillary networks, one is capillary beds of stomach, intestine, spleen and pancreas, the another from hepatic sinus.

32.3.2 Ortalsystemic anastomoses

The most serious symptoms are caused by enlargement and collateralizaion of the vessels that connect the portal and the systemic venous systems. Normally these collateralization veins are small and carry minute amounts of blood under low pressure. The naturally occurring portasystemic venous shunts are as follows:

(1) Esophageal veins which carry portal blood into the azygos system and superior vena cava through gastric coronary vein, short gastric vein, and esophogeal plexus.

(2) Hemorrhoidal veins which carry portal blood into the pudendal and iliac veins through superior and inferior hemorrhoidal veins.

(3) Umbilical veins which carry portal blood to the anterior abdominal wall veins.

(4) There are numerous small retzius veins connecting the retroperitoneal viscera with the posterior abdominal wall.

32.4 Pathophysiology

32.4.1 Obstruction can occur at three principal sites

(1) Hepatic (intrahepatic) obstruction

Portal hypertension is mainly caused by cirrhosis of the liver due to hepatitis B (90%), some are caused by schistosomiasis and alcoholic cirrhosis. The fibrosis and scarring that occur with any type of cirrhosis inhibits the transport of blood into the central veins of the hepatic lobes, leading to stasis and increased pressure within the port al venous system.

(2) Prehepatic (subhepatic or portal vein obstruction)

Portal vein obstruction may result from a congenital malformation (atresia, stenosis and cavernous transformation) and thrombosis (peritoneal cavity infection, e. g., caused by acute appendicitis) of the portal vein, and extrinsic compression (e. g., tumor). Whatever the cause, the portal vein obstruction inhibits passage of its blood to the liver.

(3) Posthepatic (suprahepatic or hepatic vein) obstruction

The obstruction may result from thrombosis (Budd-Chiari syndrome), tumors or constrictive pericarditis. It is the least common of all causes for portal hypertension, accounting for about 1% of cases.

In posthepatic cirrhosis, the abnormal resistance is predominantly at the sinusoidal and postsinusoidal position. The causes of increased resistance in this disease are: ①distortion of the hepatic veins by regenerative nodules, ② fibrosis of the hepatic veins and perisinusoidal areas, and ③ opening of arteriavenous shunts.

Schistosomiasis alone produces a presinusoidal block as a consequence of deposition of parasite ova in small portal venules.

32.4.2 Pathological changes

The elevated pressure of portal vein can cause the following pathological changes:

(1) Splenomegaly and hypersplenism

Increased resistance of portal vein can cause the increased splenic blood flow accompanying "congestive" splenomegaly, fibrosis and regeneration of pulpar cells, then, hyperfunction of damaging blood cells (hypersplenism).

(2) Dilation of portal-systemic collaterals

The dilation and increase in venous pressure within all of these systems may then result in several conditions. Esophageal varices protrude into the lumen of the esophagus, where ulceration results from irritation of food, tubes, or acid-peptic factors. Massive and potentially lethal upper gastrointestinal bleeding is a dreaded result. Hemorrhoids may prolapse and bleed. The abdominal wall collaterals may increase in size, radiating outward from the umbilicus. This condition is called caput medusae.

(3) Ascites

This condition results from increased hydrostatic pressure of portal capillaries, increased formation of hepatic lymph and splanchnic lymph, hypoalbuminemia due to primary liver disease, sodium and water retention because of endocrine and renal factors, hormones such as aldosterone and antidiuretin degraded in the liver.

About 20% of patients with portal hypertension are complicated with portal hypertensive gastropathy, which accounts for 5% of upper gastrointestinal tract bleeding of portal hypertension. Dilation of the gastric veins, edema and congestion of gastric wall result in portal hypertensive gastropathy which affects mainly the fundus and body of the stomach and produces an erythematous appearance at endoscopy. Hepatic encephalopathy or portosystemic encephalophy may occur due to toxic substances into circulation resulted from portalsystemic shunts spontaneously or operatively.

32.5 Clinical Manifestation

It is more common in man than in woman and slow progressive. The main symptoms are splenomegaly, hypersplenism, hematemesis or melena, ascites and non-specific systemic symptoms (e.g., weakness, lethargy and anorexia).

32.5.1 Splenomegaly and hypersplenism

The spleen is impalpable in the normal condition. The enlarged spleen is soft, mobile in the early stage. Later it becomes stiff and immobile due to fibrosis and adhesion. Hypersplenism develops with leukopenia (WBC count $<3\times10^9/L$), thrombocytopenia (platelet $< 70\times10^9/L$) and anemia.

32.5.2 Hematemesis (vomiting of blood) or melena (tarry stool)

Massive upper gastrointestinal tract bleeding is the most frightening manifestation of portal hypertension. It is difficult to stop automatically because of impediment in blood coagulation (severe liver disease) and decrease of platelet count (hypersplenism); consequently, hypovolemia, hypoxia and hyperammonemia and hepatic coma.

32.5.3 Ascites

It develops suddenly in association with severe hepatocellular damage and is a manifestation of hepatic decompensation. Massive bleeding can induce or increase the formation of ascites. The patient may have abdominal discomfort, flatulence and anorexia.

32.5.4 Others

The patient may have hepatomegaly, jaundice, caput medusae, spider nevus, reddened palms and hemorrhoidal varices.

32.6 Diagnosis and Differential Diagnosis

History(hepatitis, alcoholism or schistosomiasis) and three main clinical manifestations (splenomegaly and hypersplenism, hematemesis or melena, ascites) can make a correct diagnosis without difficulty. It should be remembered that above three manifestations are not always found in all patients. Laboratory tests are necessary.

(1) Blood test

In hypersplenism, blood cell count, WBC and platelets are reduced. Anemia is caused by hemorrhage, malnutrition, hemolysis, and bone marrow depression.

(2) Compromised liver function

Most alcoholics with acute upper gastrointestinal bleeding have compromised liver function. The ratio of A/G is reversed due to reduced serum albumin and increased globulin. Increased serum aminotransferase and bilirubin, prolonged PT may exist in some patients.

(3) Upper gastrointestinal series

A barium swallow outlines the varices in 70%–80% of affected patients showing intraluminal worm-like filling defects in the esophagus.

(4) BUS and CT

Ultrasoundgraphy and CT are of limited value although ultrasound may demonstrate the patency of the portal vein, cirrhosis, splenomegaly, and ascites.

(5) Esophagogastroscopy

Emergency esophagogastroscopy is the most useful procedure for diagnosing bleeding varices and should be scheduled as soon as the patient's general condition is stabilized by blood transfusion and other supportive measures. Varices appear as three or four large, tortuous submucosal bluish vessels running longitudinally in the distal esophagus. The bleeding site may be identified.

Massive upper gastrointestinal tract bleeding from esophageal varices must be distinguished from blood originating within the stomach and duodenum (peptic ulcer, gastritis, gastric carcinoma). Cirrhotic patients have a 7–10 times greater incidence of peptic ulcer than the general population does. They may coexist.

32.7 Treatment

Only 40% of patients with cirrhosis have esophageal varices that have 50%–60% chance of massive bleeding. Patients who have bled once from esophageal varices have a 70% chance of bleeding again, and about 2/3 of repeat bleeding episodes are fatal.

The general goal of treatment is to control the bleeding as quickly and reliably as possible using methods with the fewest possible side effects. Disease severity is assessed by a combination of clinical parameters and standard laboratory tests. The Child-Pugh classification is used to assess hepatic functional reserve. The combination of two clinical parameters, two biochemical criteria and one haematological criterion is evaluated and scored. A total score from the five parameters classifies the patients as Child-Pugh grade A (score 5–6 points), B (score 7–9 points) or C (score 10–15 points) (Table 32-1-1). In most clinical series, operative mortality rates for Child's class A, B and C patients are in the range of 0–5%, 10%–15%, and greater than 25% ,respectively.

Table 32-1-1 Child-Pugh classification

Classification	Number of points		
	1	2	3
Bilirubin(μmol/L)	<34	34-51	>51
Albumin(g/L)	>35	28-35	<28
Ascites	None	Slight	Moderate
Encephalopathy	None	Slight	Severe
Prothrombin time prolonged by(s)	<3	3-6	>6

32.7.1 Non-surgical management

Nonoperative treatments are generally preferred for acutely bleeding patients since they are often high operative risks because of decompensated liver function, jaundice, and massive with hepatic functional reserve of Child's Class C. The therapeutic options include blood transfusion, administration of vasopressin and insertion of a SB tube.

32.7.2 Initial treatment

The initial treatment of bleeding esophageal varices is aimed at stabilization of the circulating blood volume with fluid and blood. Fresh blood is preferable to stored blood because of its higher platelet content and other support of the blood coagulation mechanism. Other therapy should include measures to treat or prevent encephalopathy, parenteral vitamin K to correct a prolonged prothrombin time, and electrolytes and fluid as required to restore electrolyte balance and prevent shock.

32.7.3 Vasopressin infusion(pituitrin)

It lowers portal blood flow and portal pressure by a direct constricting action on splanchnic arterioles. Vasopressin is given as a peripheral intravenous infusion(at about 0.4 units/min) ,which is safer than bolus injections. The adverse systemic effects of vasopressin can be effectively counteracted by simultaneous infusion of nitroglycerin or nitroprusside. The combination of vasopressin and nitroglycerin may also be more effective in controlling variceal hemorrhage than vasopressin alone.

32.7.4 Octreotide acetate

Somatostatin and the synthetic longer-lasting analogue octreotide have the same effect on the splanchnic circulation as vasopressin but without significant side effects. These drugs are as effective as vasopressin in controlling acute variceal bleeding and now the first choice for the pharmacologic control of acutely bleeding varices. Octreotide is given as an initial bolus of 100 μg followed by a continuous infusion of 25 μg/h for 24 hours.

32.7.5 Balloon tamponade

Tubes designed for tamponade have two balloons that can be inflated in the lumen of the gut to compress bleeding varices. There are three or four lumens in the tube: two are for filling the balloons and the third permits aspiration of gastric contents. A fourth lumen in the Minnesota tube is used to aspirate the esophagus orad to the esophageal balloon. The main effect is due to traction applied to the tube which forces the gastric balloon to compress the collateral veins at the cardia of the stomach. Inflating the esophageal balloon probably contributes little, since barium X-rays suggest that it does not actually compress the varices (Figure 32-1-1).

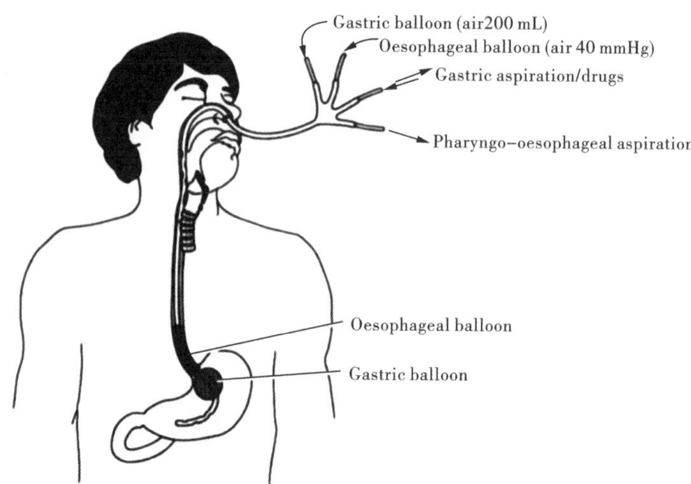

Figure 32-1-1 Compression hemostasis with Sengstaken-Blakemore tube

A new tube is used for each patient and both balloons are tested for leaks prior to insertion. The nasal route for insertion is preferred as this is ultimately more comfortable for the patient. Once in the stomach, the gastric balloon is filled with 150-200 mL of air and pulled back to impinge on the cardia. The oesophageal balloon is then inflated with 100-150 mL (the intraluminal pressure of approximately 40 mmHg) of air if bleeding continued.

70%-90% of actively bleeding patients can be controlled by balloon tamponade. The oesophageal balloon is generally deflated after 12-24 hours to has been stopped oesophageal ulceration, but the gastric balloon position may be maintained. When bleeding has stopped, the balloons are left inflated for another 24 hours. They are then decompressed, leaving the tube in place. If bleeding does not recur, the tube should be withdrawn.

Complications occur in 10%-20% of patients who require balloon tamponade. The most common serious complication is the aspiration of pharyngeal secretions and pneumonitis. Another serious hazard is the occasional instance of esophageal rupture caused by inflation of the esophageal balloon. To avoid this risk, the instructions packaged with the tube must be followed carefully.

32.7.6 Endoscopic sclerotherapy or ligation

Via fiberoptic endoscopy, 1-3 mL of sclerosant solution (sodium morrhuate) is injected into the lumen of each varix, causing it to become thrombosed. Sclerotherapy controls acute bleeding in 80%-95% of patients, and rebleeding during the same hospitolization is about half (25% versus 50%) the rebleeding rate of patients treated with a combination of vasopressin and balloon tamponade. The main complications are esophageal ulcer, stricture and perforation which is serious with high mortality rate of 50%.

A somewhat similar effect can be achieved by endoscopic rubber band ligation of the varices. The varix is lifted with a suction tip, and a small rubber band is slipped around the base. The varix necroses to leave a superficial ulcer. A controlled trial has reported rubber band ligation to be more effective in controlling bleeding (e. g., fewer episodes of rebleeding; lower mortality rate) than sclerotherapy. Both procedures are ineffective for gastric bleeding.

32.7.7 Transjugular intrahepatic portasystemic shunt(TIPS)

This is a minimally invasive way of creating a shunt between the portal vein and the hepatic vein through the liver. A catheter is introduced through the jugular vein and, under radiologic control, positioned in the hepatic vein. From this point, the portal vein is accessed through the liver, the tract is dilated, and the channel is kept open by inserting an expandable metal stent, which is left in place. This technique is of great value in controlling portal hypertension and variceal bleeding and can be used to stop acute bleeding or to prevent rebleeding in a patient who has recovered from an acute episode. The main complications include hepatic endephalopathy and stricture or occlusion.

32.7.8 Surgery

The objective of the surgical procedures used to treat portal hypertension is either to obliterate the varices or to reduce blood flow and pressure within the varices. Operation should be done after a proper preparation for emergent bleeding patients or for patients without bleeding to prevent rebleeding.

32.7.8.1 Portasystemic shunts

Many types of portasystemic shunts have been developed. Basically they can be grouped into two main categories: nonselective(total) shunts and selective shunts.

Nonselective shunts are those shunt the entire portal system, which include the end-to-side portacaval shunt, the side-to-side portacaval shunt, large-diameter interposition shunts(H-graft), and the central splenorenal shunts(Figure 32-1-2). The end-to-side shunt completely disconnects the liver from the portal system is the prototype of nonselective shunts. The portal vein is transected near its bifurcation in the liver hilum and anastomosed to the side of the inferior vena cava. The end-to-side portacaval shunt gives immediate protection from variceal bleeding and is somewhat easier to perform than a side-to-side shunts. There is a high incidence of encephalopathy after these procedures.

32.7.8.2 Selective shunts

Selective shunts lower pressure in the gastroesophageal venous plexus while preserving blood flow through the liver via the portal vein. The distal splenorenal(Warren) shunts involves anastomosing the distal end of the transected splenic vein to the side of the renal vein, plus ligation of all major collateral vessels, such as the corollary and gastroepiploic veins, between the remaining portal and isolated gastrosplenic vinous system. It is associated with a much lower incidence of encephalopathy than the non-selective shunts while it does not improves ascites and should not be performed in patients whose ascites has been difficult to control.

32.7.8.3 Partial shunts

Partial shunts provide the similar objectives with selective shunts to reduce portal hypertension, inhibit gastroesophageal varisis bleeding and preserve partial hepatic portal perfusion. A small-diameter interposition portacaval shunts using a polytetrafluoroethylene graft, combined with ligation of corollary vein and other collateral vessels. When the prosthetic graft is 10 mm or less in diameter, hepatic portal perfusion is preserved in the majority of patients.

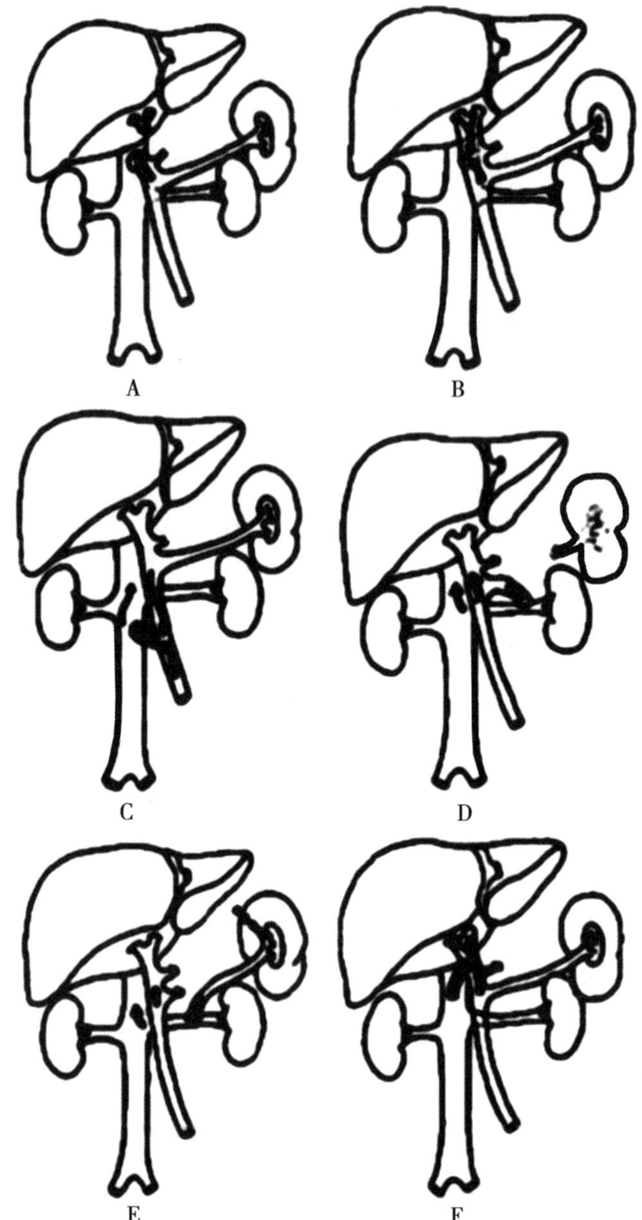

Figure 32-1-2 Types of portacaval anastomoses

A. end-to-side; B. side-to-side; C. H-mesocaval; D. central splenorenal; E. distal splenorenal(Warren); F. small-diameter H-portacaval.

32.7.9 Devascularization(extensive gastroesophageal devascularization)

The objective of devascularization is to destroy the venous collaterals that transport blood from the veins in the submucosa of the esophagus. There are different types of devascularization, of which extensive gastroesophageal devascularization is most popular used in China because of its effective result of controlling bleeding. During this procedure, four groups of pericardial veins and accompanied arteries must be ligated and separated. They are coronary veins, which include gastric branch, esophageal, superior esophageal, abnormal superior esophageal branch; short gastric veins; posterior gastric vein; left infcrior diaghram Vine.

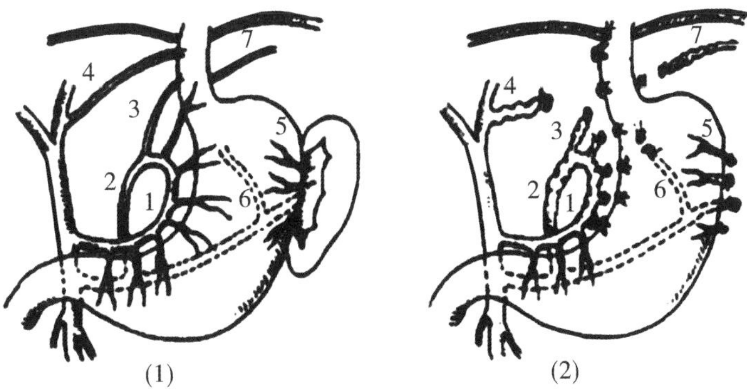

(1) Regional anatomy of pericardial vessels;(2) Transection of pericardial vessels

Figure 32-1-3 Pericardial devascularization

1. Gastric branch;2. Esophageal branch;3. High esophageal branch;4. Ectopic high esophageal branch;5. Short gastric vein;6. Posterior gastric vein;7. Left inferior phrenic vein.

32.7.10 Splenectomy

Attempts have also been made to decrease portal pressure by decreasing splanchnic inflow through splenectomy, which is suitable for severe splenomegaly patients with hypersplenism and patients with left portal hypertension caused by splenic vein thrombosis.

32.7.11 Liver transplantation

Definitive therapy for patients with advanced liver failure(Child's B or C)and poorly controlled ascites is liver transplantation. Variceal hemorrhage is the most clinical manifestation of portal hypertension prompting liver transplant evaluation.

Budd-chiari syndrome

It is produced by restriction to flow through the hepatic veins or the inferior above the liver. The resulting sinusoidal hypertension produces prominent ascties and hepatomegaly. The causes are:

(1) Congenital malformation.

(2) Thrombosis.

(3) Tumor compression.

Symptoms usually begin with a mild prodrome consisting of vague upper quadrant abdominal pain, postprandial bloating, and anorexia. After weeks or moths, a more florid picture develops consisting of gross ascites, hepatomegaly, and hepatic failure.

Colour Doppler ultrasound shows if hepatic vein and vena cava are unobstructed direction of blood flow, which is the first choice for diagnosis. The clinical diagnosis should be confirmed by venography, which shows the hepatic veins to be obstructed, usually with a beak-like deformity at their orifice.

A side-to-side portacaval or mesocaval shunt should be constructed when the obstruction is confined to the hepatic veins. Focal membranous obstruction of the suprahepatic cava may be treated by excision of the lesion with or without the addition of a patch angioplasty. Some cases may be managed nonsurgically by percutaneous transluminal balloon dilation of the stenosis.

Liver transplantation is indicated in patient with advanced hepatic decompensation either from cirrhosis or as part of the acute syndrome. The results are excellent, and the risk of later hepatocellular carcinoma is eliminated.

Part 33

Biliary Tract Disease

Chapter 1

Anatomy and Physiology

1.1 Biliary Tract Anatomy

1.1.1 Intrahepatic bile duct anatomy

Biliary tract is composed of intrahepatic and extrahepatic components. The right and left livers are drained by the right and the left hepatic ducts, whereas the caudate lobe is drained by several ducts joining both the right and left hepatic ducts. The left hepatic duct drains the three segments (Ⅱ, Ⅲ, and Ⅳ) that constitute the left liver, the right hepatic duct drains segments Ⅴ, Ⅵ, Ⅶ, and Ⅷ and arises from the junction of two main sectoral ductal tributaries. The intrahepatic ducts are tributaries of the corresponding hepatic ducts, which form part of the major portal triads that penetrate the liver, invaginating Glisson's capsule at the hilus. Bile ducts usually are located above the corresponding portal branches, whereas hepatic arterial branches are situated inferiorly to the veins. Each branch of the intrahepatic portal veins corresponds to one or two bile duct tributaries joining to form the right and left hepatic ductal systems converging at the liver hilus to constitute the common hepatic duct.

1.1.2 Extrahepatic biliary and the vascular anatomy

The extrahepatic bile ducts are represented by the extrahepatic segments of the right and left hepatic ducts joining to form the biliary confluence and the main biliary channel draining to the duodenum. The accessory biliary apparatus, which constitutes a reservoir, comprises the gallbladder and cystic duct. The confluence of the right and left hepatic ducts occurs at the right of the hilar fissure of the liver anterior to the portal venous bifurcation and overlying the origin of the right branch of the portal vein. The extrahepatic segment of the right duct is short, but the left duct has a much longer extrahepatic course (Figure 33-1-1).

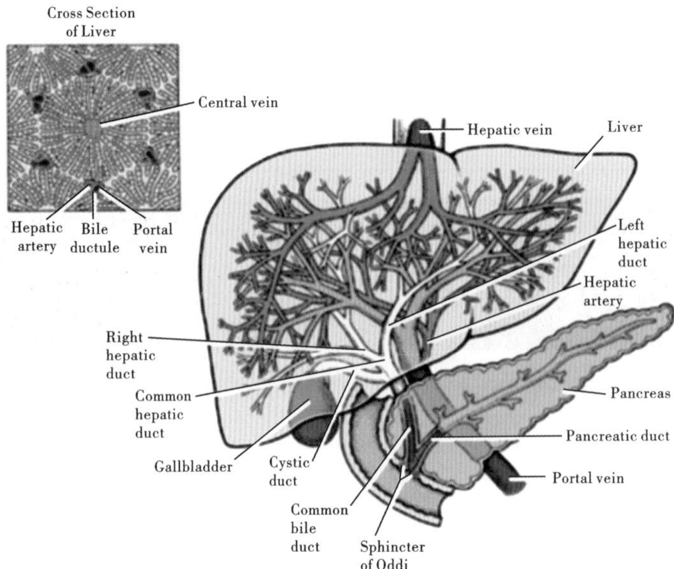

Figure 33-1-1 Biliary and the vascular anatomy

1.1.3 Main bile duct and sphincter of oddi

The main bile duct, the mean diameter of which is about 6 mm, is divided into two segments. The upper segment is called the common hepatic duct and is situated above the cystic duct, which joins it to form the common bile duct. The common duct courses downward anterior to the portal vein in the free edge of the lesser omentum and is closely applied to the hepatic artery, which runs upward on its left, giving rise to the right branch of the hepatic artery, which crosses the main bile duct usually posteriorly, although in about 20% of cases anteriorly. The cystic artery, arising from the right branch of the hepatic artery, may cross the common hepatic duct posteriorly or anteriorly. The common hepatic duct constitutes the left border of the triangle of Calot, the other corners of which were originally described as the cystic duct below and the cystic artery above. The commonly accepted definition of Calot's triangle recognizes, however, the inferior surface of the right lobe of the liver as the upper border and the cystic duct as the lower. Sphincter of Oddi is the termination of the common duct which is enveloped by a complex sphincteric muscle. It is a muscular valve that controls the flow of digestive juices (bile and pancreatic juice) through the ampulla of Vater into the second part of the duodenum (Figure 33-1-2).

1.1.4 Gallbladder and cystic duct

The gallbladder is a reservoir located on the undersurface of the right lobe of the liver within the cystic fossa and separated from the hepatic parenchyma by the cystic plate, which is composed of connective tissue closely applied to Glisson's capsule and prolonging the hilar plate. Sometimes the gallbladder is deeply embedded in the liver, but occasionally it occurs on a mesenteric attachment and may be liable to volvulus. The gallbladder varies in size and consists of a fundus, a body, and a neck. The fundus projects 1-2 cm below the hepatic edge and can often be felt when the cystic is obstructed. The gallbladder holds about 50 mL of bile when fully distended. The neck of the gallbladder tapers into the marrow cystic duct, which connects with the common duct. The lumen of the cystic duct contains a thin mucosal septum, the spiral valve of Heister, that offers mild resistance to bile flow.

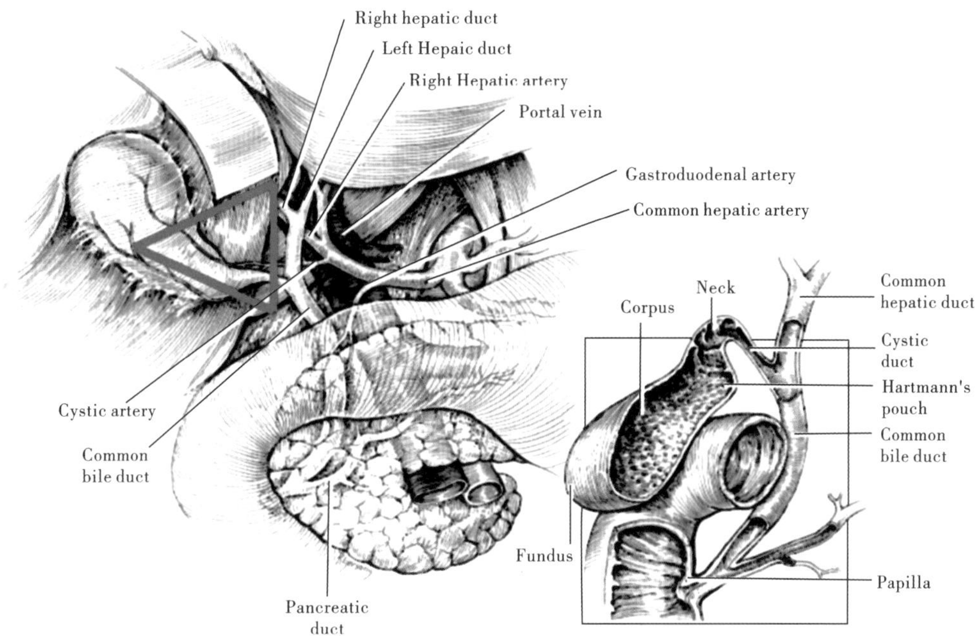

Figure 33-1-2 Extrahepatic biliary tract, Calot's triangle and sphincter of Oddi

1.1.5 Blood supply of the bile duct

The bile duct may be divided into three segments: hilar, supraduodenal, and retropancreatic. The blood supply of the supraduodenal duct is essentially axial. Most vessels to the supraduodenal duct arise from the superior pancreaticoduodenal artery, the right branch of the hepatic artery, the cystic artery, the gastroduodenal artery, and the retroduodenal artery. On average, eight small arteries measuring each about 0.3 mm in diameter supply the supraduodenal duct. The most important of these vessels run along the lateral borders of the duct and have been called the 3 o'clock and 9 o'clock arteries. The hilar ducts receive a copious supply of arterial blood from surrounding vessels, forming a rich network on the surface of the ducts in continuity with the plexus around the supraduodenal duct. The source of blood supply of the retropancreatic common bile duct is from the retroduodenal artery, which provides multiple small vessels running around the duct to form a mural plexus. The veins draining the bile ducts are satellites to the corresponding described arteries, draining into 3 o'clock and 9 o'clock veins along the borders of the common biliary channel. Veins draining the gallbladder empty into this venous system and not directly into the portal vein. The biliary tree seems to have its own portal venous pathway to the liver.

1.2 Biliary Tract Physiology

1.2.1 Bile composition and flow

Bile secretion has two major roles: ①To deliver bile acids to assist in the digestion of fats. ②To excrete certain substances, including bilirubin, specific drugs, and toxins. This multifunctional nature of bile secretion is reflected in the heterogeneous composition of bile itself. Approximately 1000 mL of bile is formed from the active secretion of organic and inorganic solutes into the canalicular space per day. The inorganic solutes(sodium, potassium, calcium, and bicarbonate) have a concentration in bile that is similar to plasma and account for the bile osmolality of approximately 300 mOsm/kg. The major organic solutes are bile acids, bilirubin, cholesterol, and phospholipids.

1.2.2 Bile salt

Bile salts, lecithin, and cholesterol comprise about 90% of the solids in bile, the remainder consisting of bilirubin, fatty acids, and inorganic salts. Gallbladder bile contains about 10% solids and has a bile salt concentration between 200 and 300 mmol/L. Bile salts are steroid molecules formed from cholesterol by hepatocytes. The rate of synthesis is under feedback control and can be increased to a maximum of about 20-fold. Two primary bile salts-cholate and chenodeoxycholate are produced by the liver. Before excretion into bile, they are conjugated with either glycine or taurine, which enhances water solubility. Intestinal bacteria alter these compounds to produce the secondary bile salts, deoxycholate and lithocholate. The former is reabsorbed and enters bile, but lithocholate is insoluble and is excreted in the stool. Bile is composed of 40% cholate, 40% chenodeoxycholate, and 20% deoxycholate, conjugated with glycine or taurine in a ratio of 3 : 1.

The functions of bile salts are①to induce the flow of bile, ②to transport lipids, and③to bind calcium ions in bile. In bile, they form multi-molecular aggregates called micelles in which the hydrophilic poles become aligned to face the aqueous medium. Water-insoluble lipids, such as cholesterol, can be dissolved within the hydrophobic centers of bile salt micelles. Molecules of lecithin, a water-insoluble but polar lipid, aggregate into hydrated bilayers that form vesicles in bile, and they also become incorporated into bile acid micelles to form mixed micelles.

Bile salts remain in the intestinal lumen throughout the jejunum, where they participate in fat digestion and absorption. Upon reaching the distal small bowel, they are reabsorbed by an active transport system located in the terminal 200 cm of ileum. Over 95% of bile salts arriving from the jejunum are transferred by this process into portal vein blood; the remainder enter the colon, where they are converted to secondary bile salts. The entire bile salt pool of 2.5-4 g circulates twice through the enterohepatic circulation during each meal, and 6-8 cycles are made each day(Figure 33-1-3). The normal daily loss of bile salts in the stool amounts to 10%-20% of the pool and is restored by hepatic synthesis.

1.2.3 Bilirubin

250-300 mg of bilirubin is excreted each day in the bile, 75% of it from breakdown of red cells in the reticuloendothelial system and 25% from turnover of hepatic heme and hemoproteins. First, heme is liberated from hemoglobin, and the iron and globin are removed for reuse by the organism. Biliverdin, the first pigment formed from heme, is reduced to unconjugated bilirubin, the indirect-reacting bilirubin of the van den Bergh test. Unconjugated bilirubin is insoluble in water and is transported in plasma bound to albumin.

Unconjugated bilirubin is extracted from blood by hepatocytes, where it is conjugated with glucuronic acid to form bilirubin diglucuronide, the water-soluble direct bilirubin. Conjugation is catalyzed by glucuronyl transferase, an enzyme on the endoplasmic reticulum. Bilirubin is transported within the hepatocyte by cytosolic binding proteins, which rapidly deliver the molecule to the canalicular membrane for active secretion into bile. Within bile, conjugated bilirubin is largely transported in association with mixed lipid micelles. After entering the intestine, bilirubin is reduced by intestinal bacteria to several compound known as urobilinogen, which are subsequently oxidized and converted to pigmented urobilins. The term urobilinogen is often used to refer to both urobilins and urobilinogen.

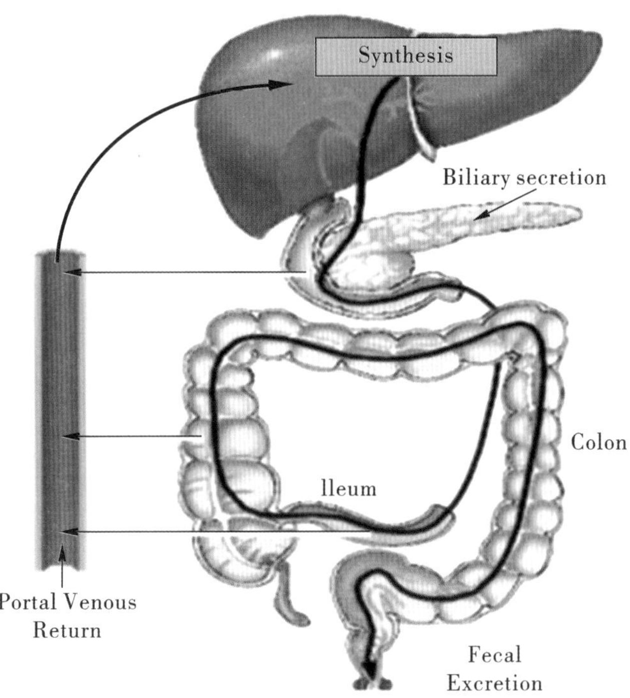

Figure 33-1-3 Enterohepatic circulation of bile salt

1.2.4 Physiology of gallbladder

The gallbladder concentrates hepatic bile by selective reabsorption of bile constituents. Sodium and chloride ions are absorbed from the gallbladder lumen by active and passive transport mechanisms. Water absorption is thought to be passive and secondary to active solute movement resulting from osmotic equilibration of transported solute within the epithelium. The secretion of water and electrolytes by the gallbladder mucosa is an active process, which can take place against hydrostatic and osmotic gradients.

During fasting, the normal gallbladder absorbs fluid at a rate corresponding to one third of the fasting gallbladder volume. After feeding, there is reversal of the direction of gallbladder transport from a net absorption to a net secretion into the gallbladder lumen. The net water transport across the gallbladder wall may be influenced by humoral factors and autonomic nerves (Figure 33-1-4). Anatomically, a prominent sphincter does not seem to be present in the cystic duct. A thin layer of smooth muscle is evident in the wall of the duct, however, and, along with the prominent mucosal folds that make up the valves of Heister, the cystic duct may act as a variable resistor to flow.

1.2.5 Physiology of common bile duct

The common bile duct does not have a primary propulsive function, the elastic fibers and the longitudinally orientated smooth muscle provide a tonic pressure, however, which may help overcome the tonic resistance of the sphincter of Oddi. The mechanism by which the sphincter of Oddi controls the flow of bile and pancreatic secretion has been clarified that have evaluated sphincter of Oddi function by sophisticated direct and indirect techniques.

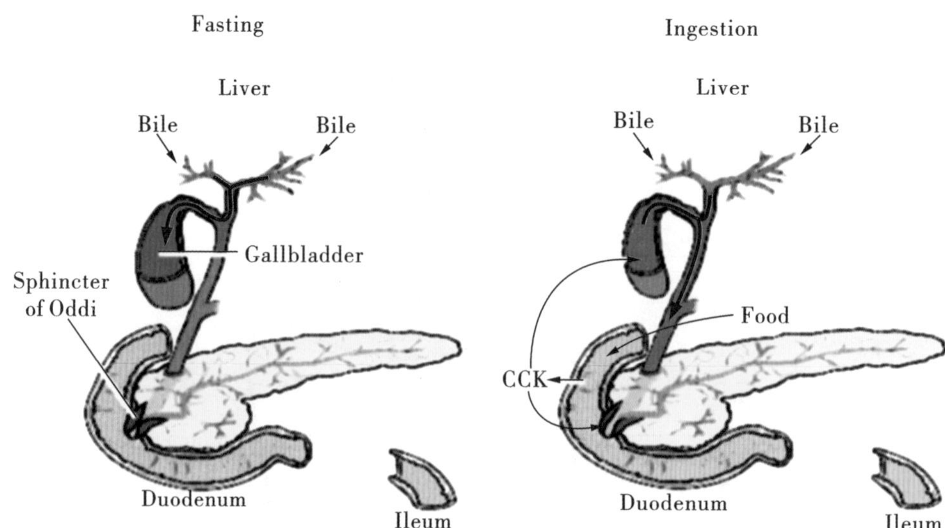

Figure 33-1-4 Storage and secretion of gallbladder bile into the intestine

Chapter 2

Special Examination of Bile System

Radiographic imaging of the biliary system and the biliary tree is commonly performed in most radiology departments. These studies include all radiology modalities especially computed tomography, magnetic resonance imaging, ultrasound, nuclear medicine, interventional procedures, and fluoroscopy imaging. In recent 20 years, with the development of radiology, imaging and ultrasound endoscopy, radiographic imaging of the biliary system offers the clinical physician many advanced diagnostic tools in the diagnosis of biliary tract disease.

2.1 Ultrasound

Transabdominal ultrasound is frequently the first imaging technique employed for patients presenting with biliary-type symptoms. Ultrasound is the ideal method for showing gallstones. They appear as strongly reflective foci with sharp acoustic shadowing (Figure 33-2-1). Unless impacted, they move rapidly with changes in posture. Demonstration of all of these features is almost totally reliable even in stones 1 mm in size. Gallstones can be differentiated from polyps, which are fixed in position, and gallbladder sludge, which is nonshadowing and moves slowly with positional variation. Ultrasound is useful for diagnosing acute cholecystitis. Gallstones in association with edema or gas in the gallbladder wall are the main findings in acute cholecystitis. Ultrasound offers the best prospect of early detection of gallbladder cancer because it is so widely used for the gallbladder-ultrasound technicians should have a low threshold for raising the possibility of gallbladder cancer whenever irregular thickening or focal masses are apparent, especially in patients older than age 60, even when no stones are present.

The sensitivity of ultrasound to dilation of the bile ducts makes it the technique of choice for the evaluation of jaundice. Nevertheless, the level of obstruction can be predicted accurately in approximately 80% of cases. Ultrasound often can determine the cause of obstruction. The demonstration of stones in the common bile duct depends on their size and position. Overall, ultrasound is reliable in the detection of biliary tree dilation and usually indicates the level of obstruction and should be the first imaging study for jaundiced patients. Demonstration of an obstructing stone, a bile duct tumor, or a pancreatic mass can inform further management. Ultrasound is also useful in other biliary disorders, including intrahepatic cholelithiasis, cholangiocarcinoma, choledochal cyst, etc.

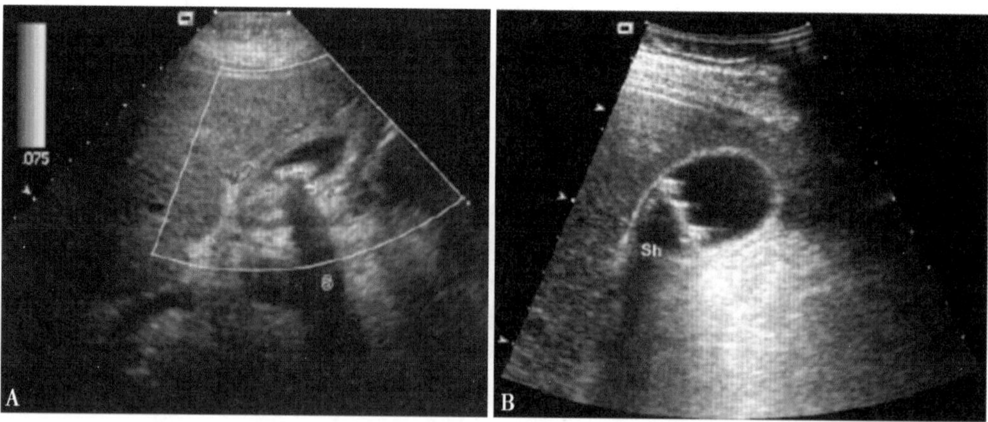

Figure 33-2-1 Gallstones

A. Echogenic foci in the gallbladder with acoustic shadowing; B. Multiple stones are layered in the dependent portion of the gallbladder, but the wall is not thickened. Sh, shadow.

2.2 Radiological Examination

2.2.1 X-ray examination

Abdominal plain film is of certain significance to the identification of biliary tract and other abdominal organs diseases, but the diagnostic value of simple abdominal plain film for biliary disease is limited (Figure 33-2-2). A few (15%) patients had higher calcium content in the gall stones, and the abdominal plain film showed the shadow of opaque stone in the hepatobiliary region. Biliary tract accumulation of air is suggestive of biliary tract and intestinal fistula or severe bacterial infection. The display part or the whole gallbladder is called porcelain gallbladder. The gas bubbles in the gallbladder wall suggest an infection of aerobe, which is called cholecystitis. Abdominal X-rays can also be used for other abdominal emergencies.

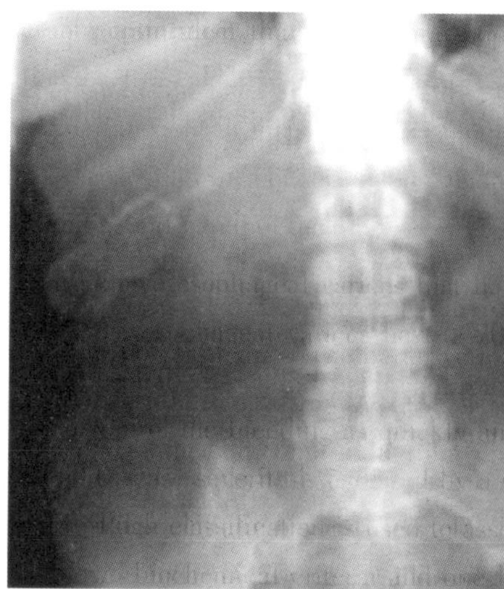

Figure 33-2-2 Abdominal plain film showing radio opaque stones in the gallbladder

2.2.2 Venous cholangiography

Venous cholangiography was injected with a slow intravenous injection of 30% biligrafin 20 mL, or 30% biligrafin 20 mL was dissolved in 10% glucose and 250 mL of slow intravenous drip. The contrast agent was secreted into the biliary tract by the liver, and the pathological changes of the bile duct were observed, such as stenosis, expansion, filling defect and so on. The development of this method is often unclear and affected by a variety of factors, and has been replaced by radionuclide cholangiography, direct cholangiography, and magnetic resonance cholangiography.

2.2.3 Computed tomography

Advances in technology have expanded the role of CT in evaluating the biliary tree. The ability to obtain high-resolution, thin-slice images in a single breath hold and the ability to view these images in cine mode are ideal for tracing the dilated bile ducts to the point of obstruction. Delineation of variant biliary anatomy is possible if the biliary tree is dilated. Additionally, the relationship of arteries to the bile ducts, information valuable for surgical planning, can be identified.

Computed tomography is not performed specifically to evaluate the gallbladder except when it is known that the gallbladder wall is diseased. CT can demonstrate some gallstones, and pancreatic disease. The specificity for biliary duct stones is low with CT, but CT can demonstrate some of them and associated acute and chronic pancreatitis. One of the advantages of CT is that the scan can help determine the type of gallstones (e. g. , cholesterol, pigmented), identify pathological dilation of the extrahepatic bile ducts, and can detect pancreatic cancer with 100% accuracy. While CT is not the imaging modality of choice for visualizing the biliary tree directly it is useful in diagnosing liver, gallbladder, and pancreatic disease. The sensitivity for identifying bile duct stones is low; however, in a few cases a stone in the bile ducts can be identified.

The CT imaging appearances of gallbladder carcinoma include a mass replacing the gallbladder (seen in 40%-65% of cases), focal or diffuse gallbladder wall thickening (seen in 20%-30% of cases), and an intraluminal polypoid mass (seen in 15%-25% of cases) (Figure 33-2-3). Additional imaging findings associated with gallbladder carcinoma reflect the pattern of disease spread.

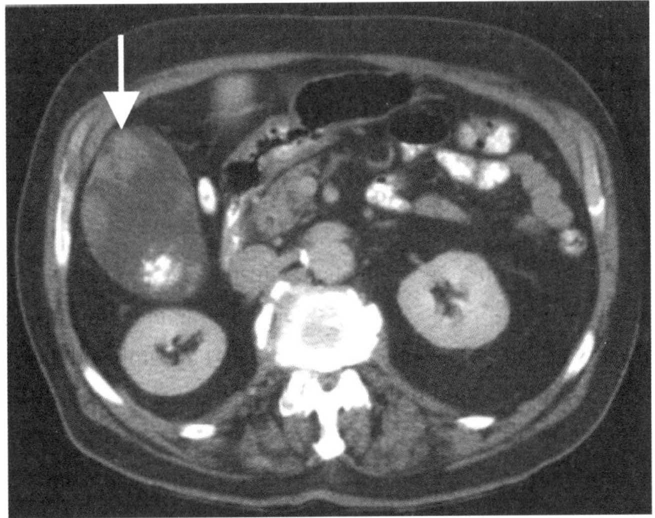

Figure 33-2-3 Gallbladder carcinoma

The gallbladder is distended and contains calcified stones. Nodular soft tissue emanates from the gallbladder wall into the lumen (arrow).

2.2.4 Precutaneous transhepatic cholangiography

Precutaneous transhepatic cholangiography(PTC)is both a diagnostic procedure in cases of suspected obstructive jaundice,and therapeutic in that dilated bile ducts could be drained during the procedure. Occasionally a stone could be removed by this procedure eliminating the risk of open surgical intervention. Today there are many other invasive procedures with lower risk than PTC. This study was a type of invasive cholangiography that involved direct puncture of the biliary ducts. A fine needle was passed from the skin surface through the liver into a biliary duct. Risk of the procedure included possible puncture of the lung, bleeding from the liver and vascular injury. This was not an easy procedure to perform so benefit of the procedure had to far outweigh its risk before it was performed.

2.2.5 Endoscopic retrograde cholangiopancreatography

The term endoscopic retrograde cholangiopancreatography(ERCP) refers to imaging the biliary ducts and pancreatic duct using a retrograde approach through an endoscope. ERCP is both a diagnostic tool and a therapeutic procedure for certain conditions. It is usually performed following other radiologic studies that are inconclusive(i. e. ,ultrasound or magnetic resonance cholangiopancreatography). ERCP provides direct opacification of bile ducts and pancreatic ducts,with success rates of 92% -97% ,and provides dynamic information during contrast medium introduction and drainage. It allows visual assessment of the duodenum and ampulla of Vater and enables biopsy and brushings,as well as interventional procedures such as sphincterotomy and stone extraction,biliary stenting and biliary stricture dilatation. Complication rates vary depending on the indication for the procedure,the presence of coexisting disease and the experience of the endoscopist,with severe complication rates of 0.9% -2.3% ,and total complication rates of 8.4% -11.1% ,the most common significant complication being acute pancreatitis. The main diagnostic pitfall with ERCP is the underfilling of ducts above a stricture.

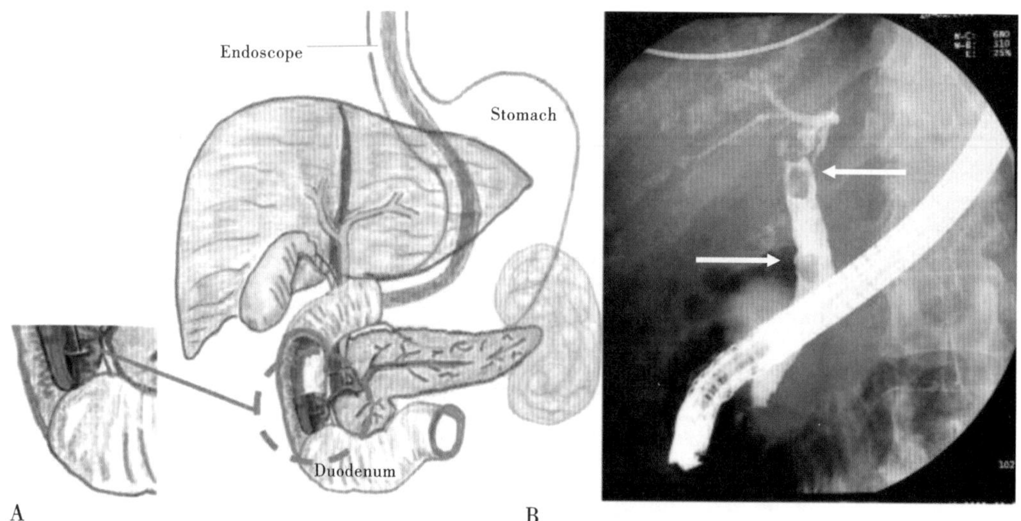

Figure 33-2-4 Diagnosis of choledocholithiasis

A. The schematic drawing of ERCP;B. an ERCP demonstrates stones in the common bile duct(arrows).

2.2.6 Intraoperative and postoperative cholangiography

The operative cholangiogram is also called the immediate cholangiogram because it is performed during cholecystectomy. It can be performed either before or after removal of the gallbladder. The cystic duct is tied off just proximal to the neck of the gallbladder and a catheter is inserted into the cystic duct near its joining the common hepatic duct. 6–10 mL of water soluble iodinated radiocontrast is injected. The surgeon is careful not to inject air since even a small quantity of air can mimic a radiolucent biliary stone. The entire biliary tree should be demonstrated with contrast spilling into the duodenum.

If the CBD has been explored at cholecystectomy a T–tube is usually left in place and cholangiography performed via this tube after about 7 days, prior to its removal. Cholangiography should confirm stone clearance and the free passage of contrast medium into the duodenum. Care must be taken to avoid the injection of air bubbles (Figure 33–2–5).

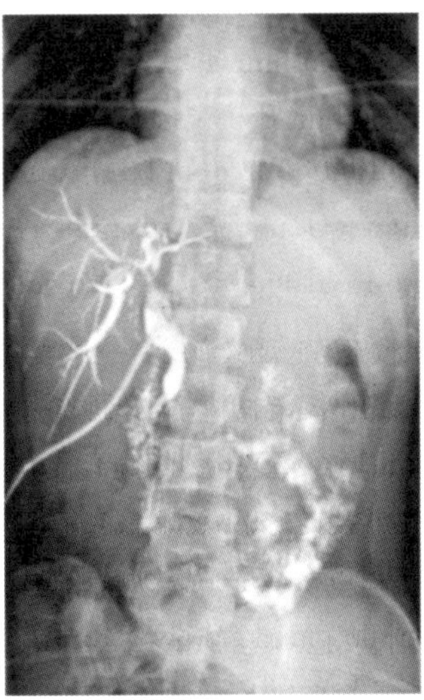

Figure 33–2–5 T–tube cholangiography

2.2.7 Hepatobiliary scintigraphy

Hepatobiliary iminodiacetic acid (HIDA) scintigraphy uses a derivative of iminodiacetic acid, a bilirubin analogue, labelled with 99mTc. It is injected intravenously and serial gamma camera images are obtained over 2–4 hours. It relies on near–normal bilirubin levels, although some agents can be excreted with moderate elevations of bilirubin. Serial image acquisitions show accumulation of the isotope in the liver, bile ducts, duodenum, small bowel and gallbladder (providing it is present and the cystic duct is patent).

2.2.8 Cholangioscopy

Cholangioscopy is a noninvasive endoscopic method used for both direct visual diagnostic evaluation and simultaneous therapeutic intervention of the bile ducts. A cholangioscope can be inserted into the bile duct directly during operation, percutaneously via the sinus tract of percutaneous transhepatic biliary drainage or via the duodenal papilla using a mother baby endoscope system. Cholangioscopy provides direct visual assessment of the bile ducts, tissue sampling, and therapeutic interventions. With the introduction of a sophisticated spyglass cholangioscope system for cholangiopancreatoscopy, most experts believe that peroral cholangioscopy will soon become a universally adopted technique for the evaluation and treatment of biliary tract diseases. It is a fact that most of cholangioscopy indications are to evaluate indeterminate biliary strictures. Currently, the established indication of cholangioscopy in therapeutic field is to treat difficult biliary stones, when associated with electrohydraulic lithotripsy (EHL) or laser lithotripsy (LL). Nevertheless, the indications continued to expand and several applications have been described, such as treatment of biliary strictures, lithotripsy of pancreatic duct stones, tumor ablation, gallbladder and biliary drainage, guidewire placement, foreign body removal, and the diagnosis and treatment of hemobilia.

2.2.9 MRI or magnetic resonance cholangiopancreatography

Magnetic resonance cholangiopancreatography (MRCP) has substantially replaced diagnostic PTC and ERCP. It relies on heavily T_2-weighted sequences that display stationary water as high signal. Multiplanar thin and thick section acquisitions are obtained using fast spin-echo techniques. Since conventional MRCP is not reliant on contrast excretion it is suitable for jaundiced patients.

More recently MR has been combined with hepatobiliary contrast agents. These agents, which include mangafodipir trisodium, gadobenate dimeglumine and gadoxetic acid disodium, shorten T_1 relaxation, providing positive contrast images on T_1-weighted sequences. Imaging is performed at least 30 minutes after IV infusion to allow hepatocyte uptake and biliary excretion. It therefore provides functional as well as anatomical information but, as with CT-IVC, depends on near-normal excretory hepatocyte function. Since T_1-weighted MR sequences are used it is possible to use near-isotropic three-dimensional gradient echo acquisitions. Contrast-enhanced MR cholangiography using hepatobiliary contrast agents has similar applications to CT-IVC, except that it is not as sensitive as conventional MRCP for the detection of choledocholithiasis.

Diagnostic pitfalls with MRCP include localised signal voids caused by surgical clips, and intraductal gas or blood. Bile flow voids may mimic small stones but the former are centrally placed and have less well-defined margins than stones. Acquisition times are longer for MRCP than CT-IVC and therefore more prone to motion artefacts (Figure 33-2-6).

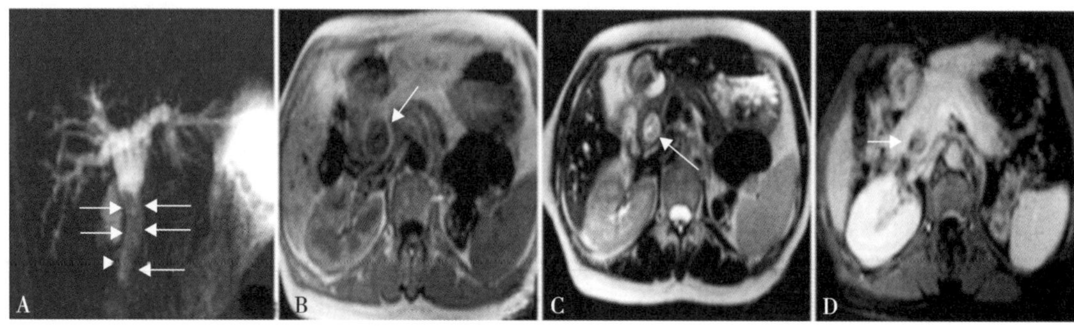

Figure 33-2-6 MRCP

The arrow shows choledocholithiasis.

2.2.10 Endoscopic ultrasound

EUS is a minimally invasive imaging modality that provides high-resolution images of the extrahepatic biliary tree and the surrounding structures. It has been shown to be accurate in the detection and staging of bile duct and gallbladder cancers and is especially useful for small tumors. Intraductal techniques, which are still in evolution, may provide even more information about the cause and extent of biliary strictures and mural tumors. EUS also has been shown to be useful for the detection of biliary stones and sludge when transabdominal ultrasound is not diagnostic. In many cases, diagnostic EUS can be followed immediately by therapeutic ERCP if needed. Although the instruments and techniques for endosonography continue to improve, at present EUS can be considered a promising minimally invasive tool for evaluating the biliary tree.

2.2.11 Positron emission computed tomography

Gallbladder cancer concentrates FDG avidly and hence appears to have a potential role in staging. FDG PET combined with diagnostic CECT helps in evaluation of the primary mass, evaluation of adjacent organ invasion, and detection of regional and nodal and peritoneal and distant metastases (Figure 33-2-7). Diagnostic accuracy of 18F-FDG PET/CT is 96% for the primary, 86% for lymph nodal metastases, and 96% for metastatic disease. 18F-FDG PET/CT has no advantage over conventional imaging modalities in diagnosis of CCA. In the detection of intrahepatic bile duct lesions, the sensitivity is in the range of 91%-95% and specificity ranging from 80 to 100%. The ability of FDG PET to detect cholangiocarcinoma also depends upon the pattern of growth of the lesion-whether mass-forming or infiltrative. PET has a lower sensitivity (SIV) (38%-43%) and greater specificity (SP) (95%-100%) in detection of involved nodes, as compared to CECT (SN 43%-54%, SP 59%-76%). PET is highly accurate for the detection of suspected as well as unsuspected distant metastases and leads to change in management in up to 30% of patients.

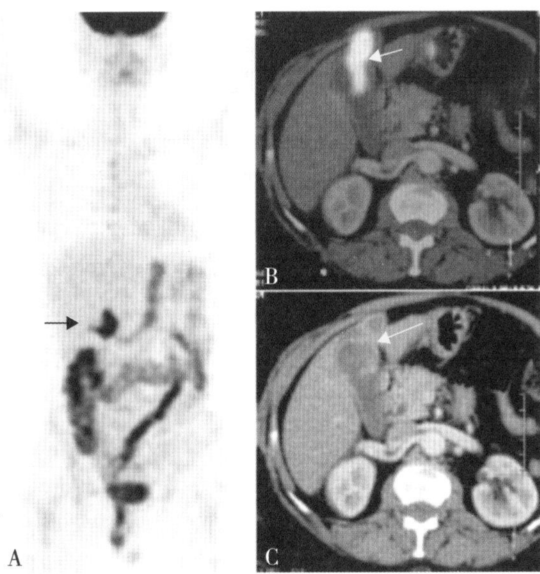

Figure 33-2-7 FDG PET-CT examination of gallbladder carcinoma

18 F-FDG PET/CT shows hyper-metabolic mass with max SUV 13.4 involving the fundus and body of the gall bladder (arrow in A-C). Histopathology post-radical cholecystectomy was adenocarcinoma of the GB.

Chapter 3

Biliarytract Malformation

3.1 Biliary Atresia

Biliary atresia, the most common condition causing obstructive jaundice in the first month of life, is defined as the atresia occurring in a whole or a part of the extrahepatic bile ducts which might lead to complete obstruction of bile flow. Biliary atresia was designated as a specific disease in 1892 and the first successful operation to correct the malformation was reported in 1928. In 1957, Kasai introduced a surgical method, hepatic portoenterostomy aiming to relieve biliary obstruction in infants considered to have uncorrected biliary atresia. Gradual confirmation of Kasai's operation was reported in the following years and it is accepted as the preferred treatment of uncorrected biliary atresia. Liver transplantation, especially reduced-size and living-related liver transplantation, provides new hope for infants who suffered from liver failure or not benefited from Kasai's operation.

3.1.1 Epidemiology

The incidence of biliary atresia is about 1 in 10 000–167 000 live birth. The ratio of male to female is 1 : (1.4–1.7). No racial differences or genetic predominance are related to the occurrence of biliary atresia. Associated malformations, such as polysplenia syndrome and congenital heart diseases were reported in about 11% of patients with biliary atresia.

3.1.2 Etiology

Biliary atresia is regarded as a development-related disorder which has not been proved scientifically. At 4 weeks of embryonic life, the biliary duct system originates from the hepatic diverticulum of the foregut and then differentiates to a caudal and cranial component. Common bile duct derives from the caudal component and proximal extrahepatic ducts derive from the cranial component. Any fault in ductal embryogenesis may lead to the failure of the extrahepatic biliary system to develop patency.

Other associated hypotheses, such as adverse environmental factors, bacteria or virus infection, reduced blood supply, anomalous bile acid metabolism, and pancreaticobiliary maljunction, have been suggested. However, all of these hypotheses need to be proved in further study.

3.1.3 Clinical classification

Biliary atresia can be classified into three categories. Type 1: atresia at the site of the common bile duct (11.9%). Type 2: atresia at the site of the hepatic duct (2.5%). Type 3: atresia at the site up to the porta hepatis (84.1%).

The subtypes according to the patterns of the distal ducts are as follows: ①patent common bile duct (20%). ②fibrous common bile duct (62%). ③aplasia of the common bile duct (15%). ④miscellaneous (3%).

The subgroups according to the patterns of hepatic radicles at the porta hepatis are as follows: ①dilated hepatic ducts (5%). ② hypoplastic hepatic ducts (6%). ③ bile lake (8%). ④ fibrous hepatic ducts (19%). ⑤fibrous mass (56%). ⑥aplasia of hepatic ducts (6%).

3.1.4 Clinical manifestations

The cardinal signs and symptoms are as follows: ① Jaundice: jaundice appears in some patients shortly after birth and persists in several weeks different from neonatal physiological jaundice fading fast within two weeks. ② Hepatomegaly: persisting obstruction of biliary ducts and difficulties of bile flow causes increase in liver size and formation of liver cirrhosis. ③ Clay-colored stools: meconium color is normal in most infant. The stools in the neonatal period are yellowish or light yellowish and clay-colored stools appear in the later period after birth. ④ Dark brown urine: increased serum bilirubin is excreted through urine. ⑤ Others: other presentations, including splenomegaly, esophageal variceal bleeding, anemia, malnutrition, and vitamins K deficiency, are also common in patients with biliary atresia.

3.1.5 Diagnosis

Jaundice infants with hepatomegaly, clay-colored stools, and dark brown urine should be suspected of biliary atresia. In addition to typical clinical characteristics, further investigations, including biochemical studies, needle biopsy of the liver, and assistant examinations are often needed.

Several valuable variants are as follows: ① Hyperbilirubinemia: conjugated bilirubin makes up more than 20% of the total fraction. ② Lipoprotein-X (Lp-X): results of a test for Lp-X are positive in patients with biliary atresia, however, results are also positive in 20% patients with neonatal hepatitis. ③ γ-glutamyl transpeptidase (γ-GTP): the levels of γ-GTP are also elevated in patients with biliary atresia. ④Duodenal fluid aspiration: it is an easy, rapid, cheap, and noninvasive method. Typical yellow bilirubin liquid is detected in duodenal fluid aspiration within 24 hours. ⑤ Hepatobiliary scintigraphy: technetium-labeled isopropyl phenyl alanine acid (DISIDA) is used to differentiate biliary atresia from other causes of cholestasis. Invisible technetium-labeled agent in intestine proves biliary atresia. ⑥ Ultrasonography: it is also a simple, inexpensive, and noninvasive method and should be used as the first step to identify the suspected infants. Morphology and patent of biliary ducts are easily demonstrated by ultrasonography.

3.1.6 Differential diagnosis

Biliary atresia needs to be differentiated from other causes of neonatal pathological jaundice, including neonatal hepatitis, cholestasis, metabolic diseases, hematologic problems, and genetic disorders.

3.1.7 Treatments

All of the patients with biliary atresia should be treated by surgery. Early diagnosis and timely operation is critical to delay liver failure. Besides general preparation for abdominal operation, vitamin K is given daily before operation(1 mg/kg of body weight) and broad-spectrum antibiotics are administrated, starting 36 hours before surgery. Blood transfusion preparation also needs to be completed.

Hepatic portoenterostomy(Kasai's procedure) is the standard surgery for treatment of biliary atresia. Fibrous messes at liver hilum are totally removed and the exposed area of the transected surface at the level of bifurcation of the portal vein is anastomosed to the hepatic branch of jejunum. Microscopic biliary ducts drain bile into the intestine and an auto approximation between the ductal and intestinal epithelium is performed.

Patients are given intravenous fluids with nasogastric drainage postoperatively. Oral feedings can be done when bowel activity is recovered. To prevent patients from cholangitis after surgery, broad-spectrum antibiotics are used routinely.

In addition to the common postoperative complications related to abdominal operation, cholangitis is the most common and serious complication after Kasai's procedure. It is thought to be due to several causes, including the reflux of intestinal contents toward the bile ducts, portal venous infection, and bacterial translocation. Suspected patients with the presence of fever, decreased quantity of bile, an increase in serum bilirubin levels, and a progressive deterioration of hepatic function should be considered as cholangitis. Intensiveuse of antibiotics and choleretics needs to be performed in patients suspected of cholangitis. Portal hypertension caused by hepatic fibrosis is a serious complication in patients with biliary atresia after Kasai's operation as well. The presence of upper or lower gastrointestinal bleeding and splenomegaly indicates the appearance of portal hypertension. Anomalies in the metabolism of fat, protein, and vitamins occur from time to time and they cause difficulties in weight gaining after surgery.

Despite patients with biliary atresia can benefit from Kasai's operation, most of them suffer from progressive deterioration of liver function and frequent occurrence of cholangitis. Liver transplantation therefore is the final hope for patients overcoming liver failure in biliary atresia. Living related liver transplantation (LRLT) resolves the problems of insufficient donors and contributes to improving patients' outcomes.

3.2 Choledochal Cyst

Choledochal cyst, or the common bile duct dilatation, was first reported by Douglas in 1852. The condition is a relatively rare abnormality with an estimated incidence in Western populations of 1 in 13,000-15,000. However, this condition is far more common in the East, with rates as high as 1 per 1,000 having been described in Japan. The etiology remains unknown, but choledochal cysts are likely to be congenital in nature. The pathologic features of the condition frequently include an anomalous junction of the pancreatic and common bile ducts(pancreaticobiliary malunion, PBMU), intrahepatic bile duct dilatation with or without downstream stenosis, and various degrees of hepatic fibrosis.

3.2.1 Etiology

A number of theories have been proposed for the etiology of the choledochal cyst. Congenital weakness of the bile duct wall, a primary abnormality of proliferation during embryologic ductal development and congenital obstruction has been given as possible causes. Unequal proliferation of epithelial cells of primitive bile ducts when they are still solid is postulated as a hypothesis. If cellular proliferation is more active than that of distal portion of the duct, canalization will give rise to an abnormally dilated proximal end. An obstructive factor in the early developmental stage was stressed as a causative factor. It is based on an experimental study in which cystic dilatation of the common bile duct was produced by ligation of the distal end of the common bile duct in the neonatal lamb, but not in a later stage of development.

In 1969, the so called "long common channel theory" was proposed as a new concept. This explained that PBMU allows reflux of pancreatic enzymes into the common bile duct, and this leads to dissolution of the ductal wall. This theory is in vogue and supported by the high amylase content in the aspirated fluid from the choledochal cyst. In addition, it is stated that the common bile duct could become obstructed at the distal end of the cyst due to edema or eventually fibrosis caused by refluxed pancreatic fluid. A diagnosis of choledochal cyst can be made antenatally as early as the 5th month of gestation, but at this time, fetal pancreas has not matured enough to produce functional enzymes, so the exact role of the pancreatic fluid is unclear. From research on human fetuses, it was demonstrated that the pancreaticobiliary ductal junction was outside the duodenal wall before the 8th week of gestation then moved inward toward the duodenal lumen, suggesting that PBMU may be caused by arrest of this migration. An anomalous pancreaticobiliary ductal junction (PBMU) combined with congenital stenosis are the basic causative factors of the choledochal cyst rather than weakness caused by reflux of the pancreatic fluid, at least in perinatal and young infants.

3.2.2 Pathology

The bile duct mucosa shows erosion, epithelial desquamation and papillary hyperplasia with regenerative atypia. Erosion, epithelial desquamation and dysplasia in the bile duct mucosa without carcinoma are frequently found in patients with choledochal cyst. Additionally, metaplastic changes, such as mucous cells, goblet cells and Paneth's cells, were observed. Such hyper plastic and metaplastic epithelia were apt to increase with age, and progress into dysplasia in adult cases, probably resulting in carcinogenic factors of the bile duct carcinoma.

The gallbladder mucosa in patients with PBMU shows cholecystitis, cholesterolosis, adenomyosis or adenomyomatosis, polyp including adenoma, and epithelial hyperplasia, which is particularly characteristic in PBMU.

Bile duct mucosa with FFCC shows non-specific changes such as mucosal ulceration/sloughing, fibrosis, and inflammatory cell infiltration, indicating that children with FFCC may be at a high risk for carcinogenesis in the extrahepatic bile duct. These changes are the same ones as seen in cystic or fusiform type choledochal cysts. The gallbladder mucosa showed diffuse epithelial hyperplasia characterized, with or without metaplasia of pyloric glands, goblet cells, and Paneth's cells.

Choledochal cysts are usually classified into three groups, based on anatomy. However, it can be classified into six types further based on the cholangiographic findings which associated with presence or absence of PBMU. Type Ⅰ, cystic dilatation of the extrahepatic bile duct; Type Ⅱ, fusiform dilatation of the extrahepatic bile duct; Type Ⅲ, forme fruste choledochal cyst without PBMU; Type Ⅳ, cystic diverticulum of the common bile duct; Type Ⅴ, choledochocele (diverticulum of the distal common bile duct); Type Ⅵ, intrahepatic bile duct dilatation alone (Caroli's disease). The majority is choledochal cysts with PBMU.

3.2.3 Diagnosis

3.2.3.1 Clinical manifestations

Choledochal cysts can present at any age, but more than half of patients within the first decade of life. Clinical manifestations of choledochal cysts differ according to the age of onset, but jaundice, abdominal mass and pain are the most common clinical characteristic symptoms.

In young infants, ranging neonates to 3 months old, the presence of obstructive jaundice, acholic stools and hepatomegaly, depending on the degree of obstruction, are the characteristic symptoms. These patients sometimes have advanced liver fibrosis. Another clinical presentation in young infants is a large upper abdominal mass without jaundice and abdominal pain due to pancreatitis. Choledochal cysts in adolescence and adulthood appear to behave differently.

Choledochal cysts undiagnosed for many years may ultimately lead to the development of cholelithiasis, liver cirrhosis, portal hypertension, hepatic abscess, and biliary carcinoma before cyst excision can be performed. Thus, surgery in this group is much more difficult than in children, and the incidence of postoperative complications is quite high even after primary cyst excision.

3.2.3.2 Ultrasonography

Currently abdominal ultrasonography is being used; this is probably the best screening method and should be applied first in patients who are suspected of having choledochal cyst. Furthermore, in recent years, the number of patients who are diagnosed by antenatal ultrasonography is increasing. This method also clearly demonstrates IHBD dilatation and the state of the liver parenchyma.

3.2.3.3 Radiological findings

For the diagnosis of choledochal cyst, it is important to detect not only dilatation of the extrahepatic bile duct, but also PBMU. ERCP can accurately visualize the configuration of the pancreaticobiliary ductal system in detail and is unlikely to be replaced by other investigations, especially in cases where fine detail is required presurgically. However, it is invasive and therefore unsuitable for repeated use and is contraindicated during acute pancreatitis. Percutaneous transhepatic drainage followed by cholangiography via the drainage tube is also valuable, especially for choledochal cyst with IHBD dilatation and severe jaundice. Intraoperative cholangiography is unnecessary if the entire biliary system has been delineated before cyst excision using the previously mentioned radiological investigations; however, it should not be omitted if the pancreaticobiliary ductal system is not visualized entirely. MRCP can provide excellent visualization of the pancreaticobiliary ducts in patients with CBD and allow detection of narrowing, dilatation, and filling defects with medium to high degrees of accuracy. MRCP is noninvasive and can partially replace ERCP as a diagnostic tool for the evaluation of anatomic anomalies of the pancreaticobiliary tract. Another advantage of MRCP over ERCP is that the pancreatic duct can be visualized upstream to an obstruction of the area of stenosis (Figure 33-3-1).

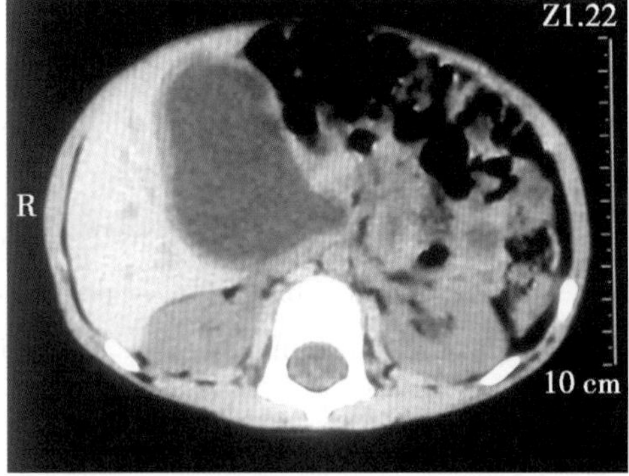

Figure 33-3-1 CT scan of choledochal cyst

3.2.4 Differential diagnosis

In prenatal period, the differential diagnosis of CBD is intra-abdominal cystic lesions, such as Type I biliary atresia, ovarian cyst, giant cystic meconium peritonitis, duplication cyst and mesenteric cyst. After birth, CBD can be differentiated by combinations of the imaging studies.

3.2.5 Management

Cyst excision is the definitive treatment of choice for choledochal cyst because of the high morbidity and high risk of carcinoma after internal drainage, a commonly used treatment in the past. Recently, more attention has been paid to treatment of intrahepatic and intrapancreatic ductal diseases such as IHBD dilatation with downstream stenosis, debris in the IHBD, and protein plugs or stones in the common channel. The transection level of the common hepatic duct and excisional level of the intrapancreatic bile duct are also highly controversial.

Operation should be performed when choledochal cyst diagnosed, but perfect pre-operative preparation should be done also, because the surgical procedure is complex. Cyst excision and Roux-en-Y hepaticojejunostomy is the treatment of choice in both children and adults with choledochal cyst.

The lesion should be resected completely and then the bile duct should be reconstructed. So the dilated CBD should be removed totally with cholecystectomy, for the biliary tract reconstruction, Roux-en-Y hepaticojejunostomy used most common. End-to-end anastomosis during Roux-en-Y hepaticojejunostomy is recommended to prevent elongation of the blind pouch. Mostly, an anti-reflux valve should be made on Roux-en-Y limb to prevent cholangitis after operation; we recommend an intussusception valve on Roux-en-Y limb to prevent cholangitis.

Chapter 4

Gallstones

4.1 Incidence

A gallstone is a stone formed within the gallbladder out of bile components, which produces the majority of surgical diseases of the gallbladder and bile ducts. The incidence of gallstones varies with different races, geographic locations, and dietary habits. In developed countries, 10% – 15% of adults have gallstones. Rates in many parts of Africa, however, are as low as 3%. Women more commonly have stones than men and they occur more commonly after the age of 40. A higher than normal incidence of gallstones occurs with pregnancy, diabetes, pancreatitis, cirrhosis, obesity, and hypothyroidism.

4.2 Gallstone Types

Gallstones are classified according to their chemical composition into cholesterol stones, mixed stones and pigment stones (Figure 33-4-1).

Cholesterol stones consist almost entirely of cholesterol and are often solitary (cholesterol solitary). Occasionally cholesterol stones present as a single, large, smooth, soft, yellow white stone containing almost pure cholesterol arranged in a radiating manner. Cholesterosis of the gallbladder is a specific pathologic entity in which many tiny plaques of cholesterol are present within heaped up mucosal folds in the gallbladder dotting its interior lining; since they resemble the seeds of a ripe strawberry, the term "strawberry gallbladder" is often used.

Pigment in bile is a result of bilirubin production. Pigment stones are multiple, soft, and black and resemble fine particles of sand. They are composed of bilirubin or biliverdin and may develop from antecedent cirrhosis, chronic hemolysis, or bile stasis with or without infection.

Mixed stones account for 90% of gallstones. Cholesterol is the major component. Other components include calcium bilirubinate, calcium phosphate, calcium carbonate, calciumpalmitate and proteins. Usually they are multiple, and they are often faceted.

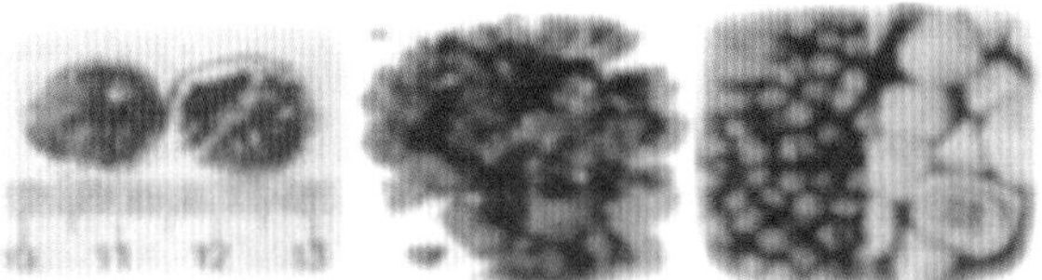

Figure 33-4-1 Three types of gallstones

4.3 Gall Bladder Stones

4.3.1 Pathogenesis

(1) Metabolic

Cholesterol, insoluble in water, is held in solution by a detergent action of bile salts and phospholipids with which it forms micelles. Bile containing cholesterol stones has an excess of cholesterol relative to bole salts and phospholipids, thus allowing crystals to form. Such bile is termed "supersaturated" or "lithogenic".

(2) Infection

The role of infection in causing stones is unclear. The bile from patients with gallstones is often sterile, but organisms have been cultured from the centers of gallstones, the radiolucent center of many gallstones may represent mucus plugs originally formed around bacteria. Helicobacter pylori antigens have been isolated within gallbladder containing stones.

(3) Bile stasis

Gallbladder contractility is reduced by oestrogens, in pregnancy and after truncal vagotomy, situations in which the incidence of gallstones is increased. Patients on long term parenteral nutrition have a high incidence of stones. Lack of good oral intake precludes the release of cholecystokinin, the hormonal stimulant of gallbladder contraction released from the duodenal mucosa.

4.3.2 Clinical manifestation and complications

(1) Silent gallstones (asymptomatic gallstones)

20% -40% of patients with gallbladder stones without symptoms or mild gastrointestinal symptoms. About 2% of patients with asymptomatic gallbladder stones develop symptoms, usually biliary colic is not one of the complications of gallstone disease. Patients with chronic colic tend to have symptoms of the same level of severity and frequency.

(2) Gastrointestinal symptoms

Most patients have a right upper abdominal pain after a meal especially fat meal with flatulent, belching and frequency.

(3) Colic pain

Biliary colic, the most characteristic symptom, is caused by transient gallstone obstruction of the cystic duct. The pain of biliary colic is usually steady, not intermittent, like that of intestinal colic. In some patient, attacks occur postprandially in others, there is no relationship to meals.

(4) Mirizzi syndrome

This syndrome is described as gallstones lodged in either the cystic duct or the Hartmann pouch of the gallbladder, which compress the common hepatic duct with or without fistulas, causing symptoms of obstructive jaundice and cholangitis. It can be divided into four types (Figure 33-4-2).

Type Ⅰ——No fistula present.

Type Ⅱ——Fistula present, defect smaller than 33% of the CBD diameter.

Type Ⅲ——Defect 33% - 66% of the CBD diameter.

Type Ⅳ——Defectlager than 66% of the CBD diameter.

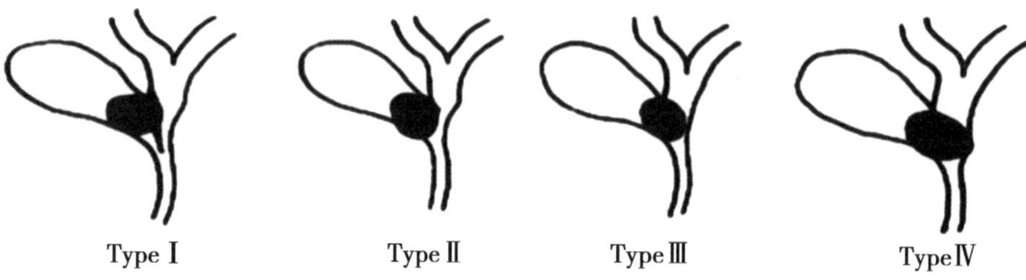

Figure 33-4-2 Mirizzi syndrome

(5) Gallbladder mucocele

Long standing obstruction to the outflow from the gallbladder results in overdistension of the gallbladder; occasionally, the gallbladder assumes massive proportions and the volume may be as much as 1.5 liters. The bile or bile pigment is slowly resorbed, and continuing secretion from the mucosa of the gallbladder results in clear and watery or mucoid content (white bile).

4.3.3 Diagnosis

The essential symptoms: Epsodic abdominal pain, dyspepsia.

Ultrasound: An ultrasound scan of the gallbladder should usually be the first test. Gallstones can be demonstrated in about 95% of cases, and a positive reading for gallstones is almost never in error.

CT, MRCP, but notroutine.

4.3.4 Treatment

Cholecystectomy is the first choice for treating patients with symptomatic gallbladder stone and complications. The presence of either of the following portends a more serious course and should probably serve as a reason for prophylactic cholecystectomy: ①Large stones (> 2-3 cm in diameter), because they produce acute cholecystitis more often than small stones. ②A porcelain gallbladder, because it is often associated with carcinoma. ③A gallbladder without contractive function. ④Gallbladder polyps>1 cm in diameter or gallbladder wall >3 mm. ⑤Patients with controlled diabetes and coexistent cardiopulmonary or other problems increase the risk of surgery, operation should be performed during the relief period after acute onset.

(1) Indications for choledochotomy

The traditional indications for choledochotomy are as follows: ① palpable duct stones; ② there is jaundice or a history of jaundice or cholangitis; ③the common bile duct is dilated more than 1 cm; ④choledocholithiasis is proved or suspected preoperatively.

(2) Laparoscopic cholecystectomy

The advantage of laparoscopic cholecystectomy (LC) over other therapies for gallstone diseases are multiple (Table 33-4-1).

Table 33-4-1 Advantages and disadvantages of laparoscopic cholecystectomy compared to open cholecystectomy

Advantages	Disadvantages
Less pain	Lack of depth perception
Smaller incisions	View controlled by camera operator
Better cosmesis	More difficult to control hemorrhage
Shorter hospitalization	Decreased tactile discrimination
Earlier return to full activity	Potential CO_2 insufflation complications
Decreased total costs	Adhesions/inflammation limit use
	Sight increase in bile duct injuries

4.4 Extrahepatic Bile Duct Stones

4.4.1 Pathology

The extrahepatic bile duct stones consist of secondary stones and primary stones.

The evidence suggests that most cholesterol stones develop within the gallbladder and reach the duct after traversing the cystic duct. These are called secondary stones. Pigment stones may have a similar pedigree or more often, develop de novo within the common duct. These are called primary common duct stones.

①Obstruction of common bile duct: the obstruction is usually intermittent with dilatation and thickness of bile duct, bile stasis, and secondary infection. ② Secondary infection: congestion and edema of common bile duct aggravate obstruction and cause obstructive suppurative cholangitis and sepsis. Hemobilia may occur due to ulceration and perforation of bile duct. ③Compromised liver function, necrotic liver cells and intrahepatic abscesses can be caused by obstruction and infection. ④ Common bile duct stones impacted within the distal duct at the ampulla of Vater may produce biliary pancreatitis.

4.4.2 Clinical manifestation

Choledocholithiasis may be asymtomatic or may produce sudden toxic cholangitis, leading to a rapid demise. The seriousness of the disease parallels the degree of obstruction, the length of time it has been present, and the extent of secondary bacterial infection. Classical symptoms are biliary colic, intermittent chills and fever, and jaundice (Charcot's triad). Nausea and vomiting, not part of Charcot's triad, are the only other frequent symptoms.

(1) Abdominal pain: Biliary colic from common duct obstruction can not be distinguished from that caused by stones in the gallbladder. The pain is felt in the right subcostal region, epigastrium, or even the substernal area and referred pain to the region of the right scapula is common, which is caused by spasm of Oddi's sphincter.

(2) Chills and fever: The most frequent symptom is chills and fever, which is intermittent and present in about 2/3. The temperature may reach to 39-40℃.

(3) Jaundice: During total obstruction, the stool is acholic or only lightly pigmented and the urine is dark.

(4) Physical examination: Deep subcostal tenderness, percussion pain on the liver and rebound pain may present. Enlarged gallbladder may be palpable.

(5) Laboratory: The work up of the jaundiced patient should include evaluation of the stool for bilirubin and the urine for urobilinogen and bilirubin. The serum bilirubin is elevated, mainly the direct fraction, as well as the serum alkaline phosphatase. In cholangitis, leukocytosis of 15,000/μL is usual, and values above 20 000/μL are common. Mild increase in AST, ALT, ALP and GGT is often seen with extrahepatic obstruction of the ducts; rarely, AST levels transiently reach 1000 units.

(6) Imaging studies: Plain abdominal radiography and CT may reveal a radiopaque stone. Ultrasound scans will usually show gallbladder stones and, depending on the degree of obstruction, dilatation of the bile duct. ERCP is indicated if the patients have had a previous cholecystectomy. If cholecystectomy has not been performed, cholangiography should be part of operative management. Preoperative ERCP would rarely be indicated in a patient scheduled for cholecystectomy. MRCP is useful for patients with extrahepatic obstruction.

4.4.3 Differential diagnosis

Biliary colic should be differential from renal colic and enteric colic. Obstructive jaundice should be differential from pancreatic head cancer or ampulla cancer.

4.4.4 Treatment

4.4.4.1 Antibiotics

Patients with cholangitis should be treated with systemic antibiotics and other measures as described in the preceding section; this usually controls the attack within 24–28 hours.

4.4.4.2 Surgical treatment

The principle of surgical treatments are removing gallbladder stones completely, relieving bile duct stricture and obstruction and keeping bile drainage free.

(1) Cholangiotomy and T tube drainage

When the common duct is explored through a choledochotomy (either during a laparoscopic or open operation), a T tube is usually left in the duct, and cholangiograms must be taken 2 weeks or so postoperatively before being removed. Any residual stones discovered on these postoperative X–rays can be extracted 4–6 weeks later through the T tube tract.

(2) Cholangiojejunostomy

A biliary enteric anastomosis should be done if the patient has had a previous common duct exploration or stricture in distal common bile duct (Figure 33–4–3).

(3) Endoscopic sphincterotomy

Patients with common duct stones who have had a previous cholecystectomy are best treated by endoscopic sphincterotomy. Using a side viewing duodenoscope, the ampulla is cannulated, and a 1 cm incision is made in the sphincter with an electrocautery wire. The opening created in the sphincter permits stones to pass from the duct into the duodenum. Endoscopic sphincterotomy is unlikely to be successful in patients with large stones (e. g., >2 cm).

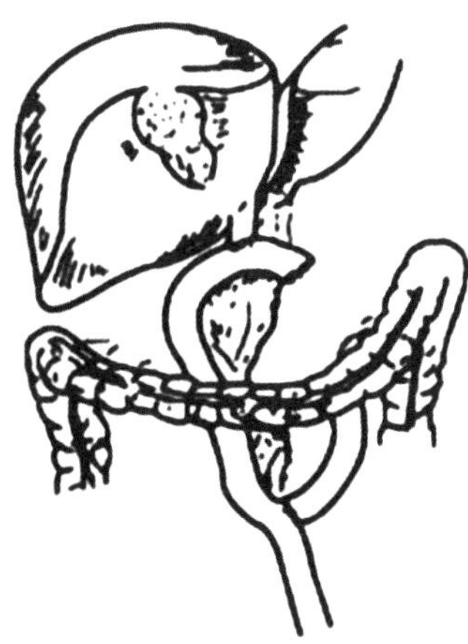

Figure 33-4-3 Roux-en-Y cholangiojejunostomy

4.5 Intrahepatic Bile Duct Stone

Most occurs in left lateral and right posterior segments. Commonly complicated with extrahepatic bile duct stone. Except for pathological change of extrahepatic duct stone, the pathology of intrahepatic bile duct stone includes stricture of intrahepatic duct, cholangitis and carcinoma of intrahepatic duct.

4.5.1 Clinical manifestation

The symptoms are similar to the extrahepatic duct stone if complicated with exrtahepatic stone. The patients may have malaise in liver area, flatulent. Painand fever may be present during acute onset. When both sides of bile ducts obstructed, the patients may have jaundice. Biliary hepatic abscesses occur in patients complicated with infection. For elderly patients with long history, frequent onset of cholangitis, jaundice, fever and weight loss, hepatobiliary carcinoma should be considered.

Laboratory: AST and ALT may increase. If CA19-9 or CEA increase, we should think about carcinoma of intrahepatic duct.

4.5.2 Physical examination

The main clinical signs include local enlargement of the liver, tenderness and percussion pain.

4.5.3 Treatment

Stones in the intrahepatic branches of the bileduct can usually be removed without difficulty during common duct exploration. In some cases, however one or more of the intrahepatic ducts have become packed with stones, and the associated chronic inflammation has produced stenosis of the duct near its junction with the common hepatic duct. It is often impossible in these cases to clear the duct of stones, and if the disease involves only one lobe (usually the left lobe), hepatic lobectomy is indicated. Cholangiojejunostomy also can adapt to hepatolithiasis.

Chapter 5

Acute Cholecystitis

Acute cholecystitis is acute chemical and(or) bacterial inflammation of gallbladder resulting from any blockage of the cystic duct, which is prevalent in women. Symptoms include right upperabdominal pain, nausea, vomiting, and occasionally fever. The differentiation of biliary colic from acute cholecystitis is unresolved blockage of the cystic duct. In biliary colic, the obstruction is temporary and self-limited. In acute cholecystitis, the obstruction does not resolve, and inflammation ensues, with edema and subserosal hemorrhage. Without resolution of the obstruction, the gallbladder will progress to ischemia and necrosis. Eventually, acute cholecystitis becomes acute gangrenous cholecystitis and, when complicated by infection with a gas-forming organism, acute emphysematous cholecystitis. Complications of acute cholecystitis include gallstone pancreatitis, common bile duct stones, or inflammation of the common bile duct.

5.1 Etiology

5.1.1 Acute calculous cholecystitis

Gallstones blocking the flow of bile consist of 90% cases of cholecystitis. Blockage of bile flow leads to an enlarged and tense gallbladder(Figure 33-5-1). The gallbladder becomes infected by bacteria especially from gastrointestinal tract, predominantly E. coli, Klebsiella, Streptococcus, and Clostridium species. Inflammation can spread to the outer covering of the gallbladder and surrounding structures such as the diaphragm, causing referred right shoulder pain.

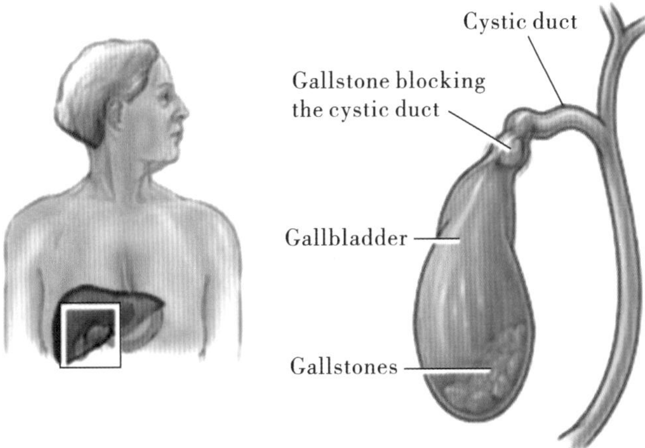

Figure 33-5-1 Nosogenesis of acute calculous cholecystitis: gallstone blocking the cystic duct

5.1.2 Acute acalculous cholecystitis

Acalculous cholecystitis, in which no stone is in the biliary tree. It accounts for 5%-10% of all cases of cholecystitis and is typically seen in people who are hospitalized and critically ill. So these patients are always associated with high morbidity and mortality rates. Males are more likely to develop acute cholecystitis following surgery in the absence of trauma. It is associated with many causes including vasculitis, chemotherapy, major trauma or burns.

5.2 Clinical Manifestation

5.2.1 Acute calculous cholecystitis

The inflammatory changes in the gallbladder manifest as fever, right upper quadrant pain, tenderness to palpation, and guarding in the right upper quadrant. This process will cause an arrest of inspiration with gentle pressure under the right costal margin, a maneuver known as Murphy's sign. Tenderness and a positive Murphy's sign help to distinguish acute cholecystitis from biliary colic, in which there is no inflammatory process. Given that the common bile duct is not obstructed, profound jaundice is uncommon in acute cholecystitis and if it happened the diagnosis of cholangitis or Mirizzi syndrome is under consideration.

5.2.2 Acute acalculous cholecystitis

The presentation of acalculous cholecystitis is similar to calculous cholecystitis, with fever, anorexia, and right upper quadrant pain. Patients are more likely to have yellowing of the skin (jaundice) than in calculous cholecystitis. Because many of these patients are critically ill, history may be impossible to obtain and the physical examination may be unreliable. The workup of fever in the intensive care patient may reveal a thickened gallbladder wall, with pericholecystic fluid.

5.3 Diagnosis

The diagnosis of cholecystitis is suggested by the accurate history(abdominal pain, nausea, vomiting, fever) and physical examinations, along with supporting laboratory and ultrasonographic testing.

5.3.1 Blood tests

In someone suspected of having cholecystitis, blood tests are performed for markers of inflammation (e.g., leucocyte count, C-reactive protein), as well as bilirubin levels in order to assess for bile duct blockage. Leucocyte count typically shows an increased white blood count(12,000-15,000/μL). C-reactive protein is usually elevated although not commonly measured. Bilirubin levels are often mildly elevated (1-4 mg/dL). If bilirubin levels are more significantly elevated, alternate or additional diagnoses should be considered such as gallstone blocking the common bile duct. Less commonly, blood aminotransferases are elevated. The degree of elevation of these laboratory values may depend on the degree of inflammation of the gallbladder.

5.3.2 Imaging

Transabdominal ultrasonography is a sensitive, inexpensive, and reliable tool for the diagnosis of acute cholecystitis, with a sensitivity of 85% and specificity of 95%. Ultrasound findings suggestive of acute cholecystitis include gallstones(Figure 33-5-2), fluid surrounding the gallbladder, gallbladder wall thickening (wall thickness over 3 mm. Figure 33-5-3), dilation of the bile duct, and sonographic Murphy's sign. Given its higher sensitivity, hepatic iminodiacetic acid(HIDA) scan can be used if ultrasound is not diagnostic. CT scan may also be used if complications such as perforation or gangrene are suspected, but CT is less sensitive than ultrasound for the diagnosis of acute cholecystitis.

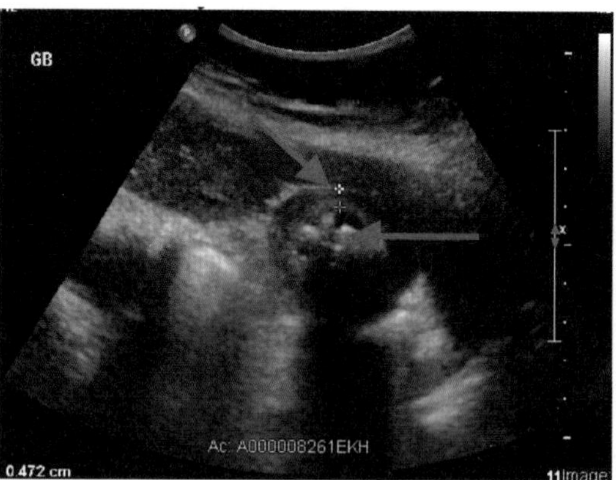

Figure 33-5-2 Acute cholecystitis as seen on ultrasound

The closed arrow points to gallbladder wall thickening. Open arrow points to stones in the gallbladder.

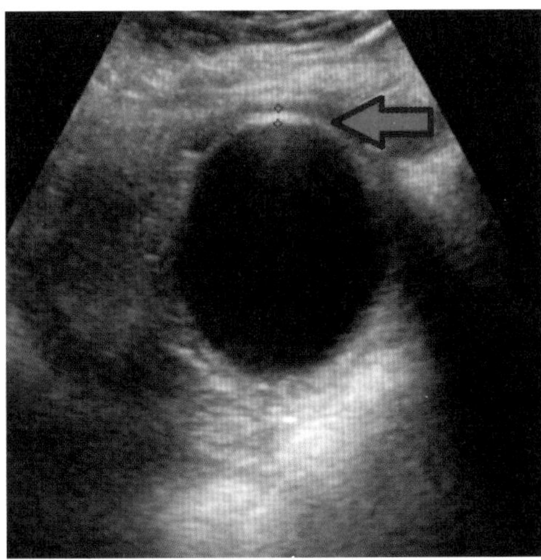

Figure 33-5-3 Mild gallbladder wall thickening of 3.5 mm in a person with acute cholecystitis as seen on ultrasound

5.3.3 Differential diagnoses

Many other diagnoses have similar symptoms as cholecystitis. Additionally the symptoms of chronic cholecystitis are commonly vague and can be mistaken for other diseases. These alternative diagnoses include but are not limited to the following:

- Acute peptic ulcer exacerbation.
- Acute pancreatitis.
- Pneumonia.
- Myocardial ischemia.
- Hiatal hernia.
- Biliary colic.
- Choledocholithiasis.
- Cholangitis.
- Appendicitis.
- Colitis.
- Kidney stone.

5.4 Complications

A number of complications may occur from cholecystitis if not detected early or properly treated. Signs of complications include high fever, shock and jaundice. Complications include the following:

- Gangrene.
- Gallbladder rupture.
- Empyema.
- Fistula formation and gallstone ileus.
- Adenomyomatosis.

5.5 Treatment

5.5.1 Acute calculous cholecystitis

Although infection following stasis and inflammation, most cases of acute cholecystitis are complicated by superinfection of the inflamed gallbladder. Therefore, patients are given nothing by mouth, intravenous injection fluids and parenteral antibiotics are started. Given that gram-negative aerobes are the most common organisms found in acute cholecystitis, followed by anaerobes and gram-positive aerobes, broad-spectrum antibiotics are warranted. Parenteral narcotics are usually required to control the pain. Cholecystectomy, whether open or laparoscopic, is the treatment of choice for acute cholecystitis. The timing of operative intervention in acute cholecystitis has long been a source of debate. Many surgeons advocated for delayed cholecystectomy, with patients managed nonoperatively during their initial hospitalization and discharged home with resolution of symptoms. An interval cholecystectomy was then performed at approximately 6 weeks following the initial episode. Given the inflammatory process occurring in the porta hepatis, early conversion to open cholecystectomy should be considered when delineation of anatomy is not clear or when progress cannot be made laparoscopically. With substantial inflammation, a partial cholecystectomy, transecting the gallbladder at the infundibulum with cauterization of the remaining mucosa, is acceptable to avoid injury to the common bile duct. Some patients present with acute cholecystitis but have a prohibitively high operative risk. For these patients, a percutaneously placed cholecystostomy tube should be considered. Frequently performed using ultrasound guidance under local anesthesia with some sedation, cholecystostomy can act as a temporizing measure by draining the infected bile. Percutaneous drainage allows improvement in symptoms and physiology, allowing for a delayed cholecystectomy, 3-6 months after medical optimization.

5.5.2 Acute acalculous cholecystitis

Treatment of acalculous cholecystitis is similar to that of calculous cholecystitis, with cholecystectomy being therapeutic. Given the substantial inflammation and high risk of gallbladder gangrene, an open procedure is generally preferred. However, many of these patients are critically ill and would not tolerate the process of a laparotomy. Accordingly, percutaneous drainage of the distended and inflamed gallbladder is carried out in patients unable to tolerate a laparotomy. The cholecystostomy tube used to drain the gallbladder can be placed by ultrasound or CT guidance. Approximately 90% of patients will improve with percutaneous drainage, and the tube can eventually be removed. If follow-up imaging continues to demonstrate no stones, interval cholecystectomy is generally unnecessary.

Part 34

Pancreas Disease

Chapter 1

Anatomy and Physiology

1.1 Anatomy

The pancreas lies within the retroperitoneum in the upper abdomen, lying in front of the second lumbar vertebra and ending in the splenic hilum. The gland can be divided into four portions head, neck, body, and tail. The head of the pancreas is intimately adherent to the medial portion of the duodenum and lies in front of the inferior vena cava and superior mesenteric vessels. A small tongue of the tissue called the uncinate process lies behind the superior mesenteric vessels. The stomach and the first portion of the duodenum lie partly in front of the pancreas. The common bile duct passes through a posterior groove in the head of the pancreas adjacent to the duodenum. Diseases in the head of the gland can obstruct the common bile duct and duodenum, giving rise to obstructive jaundice and vomiting. The neck of the pancreas overlies the portal vein, which may be invaded by carcinoma, rendering such a lesion unresectable. The body of the pancreas is in contact posteriorly with the aorta, the left adrenal gland, and the left kidney. The body overlies the vertebral column, and in blunt abdominal trauma, the pancreas can be crushed. The tail of the pancreas lies in the hilum of the spleen and can be injured during splenectomy. The blood supply of the pancreas is derived from branches of the celiac and superior mesenteric arteries. The superior pancreaticoduodenal artery arises from the gastroduodenal artery, runs parallel to the duodenum, and eventually meets the inferior pancreaticoduodenal artery, a branch of the superior mesenteric artery, to form an arcade. The splenic artery provides tributaries that supply the body and tail of the pancreas. The main branches are termed the dorsal pancreatic magna, and caudal pancreatic arteries. The venous drainage of the pancreas corresponds with the arterial anatomy. Veins draining the pancreatic parenchyma eventually terminate in the portal vein, which arises posterior to the neck of the pancreas by the union of the splenic and superior mesenteric veins. Multiple lymph node groups drain the pancreas. From the head of the gland, nodes in the pancreaticoduodenal groove communicate with subpyloric, portal, mesocolic, mesenteric, and aortocaval nodes. Lymphatic vessels in the body and tail of the pancreas drain to retroperitoneal nodes in the splenic hilum or celiac, aortocavel, mesocolic, or mesenteric nodes.

A dual sympathetic and parasympathetic innervation subserves the pancreas. Preganlionic axons arise from cell bodies within the thoracic sympathetic ganglia and travel as the splanchnic nerves to terminate within the celiac ganglia. From these structures, postganglionic sympathetic fibers traverse retroperitoneal tissue to innervate the pancreas and serve as the principal pathways for pain of pancreatic origin. This sympathetic pathway is the target during splanchnicectomy for the relief of pain of pancreatic origin. The parasympathetic innervation of the pancreas commences with preganglionic fiber cell bodies that reside within the vagal nuclei, the axons of which terminate in parasympathetic ganglia within the pancreatic parenchyma. Postganglionic parasympathetic fibers then traverse a short course to innervate the pancreatic islets, acini, and ducts, and they serve an exclusively efferent function.

The main pancreatic duct(the duct of Wirsung, 2–3 mm in diameter) courses along thih the gland from the tail to the head and joins the common bile duct just before entering the duodenum at the ampulla of Vater(85%). The opening of the pancreatic duct in some patients is separated into the duodenum from the common bile duct. The accessory pancreatic duct(the duct of Santorini) enters the duodenum 2–2.5 cm proximal to the Vater.

1.2 Physiology

1.2.1 Exocrine function

The external secretion of the pancreas consists of a clear, alkaline(pH 7.0–8.3) solution of 750–1000 mL/d containing digestive enzymes. Secretion is stimulated by the hormones Secretin and cholecystokinin(CCK) and by parasympathetic vagal discharge. Secretin and CCK are synthesized, store, and released from duodenal cells in response to specific stimuli. The acid in the duodenablumen causes the release of secretin, and luminal digestions products of fat and protein cause the release of CCK.

Pancreatic enzymes are synthesized, stored(as zymogen granules), and released by the acinar cells of the gland, principally in response to CCK and vagal stimulation. Pancreatic enzymes are proteolytic, lipolytic, and amylolytic. Lipase and amylase are stored and secreted in active forms. The proteolytic enzymes are secreted as inactive precursors and activated by the duodenal enzyme enterokinase. Other enzymes secreted by pancreas include ribonucleases and phospholipase A.

1.2.2 Endocrine function

The best known endocrine function of the pancreas involves glucose homeostasis. Insulin decreases glycogenolysis, lipolysis, proteolysis, gluconeogenesis, ureagenesis, and ketogenesis. Insulin secretion is stimulated by rising or high serum concentrations of metabolic substrates such as glucose, amino acids, and perhaps short-chain fatty acids. Insulin release is also stimulated by glucagons, secretin, CCK, vasoactive intestinal polypeptide(VIP), and gastrin.

Glucagon(29 amino acids) release is stimulated by blood glusose reduction in serum glucose. Gallstone causes hyperglycemia by promoting liver glycogenolysis and gluconeogenesis from proteins. Other effects of glucagons included inhibition of gastric acid secretion, inhibition of gastrointestinal motility, and stimulation of choleresis and triglyceride lipolysis.

Somatostatin release is stimulated by a meal, vagus, bombesin, CCK, gastrin, and secretin. Somatostatin has a broad spectrum of gastrointestinal activity, including inhibition of gastric acid and pepsin secretion, inhibition of pancreatic exocrine secretion, and inhibition of gastrointestinal motor activity, as well as reduction of gastrointestinal blood flow.

The pancreatic polypeptide, gastrin, and VIP are produced by the islet cells.

Chapter 2

Acute Pancreatitis

Acute pancreatitis is one of five acute abdomen (acute pancreatitis, acute appendicitis, intestinal obstruction, perforated gatroduodenal ulcer and cholecystitis or cholelithiasis). Acute pancreatitis is not only a local inflammation of pancreas but also a systemic disease involving multiple organs.

2.1 Etiology

Most cases of pancreatitis are caused by gallstone disease, alcoholism or hyperlipidemia, a few results form hypercalcemia, trauma, and genetic predisposition and the remainder are idiopathic.

2.1.1 Obstructive factors

The most common cause of obstruction is biliary stone. 40% –60% of cases of pancreatitis are associated with gallstone disease, which, if untreated, usually gives rise to additional acute attacks. Gallstone migrates through the ampulla of Vater, causing diversion of bile into the pancreatic duct and subsequently bile induced pancreatic parenchymal injury. Gallstone associated pancreatitis is related to the anatomic existence of a common channel between the pancreatic and bile ducts, and it occurs in the setting of gallstone migration through the ampullary region. Other factors include biliary ascariasis, edema of duodenal ampulla, spasm of ampulla sphincter, neoplasm and stricture of ampulla.

2.1.2 Alcoholic pancreatitis

Alcohol stimulates gastric acid secretion which increases CCK–PZ (cholecystokinin and pancreazymin) excretion in duodenum and then pancreatic secretion. Alcohol is a known stimulant of gastric acid secretion, and the resultant duodenal acidification is a stimulus for the increases release of secretin, which increases the exocrine secretion of pancreatic fluid and bicarbonate. Alcohol increases the resistance of the sphincter of Oddi at the ampulla of Vater, thereby causing partial obstruction to the flow of pancreatic exocrine secretion. Secondly, alcohol may initiate enzyme extravasation and cause pancreatic injury as a result of protein obstruction of the pancreatic duct. Thirdly, alcohol induces the intermediate state of hypertriglyceridemia. The toxic levels of free fatty acids, produced from the lipolysis of triglycerides, may induce pancreatic injury by causing acinar cell or capillary endothelial cell injury. Fourthly, injury generated by oxygen derived free radicals is one of the mechanisms.

2.1.3 Hyperlipidemia

In patients with primary hyperlipidemia, pancreatitis seems to be a direct consequence of the metabolie abnormality. Hyperlipidemia may occur secondary to nephritis, castration, or exogenous estrogen administration, or it may occur as hereditary hype lipidemia (FredRick Types 1 and 5), notable for hypertriglyceridemia and chylomicronemia.

2.1.4 Hypercalcemia

Hypercalcemia is associated with acute pancreatitis, generally rising as a result of hyperparathyroidism. The mechanism of hypercalcemia related pancreatitis may involve caleium induced trypsinogen activation, with subsequent parenchymal autodestruction, calcium associated stone precipitation in the pancreatic duct causing ductal obstruction, or calcium stimulated pancreatic exocrine hypersecretion.

2.1.5 Trauma

Acute pancreatitis may also occur after pancreatic trauma, i. e., penetrating or blunt external trauma, intraoperative manipulation, or ampullary and pancreatic ductal overdistention during retrograde pancreatography.

2.1.6 Others

Drugs are probably responsible for more cases of acute pancreatitis than is generally suspected. The most commonly incriminated drugs are corticosteroids, estrogen containing contraceptives, azathioprine, thiazide diuretics, and tetracyclines. Pancreatitis associated with use of estrogens is usually the result of drug induced hypertriglyceridemia.

Acute pancreatitis can also be caused by viral infections, e. g., hepatitis virus, parotitis virus and typhoid bacillus.

In about 15% of patients there is no identifiable cause of the condition, i. e., idiopathic pancreatitis.

Operation and endoscopy (iatrogenic pancreatitis): most cases of postoperative pancrcatitis follow common bile duct exploration, especially if sphincterotomy was performed. Two practices, now largely abandoned, were often responsible: ①Use of a common duct T tube with a long arm passing through of sphincter of Oddi; ②Dilation of the sphincter to 5-7 mm during common duct exploration.

2.2 Pathogenesis

Pancreatitis due to enzymatic digestion of the gland is supported by the finding of proteolytic enzymes in drainage fluid and increased amounts of phopholipase A and lysolecithin in pancreatic tissue from patients with acute pancreatitis. Phospholipase A, in the presence of small amounts of bile salts, attacks free phospholipids (e. g., lecithin) and those bound in cellular membranes to produce extremely potent lyso compounds. Lysolecithin, which would result from the action of phospholipase A on biliary lecithin, or phospholipase A itself, plus bile salts, is capable of producing severe necrotizing pancreatitis. Trypsin is important in this scheme, because small amounts are needed to activate phospholipase A from its inactive precursor.

Elastase, which is both elastolytic and proteolytic, is secreted in an inactive form. Because it can digest the walls of blood vessels, elastase has been thought to be important in the pathogenesis of hemorrhagic pancreatitis.

Enzymatic digestion (autodigestion): The resultant local tissue injury is mediated by numerous enzymes. Trypsin not only destroys tissue but also activates other destructive enzymes such as elastase and lecithinase. Vasoactive substances including kinins, kallikrein, and histamine lead to cardiovascular dysfunction and collapse.

MODS (principally ARDS, myocardial depression, renal insufficiency, and gastric stress ulceration) may occur because of ischemia, inflammatory mediators and SIRS.

2.3 Pathology

2.3.1 Edematous pancreatitis

The pancreas represents local or diffused edema with congestion, and becomes enlargement, and hard. Microscopically, it shows acinic and interstitial edema, infiltrated with inflammatory cells with small hemorrhage and small foci of necrosis.

2.3.2 Hemorrhagic and necrotic pancreatitis

Pancreatic hemorrhage and necrosis are the characteristics of this stage. Swollen, soft-black pancreas with unclear structure is appeared. Bloody ascites, fat necrosis with saponifying patches in omentum, mesentery, retroperitoneal areas are also the feature. Microscopically, hemorrhagic pancreatitis is characterized by bleeding into the parenchyma and surrounding retroperitoneal structures and extensive pancreatic necrosis.

In both forms, the peritoneal surfaces may be studded with small calcifications representing areas of fat necrosis.

2.4 Clinical Manifestation

2.4.1 Abdominal pain

The acute attack begins following a large meal and consist of severe epigastric pain that radiates through to the back, persistent with vomiting and retching.

When inflammation is located in the head of pancreas, the patient may only have right upper abdominal pain, which radiates to right shoulder; in the tail, left upper abdominal pain and radiating to left shoulder may occur. Generalized nonlocalized abdominal pain may also be observed. In patients with alcohol associated pancreatitis, pain often commences between 12 and 48 hours after an episode of inebriation. In contrast, patients with gallstone pancreatitis typically experience the onset of pain after a large meal.

Nausea and vomiting frequently accompany the abdominal pain. The vomiting may be severe and protracted. Vomitus is usually gastrointestinal content, sometimes with coffee like. The pain can not be relieved after vomiting.

2.4.2 Abdominal distention

Abdominal distention may be the result of a paralytic ileus arising from retroperitoneal irritation or may occur secondary to a retroperitoneal phlegmon and large amount of ascites. Decreased or absent bowel sounds, silent abdomen, and failure to pass gas or feces.

2.4.3 Peritoneal irritation

Tenderness, rebound pain, rigidity, guarding.

2.4.4 Systemic symptoms

Most patients have increased temperature without chilling, except for completing with acute cholangitis. Patients with severe pancreatitis may manifest major circulatory derangements such as hypotension, hypovolemia, hypoperfusion and shock.

2.4.5 Bleeding

Severe pancreatitis associated with hemorrhage into the retroperitoneum may produce two distinctive physical signs: Turner's sign (bluish discoloration in the flank) and Cullen's sign (bluish discoloration in the periumbilical region). These physical signs are results of the tracking of blood stained retroperitoneal fluid through the tissue planes of the abdominal wall to the flank or along the falciform ligament to the umbilical area. These signs signal the presence of a severe episode of acute hemorrhagic pancreatitis, with an overall mortality that may exceed 30%.

Gastrointestinal bleeding leads to hematemesis and melena.

2.5 Laboratory Studies

2.5.1 Amylase

The determination of serum amylase is the most widely used laboratory test in the diagnosis of acute pancreatitis. In most cases, hyperamylasemia is observed within 24 hours of the onset of symptoms, and the value of serum amylase markedly increases more than 500 U/dL (normal range 40 – 180 U/dL, Somogyi test), with gradual return to normal during the subsequent 7 days.

The measurement of urinary amylase (normal value 80 – 300 U/dL, Somogyi test) excretion has also been proposed as a sensitive index of the disease. Urinary amylase elevations persist for a longer period of time than serum elevations, with the magnitude of urinary elevations frequently surpassing the magnitude of serum elevations.

2.5.2 Serum lipase

The elevation of serum lipase (normal value 23–300 U/L) is a more accurate indicator of acute pancreatitis than is the elevation of serum amylase, because lipase is solely of pancreatic origin.

2.5.3 Additional tests

Hematologic evaluation may reveal hemoconcentration from third space fluid sequestration. An elevated white blood cell count above 10,000 cells/μL is typical. Serum chemistries often reveal hyperglycemia, abnormalities of liver function tests, and hypocalcemia. Hyperglycemia appears to be the result of relative hypoinsulinemia and relative hyperglucagonemia, and it is associated with the degranulation of beta cells. Mild azotemia is related to fluid sequestration, resultant hypovolemia, and diminished cardiac output. Hypocalcemia is the consequence of dilutional hypoalbuminemia, calcium deposition in areas fat necrosis, and resistance of skeletal bone to parathyroid hormone stimulation.

Diagnostic paracentesis is occasionally utilized to confirm the diagnosis of acute pancreatitis. Elevations in peritoneal fluid amylase and lipase may be found in settings where their respective serum levels are normal. However, diagnostic paracentesis is not an ideal test for the confirmation of the diagnosis of acute pancreatitis due to its invasive nature, its potential for complications, and the lack of complete specificity of peritoneal fluid enzyme elevations for acute pancreatits.

2.6 Imaging Study

2.6.1 X-ray

Chest film findings supportive of the diagnosis of acute pancreatitis, but not specific for the disease, include left basal atelectasis, elevation of the left hemidiaphragm, and left pleural effusion, which reflect the presence of a significant peridiaphragmatic, retroperitoneal inflammation.

Abdominal radiographs reveal nonspecific abnormalities in the majority of patients. Most frequently seen on the abdominal plain film is the presence of air in the duodenal loop, representing a local duodenal ileus secondary to the adjacent inflammatory reaction in the head of the gland. Also common is the abnormality referred to as therainage loop sign, representing a dilated proximal raina loop localized to the upper abdomen, adjacent to the pancreatic bed. The colon cutoff sign may also be observed, indicative of distention of the colon to the level of the transverse colon, with little to no air being present in the splenic flexure and more distal colon. Abdominal film reveals gallstones in the gallbladder, pancreatic calcification, and obliteration of the psoas margin secondary to retroperitoneal edema.

2.6.2 Sonography

Abdominal sonography may be used to detect pancreatic edema and acute peripancreatic fluid collections. In addition, in patients with suspected gallstone associated pancreatitis, the gallbladder can be assessed for gallstones, and the common bile duct can be evaluated for size and the presence of stones.

2.6.3 CT scanning

CT is the most widely accepted and sensitive method used to confirm the diagnosis of acute pancreatitis. Pancreatic changes include diffuse or focal parenchymal enlargement, edema, or necrosis with liquefaction. Peripancreatic changes include blurring or thickening of the surrounding tissue planes and the presence of fluid collections. An approximate correlation exists between the degree of CT abnormality and the clinical course and severity of the acute pancreatitis. CT is useful for the demonstration of structural complications, such as pancreatic abscess, pseudocyst, or necrosis.

2.7 Diagnosis

Acute pancreatitis is often suspected on the basis of clinical presentation, with the diagnosis supported by appropriate laboratory determinations and radiographic findings.

2.8 Clinical Classifications

Acute pancreatitis can be divided into three major categories including mild acute pancreatitis(MAP), moderately severed acute pancreatitis(MSAP) and severe acute pancreatitis(SAP). The diagnostic criteria are as follows:

MAP: No local or systemic complications, no organ failure. MAP accounts for 60%-80% of acute pancreatitis and the mortality rate of MAP is extremely low.

MSAP: Accompanied by local or systemic complications, MSAP may be associated with a transient organ failure(recoverable within 48 h). MSAP accounts for 10%-30% of acute pancreatitis and the mortality was under 5%.

SAP: With one or multiple organ failure(lasting more than 48 hours), SAP accounts for 5%-10% of acute pancreatitis, and the mortality rate is as high as 30%-50%.

2.9 Complications

The local complications include pancreatic necrosis, peripancreatic abscess and pseudocyst.

2.10 Differential Diagnosis

Acute pancreatitis should be differentiated from cholecystitis, peptic ulcer perforation, acute abdominal obstruction, renal colic, acute gastroenteritis and coronary disease.

2.11 Treatment

2.11.1 Medical treatment

The goals of medical therapy are reduction of pancreatic secretory stimuli and correction of fluid and electrolyte derangements.

(1) Gastric suction and diet control

Oral intake is withheld, and a nasogastric tube is inserted to aspirate gastric secretions, although the latter has no specific therapeutic effect.

(2) Fluid replacement and preventing shock

Patients with acute pancreatitis sepuester fluid in the retroperitoneum, and large volumes of intravenous fluids are necessary to maintain circulating blood volume, electrolyte balancc and renal function. In severe hemorrhagic pancreatitis, blood transfusions may also be required.

(3) Spasmolytic and painkiller

Abdominal pain is treated with careful administration of narcotic analgesics accompanied with spasmolytic. Morphine is avoided because of its potential for causing sphincter of Oddi spasm, an entity that could theoretically potentiate ongoing pancreatic parenchymal injury.

(4) Pancreatic exocrine secretion suppression

Therapeutic attempts to suppress pancreatic enzyme secretion have included nasogastric suction, histamine H_2 receptor antagonists, antacids, anticholinergics, glucagons, calcitonin, somatostatin and cholecystokinin receptor antagonists such as proglumide. Somatostatin is a potent inhibitor of ncreatic exocrine secretion and gastric acid output.

(5) Nutrition

Total parenteral nutrition avoids pancreatic stimulation and should be used for nutritional support in any severely ill patient who will be unable to eat for more than 1 week.

(6) Antibiotics

Prophylacitic broad spectrum antibiotics are often used in patients with severe pancreatitis to reduce bacterial translocation, local complications and systemic sepsis.

(7) Elimination of toxic intrapetitoneal contents

Toxic intraperitoneal compounds exudated from acute pancreatitis mediate many adverse systemic effects such as hypotension, pulmonary failure, hepatic failure, and altered vascular permeability. Peritoneal lavage may be of benefit in reducing the early systemic complications of severe pancreatitis.

2.11.2 Surgical treatment

Operative intervention in patients with acute pancreatitis is indicated in four specific circumstance: ① Uncertainty of diagnosis; ②Treatment of secondary pancreatic infections; ③Correction of associated biliary tract disease. ④Progressive clinical deterioration despite optimal supportive care.

(1) Treatment of secondary pancreatic infections

Treatment of secondary pancreatic infections combines antibiotic therapy with prompt drainage. The management of infected pancreatic necrosis and abscesses are as follows: ①Laparotomy with debridement and wide sump drainage. ②Laparotomy with debridement and open packing. In either case, the anterior transperitoneal approach to the abdomen is used to facilitate exposure. The gastrocolic omentum is divided, and the retroperitoneum is debrided of devitalized tissues. Anatomic resection is usually avoided. The peripancreatic region is copiously irrigated with saline and topical antibiotic solutions. Subsequently, wide sump drainage of the retroperitoneum or open packing is instituted. The wide sump drainage technique allows fascial closure of the abdomen and places multiple large bore drains in dependent positions to drain the infected areas. ③Patients with abscesses or infected pseudocysts may be managed via percutaneous drainage techniques.

(2) Management of biliary pancreatitis

Treatment option for operative intervention in patients with gallstone associated pancreatitis involves early surgical intervention within the first 72 hours after the onset of the disease. The rationale for such early intervention is that early elimination of ampullary struction by a common duct calculus can theoretically reduce the severity of the episode of pancreatitis ERCP can be used to retrieve choleocholithiasis, and impacted ampullary stones.

2-4 weeks are allowed to elapse between hospitalization for acute pancreatitis and admission for definitive biliary tract surgery.

Chapter 3

Chronic Pancreatitis

3.1 Etiology

Chronic pancreatitis is a clinical entity that includes recurrent or persistent abdominal pain and evidence of exocrine and endocrine pancreatic insufficiency. The most common cause of chronic pancreatitis in industrialized countries is alcohol abuse while biliary disease is a predominant reason in China. In underdeveloped or developing countries, chronic pancreatitis appears to be related to nutritional deficiencies or toxin ingestion. In patients with hyperparathyroidism, the associated hypercalcemia is responsible for chronic pancreatitis, possibly due to overstimulation of the gland's exocrine and precipitate of protein aggregates in the main pancreatic duct system. Acute pancreatitis may play a role in the development of chronic pancreatitis. In some patients with idiopathic chronic pancreatitis, the etiology of the disease is unknown.

3.2 Pathology

Pathologic findings in chronic pancreatitis include evidence of acinar loss, glandular shrinkage, proliferative fibrosis, calcification, and ductal structuring. Electron microscopic findings in chronic pancreatitis reveal evidence of dense collagen and fibroblastic proliferation in the parenchyma: this fibroproliferative response separates large clusters of islet cells with normal or nearly normal ultrastructural features.

3.3 Clinical Manifestation

Abdominal pain is the feature that prompts consultation. The pain is commonly epigastric in location but may be localized to the right or left side of the midline. Radiation of the pain to the back is common. Some patients have continuous pain, whereas others have recurrent episodes of pain that entirely resolve between attacks.

Anorexia and weight loss may be present. Insulin-dependent diabetes mellitus occurs in up to 1/3 of patients. Up to one quarter have steatorrhea, indicative of a major reduction in pancreatic exocrine function. Abdominal pain, weight loss, diabetes, and steatorrhea serve as a classical presentation in patients with chronic pancreatitis.

3.4 Diagnosis

Chronic pancreatitis is usually suspected on clinical findings. Routine laboratory tests are rarely helpful. Radiographic evaluation may reveal pancreatic calcifications on plain abdominal films.

A CT scan of the abdomen is useful in the evaluation of both parenchymal and ductal disease. The size texture of the gland is evaluated and inspected for pancreatic parenchymal calcifications, nodularity, and inhomogeneous densities, as well as pseudocyst formation and dilation of the pancreatic ductal system. Important information is gained by the use of ERCP.

Characteristic early changes in chronic pancreatitis observed via ERCP include ductal dilatation and filling of secondary and tertiary branches, which ordinarily are not visualized. Patients with well established chronic pancreatitis demonstrate ductal strictures and calculi and often show pseudocyst formation.

3.5 Treatment

3.5.1 Nonoperative management

Three areas are encompassed in the nonoperative management of chronic pancreatitis: control of abdominal pain, treatment of endocrine insufficiency, and treatment of exocrine insufficiency.

①The control of abdominal pain can be a major problem, and it is generally the sole indication for operative intervention. ②In the typical setting of alcohol-related chronic pancreatitis, total abstinence from alcohol is mandatory for nonoperative pain relief and is successful in some patients. Dietary manipulation, including small volume, frequent, low-fat meal, is recommended. High dosage regimens of exogenous pancreatic enzyme supplements, which theoretically decrease pancreatic secretion and thereby reduce pain, have had variable outcomes. ③Exogenous insulin therapy in patients with chronic pancreatitis associated diabetes must be used cautiously; one must attempt to control glycosuria and avoid hypoglycemia.

3.5.2 Surgical treatment

The primary goal of operative management is the relief of pain, the secondary consideration being to preserve maximal endocrine and exocrine function. Surgical treatment of chronic pancreatitis can be broadly categorized into three groups; ampullary procedures, ductal drainage procedures, and ablative procedures.

Celiac plexus block: It may be used to obtain relief. Thoracoscopic splanchnicectomy resection of segments of the greater and lesser splanchnic nerves as they enter the thorax from the abdomen has been used.

Chapter 4

Carcinoma of the Pancreas

Cancer of the pancreas is more common in smokers than in nonsmokers, more common in males than in females, and appears to be linked to the presence of diabetes mellitus. Cancer of the pancreas is possibly linked to both a history of previous chronic pancreatitis and the ingestion of a high fat diet. A small percentage of patients appear to have an inherited or familial form of pancreatic cancer.

4.1 Pathology

Over 90% of malignant pancreatic tumors are classified as duct cell adenocarcinomas. The most common site of origin of duct cell adenocarcinomas is the pancreatic head, where 2/3 of the cases are localized. Subtypes of duct cell adenocarcinoma include mucinous and adenosquamous varieties. Less common types of pancreatic cancer include cystadenocarcinoma and acinar cell carcinoma. Recent studies have identified recurrent chromosome abnormalities in pancreatic adenocarcinoma, which can provide clues to the specific genes involved in the pathogenesis of this tumor.

Metastasis and spread are mainly from lymphatic metastasis and direct invasion.

4.2 Diagnosis

4.2.1 Clinical manifestation

The most common clinical features in patients with pancreatic carcinoma are jaundice, weight loss, and abdominal pain.

(1) About 75% of patients with carcinoma of the head of the pancreas present with abdominal pain, generally reflected as a dull, aching pain in the mid epigastrium or the right upper quadrant, with possible radiation to the back. Back pain occurs in 25% of patients and is associated with a worse prognosis.

(2) Approximately three quarters of patients present with jaundice. Hepatomegaly and a palpable gallbladder may also be noted.

(3) Weight loss, faint and cachexia.

(4) Alimentary symptoms include poor appetite, anorexia, dyspepsia diarrhea or constipation, nausea and vomiting if invasion to duodenum or stomach.

(5) Others: Fever, mass, ascites. Some patients may present with symptoms of diabetes mellitus.

4.2.2 Laboratory tests

The majority of patients have laboratory abnormalities marked by increased amylase, blood sugar, positive sugar tolerance test, increased ALP, bilirubin, and transaminase if there is hepatic metastasis or CBD obstruction. Serologic markers for pancreatic carcinoma have been evaluated, including CEA, CA19-9, and pancreatic carcinoma associated antigen (PCAA). The levels are elevated in most patients with pancreatic cancer and also in other gastrointestinal cancers. No currently available serologic test is completely accurate for diagnosis. At present, CA 19-9 is used most frequently to assist in diagnosis and follow-up.

4.2.3 Imaging study

In patients with suspected pancreatic carcinoma, radiologic intervention is extremely important for diagnosis, staging, and management.

(1) Barium upper gastrointestinal series may be positive in patients with large tumors, showing widening of the duodenal sweep or the inverted "3" sign.

(2) Sonography is a useful screening examination, who are more likely to have cholestatic jaundice.

(3) CT scanning is an essential procedure for the evaluation of pancreatic neoplasms. Dynamic, thin section, contrast enhanced CT scanning allows visualization of the entire pancreas, without distortion from overlying bowel gas, and it provides better accuracy in detecting hepatic metastases, determining the size of the pancreatic neoplasm, and locally staging the tumor.

(4) MRI or MRCP: MRI appears to offer no advantage over CT. Magnetic resonance cholangiopancreatography which has the ability to image the bile duct and pancreatic duct without the need for instillation of contrast and the attendant risks of endoscopic cannulation.

(5) ERCP is particularly valuable in the diagnosis of duodenal or ampullary carcinoma, and may also be useful in cases of partial biliary obstruction, where the endoscopically injected contrast can fill the proximal biliary anatomy for subsequent biliary enteric reconstruction. Biliary stent may be placed at the time of ERCP as a short or long term maneuver to palliate biliary obstruction and allow for reduction in the degree of jaundice.

Endoscopic ultrasound has been applied to the staging of pancreatic neoplasm, with early results in skilled hands appearing to be comparable to those obtained with CT and angiography.

(6) Percutaneous transhepatic cholangialrainage (PTCD) can visualize the biliary tree through injected contrast. In the setting of an obstructing pancreatic neoplasm is generally combined with catheter drainage of the biliary tree via the percutaneous transhepatic route.

4.3 Treatment

The majority of patients presenting with pancreatic neoplasms are operative candidates and are treated surgically. In a minority of patients, nonoperative therapy may be appropriated.

4.3.1 Operative therapy

Pancreatic resection for pancreatic cancer is appropriate only if all gross tumor can be removed with a standard resection.

(1) Pancreaticoduodenectomy

For curable lesions of the head, Pancreaticoduodenectomy is required. This involves resection of the common bile duct, the gallbladder, entire duodenum, head of pancreas to the level of the superior mesenteric vein, pylorus, and distal stomach. Restoration of gastrointestinal tract continuity utilizes the proximal jejunum brought through the transverse mesocolon for pancreaticojejunostomy, hepaticojejunostomy, and gastrojejunostomy.

In last ten years, the utility of minimally invasive procedure in pancreatic surgery has been gradually rising. There has been growing interest in performing pancreatectomy by the laparoscopic approach.

(2) Palliative surgery

Palliative surgery for pancreatic carcinoma is performed in patients with unresectable disease or in patients with prohibitive risk for resection. Palliative surgical treatment seeks to alleviate biliary obstruction, duodenal obstruction, and tumor associated pain.

4.3.2 Adjuvant therapy

After procedure, standard of adjuvant therapy includes chemotherapy or chemoradiation.

Chapter 5

Insulinoma

The most common endocrine tumor of the pancreas is the insulinoma. Insulinoma is associated with whipple's triad, which consists of symptoms of hypoglycemia at fasting, documentation of blood glucose levels of less than 2.8 mmol/L, and relief of symptoms following administration of glucose.

The symptoms can be categorized into two groups: hypoglycemia induced catecholamine surge symptoms (shaking, irritability, weakness, diaphoresis, tachycardia, and hunger) and neuroglycopenic symptoms (personality change, confusion, obtundation, seizure, and coma). Typically, the relief of symptoms is achieved by the condumption of carbohydrate rich foods.

5.1 Laboratory Study

The most reliable method for diagnosing insulinomas involves a monitored 72 hours fasting. Blood for glucose and insulin determinations is sampled every 4–6 hours during the fasting and particularly when symptoms develop. Symptomatic hypoglycemia with fasting is usually associated with concurrent serum insulin levels greater than 25 U/mL. Additional support for the diagnosis of insulinoma is derived from the calculation of the insulin to glucose ratio. Normal values are less than 0.3, whereas nearly all patients with insulinomas demonstrate insulin to glucose ratios greater than 0.4 after an overnight fasting.

5.2 Imaging Study

High resolution CT and MR scans are successful demonstrated in 40%–50% of tumors. Endoscopic ultrasound examination of the pancreas may be able to show a much higher percentage. Transhepatic portal venous sampling has proved to be the most accurate preoperative localizing method, demonstrating the position in the pancreas of above 90% of lesions.

5.3 Treatment

Surgery should be done promptly, because with repeated hypoglycemic attacks, permanent cerebral damage occurs and the patient becomes progressively more obese. Moreover, the tumor may be malignant.

Part 35

Upper Gastrointestinal Hemorrhage

35.1 Definition

Upper Gastrointestinal(GI) tract includes esophagus, stomach, duodenum, proximal jejunum and biliary tract. Clinical manifestation of massive hemorrhage from the upper GI tract is a large volume of hematemesis or hematochezia. Vomiting of bright red or dark blood indicates that the source of bleeding lies proximal to the ligament of Treitz. The characteristic coffee-grounds nature of "changed" blood is due to the conversion of hemoglobin to methemoglobin by gastric acid. Melena(black, tarry stool) is usually due to bleeding from a source in the proximal GI tract; however, hematin(the black pigment produced by oxidation of heme) can be seen in the stool when the bleeding point is as far distal as the cecum, if transit time is prolonged. Melena can be caused by as little as 100 mL of blood in the stomach and can persist for up to 5 days after bleeding has ceased.

In adult, if bleeding over 800 mL once, accounting for 20% of circulation, symptoms and signs of shock would appear. The volume and rate of bleeding loss must be determined since therapy will have to be instituted immediately in the patient with massive bleeding. The triad including hematemesis, hematochezia, and hypovolemia indicates massive GI bleeding and requires urgent treatment. Signs and symptoms of hypovolemia, including weakness, pallor, sweating, dizziness, tachycardia, and extreme thirst, signify massive bleeding.

35.2 Causes

There are five common causes of massive upper GI bleeding:

(1) Peptic ulcer(50%-60%, 3/4 duodenal ulcer). Most are chronic ulcer located in postbulbar part of duodenum or lesser curvature of stomach. Bleeding cannot stop automatically due to invasion and rupture of the artery within the ulcer.

(2) Portal hypertension (25%). Most are caused by hepatic cirrhosis with esophageal varices. The esophageal and gastric mucosa become thinner due to varices and easy to be damaged by rough food and erosion of reflux of gastric juice, and portal hypertension that result in ruptured varix and massive hemorrhage.

(3) Stress ulcer and acute erosive gastritis. It is a lesion with shallow, multiple, disseminated erosion of the gastric mucosa. Most are located in antrum pylori and result in massive hemorrhage. The patient may have a history of alcohol abuse, ingestion of salicylates or nonsteroidal anti-inflammatory drugs(NSAIDs) or adrenocortisteroids.

(4) Intrahepatic local infection, hepatic tumor and trauma. Intrahepatic infection can cause intrahepatic duct dilation and multiple liver abscesses; the abscesses rupture into portal vein or branches of artery and result in large amount of blood going into biliary tract, and then duodenum.

(5) Gastric carcinoma. Due to ischemia and necrosis of tumor, the surface become erosion and ulceration, and then blood vessel erosion cause massive hemorrhage.

35.3 Clinical Manifestation

The position of upper GI bleeding can be divided in three parts:

(1) Esophagus and gastric fundus(ruptured varix bleeding). Rapid massive bleeding, volume of 500–1000 mL blood, and shock. The main clinical manifestation is hematemesis, and single hematochezia is rare. Recurrent bleeding is common after nonoperative management.

(2) Stomach and bulbar of duodenum(ulcer, hemorrhagic gastritis, and gastric cancer). Rapid but < 500 mL once, less patient with shock. Either hematemesis or hematochezia can be the main symptom. Most stop bleeding by nonoperative treatment, but it may occur afterwards.

(3) Distal duodenum and proximal jejunum(intrahepatic duct bleeding). Less volume, 200–300 mL, seldom with shock. Hematochezia is the main symptom. Transient stopping bleeding after nonoperative treatment with periodic recurrence, the duration normally is 1–2 weeks.

Generally speaking, other hematemesis or hematochezia depends on the rate and volume of bleeding, while the area of bleeding is on a minor position.

After admitting the patient to the hospital and initiating the steps for assessing the status of the circulatory system and the magnitude of the bleed, a history should be taken and physical examination performed. Of the commonly encountered causes of upper GI bleeding, only portal hypertension with esophageal varices is associated with characteristic physical findings. However, over half of cirrhotic patients who bleed from an upper GI site do so fro nonvariceal lesion.

35.3.1 Esophageal varices

Ruptured varix is considered in the patient with upper GI hemorrhage who has a history of chronic alcoholism or liver disease. Frequently the patient is in a precomatose state, and physical examination reveals hepatomegaly, splenomegaly, caput medusae, spider hemangiomas, reddened palms, mild jaundice, ascites, and muscle wasting. Definitive diagnosis of variceal hemorrhage is diagnosed by esophagoscopy. A barium swallow that will outline the extent of the varices (filling defect) is more useful when the patient is not bleeding. Patients with portal hypertension may bleed from hemorrhagic gastritis or peptic ulcer disease rather than from varices; endoscopy will establish the diagnosis.

35.3.2 Gastritis

Massive hemorrhage from erosive gastritis was once a common cause of upper GI bleeding in critically ill patients. In recent years, the routine use of prophylactic acid-reducing medical therapy has diminished the incidence of this entity. Bleeding from stress gastritis is most frequently encountered in patients with extensive burns, trauma, or sepsis. In fact, the development of hemorrhagic gastritis in a postoperative patient should alert the physician to the possibility of an occult source of sepsis. In other patients with bleeding gastritis, the history may reveal ingestion of substances that are toxic to gastric mucosa such as aspirin, indomethacin, steroids, or alcohol. Diagnosis is made exclusively with gastroscopy and more often than not reveals diffuse disease that precludes both endoscopic coagulation and limited gastric resection.

35.3.3 Peptic ulcer

The cause of 40%–50% of all cases of massive upper GI bleeding is peptic ulcer, nearly equally distributed between gastric and duodenal ulcer. When hemorrhage occurs from a peptic ulcer, whether the source is in the stomach or the duodenum, the immediate aim is to control the bleeding. The diagnosis is often suggested by history, unless bleeding is occurring for the first time as the symptom of an acute stress ulcer. Physical examination and laboratory studies are usually of little help.

If the bleeding stops as a result or gastric lavage or if bleeding has stopped before admission to the hospital so that a nasogastric tube aspirate yields only old or changed blood, gastroscopy may be deferred and angiography will not be helpful. The patient should be managed with gastric suction to decompress the stomach and gastric pH neutralization, as outlined previously. Most patients should undergo elective endoscopy, but an upper GI contrast radioguaphic study may be safely performed if bleeding has not recurred for 12 hours. If bleeding recurs, emergency endoscopy with or without subsequent angiography, should be used to identify the precise source of bleeding.

Once the diagnosis of peptic ulcer is made by any of these measures, it is treated medically, endoscopically, or operatively, depending on the previous history of bleeding, pain, and chronicity. Emergency operation is indicated for patients whose estimated blood loss exceeds 2500 mL in the first 24 hours or 1500 mL in the second 24 hours, or for those whose bleeding recurs while they are hospitalized; according to these criteria, approximately 25% of patients require emergency surgery. The choice of operation is designed to reduce gastric acidity and prevent recurrence of peptic ulcer disease.

35.4 Initial Management

After placing large-bore (14-gauge of larger) intravenous catheters, a large-bore nasogastric tube is passed into the stomach for lavage with large volumes of saline. The temperature of the lavage fluid probably is not important; in fact, ice-cold saline lavage may be injurious to the gastric mucosa. Gastric lavage performs several functions: the rate of hemorrhage is monitored, blood clots are evacuated, and hemostasis may be augmented. Bleeding ceases during gastric lavage about 90% of the time. When active hemorrhage stops, the Ewald tube may be replaced with a standard (16 Fr) nasogastric tube.

Although it was never proven to be of benefit, empiric therapy with histaminc H_2 rcccptor antagonists is usually begun at this time. Preliminary data suggest that intravenous somatostatin may cease nonvariceal bleeding.

The most important diagnostic maneuver in the patient with massive upper GI bleeding is endoscopy, preferably with a flexible fiberoptic esophagogastroscope. Endoscopy should be performed within 12-24 hours of admission. If bleeding is present during the examination, its source and magnitude can be determined simultaneously, and in some cases hemostasis can also be attempted. For example, if bleeding esophageal varices are encountered, not only is the diagnosis made with certainty but definitive therapy can be administered by injection of sclerosing agents. In the presence of somewhat localized gastritis, angiodysplasia, or bleeding peptic ulcer, the endoscopist can attempt control of hemorrhage by using electrocautery, neodymium YAG laser, or heater probe application under the endoscope. It should be emphasized that these procedures have the potential hazard of perforation if applied inappropriately.

Once diagnosis is established, subsequent management is instituted as follows (Figure 35-1-1):

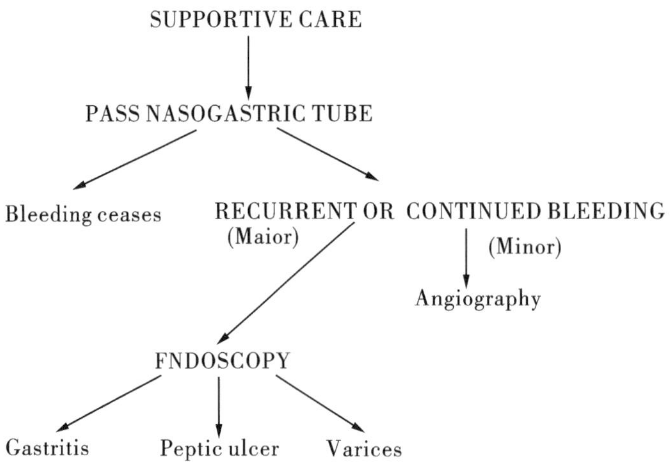

Figure 35-1-1 Diagnosis and treatment procedure of upper gastrointestinal bleeding

▶Supportive care:①Monitor vital signs and central venous pressure. ②Type and cross-match blood. ③Large-bore intravenous catheter. ④Crystalloid, plasma expanders, and blood.

▶Pass nasogastric tube: ①Evacuate blood and clots. ②Saline lavage. ③Constant antacid infusion and/or intravenous histamine H_2-blockers.

▶Bleeding ceases

(1) Antacid therapy.

(2) Next day, make diagnosis:①Endoscopy. ②Upper gastrointestinal series, enteroclysis.

(3) Elective surgery if indicated.

▶Recurrent or continued bleeding

· Angiography:①Intra-arterial vasopressin. ②Embolization. ③Urgent operation. ④Localization.

▶Endoscoty

Gastritis:①Medical management. ②Vagotomy and subtotal gastrectomy. ③Vagotomy, pyloroplasty and ligation of bleeding points.

Peptic ulcer:①Endoscopic therapy. ②Continued medical management. ③Urgent operation.

Varices:①Sclerotherapy. ②Vasopressin infusion. ③Balloon tamponade. ④Urgent portacaval shunt or devascularization procedure.

Part 36

Spleen Diseases

36.1 Anatomy

The abdominal surface of the diaphragm separates the spleen from the lower left lung and pleura and the ninth to eleventh ribs. The visceral surface faces the abdominal cavity and contains gastric, colic, renal, and pancreatic impressions. Spleen size and weight vary with age, with both diminishing in the elderly and those with underlying pathologic conditions. The average adult spleen is 7–11 cm in length and weighs 150 g (range 70–250 g). Splenomegaly is described variably within the surgical literature as moderate, massive, and hyper, which reflects a lack of consensus. Most would agree, however, that splenomegaly applies to organs weighing 500 g and/or average 15 cm in length.

The spleen's superior border separates the diaphragmatic surface from the gastric impression of the visceral surface and often contains one or two notches, which are particularly pronounced when the spleen is greatly enlarged.

Of particular clinical relevance, the spleen is suspended in position by several ligaments and peritoneal folds to the colon (splenocolic ligament), the stomach (gastrosplenic ligament), the diaphragm (phrenicosplenic ligament), and the kidney, adrenal gland, and tail of the pancreas (splenorenal ligament). The gastrosplenic ligament contains the short gastric vessels; the remaining ligaments are avascular, with rare exceptions, such as in patients with portal hypertension. The relationship of the pancreas to the spleen also has important clinical implications. In cadaveric anatomic series, the tail of the pancreas has been demonstrated to lie within 1 cm of the splenic hilum 75% of the time and in 30% of patients actually to abut the spleen.

The spleen derives most of its blood from the splenic artery, the longest and most tortuous of the three main branches of the celiac artery. The splenic artery can be characterized by the pattern of its terminal branches. The distributed type of splenic artery is the most common (70%) and is distinguished by a short trunk with many long branches entering over three quarters of the spleen's medial surface. The less common magistral type of splenic artery (30%) has a long main trunk dividing near the hilum into short terminal branches, and these enter over 25%–30% of the spleen's medial surface. The spleen also receives some of its blood supply from the short gastric vessels that branch from the left gastroepiploic artery running within the gastrosplenic ligament. The splenic vein joins the superior mesenteric vein to form the portal vein and accommodates the major venous drainage of the spleen (Figure 36–1–1).

The red pulp is comprised of large numbers of venous sinuses, which ultimately drain into tributaries of the splenic vein. The sinuses are surrounded and separated by the reticulum, a fibrocellular network of collagen fibers and fibroblasts. Within this network or mesh lie splenic macrophages. These intersinusoidal regions appear as splenic cords. The venous sinuses are lined by long, narrow endothelial cells that are variably in close apposition to one another or are separated by intercellular gaps in a configuration unique to the spleen. The red pulp serves as a dynamic filtration system, enabling macrophages to remove microorganisms, cellular debris, antigen–antibody complexes, and senescent erythrocytes from the circulation.

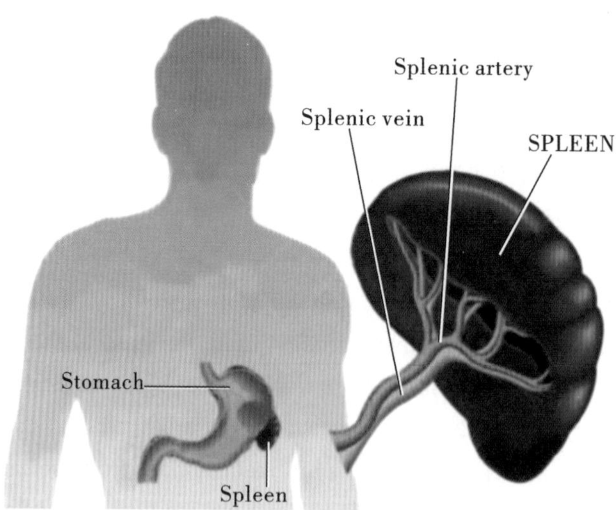

Figure 36-1-1 Anatomy of spleen

36.2 Physiology

The cellular functions include hematopoiesis, storage, "pitting", and "culling". Hematopoiesis, which supplies erythroid, myeloid, lymphoid cells, and platelets in fetal life, essentially ceases by the seventh intrauterine month. In human beings, the spleen does not serve as an important reservoir for blood cells, except platelets. At any given time, about one third of the total platelet mass is in the spleen.

Pitting refers to the removal of rigid structures such as Heinz bodies, Howell-Jolly bodies, and hemosiderin granules from red cells. The process involves the removal of nondeformable intracellular substances from deformable cells. The rigid body is phagocytized while the deformable cytoplasmic mass passes into the sinus and returns to the general circulation. The post-splenectomy blood smear is characterized by the presence of circulating erythrocytes with Howell-Jolly and Pappenheimer bodies (siderotic granules). Nucleated cells also have their nuclei removed in the same fashion.

Culling is the term applied to the spleen's ability to remove red cells that are aged or abnormal. Normally, as the red cell ages after a life span of approximately 120 days, it loses osmotic balance and membrane integrity, and therefore deformability. When these cells lose their deformability they are phagocytized by native macrophages. The spleen does not represent the only site for red cell destruction, and there is no difference in red cell survival following splenectomy. Naturally deformed cells and red cells that are affected by disease states also are removed by phagocytosis. In those circumstances in which there is a superabundance of reticulocyte formation, these cells are remodeled in the spleen and exit as mature cells. In the normal adult, the spleen is the most important site of selective erythrocyte sequestration. During its 120 days life cycle, the red cell spends an estimated minimum of 2 days within the spleen which, when normal, contains about 25 mL RBCs.

The neutrophil has a half-life of about 6 hours; hence 85% of neutrophils either emigrate at random into tissues or are destroyed within 24 hours. Although the role of the spleen in the destruction of neutrophils under normal conditions is not well quantified, the role of the spleen is amplified in some hypersplenic states, with resulting neutropenia. This augmented removal can occur because of splenic enlargement and accelerated sequestration of granulocytes or because of enhanced splenic removal of altered granulocytes, as seen in immune neutropenia.

In addition to the phagocytosis of antibody-coated cells, the immunologic functions of the spleen include antibody synthesis[especially immunoglobulin M (IgM)], generation of lymphocytes, and production of tuftsin, opsonins, properdin, and interferon.

36.3 Diseases

36.3.1 Hereditary spherocytosis

Hereditary spherocytosis(HS) results from an inherited dysfunction or deficiency in one of the erythrocyte membrane proteins(spectrin, ankyrin, band 3 protein, or protein 4.2). The resulting destabilization of the membrane lipid bilayer allows a pathologic release of membrane lipids. The red blood cell assumes a more spherical, less deformable shape, and the spherocytic erythrocytes are sequestered and destroyed in the spleen. Hemolytic anemia ensues; in fact, HS is the most common hemolytic anemia for which splenectomy is indicated. 26 HS is inherited primarily in an autosomal dominant fashion; the estimated prevalence in Western populations is 1 in 5000.

Patients with typical HS forms may have mild jaundice. Splenomegaly usually is present on physical examination. Laboratory examination reveals varying degrees of anemia: patients with mild forms of the disease may have no anemia; patients with severe forms may have hemoglobin levels as low as 4-6 g/dL. The mean corpuscular volume is typically low to normal or slightly decreased. For screening, a combined elevated mean corpuscular hemoglobin concentration and elevated erythrocyte distribution width are excellent predictor. Other laboratory indicators of HS include those providing evidence of rapid red blood cell destruction, including elevated reticulocyte count, elevated lactate dehydrogenase level, and increased level of unconjugated bilirubin. Spherocytes are readily apparent on peripheral blood film.

Dramatic clinical improvement-even despite persistent hemolysis-often occurs after splenectomy in patients with severe disease. Because children can be affected with HS, the timing of splenectomy is important and is aimed at reducing the quite small possibility of overwhelming post-splenectomy sepsis. Delaying such an operation until the patient is between the ages of 4 and 6-unless the anemia and hemolysis accelerate-is recommended by most.

Gallstones are more likely to develop in patients with HS, and over half of patients between the ages of 10 and 30 with HS have cholelithiasis. 27 For children with cholelithiasis prophylactic cholecystectomy is recommended at the time of splenectomy.

Hereditary elliptocytosis(HE) merits a brief discussion to distinguish it from HS. Both HS and HE are conditions of the red blood cell membrane that result from genetic defects in skeletal membrane proteins. With the HE defect, the red blood cell elongates as it circulates, so that far fewer red blood cells are sequestered or destroyed when transiting the splenic parenchyma. Unless >50% of red blood cells are affected(a scenario that could permit development of a clinical syndrome like HS) HE may be considered harmless.

36.3.2 Aneurysms of the splenic artery

Splenic artery aneurysm was first described by Baussier in 1770. St. Leger Brockman described one of the first surgical cases in 1930. The first radiologic diagnosis was made by Lindboe in 1932.

The splenic artery is the most common visceral artery aneurysm and the second most common site of intra-abdominal aneurysms secondary to the abdominal aorta. The incidence in autopsy series ranges between 0.02% and 0.16%. Splenic artery aneurysms may occur as a complication of acute pancreatitis or pancreatic pseudocysts. An incidence as high as 10% has been reported. 17 A splenic artery aneurysm should be suspected in a patient with pancreatitis who develops gastrointestinal(GI) bleeding without an obvious source. Arteriography should be performed and is usually diagnostic as well as therapeutic. Embolization is successful in 73%. 18 In those patients with a pancreatic pseudocyst, drainage of the cysts is necessary to prevent subsequent hemorrhage.

Splenic artery aneurysms may be more prevalent in women, usually as a consequence of atherosclerosis. In a series of 125 cases reported by Sherlock and Learmonth, the average diameter was 3.4 cm and the largest was 15 cm. The main splenic artery was involved in 81% of the cases, while 26% were multiple. 87% of splenic artery aneurysms occurred in women, and 92% of the women had been pregnant an average of 4.5 times. Rupture in the pregnant female, however, has been associated with 70% maternal and 95% fetal mortality. Rupture during pregnancy occurs in 69% of the patients during the third trimester.

A splenic artery aneurysm usually is discovered in the sixth decade as an incidental finding. 83% of the patients are asymptomatic at the time of diagnosis. The remainder present with epigastric, left upper quadrant, or left flank pain. The pain usually can not be attributed conclusively to the aneurysm. The physical examination is usually normal, and a bruit is detectable in <10% of cases. A calcified lesion is noted on plain film of the abdomen in 70% of the patients.

Rupture of the aneurysm is manifested by sudden abdominal pain. In 12.5% a warning hemorrhage occurs, with temporary cessation of bleeding. Rupture into the colon, stomach, and intestine may take place, but intraperitoneal rupture is by far the most common presentation. The risk of rupture in a calcified aneurysm is low, occurring in 1 of 34 patients; the patient was followed for 1-19 years, and that aneurysm was 7 cm in diameter. When rupture occurs in the nonpregnant female, it is usually contained in the lesser sac, resulting in a patient mortality rate of <5%.

Criteria for elective operation are not firm, but it is generally believed that removal is not required for the asymptomatic lesion that is <2 cm in diameter. Symptomatic aneurysms and those greater than 2 cm should be removed if the patient is a reasonable operative risk. Lesions proximal to the hilus of the spleen can be managed by resection and primary end-to-end anastomosis or proximal and distal ligation with resection of the involved segment. Proximal ligation is reasonable because the spleen will not become ischemic following central ligation of the main splenic artery. Distal lesions and multiple lesions generally require splenectomy and resection of the involved splenic artery. An aneurysm detected in a female who anticipates pregnancy should be removed and one detected during pregnancy should be removed before the third trimester.

36.4 Surgery

36.4.1 Step 1

The standard supine position is employed with an optional small roll/bump under the left flank. Mechanical retractors greatly enhance exposure and the primary surgeon should stand on the right side of the patient; the first assistant opposite the surgeon on the left side of the patient. There are two standard incisions for open splenectomy: a supraumbilical midline or left subcostal with or without midline extension. A midline incision is usually employed in trauma cases. Examine each patient following induction of anesthesia to estimate the location of the splenic hilum and the tip of the spleen, so the incision location optimizes exposure. The principle of retraction is that of moving the incision over the operative field. Two points of retraction include one retractor to gently hold the colon in the lower abdomen and counter retraction to lift the left portion of the incision superiorly and out of the operative field. The standard order of steps is arranged to minimize blood loss, minimize the size of the spleen and maintain adequate exposure while performing the deepest and most challenging dissection. Identify the splenic artery near its origin from the celiac axis, which is accessed through the gastrohepatic ligament.

36.4.2 Step 2

Upon entering the peritoneal cavity and again before closing, a thorough search for accessory spleens should be conducted, especially if the indication for splenectomy is hematological. Open the gastrosplenic ligament through an avascular area and then proceed to dissect the short gastric vessels. These may be secured with hemoclips or ligatures. The last several vessels in the gastrosplenic ligament are of particular note. These branches are often quite short, so care must be taken to utilize adequate tissue for hemostasis without injuring the greater curvature of the stomach. The LigaSure (R) device, the harmonic/ultrasonic scalpel or a linear stapler can also be utilized for dividing the gastrosplenic ligament as is employed during laparoscopic splenectomy.

36.4.3 Step 3

While dividing splenic attachments, always attempt to stay closer to the spleen than to the opposite structure. Proceeding inferiorly along the gastrosplenic ligament typically includes dividing the left gastroepiploic artery. Taking down the splenic flexure and the splenocolic attachment usually facilitates this dissection. The spleen is then gently and progressively retracted medially with the surgeon's left hand. Using a laparotomy pad under the retracting hand, it is a relatively simple maneuver for the surgeon to identify the peritoneal attachments and provide exposure with the left index finger. The attachments are divided with curved scissors proceeding from the inferior pole to the superior pole and then dividing the splenorenal ligament as the spleen is gradually rotated medially and anteriorly. Care should be taken with any blunt dissection as the splenic capsule is relatively thin and even small tears can result in moderate bleeding. Likewise, care should be taken as proceeding posteriorly around the inferior pole in order to avoid the adrenal gland.

36.4.4 Step 4

Once all of the splenic attachments have been divided the splenic hilum can be addressed definitively. Lift the spleen up and out of the retroperitoneum. This maneuver serves to clearly identify and separate the splenic vessels from the tail of the pancreas as shown. Laparotomy pads packed into the retroperitoneum can assist with elevating the spleen into the incision while controlling oozing in the retroperitoneum. With the assistant holding the spleen, the surgeon can separate the tail of the pancreas from the splenic vessels in order to protect the tail of the pancreas prior to dissecting and applying curved clamps. The surgeon divides the splenic artery and vein proximal to their bifurcation between clamps and applies a suture ligature to each after removing the spleen. We first clamp the artery, which is typically anterior to the splenic vein, and then squeeze the spleen in order to promote autotransfusion of splenic blood prior to clamping the vein. Once the spleen is removed and all of the named vessels have been doubly ligated, the operative field can be inspected for hemostasis. The abdomen is closed with or without a closed.

Part 37

Arterial Aneurysms

An aneurysm is defined as a permanent localized dilation of an artery to more than 1.5 times its expected diameter. Aneurysmsmay develop at any position in the artery tree, but are most commonly found in the distal abdominal aorta, the iliac arteries, the popliteal artery, the common femoral artery, the arch and descending portions of the thoracic aorta and the carotid arteries, the frequency is decreasing in the vessels above. A true aneurysm involves all the wall layers of the artery. False aneurysms are caused by rupture of the anastomotic site between graft and vessel or the vessel wall, with containment of blood by surrounding tissue.

The main clinical significance of central aneurysms (intrathoracic and intra-abdominal) is associated with the risk of aneurysm rupture, whereas the main clinical manifestations of peripheral aneurysms are associated with the risk of thrombosis or embolism. Aneurysms are classified according to the anatomical location, morphology, and etiology. The most common aneurysm morphology is a fusiform, symmetrical circumferential enlargement that involves all layers of the artery wall. Aneurysms may also be saccular that affect only part of the arterial circumference.

The most common cause of aneurysms is atherosclerotic degeneration of the arterial wall. The pathogenesis is multifactorial, which involves genetic susceptibility, aging, inflammation, atherosclerosis, and activation of local proteolytic enzymes. Most aneurysms occur in elderly people, and the prevalence of aneurysms increases with age.

Chapter 1

Abdominal Aortic Aneurysms

1.1 Epidemiology and Etiology

Most aneurysms of the abdominal aorta involve the aortic segment between the onset of the renal artery and the bifurcation of the aorta, but the variable portions of the common iliac artery could also be involved. Abdominal aortic aneurysms are present in 2% of the elderly population. The prevalence of abdominal aortic aneurysm was 1.8%–6.6% at autopsy. In a large autopsy study, the prevalence of male abdominal aortic aneurysms was 4.3%, increasing rapidly beyond the age of 55 years and peaking at the age of 80. The prevalence of female was 2.1%, increasing beyond the age of 70 years. The abdominal aorta is the most common and most dangerous site for atherosclerotic aneurysms because aneurysms here are more likely to rupture than aneurysms of smaller peripheral arteries.

Smoking is the main risk factor for the abdominal aortic aneurysms. The presence of abdominal aortic aneurysms is 8 : 1 between smokers and nonsmokers. In the ADAM (Aneurysm Detection and Management) study, smoking-related prevalence accounted for 78% of all abdominal aortic aneurysms. 40% of patients with abdominal aortic aneurysms have hypertension. Surprisingly, diabetes seems to play a protective role in abdominal aortic aneurysm formation.

1.2 Clinical Manifestation

Most abdominal aortic aneurysms are asymptomatic before rupture. Because there is no large-scale screening program for abdominal aortic aneurysms, most aneurysms are foundin routine physical examinations with the palpation of a pulsatile abdominal mass or on imaging while investigating an unrelated problem. The main clinical manifestations are abdominal pulsatile mass, pain, compression symptoms, embolism, and symptoms of rupture. Most patients feel abnormal fluctuations in the position near umbilical or cardiac cavities. The physical finding is a palpable fusiform or globular pulsatile abdominal mass. For smaller aneurysms, masses always concentrate in the upper abdomen above the umbilicus, and the normal location is the infrarenal portion of the abdominal aorta. Larger aneurysms protrude distally into the abdomen below the umbilicus or proximally into the space behind the rib cage. The pain caused by an abdominal aortic aneurysm is often abdominal, low back pain. Abrupt abdominal pain is a precursor of rapid expansion or even rupture to the aneurysm mass. Abdominal distension and anorexia are the manifestations that the gastrointestinal tract has been squeezed. When the renal pelvis and ureter are squeezed, it will cause urinary tract obstruction-related symptoms. Compression of bile ducts will lead to obstructive jaundice. Once the thrombus or atheroma in the aneurysm cavity falls off, it can be rushed to the distal end with the blood flow, resulting in arterial embolism of the lower extremities, leading to limb ischemia or even necrosis.

The most feared complication of abdominal aortic aneurysm is aneurysm rupture. Aneurysms can rupture freely into the peritoneal cavity or into the retroperitoneum. Free intraperitoneal rupture is usually anterior rupture, accompanied by immediate hemodynamic collapse and high mortality rate. The retroperitoneal rupture is usually posterior and may be contained by the psoas, the periaortic tissues or the perivertebral tissues.

1.3 Diagnosis

1.3.1 Physical examination

Physical examination is important for the diagnosis of abdominal aortic aneurysms, especially in thin patients and patients with large aneurysms. An important feature on physical examination is detection of expansile pulsationin which the gap between both hands placed on either side of the aneurysm widens with each systole. However, most patients with aneurysms are not thin. Therefore, physical examination is sometimes unreliable, resulting in 50% false-positive and 50% false-negative.

1.3.2 Abdominal ultrasound

Ultrasound is the most useful andcheapest method to diagnose and follow up abdominal aortic aneurysms. It can accurately measure the size and position of the inferior aneurysm. Ultrasound can detect abdominal aortic aneurysms whose diameter is more than 3 cm. It can display the size of the aneurysm, with or without plaque and thrombus, and can also provide hemodynamic parameters. Due to its low cost, wide availability, and lack of risk, ultrasound is particularly useful for screening and monitoring aneurysms and may be useful for follow-up after endovascular repair.

1.3.3 CT and MRI

CT is the most precise test for aortic aneurysms imaging. CT plain scan and enhanced scan can accurately display the morphology of the aneurysm and its adjoining relationship with surrounding organs, and can also determine whether there is anatomical abnormality. CT scans provide valuable information about aneurysm architecture and have been used to predict aneurysm expansion rates. In addition, CT scans show important adjacent structures that affect abdominal aortic aneurysm repair, such as colonic or pancreatic masses, horseshoe kidneys or other renal abnormalities, and abnormal vein including retroaortic renal vein, and left-sided or duplicated vena cava. Magnetic resonance angiography can clearly show the location, shape, size of lesions in the absence of contrast agents, and can provide realistic images.

1.4 Treatment

Abdominal aortic aneurysm is unlikely to heal without treatment. Once the mortality rate of rupture is as high as 70% -90% ,and the mortality rateafter elective surgery has fallen below 5%. So it should be diagnosed and treated early. Surgery is still the main treatment method. For high-risk patients, endovascular repair can be used.

1.4.1 Surgical treatment

The selection of aneurysm repair for patients is based on assessments of the risks of rupture. Surgical indications include the following: The diameter of the aneurysmal sac is greater than 5 cm; Pain, especially persistent severe abdominal pain; Gastrointestinal tract, urinary system oppression leading to obstructive symptoms; Concurrent infection. Patients with ruptured aortic aneurysms need immediate surgical repair.

Patients with aneurysms are usually elderly and frequently have coexisting pulmonary, cardiac, or renal disease, which increase the risk of aneurysm repair. Adequate preoperative evaluation and appropriate patient selection can reduce the risk of perioperative period.

The most important step in preparing for invasive treatment of aortic lesions is the cardiac assessment. Severe coronary artery disease is present in 50% of patients in whom it is suspected and in 20% of patients without clinical manifestation of the disease. The presence of uncorrected coronary artery disease increases the risk of death from 3% to 10%. Because not all the patients at risk could be indentified through history, physical examinations, and electrocardiography (ECG), non-invasive tests have been used to identify patients who may benefit from strategic changes or coronary revascularization. Exercise ECG testing has largely been replaced by the stress or dipyridamole thallium cardiac scintillation scan and the dobutamine echocardiogram. Other important risk factors for surgical repair of abdominal aortic aneurysms include chronic obstructive pulmonary disease and impaired renal function. Pulmonary function can serve as a initial prognostic guide and should be selected before surgical intervention. Preoperative renal function is an important determinant of perioperative morbidity and affects the use of contrast agents in diagnostic tests or endovascular treatment.

Conventional surgical repair of abdominal aortic aneurysm involves the replacement of the aneurysmal segment with a synthetic fabric graft. Open surgical repair of abdominal aortic aneurysms is performed by transperitoneal or retroperitoneal exposure of the aorta under general endotracheal anesthesia. Traditionally, transperitoneal approach through midline laparotomy has been most commonly used for abdominal aortic aneurysm repair, but retroperitoneal operations via flank incision may reduce perioperative pulmonary and gastrointestinal complications. Preoperative preparation to optimize cardiopulmonary function, and careful intraoperative hemodynamic monitoring with fluid management and appropriate blood transfusion can significantly reduce the operational risk. The operative death rate for patients accept the selective infrarenal abdominal aneurysmectomy is 2% -4% ,and there is also a possibility of 5% -10% of complications, such as hemorrhage, renal failure, myocardial infarction, graft infection, limb ischemia, intestinal ischemia, and erectile dysfunction. The long-term outcomes of aneurysmectomy are excellent because the success rate of transplantation is very high and the formation of pseudoaneurysms at the anastomosis is rare.

1.4.2 Endovascular therapy

Traditional surgical repair requires a major surgical procedure with substantial morbidity and mortality.

Endovascular aneurysm repair differs from open surgical repair in that the prosthetic graft is introduced into the aneurysm through the femoral arteries and fixed to the non aneurysmal infrarenal neck and iliac arteries with a self-expanding or balloon-expanding stent rather than sutures. As a result, a major abdominal incision is avoided, and for patient, the morbidity associated with the procedure is much reduced. Endovascular therapy introduced in 1991 is rapidly gaining popularity. Although endovascular therapy reduces the time of ICU and hospital stay, and reduces the surgery-related morbidity and mortality, it is associated with higher failure rates and equipment-related expenses. Due to little operative trauma of endovascular therapy, many high-risk patients who can not tolerate traditional surgery could access treatment.

The average failure rate for the initial placement of the graft was 5%-10%, and many technical problems may occur, including iliac and aortic rupture from the deployment device. The most important intermediate or long-term adverse outcome is continuous perfusion of the aneurysm ("endoleak"), caused by ineffective proximal or distal sealing, continuous retrograde flow through lumbar or inferior mesenteric arteries, and erosion of the graft material or modular separation in the device itself.

Chapter 2

Ruptured Aortic Aneurysms

2.1 Etiology

As the size increases, lateral pressure within the aneurysm may eventually lead to spontaneous rupture of the aneurysmal wall. Although bleeding may occur immediately, there is usually an interval of several hours between the first episode of bleeding and later retroperitoneal haematoma. This phenomenon is called "contained rupture". When periaortic tissue no longer contains the expanding hematoma, "free rupture" occurs with exsanguination into the free peritoneal cavity. Interestingly, ruptured aneurysms are more likely to occur in the autumn and winter.

The most important factor associated with rupture is the diameter of the maximal cross-sectional of aneurysm. The largest diameter of the aneurysm is most related to the possibility of rupture. The biggest factors that increase the risk of rupture are chronic obstructive pulmonary disease and pain. Even obscure and atypical pain has been found to be closely related to subsequent rupture. Advanced age, female gender, and renal failure are associated with an increased risk of rupture.

2.2 Clinical Manifestation

Most aortic aneurysms are asymptomatic until rupture begins. The patient experienced abrupt and severe abdominal pain that usually radiates to the back and occasionally to the inguinal region. 75% of patients were accompanied by high blood pressure and tachycardia. The patient was more restless and sweating. Blood loss causes vertigo or syncope. After the first hemorrhage, the pain may become reduced or blurred and may disappear. It will only appear again and progress to shock when the bleeding continues.

When perivascular tissue is bleeding, a separate pulsatile abdominal mass may appear. In contrast to intact aneurysms, the ruptured aneurysm at this stage is usually tender. As the bleeding continues (usually after entering the peritoneum), the discrete mass will be replaced by a poorly defined mid-abdominal fullness, which often extend to the left flank. Shock becomes profound, manifest as hypotension, peripheral vasoconstriction, and anuria. Less than 2/3 of patients with this disorder show the classic triad of pain, pulsatile abdominal masses, and hypotension associated with a ruptured abdominal aortic aneurysm.

2.3 Diagnosis

Definitive diagnosis mainly depends on imaging studies. There is no time for X-rays, ECG, CT scans, blood examinations, or other examinations except the emergency abdominal ultrasound examination to confirm an aneurysm, if ultrasound is readily available. An emergency abdominal ultrasound performed in the emergency room could confirm the presence of aortic aneurysms but will not disclose the bleeding. CT scans could reliably confirm hemorrhage from an aneurysm, but the delay in obtaining them usually can not be used in unstable patients.

2.4 Treatment and Prognosis

Aneurysm ruptureis often accompanied by hemorrhagic shock, so anti-shock therapy is essential. Laparotomy must be performed as soon as the intravenous infusion has been started and the blood has been sent for cross-matching. Control of the aorta proximal to the aneurysm must be obtained immediately. Through a midline incision, the aorta is cross-clamped or compressed at the diaphragmatic hiatus. After obtaining distal control of the iliac and collateral arteries, a proximal clamp should be placed immediately above the aneurysm to allow perfusion of the visceral and renal arteries. Subsequent management is similar to the elective aortic aneurysm repair.

The successful outcome of the operation is related to the patient's condition on arrival, the promptness of diagnosis, and the speed of controlling bleeding and blood replacement. The surgical mortality is 60% - 80%. Unfortunately, as many patients with ruptured aneurysms dying before reaching the hospital, the overall mortality rate is close to 90%. The main factors responsible for improved survival are immediate surgery with rapid proximal aortic control, avoidance of technical errors, and expeditious completion of the operation. Without operation, the outcome is uniformly fatal.

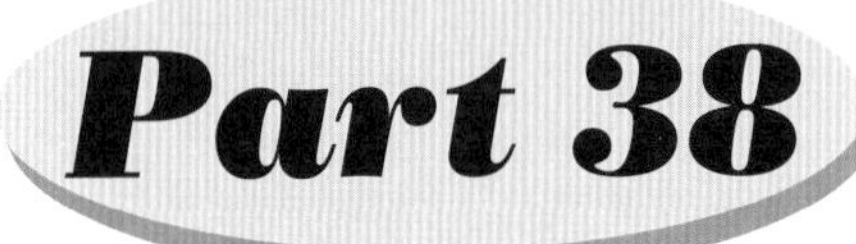

Part 38

The Diseases of Veins and Lymphoduct

Chapter 1

Venous Anatomy and Hemodynamic

1.1 Venous Anatomy

Vein disease always occurs in legs. Abnormal anatomy and hemodynamics of veins play an important role in the pathogenesis of venous diseases. A clear understanding of the anatomy and hemodynamic of the venous system in legs is essential to understanding pathophysiology and treatment.

The venous anatomy of legs is divided into the deep veins, the superficial veins and the perforating veins. The superficial veins have two major trunks, the greater saphenous vein and the lesser saphenous vein. The greater saphenous vein ascends in the superficial compartment and drains into the common femoral vein after entering the fossa ovalis. Before the greater saphenous vein entries the common femoral vein, it receives media and lateral accessory saphenous veins, as well as small tributaries from the inguinal region, pudendal region, and anterior abdominal wall. The lesser saphenous vein originates from the lateral side of the dorsal venous plexus at the lateral aspect of foot and ascends posterior to the lateral malleolus, and it drains into the popliteal vein after penetrating the fascia. The deep veins in legs are named according to their paired arteries. Perforating veins connect the superficial venous system to the deep venous system at various in the leg–the foot, the medial and lateral calf, the mid and distal thigh. The perforating veins in the foot are either valveless or with valves directing blood from the deep to the superficial venous system.

1.2 Venous Hemodynamic

Blood is pushed to the heart by compression of the deep veins through calf muscle contractions during walking, and flow is unidirectional due to a series of one-way valves. The calf muscles augment venous return by functioning as a pump. In the supine state, the resting venous pressure in the foot is the difference between the residual kinetic energy and the resistance that comes from arterioles and precapillary sphincters. There is thus generated a pressure gradient to the right atrium of 10–12 mmHg. In the upright position, the resting venous pressure of the foot is a reflection of the hydrostatic pressure from the upright blood column extending of the right atrium to the foot. The return of the blood to the heart from the legs is facilitated by the pump function of the calf muscle.

Chapter 2

Varicose Veins

2.1 Etiology and Epidemiology

Varicose veins are common diseases. Abnormally dilated veins occur in several locations in the body: the spermatic chord, esophagus, and the legs. Modern studies have identified female gender, pregnancy, family history, prolonged standing, and history of phlebitis as the risk factors for varicose veins.

Varicose veins are classified as primary varicose veins and secondary varicose veins. Primary varicose veins are thought to be caused by the diminished elasticity and valvular incompetence of the vein wall due to genetic or developmental defects. Most isolated superficial venous insufficiency are primary varicose veins. Secondary varicose veins are caused by deep venous thrombosis, arteriovenous fistula, destruction of valves caused by trauma, or nontraumatic proximal venous obstruction. The result of varicose veins can range from heaviness, pain, and swelling after prolonged standing, to severe lipodermatosclerosis, edema, and ulceration.

2.2 Pathogenesis

The pathogenesis of varicose veins includes the fundamental defects in the strength and the abnormal characteristics of the venous wall. These defects may be generalized or localized and are consist of defects in elastin and collagen. Anatomic differences in the location of the superficial veins of the lower extremities may be related to the pathogenesis of varicose veins. For example, the main trunk of saphenous vein is not always involved in varicose veins. Perhaps this is because it contains a well-developed medial fibromuscular layer and is supported by the fibrotic connective tissue that is associated with the deep fascia. In contrast, tributaries of the long saphenous vein are less supported by the subcutaneous fat and are located in the superficial layer of the superficial fascia. These tributaries also contain less muscle tissue in the venous walls. Thus, these, not the main trunk of saphenous vein, may become selectively varicose.

2.3 Clinical Manifestation

The clinical manifestation of patients with varicose veins can be quite variable. The varicosities appear as dilated, tortuous, elongated veins and predominantly occur in the medial aspect of the lower extremity along the course of the greater saphenous vein.

The patients with symptomatic varicose veins shows, most often, the symptoms of local aching, heaviness, discomfort, and sometimes outright pain in the calf of the affected limb. And the symptoms are particularly worse at the end of the day. it is most likely that the prolonged sitting or standing causes venous distention and associated pain. The symptoms usually decrease or disappear in the morning.

Primary varicose veins consist of elongated, tortuous, superficial veins which are bulging and contain incompetent valves. Varicose veins refer to any dilated, tortuous, slender vein of any caliber. Telangiectasia refers to small intradermal varicosities. Reticular veins are subcutaneous dilated veins that enter the tributaries of the main shaft or trunk veins. Trunk veins are the designated veins, such as the greater or lesser saphenous veins or their tributaries. These cause the symptoms of mild swelling, heaviness, and easy fatigability. Moderate swelling, increased heavy sensation appeares in larger varicosities, and early skin changes of mild pigmentation and subcutaneous induration appear at the same time. When varicose veins become severe, significant swelling and calf pain occur after standing, sitting, or walking, and multiple dilated veins are clusters like distribution, heavy medial and lateral supramalleolar pigmentation could also be found.

Physical examination begins with inspection of all extremities to determine the distribution and severity of the varicosities. Bimanual circumferential palpation of the thighs and calves is helpful and any signs of infection in the legs should be noted. Arterial pulses should be examined and are usually sufficient. The Brodie-Trendelenburg test is a useful physical examination for identifying the sites of valvular incompetence. With the patient lying supine, the leg is elevated until all varicose veins collapse, then, a tourniquet is placed at the mid thigh, and the patient is instructed to stand. If the varicose veins continue to collapse, this indicates valvular insufficiency at the saphenofemoral junction. If varicose veins refill quickly, perforator vein incompetence is implicated. Today, the Perthes test for deep venous occlusion and the Brodie-Trendelenburg test of axial reflux have been virtually replaced by hand-held Doppler instrument supplemented by duplex evaluation. The hand-held Doppler instrument can detect the phenomenon of saphenous vein regurgitation.

2.4 Diagnosis

According to the clinical manifestations of varicose veins of the lower extremities, the diagnosis is not difficult, and if it is necessary, auxiliary examinations such as ultrasound and venography can be used to determine the nature of the lesions more accurately.

2.5 Differential Diagnosis

Ulceration, brawny induration, and hyperpigmentation are often the symptoms of chronic deep venous insufficiency. It is important to recognize it because the changes cannot be resolved by saphenous vein stripping.

If young patients have extensive varicose veins, especially unilateral and atypical distributions, Klippel-Trenaunay syndrome must be considered. The classic triad is varicose veins, limb hypertrophy, and skin birthmarks. Because the deep veins are often anomaly or absent, saphenous vein stripping can be dangerous.

2.6 Treatment

Indications for treatment are pain, heaviness, easy fatigability, external bleeding, recurrent superficial thrombophlebitis, and appearance changes.

2.6.1 Nonsurgical treatment

Treatment for varicose veins initially involves a program directed at management of venous insufficiency, including elastic stocking support, periodic leg elevation, and regular exercise. Prolonged sitting and standingshould be avoided, and the compression stockings should be worn all day to diminish venous distention during standing and removed at night.

2.6.2 Sclerotherapy

Compression sclerotherapy is mainly applied to spider veins, telangiectasias, and small varicosities that persist after vein stripping. In the supine position, a small volume of sclerosing solution (0.2% –3% sodium tetradecyl) was injected into the varicose veins. The direct pressure of compression socks is maintained for 1 week at the thigh and 6 weeks at the calf.

2.6.3 Surgical treatment

Indications for surgical treatment include persistent pain, recurrent superficial thrombophlebitis, erosion of the overlying skin with bleeding, and signs of chronic venous insufficiency. High ligation of the great saphenous vein or the small saphenous vein and varicose vein stripping are the main surgical methods. This is performed by ligating the saphenofemoral junction and the branches of the major proximal saphenous vein through a small incision in the groin, isolating the saphenous vein at the medial malleolus, passing a stripper trough the vein from bottom to top and fixing it proximally to the ligated vein and then stripping the entire vein by withdrawing the stripper. In recent years, venous laser closure has been used to treat varicose veins, but the long-term efficacy remains to be seen.

Chapter 3

Deep Venous Thrombosis

Deep venous thrombosis(DVT)has significant morbid consequences. The thrombotic process initiating in a venous segment can spread to involve more proximal segments of the deep venous system,and thus resulting in edema,immobility,and pain. Pulmonary embolism is the most terrible sequela of acute DVT and has a high mortality rate. Deep vein thrombosis occurs most often in the lower extremities.

3.1 Etiology

Virchow's triad(hypercoagulability, vascular injury, and stasis) should be the basis of assessing risk factors for deep venous thrombosis. Causes of deep vein thrombosis include venous insufficiency,paralysis, severe heart failure,long-term bed rest,pelvic or limb fracture,or lengthy operation. Damaged endothelium causes platelet aggregation,degranulation,and formation of thrombus. Hypercoagulability is common in pregnancy,postpartum or postoperative,trauma,malignancy.

3.2 Clinical Manifestation

The diagnosis of deep vein thrombosis can not rely solely on symptoms and signs,half of patients with acute thromboses have no abnormality detectable in the involved extremity. Homans' sign(pain on passive dorsiflexion of the ankle)is positive in only half of cases. Some patients develope acute pulmonary embolism unaccompanied by leg pain or edema.

Typical symptoms of DVT are dull pain in the calf or leg associated with mild edema. With extensive proximal deep venous thrombosis,there can be massive edema,dilated superficial collateral veins,and cyanosis. In phlegmasia alba dolens, the leg is pulseless, pale, and cool due to the accompanying arterial spasm.

3.3 Diagnosis

The patients who experienced a sudden swelling of one limb, with pain and superficial vein dilation, should be suspected of deep venous thrombosis of the lower extremities. The following examinations will help to confirm the diagnosis and understand the extent of the lesion.

(1) Duplex ultrasound

Biphasic ultrasound has now become the preferred auxiliary test for diagnosing DVT. It is a non-invasive examination, does not expose the patient to radiation, and has specificity and sensitivity of greater than 95%. Doppler findings that suggest acute deep venous thrombosis are absence of spontaneous flow, loss of flow variation with respiration, and failure to increase flow velocity after distal expansion.

(2) Phlebography

Injecting contrast material into the venous system is one of the most accurate method of confirming DVT and its location. The superficial venous system must be occluded with a tourniquet, and inject from the veins in the foot for observing the deep venous system. Although this is a good examination for finding occlusive and nonocclusive thrombus, it is also invasive and is affected by the comparison of risks.

3.4 Differential Diagnosis

The symptoms of localized muscle strain or contusion and achilles tendon rupture are similar to those of deep vein thrombosis. Unilateral leg swelling can also be caused by lymphedema, obstruction of the popliteal vein by Baker's cyst, or obstruction of the iliac vein by retroperitoneal mass. Bilateral leg edema indicates the failure of heart, liver, or kidney, in addition, the inferior vena cava obstruction caused by tumor and pregnancy could also lead to bilateral leg edema.

3.5 Treatment

The purpose of treatment is to reduce the incidence of complications associated with deep vein thrombosis, including varicose veins, chronic venous insufficiency or postphlebitic syndrome, recurrent deep venous thrombosis, or pulmonary thromboembolism.

3.5.1 Nonsurgical treatment

Systemic anticoagulation is the primary treatment for deep venous thrombosis. It decreases the risk of pulmonary embolism and extension of venous thrombosis, and also reduces the recurrent rate of deep venous thrombosis by 80%. Systemic anticoagulation does not directly lyse thrombi but reduces blood clotting, prevent extension of venous thrombosis and facilitate recanalization. Heparin should be initiated immediately and dosed to a goal PTT of 1.5-2.5 times of normal. Achieving therapeutic heparinization within the first 24 hours after diagnosis can reduce the recurrent rate of deep venous thrombosis.

The advantages of low-molecular-weight heparin (LMWH) over standard heparin preparations include lower risk of bleeding and thrombocytopenia, less interference with proteins C and S, less complement activation, and lower risk of osteoporosis. Usually LMWH is injected intravenously or subcutaneously to achieve hypocoagulability, and then switched to oral warfarin. Warfarin is as safe and effective as LMWH in the treatment of deep venous thrombosis. The recommended treatment for anticoagulant therapy is using warfarin for 3-6 months, and maintaining the international normalized ratio (INR) at 2.0-3.0. If the patient has a known hypercoagulable state or has experienced episodes of venous thrombosis, lifetime anticoagulation is required in the absence of contraindications.

The efficacy of fibrinolytic agents in the treatment of deep venous thrombosis has been widely demonstrated. Commonly used fibrinolytic agents include urokinase, streptokinase, and recombinant tissue plasminogen activator (t-PA). Fibrinolytic agent activates fibrinogen in plasma to become fibrinogen, and then dissolves thrombus.

3.5.2 Surgical treatment

Thrombectomy is most commonly used in early cases of deep venous thrombosis of the lower extremities. The best time to take thrombectomy should be within 3 days after onset. The most used surgical method is Fogarty catheter thrombectomy. To prevent recurrence, postoperative adjuvant anticoagulation therapy is necessary for 2 months.

3.6 Prevention

Surgery significantly increases the risk of deep vein thrombosis. Therefore, it is very necessary to prevent deep venous thrombosis routinely in surgical patients. Guidelines for venous thromboembolism prophylaxis are based on specific risk factors for patients. For some low-risk patients, prophylaxis is mainly to encourage early ambulation. In higher-risk patients, appropriate prophylaxis includes the use of low-dose unfractionated heparin or LMWH. Patients with hypercoagulable state or paralysis can benefit from lifetime anticoagulation with low-dose warfarin or prophylactic inferior vena cava filter placement.

Chapter 4

Lymphedema

Lymphedema is a chronic progressive disease caused by lymphatic circulation disorders and persistent accumulation of protein-rich interstitial fluids. It usually occurs on limbs, and the lower limbs are the most common site.

4.1 Etiology and Classification

Lymphedema is usually divided into two categories: primary lymphedema and secondary lymphedema. Primary lymphedema is caused by abnormal development of lymphatic vessels. The most common cause is hypoplasia, resulting in a severe reduction in the number of lymphatic vessels and lymphatic vessel diameter.

It is classified by age at onset of the disease. Congenital lymphedema develops before 1 year of age; if familial, it is called Milroy's disease. Lymphedema praecox occurs between 1 and 35 years of age; if familial, it is called Meige's disease. Lymphedema tarda develops after age 35.

Secondary lymphedema results from various disease processes that cause obstruction to the lymphatic system. These reasons include lymphadenectomy, fibrosis after radiotherapy, tumor infiltrating lymph node. Filariasis is also an important cause of lymphedema in filariasis endemic areas.

4.2 Clinical Manifestation

Painless edema is a common symptom for primary lymphedema. Lymphedema development is usually slowly progressive and painless. In the early stages, the edema is pitting, but as the disease progresses, chronic fibrosis occurs and the edema becomes non-pitting. The distribution of edema is usually centered around the ankle and is most pronounced at the instep, and produces a buffalo hump appearance. The patient's skin is reddish, and its temperature is slightly higher, then the skin became thicker, and "rubber leg" may appear later. Secondary infection may cause symptoms of localized red, swollen, hot, pain, and even systemic infection. Mild skin lesions cause ulcers that are difficult to heal. Rarely, chronic lymphedema may develop lymphangiosarcoma.

4.3 Diagnosis

It is not difficult to make clinical diagnosis based on medical history and physical examinations. The following tests will help to confirm the diagnosis and understand the type, the location, and the cause of the lesion.

Lymphoscintigraphy is a specialized test used for the detection of lymph node metastasis and helps to make etiology and location diagnosis. CT and MRI are useful tests in patients with suspected secondary lymphedema caused by unknown malignancy. Lymphangiography is rarely used now, as it may damage the lymphatic vessels further.

4.4 Differential Diagnosis

Other multiple diseases can also lead to bilateral lower extremity edema, including congestive heart failure, chronic renal or hepatic insufficiency, and hypoproteinemia. In patients with unilateral edema, differential diagnoses include congenital vascular malformations, chronic venous insufficiency, and reflex sympathetic dystrophy.

4.5 Treatment

Currently, lymphedema is a chronic disease that can not be completely cured. However, various conservative measures can significantly reduce the risk of further complications and disability.

4.5.1 Nonsurgical treatment

The preferred treatment is external compression and meticulous skin care. Mechanical reduction of lymphedema can be achieved to the greatest degree through frequent leg elevation, manual lymphatic drainage massage, low-stretch wrapping techniques, and intermittent pneumatic compression. Graduated compression stockings maintain the limb after reduced by pneumatic compression. Diuretics can be used for acute edema caused by secondary infection or for coexisting venous stasis disease, but these agents are not recommended for long-term use in lymphedema.

Drying and cracking of the skin can be the way for bacteria to enter, so, good skin care can prevent infection. Applying a moisturizing lotion regularly is essential, especially after bathing.

4.5.2 Surgical treatment

Only 10% of patients with lymphedema have surgical indications. Operation may be considered in rare cases of severe dysfunction and recurrent lymphangitis. Surgical options include excision with skin grafting, closure of disrupted lymphatic vessels, omental transposition, and microsurgical lymphovenous anastomosis. The main goals of these operations are to reduce limb bulk, either by ablation techniques (excision of excess tissue) or physiological techniques (lymphatic reconstruction).

Part 39

Anatomy of the Genitourinary tract

Urology deals with diseases and disorders of the male genitourinary tract and the female urinary tract. Surgical diseases of the adrenal gland are also included. To understand the basic anatomy and relations involved in male genitourinary tract and the female urinary tract is of great importance for urological surgeons.

39.1 Adrenal glands

Each kidney is capped by an adrenal gland, and both organs are enclosed within Gerota's fascia. Each adrenalgland weighs about 5 g. The right adrenal gland is triangular in shape; the left one is more rounded and crescentic. Each gland is composed of a cortex, chiefly influenced by the pituitary gland, and a medulla derived from chromaffin tissue. The right adrenal gland lies between the liver and the vena cava. The left adrenal gland is close to the aorta and is covered on its lower surface by the pancreas; superiorly and laterally, it is related to the spleen. Each adrenal gland receives three arteries: one from the inferior phrenic artery, one from the aorta, and one from the renal artery. Blood from the right adrenal gland is drained by a very short vein that empties into the vena cava; the left adrenal vein terminates in the left renal vein. The lymphatic vessels accompany the suprarenal vein and drain into the lumbar lymph nodes.

39.2 Kidneys

The kidneys lie along the borders of the psoas muscles and are therefore obliquely placed. The position of the liver causes the right kidney to be lower than the left one. The adult kidney weighs about 150 g. The kidneys are supported by the perirenal fat (which is enclosed in the perirenal fascia), the renal vascular pedicle, abdominal muscle tone, and the general bulk of the abdominal viscera. The functioning unit of the kidney is the nephron, which is composed of a tubule that has both secretory and excretory functions. The secretory portion is contained largely within the cortex and consists of a renal corpuscle and the secretory part of the renal tubule. The excretory portion of this duct lies in the medulla. The renal stroma is composed of loose connective tissue and contains blood vessels, capillaries, nerves, and lymphatics. Usually there is one renal artery, a branch of the aorta, which enters the hilum of the kidney between the pelvis, which normally lies posteriorly, and the renal vein. The renal veins are paired with the arteries, but any of them will drain the entire kidney if the others are tied off. The renal nerves derived from the renal plexus accompany the renal vessels throughout the renal parenchyma. The lymphatics of the kidney drain into the lumbar lymph nodes.

39.3 Calices, renal pelvis and ureters

The tips of the minor calices (8–12 in number) are indented by the projecting pyramids. These calices unite to form 2 or 3 major calices, which join to form the renal pelvis. The pelvis may be entirely intrarenal or partly intrarenal and partly extrarenal. Inferomedially, it tapers to form the ureter. The adult ureter is about 30 cm long, varying in direct relation to the height of the individual. It follows a rather smooth S curve. Areas of relative narrowing are found at the ureteropelvic junction, where the ureter crosses over the iliac vessels, and where it courses through the bladder wall. The ureters lie on the psoas muscles, pass medially to the sacroiliac joints, and then swing laterally near the ischial spines before passing medially to penetrate the base of the bladder.

39.4 Bladder

The bladder is a hollow muscular organ that serves as a reservoir for urine. In women, its posterior wall and dome are invaginated by the uterus. The adult bladder normally has a capacity of 400–500 mL. When empty, the adult bladder lies behind the pubic symphysis and is largely a pelvic organ. The ureters enter the bladder posteroinferiorly in an oblique manner and at these points are about 5 cm apart. The orifices, situated at the extremities of the crescent-shaped interureteric ridge that forms the proximal border of the trigone, are about 2.5 cm apart. The trigone occupies the area between the ridge and the bladder neck. In males, the bladder is related posteriorly to the seminal vesicles, vasa deferentia, ureters, and rectum. In females, the uterus and vagina are interposed between the bladder and rectum. In both males and females, the bladder is related to the posterior surface of the pubic symphysis, and, when distended, it is in contact with the lower abdominal wall. The blood supply of bladder is from the superior, middle, and inferior vesical arteries, which arise from the anterior trunk of the internal iliac (hypogastric) artery, and by smaller branches from the obturator and inferior gluteal arteries. In females, the uterine and vaginal arteries also send branches to the bladder.

39.5 Prostate gland

The prostate is a fibromuscular and glandular organlies just inferior to the bladder. The normal prostate weighs about 20 g and contains the posterior urethra, which is about 2.5 cm in length. It is supported anteriorly by the puboprostatic ligaments and inferiorly by the urogenital diaphragm. The prostate is perforated posteriorly by the ejaculatory ducts, which pass obliquely to empty through the verumontanum on the floor of the prostatic urethra just proximal to the striated external urinary sphincter. The prostate gland lies behind the pubic symphysis. Located closely to the posterosuperior surface are the vasa deferentia and seminal vesicles. Posteriorly, the prostate is separated from the rectum by the 2 layers of Denonvilliers' fascia, serosal rudiments of the pouch of Douglas, which once extended to the urogenital diaphragm.

39.6 Seminal vesicles

The seminal vesicles lie just cephalic to the prostate under the bottom of the bladder. They are about 6 cm long and quite soft. Each vesicle joins its corresponding vas deferens to form the ejaculatory duct. The ureters lie medial to each, and the rectum is contiguous with their posterior surfaces.

39.7 Spermatic cord

The two spermatic cords extend from the internal inguinal rings through the inguinal canals to the testicles. Each cord contains the vas deferens, the internal and external spermatic arteries, the artery of the vas, the venous pampiniform plexus, which forms the spermatic vein superiorly, lymph vessels, and nerves. All of the preceding are enclosed in investing layers of thin fascia. A few fibers of the cremaster muscle insert on the cords in the inguinal canal.

39.8 Epididymis

The upper portion of the epididymis is connected to the testis by numerous efferent ducts from the testis. The epididymis consists of a markedly coiled duct that, at its lower pole, is continuous with the vas deferens. An appendix of the epididymis is often seen on its upper pole; this is a cystic body that in some cases is pedunculated but in others is sessile. The epididymis lies posterolateral to the testis and is nearest to the testis at its upper pole. Its lower pole is connected to the testis by fibrous tissue. The vas lies posteromedial to the epididymis.

39.9 Testis

The average testicleis measureed about 4 cm× 3 cm× 2.5 cm. It has a dense fascial covering called the tunica albuginea testis, which, posteriorly, is invaginated somewhat into the body of the testis to form the mediastinum testis. This fibrous mediastinum sends fibrous septa into the testis, thus separating it into about 250 lobules. The testis is covered anteriorly and laterally by the visceral layer of the serous tunica vaginalis, which is continuous with the parietal layer that separates the testis from the scrotal wall. At the upper pole of the testis is the appendix testis, a small pedunculated or sessile body similar in appearance to the appendix of the epididymis. The blood supply to the testes is closely associated with that to the kidneys because of the common embryologic origin of the two organs. The lymphatic vessels from the testes pass to the lumbar lymph nodes, which in turn are connected to the mediastinal nodes.

39.10 Penis and male urethra

The penis is composed of 2 corpora cavernosa and the corpus spongiosum, which contains the urethra, whose diameter is 8–9 mm. These corpora are capped distally by the glans. Each corpus is enclosed in a fascial sheath, and all are surrounded by a thick fibrous envelope known as Buck's fascia. A covering of skin, devoid of fat, is loosely applied about these bodies. The prepuce forms a hood over the glans. Beneath the skin of the penis (and scrotum) and extending from the base of the glans to the urogenital diaphragm is Colles' fascia, which is continuous with Scarpa's fascia of the lower abdominal wall. The proximal ends of the corpora cavernosa are attached to the pelvic bones just anterior to the ischial tuberosities. Occupying a depression of their ventral surface in the midline is the corpus spongiosum, which is connected proximally to the undersurface of the urogenital diaphragm, through which emerges the membranous urethra. This portion of the corpus spongiosum is surrounded by the bulbospongiosus muscle. Its distal end expands to form the glans penis.

The urethral mucosa that traverses the glans penis is formed of squamous epithelium. Proximal to this, the mucosa is transitional in type. Underneath the mucosa is the submucosa, which contains connective and elastic tissue and smooth muscle. In the submucosa are the numerous glands of Littre, whose ducts connect with the urethral lumen. The urethra is surrounded by the vascular corpus spongiosum and the glans penis.

39.11 Female urethra

The adult female urethra is about 4 cm long and 8 mm in diameter. It is slightly curved and lies beneath the pubic symphysis just anterior to the vagina. The epithelial lining of the female urethra is squamous in its distal portion and pseudostratified or transitional in the remainder. The submucosa is made up of connective and elastic tissues and spongy venous spaces. Embedded in it are many periurethral glands, which are most numerous distally; the largest of these are the periurethral glands of Skene, which open on the floor of the urethra just inside the meatus.

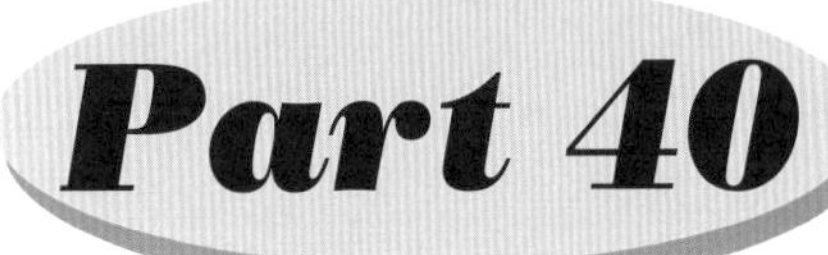

Development Anomalies of the urologic and Male Genital Tract

Genitourinary tract anomalies constitute about 1/3 of all congenital abnormalities and occur in about 10% of the population. Although those congenital anomalies are not life-threatening, they may cause infection, stone formation, or chronic renal insufficient.

Chapter 1

Renal Anomalies

Congenital anomalies occur more frequently in the kidney than in any other organ. Some cause no difficulty, but many (e. g., hypoplasia, polycystic kidneys) cause impairment of renal function.

1.1 Adult Polycystic Kidney Disease

Adult polycystic kidney disease is an autosomal dominant hereditary condition and almost always bilateral (95% of cases). Cysts of the liver, spleen, and pancreas may be noted in association with both forms. The kidneys are larger than normal and are studded with cysts of various sizes.

Pain over one or both kidneys may occur because of the drag on the vascular pedicles by the heavy kidneys, from obstruction or infection, or from hemorrhage into a cyst. Infection (chills, fever, and low-back pain) commonly complicates polycystic disease. When renal insufficiency ensues, headache, nausea and vomiting, weakness, and loss of weight occur. Hypertension is found in 60%–70% of these patients. Fever may be present if pyelonephritis exists or if cysts have been infected. In the stage of uremia, anemia and loss of weight may be evident.

Anemia may be noted, caused either by chronic loss of blood or, more commonly, by the hematopoietic depression accompanying uremia. Proteinuria and microscopic hematuria are the rule. Pyuria and bacteriuria are common. Progressive loss of concentrating power occurs. Renal clearance tests show varying degrees of renal impairment.

Except for unusual complications, the treatment is conservative and supportive. Hypertension should be controlled. Hemodialysis may be indicated. There is no evidence that excision or decompression of cysts improves renal function. If a large cyst is found to be compressing the upper ureter, causing obstruction and further embarrassing renal function, it should be resected or aspirated. When the degree of renal insufficiency becomes life-threatening, chronic dialysis or renal transplantation should be considered.

1.2 Renal Fusion

About 1 in 1000 individuals has some types of renal fusion, the most common being the horseshoe kidney. The fused renal mass almost always contains two excretory systems and therefore two ureters. The renal tissue may be divided equally between the two flanks, or the entire mass may be on one side. Even in the latter case, the two ureters open at their proper places in the bladder. It appears that this fusion of the two metanephroi occurs early in embryologic life, when the kidneys lie low in the pelvis. For this reason, they seldom ascend to the high position that normal kidneys assume.

Most patients with fused kidneys have no symptoms. Some, however, develop ureteral obstruction. Gastrointestinal symptoms (renodigestive reflex) mimicking peptic ulcer, cholelithiasis, or appendicitis may be noted. Infection is apt to occur if ureteral obstruction and hydronephrosis or calculus develops.

Fused kidneys are prone to ureteral obstruction because of a high incidence of aberrant renal vessels and the necessity for one or both ureters to arch around or over the renal tissue. Hydronephrosis, stone, and infection, therefore, are common. A large fused kidney occupying the concavity of the sacrum may cause dystocia. No treatment is necessary unless obstruction or infection is present. Drainage of a horseshoe kidney may be improved by dividing its isthmus. If one pole of a horseshoe is badly damaged, it may require surgical resection.

In most cases, the outlook is excellent. If ureteral obstruction and infection occur, renal drainage must be improved by surgical means so that antimicrobial therapy will be effective.

1.3 Ectopic Kidney

Congenital ectopic kidney usually causes no symptoms unless complications such as ureteral obstruction or infection develop. Simple congenital ectopy usually refers to a low kidney on the proper side that failed to ascend normally. It may lie over the pelvic brim or in the pelvis. It takes its blood supply from adjacent vessels, and its ureter is short. It is prone to ureteral obstruction and infection, which may lead to pain or fever. Excretory urograms reveal the true position of the kidney. Hydronephrosis, if present, is evident. There is no redundancy of the ureter, as is the case with nephroptosis or acquired ectopy (e. g., displacement by large suprarenal tumor). Obstruction and infection may complicate simple ectopy and should be treated by appropriate means.

In crossed ectopy without fusion, the kidney lies on the opposite side of the body but is not attached to its normally placed mate. Unless two distinct renal shadows can be seen, it may be difficult to differentiate this condition from crossed ectopy with fusion. Sonography, angiography, or CT should make the distinction.

Chapter 2

Obstruction of Pelvi-ureteric Junction and Hydronephrosis

Obstruction of pelvico-ureteric junction (OPUJ), the most common congenital upper urinary tract disorder, is one of the most common causes of hydronephrosis. The recognition and relief of significant obstruction is important to prevent irreversible damage to the kidneys.

2.1 Incidence

The overall incidence of neonatal hydronephrosis which leads to the diagnosis of OPUJ approximates 1 in 500 births. The ratio of males to females is 2 : 1 in the neonatal period, with the 60% occurring in left sided lesions. In the newborn period, a unilateral process is most common, but bilateral OPUJ was found in 10%–49% of neonates in some reported series.

2.2 Classification

OPUJ is classified as intrinsic, extrinsic, or secondary.

Intrinsic obstruction results from failure of transmission of the peristaltic waves across the pelvi-ureteric junction with failure of urine to be propulsed from the renal pelvis into the ureter which results in multiple ineffective peristaltic waves that eventually causes hydronephrosis by incompletely emptying the pelvic contents.

Extrinsic mechanical factors include aberrant renal vessels, bands, adventitial tissues and adhesions that cause angulation, kinking or compression of the pelvi-ureteric junction. Extrinsic obstruction may occur alone but usually coexists with intrinsic ureteropelvic junction pathology.

Secondary OPUJ may develop as a consequence of concomitant severe vesico-ureteric reflux (VUR) which occurs in 15%–30% of children who have ipsilateral OPUJ which a tortuous ureter may kink proximately.

2.3 Grading System of Postnatal Hydronephrosis

In the Society for Fetal Urology(SFU),hydronephrosis is divided into 5 grads.

There is no hydronephrosis in Grade 0. The renal pelvis is only visualized at Grade 1. Grade 2 of hydronephrosis is diagnosed when a few(but not all) renal calices are identified in addition to the renal pelvis. Grade 3 hydronephrosis requires that virtually all calices are depicted. Grade 4 hydronephrotic kidneys will exhibit similar caliceal status with the involved kidney exhibiting parenchymal thinning.

Grades 3-4 prenatal bilateral hydronephrosis indicates that the majority of the children will require surgical correction during postnatal period. Fetal urinary sodium level less than 100 mmol/L,chloride level less than 90 mmol/L and an osmolality of less than 210 mOsm/kg are considered as prognostic features for good renal function.

2.4 Clinical Presentation

With the advent of prenatal ultrasonographic screening only sporadic cases present with clinical symptoms. Before the routine fetal ultrasonography,the commonest presentation was with abdominal flank mass. 50% abdominal masses in newborns are of renal origin and with 40% being secondary to pelvi-ureteric junction obstruction. Some patients present with urinary tract infection. Other clinical presentations include irritability,vomiting and failure to thrive. 10%-35% of OPUJ are bilateral and associated abnormalities of urinary tract are seen in about 30%. OPUJ problems are often associated with other congenital anomalies,including imperforated anus,contralateral dysplastic kidney,congenital heart disease,Vater syndrome,and esophageal atresia. A renal ultrasound examiration should be performed when these diseases diagnosed.

2.5 Diagnosis

With the increasing number of antenatally diagnosed hydronephrosis,it is difficult to interpret the underlying pathology and its significance. Severe obstructive uropathies are detrimental to renal function. However,on the other hand hydronephrosis without ureteral or lower tract anomaly is common. The important aspect of postnatal investigations is to identify the group of patients who will benefit from early intervention and those who need to be carefully followed up.

2.5.1 Prenatal diagnosis

Beyond 20 weeks of gestation,fetal urine production is the main source of amniotic fluid. Therefore, major abnormalities of the urinary tract may result in oligohydramnios. Because of the distinct urine tissue interface,hydronephrosis can be detected as early as 16th week of gestation. An obstructive anomaly is recognized by demonstrating dilated renal calyces and pelvis. A multitude of measurement and different gestational age cut-off points have been recommended in the assessment of fetal obstructive uropathy. Routine estimation of anteroposterior(AP) diameter of renal pelvis in fetus with hydronephrosis is considered as a useful marker for classification of renal dilatation and possible obstruction. AP renal pelvis threshold values ranged between 2.3 mm and 10 mm. Positive predictive values for pathological dilatation confirmed in the neonate ranged between 2.3% and >40% for AP renal measurements of 2–3 mm and 10 mm, respectively.

2.5.2 Postnatal diagnosis

Follow-up ultrasound examination is necessary in postnatal period in antenatally detected hydronephrosis. If the bilateral hydronephrosis is diagnosed in utero in a male infant, postnatal evaluation should be carried out within 24 h primarily because of the possibility of posterior urethral valves. If the ultrasound scan is negative in the first 24–48 h in any patient with unilateral or bilateral hydronephrosis, a repeat scan should be performed after 5–10 days, recognizing that neonatal oliguria may mask a moderately obstructive lesion. Further careful scan of the kidney, ureter and bladder in boys is essential after the diagnosis of hydronephrosis is confirmed on the postnatal scan.

Ultrasonography depicts the dilated calyces as multiple intercommunicating cystic spaces of fairly uniform size that lead into a larger cystic structure at the hilum, representing the dilated renal pelvis. Peripheral to the dilated calyces, the renal parenchyma is usually thinned with the normal or increased echogenicity. Typically, the ureter is of normal calibre and not seen. But if it is dilated the size of ureter is also assessed ultrasonographically and graded 1–3 according to ureteral width <7 mm, 7–10 mm, >10 mm respectively.

2.5.3 Radionucleide scans

Diuretic renograms using 99mTc DTPA augmented with furosemide were useful in the diagnosis of urinary tract obstructions for a long time. DTPA is completely filtered by the kidneys a maximum concentration of 5% being reached in 5 min, falling to 2% at 15 min. ^{123}I-Hippuran and ^{99}Tc MAG3 may improve diagnostic accuracy. The kidney of the young infant is immature; renal clearance, even when corrected for body surface, progressively increases until approximately 2 years of age. Therefore, the renal uptake of tracer is particularly low in infants, and there is a high background activity. Thus, the traces such as ^{123}I-Hippuran and ^{99}Tc MAG3 with a high extraction rate provide reasonable images enabling estimation of the differential kidney function during the first few weeks of life. It is also helpful in assessing the size, shape, location and function of the kidney.

Diuretic augmented renogram is a provocative test and is intended to demonstrate or exclude obstructive hydronephrosis by stressing an upper urinary tract with a high urine flow. Obstruction usually is defined as a failure of tracer washout after diuretic stimulation. If unequivocal, it eliminates the need for further investigations. In equivocal cases, F15 in which furosemide is given 15 min before the test provides a better assessment of the drainage of upper urinary tract. Forced hydration prior to scan increases predictive value of non-obstructed pattern up to 94%. Since glomerular filtration and glomerular blood flow are still low in the newborn, the handling of isotype is unpredictable and can be misleading.

Diagnosis of OPUJ can be made also by intravenous urography. This investigation is unreliable because no helpful the concentration of contrast although shows a dilated renal pelvis with clubbed calyces often, therefore, its routine use is abounded in the paediatric urology.

2.5.4 Pressure-flow study

In the equivocal cases and in the presence of impaired function, the pressure flow study (Whitaker test) and antegrade pyelography may be necessary to confirm or exclude obstruction. Whitaker test is based on the hypothesis that if the dilated upper urinary tract can transport 10 mL/min without an inordinate increase in pressure, the hydrostatic pressure under physiological conditions should not cause impairment of renal function and the degree of obstruction if present is insignificant. However, it is an invasive test and is seldom required.

Antegrade pyelography may be performed with ultrasound guidance in patients where diagnosis is difficult and it is seldom required to determine the status of ureters. The disadvantages include difficulty in ureteral catheterization in neonates, trauma and edema may change partial obstruction to the complete one.

In patients where diagnosis is equivocal, serial examinations may be necessary. A routine use of micturating cystourethrogram (MCUG) in patients with antenatal unilateral hydronephrosis is controversial. Some authors advocate a routine use of MCUG as a part of postnatal evaluation citing 15%–30% of incidence of concomitant vesicoureteric reflux (VUR) either uni- or contra-lateral. Others recommend performing MCUG only in patients with SFU Gr Ⅲ and Ⅳ hydronephrosis.

The role of dynamic contrast enhanced MR urography in the evaluation of antenatal hydronephrosis has become appreciated. This method allows precise understanding of the kidney anatomy while providing information regarding renal functioning without radiation exposure obviating need in the use of contrast media.

2.6 Treatment

A considerable controversy exists regarding the management of newborn urinary tract obstructions. During late prenatal and early postnatal life, there is progressive increase in glomerular filtration rate. Additionally, this transition is associated with an abrupt decline in urine output from what appears to be a quite high in utero output to a rather low early neonatal level of urine production. These physiological observations may explain the common observation of hydronephrosis detected antenatally, which on postnatal follow-up reverts to an unobstructed pattern. Surgery is usually undertaken in infants whose renal function deteriorates during observation period. SFU Grades 3–4 of postnatal hydronephrosis, RRF <40% are significant independent risk factors for surgery.

A number of different operations have been described for surgical correction of OPUJ. Dismembered Anderson-Hynes pyeloplasty is considered as a gold standard in the surgical treatment of OPUJ which can be performed through extraperitoneal approach via lateral flank incision or utilizing posterior lumbotomy incision, and recently, laparoscopic approach advocated. The basic principle of these operations is an excision of pelvi-ureteric junction with a subsequent oval shaped anastomosis between ureter and lower part of pelvis. Different types of stent are place for drainage usually for 6 weeks. The most popular are Double J Pediatric Stents or Pipi Salle Stent nephrostomy (Cook, USA).

Although antegrade and retrograde endopyelotomy have been shown to be effective in children, but should be considered in older children or in those with failed primary dismembered pyeloplasty.

(1) Bilateral OPUJ: Surgical correction of the symptomatic side or side with better function should take precedence. If a nephrectomy is considered on one side, the pyeloplasty should precede this.

(2) Postoperative complications: Include infection, adhesive obstruction (transperitoneal approach), temporary obstruction at the anastomosis resulting in excessive urine leakage and failures due to postoperative stricture at anastomotic sites.

(3) Follow-up and results: Follow-up ultrasound may be performed 3–6 months after operation when maximum improvement can be seen. Follow up radionuclide scan should be done 6–8 months following pyeloplasty, in order to evaluate an improvement in the renal function and drainage. Pyeloplasty in the neonatal period when indicated gives excellent results.

Chapter 3

Ureterocele

Ureterocele is a sacculation of the terminal portion of the ureter. It may be either intravesical or ectopic; in the latter case, some portion is located at the bladder neck or in the urethra. Intravesical ureteroceles are associated most often with single ureters, whereas ectopic ureteroceles nearly always involve the upper pole of duplicated ureters.

Clinical findings vary considerably. Patients commonly present with infection, but bladder outlet obstruction or incontinence may be the initial complaint. Calculi can develop secondary to urinary stasis and are often seen in the distal ureter. Although excretory urography is usually diagnostic, sonography has replaced the excretory urogram in most centers. Voiding cystourethrography should always be part of the work-up. It may demonstrate reflux into the lower pole or contralateral ureter and occasionally shows eversion of the ureterocele during urination, in which case the ureterocele has the appearance of a diverticulum.

Treatment must be individualized. Transurethral incision was used previously only in very ill children with pyohydronephrosis; however, it has been recognized as the definitive procedure in many instances. When an open operation is needed, the procedure must be chosen on the basis of the anatomic location of the ureteral meatus, the position of the ureterocele, and the degree of hydroureteronephrosis and impairment of renal function. In general, choices range from heminephrectomy and ureterectomy to excision of the ureterocele, vesical reconstruction, and ureteral reimplantation.

Chapter 4

Congential Anomalies of the Bladder and Urethra

4.1 Exstrophy of the Bladder

Exstrophy of the bladder is a complete ventral defect of the urogenital sinus and the overlying skeletal system. Other congenital anomalies are frequently associated with it. The lower central abdomen is occupied by the inner surface of the posterior wall of the bladder, whose mucosal edges are fused with the skin. Urine spurts onto the abdominal wall from the ureteral orifices.

Many untreated exstrophic bladders reveal fibrosis, derangement of the muscularis mucosae, and chronic infection. These changes tend to defeat efforts to form a bladder of proper capacity. Renal infection is common, and hydronephrosis caused by ureterovesical obstruction may be found on urography. These films also reveal separation of the pubic bones.

During the last few years, there have been encouraging reports of complete reconstruction of this defect. Earlier, urinary diversion and resection of the bladder, with later repair of the epispadiac penis, was usually accomplished. With improved techniques and early surgery before the bladder deteriorates, however, good results are being obtained with complete reconstruction. When the bladder is small, fibrotic, and inelastic, functional closure becomes inadvisable, and urinary diversion with cystectomy is the treatment of choice. Some physicians perform ureteroileocutaneous anastomosis, while others prefer to use the colon for the diversion.

4.2 Persistent Urachus

Embryologically, the allantois connects the urogenital sinus with the umbilicus. Normally, the allantois is obliterated and is represented by a fibrous cord (urachus) extending from the dome of the bladder to the navel. If obliteration is complete except at the superior end, a draining umbilical sinus may be noted. If it becomes infected, the drainage will be purulent. If the inferior end remains open, it will communicate with the bladder, but this does not usually produce symptoms. Rarely, the entire tract remains patent, in which case urine drains constantly from the umbilicus. If only the ends of the urachus seal off, a cyst of that body may form and may become quite large, presenting a low midline mass. If the cyst becomes infected, signs of general and local sepsis will develop. Adenocarcinoma may occur in a urachal cyst, particularly at its vesical extremity, and tends to invade the tissues beneath the anterior abdominal wall. Stones may develop in a cyst of the urachus. Treatment consists of excision of the urachus, which lies on the peritoneal surface. If adenocarcinoma is present, radical resection is required.

4.3 Hypospadias

In hypospadias, the urethral meatus opens on the ventral side of the penis proximal to the tip of the glans penis. The urethra is formed by the fusion of the urethral folds along the ventral surface of the penis, which extends to the corona on the distal shaft. The glandular urethra is formed by canalization of an ectodermal cord that has grown through the glans to communicate with the fused urethral folds. Hypospadias results when fusion of the urethral folds is incomplete. There are several forms of hypospadias, classified according to location: ①glandular, that is, opening on the proximal glans penis; ②coronal, that is, opening at the coronal sulcus; ③penile shaft; ④penoscrotal; ⑤perineal. About 70% of all cases of hypospadias are distal penile or coronal.

Although newborns and young children seldom have symptoms, older children and adults may complain of difficulty directing the urinary stream and stream spraying. Chordee (curvature of the penis) causes ventral bending and bowing of the penile shaft, which can prevent sexual intercourse. For psychological reasons, hypospadias should be repaired before the patient reaches school age; in most cases, this can be done before age 2. More than 150 methods of corrective surgery for hypospadias have been described. Currently, one-stage repairs using island flap grafts are performed by more and more urologists.

Chapter 5

Cryptochidism

Cryptorchidism is the absence of one or both testes from the scrotum. It is the most common birth defect of the male genital. About 3% of full-term and 30% of premature infant boys are born with at least one undescended testis. However, about 80% of cryptorchid testes descend by the first year of life (the majority within 3 months), making the true incidence of cryptorchidism around 1% overall.

Many men who were born with undescended testes have reduced fertility, even after orchiopexy in infancy. The reduction with unilateral cryptorchidism is subtle, with a reported infertility rate of about 10%. The fertility reduction after orchiopexy for bilateral cryptorchidism is more marked, about 6 times that of the general population. The basis for the universal recommendation for early surgery shows degeneration of spermatogenic tissue and reduced spermatogonia counts after the second year of life in undescended testes. The degree to which this is prevented or improved by early orchiopexy is still uncertain.

One of the strongest arguments for early orchiopexy is reducing the risk of testicular cancer. The peak incidence occurs in the 3rd and 4th decades of the life. The risk is higher for intra-abdominal testes and somewhat lower for inguinal testes, but even the normally descended testis of a man whose other testis was undescended has about a 20% higher cancer risk than those of other men. It was demonstrated that orchi dopexy performed before puberty resulted in a significantly reduced risk of testicular cancer than if done after puberty.

Scrotal ultrasound or magnetic resonance imaging performed and interpreted by a radiologist can often, but not invariably, locate the testes while confirming absence of a uterus. At ultrasound, the undescended testis usually appears small, less echogenic than the contralateral normal testis and usually located in the inguinal region. With color Doppler ultrasonography, the vascularity of the undescended testis is poor.

The primary management of cryptorchidism is watchful waiting, due to the high likelihood of self-resolution. Where this fails, a surgery, called orchiopexy, is effective if inguinal testes have not descended after 4-6 months. When the undescended testis is in the inguinal canal, hormonal therapy is sometimes attempted and very occasionally successful. The most commonly used hormone therapy is human chorionic gonadotropin (HCG). In patients with intraabdominal maldescended testis, laparoscopy is useful to see for oneself the pelvic structures, position of the testis and decide upon surgery (single or staged procedure).

Chapter 6

Phimosis and Paraphimosis

Phimosis is a condition in which the contracted foreskin can not be retracted over the glans. Chronic infection from poor local hygiene is its most common cause. Most cases occur in uncircumcised males, although excessive skin left after circumcision can become stenotic and cause phimosis. Calculi and squamous cell carcinoma may develop under the foreskin. Phimosis can occur at any age. In diabetic older men, chronic balanoposthitis may lead to phimosis and may be the initial presenting complaint. Children under two years of age seldom have true phimosis; their relatively narrow preputial opening gradually widens and allows for normal retraction of foreskin over the glans. Edema, erythema, and tenderness of the prepuce and the presence of purulent discharge usually cause the patient to seek medical attention. Inability to retract the foreskin is a less common complaint. The initial infection should be treated with broad-spectrum antimicrobial drugs. The dorsal foreskin can be slit if improved drainage is necessary. Circumcision for phimosis should be avoided in children requiring general anesthesia; except in cases with recurrent infections, the procedure should be postponed until the child reaches an age when local anesthesia can be used.

Paraphimosis is the condition in which the foreskin, once retracted over the glans, can not be replaced in its normal position. This is due to chronic inflammation under the redundant foreskin, which leads to contracture of the preputial opening (phimosis) and formation of a tight ring of skin when the foreskin is retracted behind the glans. The skin ring causes venous congestion leading to edema and enlargement of the glans, which make the condition worse. As the condition progresses, arterial occlusion and necrosis of the glans may occur. Paraphimosis usually can be treated by firmly squeezing the glans for 5 min to reduce the tissue edema and decrease the size of the glans. The skin can then be drawn forward over the glans. Occasionally, the constricting ring requires incision under local anesthesia. Antibiotics should be administered and circumcision should be done after inflammation has subsided.

Part 41

Urinary Tract Trauma

About 10% of injuries seen in the emergency room involve the genitourinary system to some extent. Many of them are subtle and difficult tobe defined and require great diagnostic expertise. Initial assessment should include control of hemorrhage and shock along with resuscitation as required. The abdomen and genitalia should be examined for evidence of contusions or subcutaneous hematomas, which might indicate deeper injuries to the retroperitoneum and pelvic structures. Patients who do not have life-threatening injuries and whose blood pressure is stable can undergo more deliberate radiographic studies. This provides more definitive staging of the injury.

Chapter 1

Injuries to the Kidney

Renal injuries are the most common injuries of the urinary system. Most injuries occur from automobile accidents or sporting mishaps. Kidneys with existing pathologic conditions such as hydronephrosis or malignant tumors are more readily ruptured from mild trauma.

1.1 Etiology

Blunt trauma directly to the abdomen, flank, or back is the most common mechanism, accounting for 80% -85% of all renal injuries. Trauma may result from motor vehicle accidents, fights, falls, and contact sports. Vehicle collisions at high speed may result in major renal trauma from rapid deceleration and cause major vascular injury. Gunshot and knife wounds cause most penetrating injuries to the kidney. Any such wound in the flank area should be regarded as a cause of renal injury until proved otherwise. Associated abdominal visceral injuries are presented in 80% of renal penetrating wounds.

1.2 Pathology and Classification

1.2.1 Early pathologic findings

Lacerations from blunt trauma usually occur in the transverse plane of the kidney. The mechanism of injury is thought to be force transmitted from the center of the impact to the renal parenchyma. In injuries from rapid deceleration, the kidney moves upward or downward, causing sudden stretch on the renal pedicle and sometimes complete or partial avulsion. Pathologic classification of renal injuries is as follows:

Grade 1 (the most common)—Renal contusion or bruising of the renal parenchyma.

Grade 2—Renal parenchymal laceration into the renal cortex. Perirenal hematoma is usually small.

Grade 3—Renal parenchymal laceration extending through the cortex and into the renal medulla. Bleeding can be significant in the presence of large retroperitoneal hematoma.

Grade 4—Renal parenchymal laceration extending into the renal collecting system; also, main renal artery thrombosis from blunt trauma, segmental renal vein, or both; or artery injury with contained bleeding.

Grade 5—Multiple Grade 4 parenchymal lacerations, renal pedicle avulsion, or both; main renal vein or artery injury from penetrating trauma.

1.2.2 Late pathologic findings

Urinoma—Deep lacerations that are not repaired may result in persistent urinary extravasation and late complications of a large perinephric renal mass and, eventually, hydronephrosis and abscess formation.

Hydronephrosis—Large hematomas in the retroperitoneum and associated urinary extravasation may result in perinephric fibrosis engulfing the ureteropelvic junction, causing hydronephrosis. Follow-up excretory urography is indicated in all cases of major renal trauma.

Arteriovenous fistula—Arteriovenous fistulas may occur after penetrating injuries but are not common.

Renal vascular hypertension—The blood flow in tissue rendered nonviable by injury is compromised; this results in renal vascular hypertension in less than 1% of cases. Fibrosis from surrounding trauma has also been reported to constrict the renal artery and cause renal hypertension.

1.3 Clinical Findings and Indications for Studies

Microscopic or gross hematuria following trauma to the abdomen indicates injury to the urinary tract, but the degree of renal injury does not correspond to the degree of hematuria. It bears repeating that stab or gunshot wounds to the flank area should alert the physician to possible renal injury whether or not hematuria is present. Some cases of renal vascular injury are not associated with hematuria.

1.3.1 Symptoms

There is usually visible evidence of abdominal trauma. Pain may be localized to one flank area or over the abdomen. Associated injuries such as ruptured abdominal viscera or multiple pelvic fractures also cause acute abdominal pain and may obscure the presence of renal injury. Catheterization usually reveals hematuria. Retroperitoneal bleeding may cause abdominal distention, ileus, and nausea and vomiting.

1.3.2 Signs

Initially, shock or signs of a large loss of blood from heavy retroperitoneal bleeding may be noted. Ecchymosis in the flank or upper quadrants of the abdomen is often noted. Lower rib fractures are frequently found. Diffuse abdominal tenderness may be found on palpation. A palpable mass may represent a large retroperitoneal hematoma or perhaps urinary extravasation. If the retroperitoneum has been torn, free blood may be noted in the peritoneal cavity but no palpable mass will be evident. The abdomen may be distended and bowel soundsis absent.

1.3.3 Laboratory findings

Microscopic or gross hematuria is usually present. The hematocrit may be normal initially, but a drop may be found when serial studies are done. This finding represents persistent retroperitoneal bleeding and development of a large retroperitoneal hematoma. Persistent bleeding may necessitate operation.

1.3.4 Staging and X-ray findings

Staging of renal injuries allows a systematic approach to these problems. Adequate studies help define the extent of injury and dictate appropriate management. Staging begins with an abdominal CT scan, the most direct and effective means of staging renal injuries. This noninvasive technique clearly defines parenchymal lacerations and urinary extravasation, shows the extent of the retroperitoneal hematoma, identifies nonviable tissue, and outlines injuries to surrounding organs such as the pancreas, spleen, liver, and bowel. Arteriography defines major arterial and parenchymal injuries when previous studies have not fully done so. Arterial thrombosis and avulsion of the renal pedicle are best diagnosed by arteriography and are likely when the kidney is not visualized on imaging studies.

1.4 Complications

1.4.1 Early complications

Hemorrhage is perhaps the most important immediate complication of renal injury. Heavy retroperitoneal bleeding may result in rapid exsanguination. Patients must be observed closely, with careful monitoring of blood pressure and hematocrit. Complete staging must be done early. The size and expansion of palpable masses must be carefully monitored. Bleeding ceases spontaneously in 80%-85% of cases. Persistent retroperitoneal bleeding or heavy gross hematuria may require early operation. Urinary extravasation from renal fracture may show as an expanding mass (urinoma) in the retroperitoneum. A perinephric abscess may form, resulting in abdominal tenderness and flank pain.

1.4.2 Late complications

Hypertension, hydronephrosis, arteriovenous fistula, calculus formation, and pyelonephritis are important late complications. Careful monitoring of blood pressure for several months is necessary to watch for hypertension. At 3-6 months, a follow-up excretory urogram or CT scan should bedone to be certain that perinephric scarring has not caused hydronephrosis or vascular compromise; renal atrophy may occur from vascular compromise and is detected by follow-up urography.

1.5 Treatment

1.5.1 Emergency measures

The objectives of early management are prompt treatment of shock and hemorrhage, complete resuscitation, and evaluation of associated injuries.

1.5.2 Surgical measures

Blunt injuries—Minor renal injuries from blunt trauma account for 85% of cases and do not usually require operation. Bleeding stops spontaneously with bed rest and hydration. Cases in which operation is indicated include those associated with persistent retroperitoneal bleeding, urinary extravasation, evidence of nonviable renal parenchyma, and renal pedicle injuries. Aggressive preoperative staging allows complete definition of injury before operation.

Penetrating injuries—Penetrating injuries should be surgically explored. A rare exception to this rule is when staging has been complete and only minor parenchymal injury, with no urinary extravasation, is noted. In 80% of cases of penetrating injury, associated organ injury requires operation; thus, renal exploration is only an extension of this procedure.

1.5.3 Treatment of complications

Retroperitoneal urinoma or perinephric abscess demands prompt surgical drainage. Malignant hypertension requires vascular repair or nephrectomy. Hydronephrosis may require surgical correction or nephrectomy.

Chapter 2

Injuries to the Ureter

Ureteral injury is rare but may occur, usually during the course of a difficult pelvic surgical procedure or as a result of gunshot wounds. Rapid deceleration accidents may avulse the ureter from the renal pelvis. Endoscopic basket manipulation of ureteral calculi may result in injury.

2.1 Etiology

Large pelvic masses (benign or malignant) may displace the ureter laterally and engulf it in reactive fibrosis. This may lead to ureteral injury during dissection, since the organ is anatomically malpositioned. Inflammatory pelvic disorders may involve the ureter in a similar way. Devascularization may occur with extensive pelvic lymph node dissections or after radiation therapy to the pelvis for pelvic cancer. In these situations, ureteral fibrosis and subsequent stricture formation may develop along with ureteral fistulas. Endoscopic manipulation of a ureteral calculus with a stone basket or ureteroscope may result in ureteral perforation or avulsion.

2.2 Pathogenesis and Pathology

The ureter may be inadvertently ligated and cut during difficult pelvic surgery. In such cases, sepsis and severe renal damage usually occur postoperatively. If a partially divided ureter is unrecognized at operation, urinary extravasation and subsequent buildup of a large urinoma will ensue, which usually leads to ureterovaginal or ureterocutaneous fistula formation.

2.3 Clinical Findings

(1) Symptoms

If the ureter has been completely or partially ligated during operation, the postoperative course is usually marked by fever of 38.3–38.8 ℃ (101–102 °F) as well as flank and lower quadrant pain. Such patients often experience paralytic ileus with nausea and vomiting. Ureteral injuries from external violence should be suspected in patients who have sustained stab or gunshot wounds to the retroperitoneum. The mid portion of the ureter seems to be the most common site of penetrating injury. There are usually associated vascular and other abdominal visceral injuries.

(2) Signs

The acute hydronephrosis of a totally ligated ureter results in severe flank pain and abdominal pain with nausea and vomiting early in the postoperative course and with associated ileus. Signs and symptoms of acute peritonitis may be present if there is urinary extravasation into the peritoneal cavity. Watery discharge from the wound or vagina may be identified as urine by determining the creatinine concentration of a small sample.

(3) Laboratory findings

Ureteral injury from external violence is manifested by microscopic hematuria in 90% of cases. Urinalysis and other laboratory studies are of little use in diagnosis when injury has occurred from other causes.

(4) Imaging findings

Diagnosis is by excretory urography. A plain film of the abdomen may demonstrate a large area of increased density in the pelvis or in an area of retroperitoneum where injury is suspected. After injection of contrast medium, delayed excretion is noted with hydronephrosis. Partial transection of the ureter results in more rapid excretion, but persistent hydronephrosis is usually present, and contrast extravasation at the site of injury is noted on delayed films. Retrograde ureterography demonstrates the exact site of obstruction or extravasation.

2.4 Complications

Ureteral injury may be complicated by stricture formation with resulting hydronephrosis in the area of injury. Chronic urinary extravasation from unrecognized injury may lead to formation of a large retroperitoneal urinoma. Pyelonephritis from hydronephrosis and urinary infection may require prompt proximal drainage.

2.5 Treatment

Prompt treatment of ureteral injuries is required. The best opportunity for successful repair is in the operating room when the injury occurs. If the injury is not recognized until 7–10 days after the event with no infection, abscess, or other complications, immediate reexploration and repair are indicated. Proximal urinary drainage by percutaneous nephrostomy or formal nephrostomy should be considered if the injury is recognized late or if the patient has significant complications that make immediate reconstruction unsatisfactory. The goals of ureteral repair are to achieve complete debridement, a tension-free spatulated anastomosis, watertight closure, ureteral stenting and retroperitoneal drainage.

Chapter 3

Injuries to the Urinary Bladder

Bladder injuries occur most often from external force and are often associated with pelvic fractures. Iatrogenic injury may result from gynecologic and other extensive pelvic procedures as well as from hernia repairs and transurethral operations.

3.1 Pathogenesis and Pathology

When the pelvis is fractured by blunt trauma, fragments from the fracture site may perforate the bladder. These perforations usually result in extraperitoneal rupture. If the urine is infected, extraperitoneal bladder perforations may result in deep pelvic abscess and severe pelvic inflammation. When the bladder is filled to near capacity, a direct blow to the lower abdomen may result in bladder disruption. This type of disruption ordinarily is intraperitoneal. Since the reflection of the pelvic peritoneum covers the dome of the bladder, a linear laceration will allow urine to flow into the abdominal cavity. If the diagnosis is not established immediately and if the urine is sterile, no symptoms may be noted for several days. If the urine is infected, immediate peritonitis and acute abdomen will develop.

3.2 Clinical findings

(1) Symptoms

There is usually a history of lower abdominal trauma. Blunt injury is the usual cause. Patients ordinarily are unable to urinate, but when spontaneous voiding occurs, gross hematuria is usually present. Most patients complain of pelvic or lower abdominal pain.

(2) Signs

Evidence of external injury from a gunshot or stab wound in the lower abdomen should make one suspect bladder injury, manifested by marked tenderness of the suprapubic area and lower abdomen. An acute abdomen may occur with intraperitoneal bladder rupture. On rectal examination, landmarks may be indistinct because of a large pelvic hematoma.

(3) Laboratory Findings

Catheterization usually is required in patients with pelvic trauma but not if bloody urethral discharge is noted. Bloody urethral discharge indicates urethral injury, and a urethrogram is necessary before catheterization. When catheterization is done, gross or, less commonly, microscopic hematuria is usually present. Urine taken from the bladder at the initial catheterization should be cultured to determine whether infection is present.

(4) X-ray Findings

Bladder disruption is shown on cystography. The bladder should be filled with 300 mL of contrast medium and a plain film of the lower abdomen obtained. Contrast medium should be drained out completely, and a second film of the abdomen should be obtained. The drainage film is extremely important, because it demonstrates areas of extraperitoneal extravasation of blood and urine that may not appear on the filling film. With intraperitoneal extravasation, free contrast medium is visualized in the abdomen, highlighting bowel loops. CT cystography is an excellent method for detecting bladder rupture; however, retrograde filling of the bladder with 300 mL of contrast medium is necessary to distend the bladder completely.

3.3 Complications

A pelvic abscess may develop from extraperitoneal bladder rupture; if the urine becomes infected, the pelvic hematoma becomes infected too. Intraperitoneal bladder rupture with extravasation of urine into the abdominal cavity causes delayed peritonitis. Partial incontinence may result from bladder injury when the laceration extends into the bladder neck. Meticulous repair may ensure normal urinary control.

3.4 Treatment

(1) Emergency measures

Shock and hemorrhage should be treated.

(2) Surgical measures

A lower midline abdominal incision should be made. As the bladder is approached in the midline, a pelvic hematoma, which is usually lateral, should be avoided. The bladder should be opened in the midline and carefully inspected. After repair, a suprapubic cystostomy tube is usually left in place to ensure complete urinary drainage and control of bleeding.

Extraperitoneal bladder rupture can be successfully managed with urethral catheter drainage only (typically 10 days will provide adequate healing time). Large blood clots in the bladder or injuries involving the bladder neck should be managed surgically. Extraperitoneal bladder lacerations occasionally extend into the bladder neck and should be repaired meticulously. Such injuries are best managed with indwelling urethral catheterization and suprapubic diversion.

Intraperitoneal rupture should be repaired via a transperitoneal approach after careful transvesical inspection and closure of any other perforations. The peritoneum must be closed carefully over the area of injury. The bladder is then closed in separate layers by absorbable suture. All extravasated fluid from the peritoneal cavity should be removed before closure.

With appropriate treatment, the prognosis is excellent. The suprapubic cystostomy tube can be removed within 10 days, and the patient can usually void normally. Patients with lacerations extending into the bladder neck area may be temporarily incontinent, but full control is usually regained.

Chapter 4

Injuries to the Urethra

Urethral injuries are uncommon and occur most often in men, usually associated with pelvic fractures or straddle-type falls. They are rare in women. Various parts of the urethra may be lacerated, transected, or contused. Management varies according to the level of injury. The urethra can be separated into two broad anatomic divisions: the posterior urethra, consisting of the prostatic and membranous portions, and the anterior urethra, consisting of the bulbous and pendulous portions.

4.1 Injuries to the Posterior Urethra

4.1.1 Etiology

The membranous urethra passes through the pelvic floor and voluntary urinary sphincter and is the portion of the posterior urethra most likely to be injured. When pelvic fractures occur from blunt trauma, the membranous urethra is sheared from the prostatic apex at the prostatomembranous junction. The urethra can be transected by the same mechanism at the interior surface of the membranous urethra.

4.1.2 Clinical findings

Patients usually complain of lower abdominal pain and inability to urinate. A history of crushing injury to the pelvis is usually obtained. Blood at the urethral meatus is the single most important sign of urethral injury. The presence of blood at the external urethral meatus indicates that immediate urethrography is necessary to establish the diagnosis. Suprapubic tenderness and the presence of pelvic fracture are noted on physical examination. A large developing pelvic hematoma may be palpated. Perineal or suprapubic contusions are often noted. Rectal examination may reveal a large pelvic hematoma with the prostate displaced superiorly. Partial disruption of the membranous urethra (currently 10% of cases) is not accompanied by prostatic displacement.

Fractures of the bony pelvis are usually present. A urethrogram shows the site of extravasation at the prostatomembranous junction. Ordinarily, there is free extravasation of contrast material into the perivesical space. Incomplete prostatomembranous disruption is seen as minor extravasation, with a portion of contrast material flowing into the prostatic urethra and bladder.

The only instrumentation involved is urethrography. Catheterization or urethroscopy should not be done, because these procedures pose an increased risk of hematoma, infection, and further damage to partial urethral disruptions.

4.1.3 Complications

Stricture, impotence, and incontinence as complications of prostatomembranous disruption are among the most severe and debilitating mishaps that result from trauma to the urinary system. If the preferred suprapubic cystostomy approach with delayed repair is used, the incidence of stricture can be reduced to about 5%. The incidence of impotence after primary repair is 30%–80%. Incontinence in primary reanastomosis is noted in 1/3 of patients. Delayed reconstruction reduces the incidence to less than 5%.

4.1.4 Treatment

Emergency measures: Shock and hemorrhage should be treated. Urethral catheterization should be avoided.

Initial management should consist of suprapubic cystostomy to provide urinary drainage. This approach involves no urethral instrumentation or manipulation. The suprapubic cystostomy is maintained in place for about 3 months. This allows resolution of the pelvic hematoma, and the prostate and bladder will slowly return to their anatomic positions. Incomplete laceration of the posterior urethra heals spontaneously, and the suprapubic cystostomy can be removed within 2–3 weeks. The cystostomy tube should not be removed before voiding cystourethrography shows that no extravasation persists.

Delayed urethral reconstruction can be undertaken within 3 months, assuming there is no pelvic abscess or other evidence of persistent pelvic infection. The preferred approach is a single-stage reconstruction of the urethral rupture defect with direct excision of the strictured area and anastomosis of the bulbous urethra directly to the apex of the prostate. A 16F silicone urethral catheter should be placed along with a suprapubic cystostomy. Catheters are removed within a month, and the patient is then able to void.

4.2 Injuries to the Anterior Urethra

4.2.1 Etiology

The anterior urethra is the portion distal to the urogenital diaphragm. Straddle injury may cause laceration or contusion of the urethra. Self-instrumentation or iatrogenic instrumentation may cause partial disruption.

4.2.2 Pathogenesis and pathology

Contusion of the urethra is a sign of crush injury without urethral disruption. Perineal hematoma usually resolves without complications. A severe straddle injury may result in laceration of part of the urethral wall, allowing extravasation of urine. If the extravasation is unrecognized, it may extend into the scrotum, along the penile shaft, and up to the abdominal wall. It is limited only by Colles' fascia and often results in sepsis, infection, and serious morbidity.

4.2.3 Clinical findings

There is usually a history of a fall, and in some cases a history of instrumentation. Bleeding from the urethra is usually present. There is local pain into the perineum and sometimes massive perineal hematoma. If voiding has occurred and extravasation is noted, sudden swelling in the area will be present. If diagnosis has been delayed, sepsis and severe infection may be present.

The perineum is very tender, and a mass may be found. Rectal examination reveals a normal prostate. No attempt should be made to pass a urethral catheter, but if the patient's bladder is overdistended, percutaneous suprapubic cystostomy can be done as a temporary procedure. When presentation of such injuries is delayed, there is massive urinary extravasation and infection in the perineum and the scrotum.

Blood loss is not usually excessive, particularly if secondary injury has occurred. The white blood cell count may be elevated with infection. A urethrogram, with instillation of 15–20 mL of water-soluble contrast material, demonstrates extravasation and the location of injury. A contused urethra shows no evidence of extravasation.

4.2.4 Treatment

General measures: Major blood loss usually does not occur from straddle injury. If heavy bleeding does occur, local pressure for control, followed by resuscitation, is required.

The patient with urethral contusion shows no evidence of extravasation, and the urethra remains intact. After urethrography, the patient is allowed to void; and if the voiding occurs normally, without pain or bleeding, no additional treatment is necessary. If bleeding persists, urethral catheter drainage can be done.

Instrumentation of the urethra following urethrography should be avoided for patients with urethral laceration. A small midline incision in the suprapubic area readily exposes the dome of the bladder so that a suprapubic cystostomy tube can be inserted, allowing complete urinary diversion while the urethral laceration heals. Percutaneous cystostomy may also be used in such injuries.

After major urethral laceration, urinary extravasation may involve the perineum, scrotum, and lower abdomen. Drainage of these areas is indicated. Suprapubic cystostomy for urinary diversion is required. Infection and abscess formation are common and require antibiotic therapy. Immediate repair of urethral lacerations can be performed, but the procedure is difficult and the incidence of associated stricture is high. Strictures at the site of injury may be extensive and require delayed reconstruction.

Part 42

Urinary Tract and Male Genital Infections

Urinary tract infection(UTI) is a term that is applied to a variety of clinical conditions ranging from the asymptomatic presence of bacteria in the urine to severe infection of the kidney with resultant sepsis. UTI is one of the most common medical problems. UTIs are at times difficult to diagnose; some cases respond to a short course of a specific antibiotic, while others require a longer course of a broad-spectrum antibiotic.

Chapter 1

Introduction

1.1 Epidemiology

From newborns up to 1 year of age, bacteriuria is present in 2.7% of boys and 0.7% in girls. In children between 1 and 5 years of age, the incidence of bacteriuria in girls increases to 4.5%, while it decreases in boys to 0.5%. Most UTIs in children younger than 5 years are associated with congenital abnormalities of the urinary tract, such as vesicoureteral reflux or obstruction. The incidence of bacteriuria remains relatively constant in children 6–15 years of age. During adolescence, the incidence of UTI significantly increases to 20% in young women, while remaining constant in young men. Approximately 7 million cases of acute cystitis are diagnosed yearly in young women. Later in life, the incidence of UTI increases significantly for both males and females. For women between 36 and 65 years of age, gynecologic surgery and bladder prolapse appear to be important risk factors. In men of the same age group, prostatic hypertrophy/obstruction, catheterization, and surgery are relevant risk factors. For patients older than 65 years, the incidence of UTI continues to increase in both sexes. Incontinence and chronic use of urinary catheters are important risk factors in these patients.

1.2 Pathogenesis

1.2.1 Bacterial entry

There are four possible pathways of bacterial entry into the genitourinary tract. It is generally accepted that periurethral bacteria ascending into the urinary tract causes most UTI. The short nature of the female urethra combined with its close proximity to the vaginal vestibule and rectum likely predisposes women to more frequent UTIs than men. Other pathways of bacterial entry are uncommon causes of UTI. Hematogenous spread can occur in immunocompromised patients and in neonates. Lymphatogenous spread through the rectal, colonic, and periuterine lymphatics has been postulated as a cause for UTI; however, currently there is little scientific support to suggest that dissemination of bacteria through lymphatic channels plays a role in the pathogenesis of UTI. Direct extension of bacteria from adjacent organs into the urinary tract can occur in patients with intraperitoneal abscesses or vesicointestinal or vesicovaginal fistulas.

1.2.2 Host defenses

Host factorsplay an essential role in the pathogenesis of UTI. Unobstructed urinary flow with the subsequent washout of ascending bacteria is essential in preventing UTI. In addition, the urine itself has specific characteristics that inhibit bacterial growth and colonization. It also contains factors that inhibit bacterial adherence, such as Tamm-Horsfall glycoprotein. Urinary retention, stasis, or reflux of urine into the upper urinary tract can promote bacterial growth and subsequent infection. Consequently, any anatomic or functional abnormalities of the urinary tract that impede urinary flow can increase the host's susceptibility to UTI. These abnormalities include obstructive conditions at any level of the urinary tract, neurological diseases affecting the function of the lower urinary tract, diabetes, and pregnancy. Similarly, the presence of foreign bodies (such as stones, catheters, and stents) allows the bacteria to hide from these host defenses.

Other important host factors include the normal flora of the periurethral area or the prostate and the presence of vesicoureteral reflux. In women, the normal flora of the periurethral area composed of organisms such as lactobacillus provides a defense against the colonization of uropathogenic bacteria. Aging is associated with an increased susceptibility to UTI, in part because of the increased incidence of obstructive uropathy in men and alteration in the vaginal and periurethral flora from menopause in women.

1.3 Diagnosis

The diagnosis of UTI is sometimes difficult to establish and relies on urinalysis and urine culture. Occasionally, localization studies may be required to identify the source of the infection. Most often, the urine is often obtained from a voided specimen.

1.3.1 Urinalysis

Urinalysis provides a rapid screen for UTIs. The urine can be immediately evaluated for leukocyte esterase, a compound produced by the breakdown of white blood cells in the urine. Urinary nitrite is produced by reduction of dietary nitrates by many gram-negative bacteria. Esterase and nitrite can be detected by a urine dipstick and are more reliable when the bacterial count is greater than 100,000 colony-forming units per milliliter. The urinary nitrite test is highly specific but not sensitive. A combination of these tests may help to identify those patients in whom urine culture will be positive.

1.3.2 Urine culture

The gold standard for identification of UTI is the quantitative culture of urine for specific bacteria. The urine should be collected in a sterile container and cultured immediately after collection. The sample is then diluted and spread on culture plates. Each bacterium will form a single colony on the plates. The number of colonies is counted and adjusted per milliliter of urine.

1.3.3 Localization studies

Occasionally, it is necessary to localize the site of infection. For upper urinary tract localization, the bladder is irrigated with sterile water and a ureteral catheter is placed into each ureter. A specimen is collected from the renal pelvis. Culture of this specimen will indicate whether infection in the upper urinary tract is present. In men, infection in the lower urinary tract can be differentiated. A specimen is collected at the beginning of the void and represents possible infection in thc urcthra. A midstream specimen is next collected and represents possible infection in the bladder. The prostate is then massaged and the patient is asked to void again. This specimen represents possible infection of the prostate.

1.4 Treatment

Treatment with antimicrobial agents has minimized the morbidity and mortality associated with UTIs. The goal in treatment is to eradicate the infection by selecting the appropriate antibiotics that would target specific bacterial susceptibility. However, choosing the appropriate antimicrobial agents is often difficult. Many antibiotics are available, and the lowest effective dose and length of therapy are not well defined. Many conventions for the treatment of UTI are arbitrary. The general principles for selecting the appropriate antibiotics include consideration of the infecting pathogen, the patient and the site of infection. In patients with recurrent UTIs or those who are at risk for UTI, prophylactic antibiotics may be used.

Chapter 2

Upper Urinary Tract Infections

2.1 Acute Pyelonephritis

Acute pyelonephritis is defined as inflammation of the kidney and renal pelvis, and its diagnosis is usually made clinically.

2.1.1 Clinical presentation

Patients with acute pyelonephritis present with chills, fever, and costovertebral angle tenderness. They often have accompanying lower urinary tract symptoms such as dysuria, frequency, and urgency. Sepsis may occur, with 20% –30% of all systemic sepsis resulting from a urine infection. Urinalysis commonly demonstrates the presence of WBCs and red blood cells in the urine. Leukocytosis, increased erythrocyte sedimentation, and elevated levels of C–reactive protein are commonly seen on blood analysis. Bacteria are cultured from the urine when the culture is obtained before antibiotic treatment is instituted. E. coli is the most common causative organism, accounting for 80% of the cases.

2.1.2 Radiographic imaging

Contrast–enhanced CT scans can accurately demonstrate findings, confirming the diagnosis of pyelonephritis. Acute bacterial infection causes constriction of peripheral arterioles and reduces perfusion of the affected renal segments. However, CT scan is not necessary unless the diagnosis is unclear or the patient is not responding to therapy. In patients with acute pyelonephritis, renal ultrasonography is important to rule out concurrent urinary tract obstruction but can not reliably detect inflammation or infection of the kidney.

2.1.3 Management

The management of acute pyelonephritis depends on the severity of the infection. In patients who have toxicity because of associated septicemia, hospitalization is warranted. Fever from acute pyelonephritis may persist for several days despite appropriate therapy. If bacteremia is present, parenteral therapy should be continued for an additional 7–10 days and then the patient should be switched to oral treatment for 10–14 days. In patients who are not severely ill, outpatient treatment with oral antibiotics is appropriate. Therapy should continue for 10–14 days. Some patients in whom acute pyelonephritis develops will require follow-up radiologic examination such as voiding cystourethrogram or cystoscopy.

2.2 Chronic Pyelonephritis

Chronic pyelonephritis results from repeated renal infection, which leads to scarring, atrophy of the kidney, and subsequent renal insufficiency. The diagnosis is made by radiologic or pathologic examination rather than from clinical presentation.

2.2.1 Clinical presentation

Many individuals with chronic pyelonephritis have no symptoms, but they may have a history of frequent UTIs. Because patients with chronic pyelonephritis often are asymptomatic, the diagnosis is made incidentally when radiologic investigation is initiated to evaluate for the complications associated with renal insufficiency, such as hypertension, visual impairments, headaches, fatigue, and polyuria. In these patients, urinalysis may show leukocytes or proteinuria but is likely to be normal. Serum creatinine levels reflect the severity of the renal impairment. Urine cultures are only positive when there is an active infection.

2.2.2 Radiographic imaging

Intravenous pyelogram or CT scan can readily demonstrate a small and atrophic kidney on the affected side. Focal coarse renal scarring with clubbing of the underlying calyx is characteristic. Ultrasonography similarly can demonstrate these findings.

2.2.3 Management

The management of chronic pyelonephritis is somewhat limited because renal damage incurred by chronic pyelonephritis is not reversible. Eliminating recurrent UTIs and identifying and correcting any underlying anatomic or functional urinary problems such as obstruction or urolithiasis can prevent further renal damage. Long-term use of continuous prophylactic antibiotic therapy may be required to limit recurrent UTIs and renal scarring.

2.3 Renal Abscesses

Renal abscesses result from a severe infection that leads to liquefaction of renal tissue; this area is subsequently sequestered, forming an abscess. They can rupture out into the perinephric space, forming perinephric abscesses. When the abscesses extend beyond the Gerota's fascia, paranephric abscesses develop. With the development of effective antibiotics and better management of diseases such as diabetes and renal failure, renal/perinephric abscesses due to gram-positive bacteria are less prevalent; those caused by E. coli or Proteus species are becoming more common.

2.3.1 Clinical presentation

The most common presenting symptoms in patients with renal/perinephric abscesses include fever, flank or abdominal pain, chills, and dysuria. Many of the symptoms have lasted for more than two weeks. A flank mass may be palpated in some patients. Urinalysis usually demonstrates white blood cells; however, it may be normal in approximately 25% of the cases. Urine cultures only identify the causative organisms in about 1/3 of cases and blood cultures in only about half of cases.

2.3.2 Radiographic imaging

Renal abscesses can be accurately detected using ultrasonography or CT scans. There is a wide range of ultrasonographic findings ranging from an anechoic mass within or displacing the kidney to an echogenic fluid collection that tends to blend with the normally echogenic fat within Gerota's fascia. With high sensitivity, CT scans can demonstrate an enlarged kidney with focal areas of hypoattenuation early during the course of the infection. Once the inflammatory wall forms around the fluid collection, the abscess appears as a mass with a rim of contrast enhancement, the "ring" sign. CT scans may also demonstrate thickening of Gerota's fascia, stranding of the perinephric fat, or obliteration of the surrounding soft-tissue planes.

2.3.3 Management

The appropriate management of renal abscess must require appropriate antibiotic therapy. Because it is often very difficult to identify the correct causative organisms from the urine or blood, empiric therapy with broad-spectrum antibiotics is usually recommended. If the patient does not respond within 48 h of treatment, percutaneous drainage under CT or ultrasound guidance is indicated. The drained fluid should be cultured for the causative organisms. If the abscess still does not resolve, then open surgical drainage or nephrectomy may be necessary. Follow-up imaging is needed to confirm resolution of the abscesses. These patients will also require evaluation for underlying urinary tract abnormalities such as stone or obstruction after the infection has been resolved.

Chapter 3

Lower Urinary Tract Infections

3.1 Acute Cystitis

Acute cystitis refers to urinary infection of the lower urinary tract, principally the bladder. Acute cystitis more commonly affects women than men. The primary mode of infection is ascending from the periurethral/vaginal and fecal flora. In general, those in whom acute cystitis developed do not usually require any extensive radiologic investigation, such as a voiding cystourethrogram.

3.1.1 Clinical presentation

Patients with acute cystitis present with irritative voiding symptoms such as dysuria, frequency, and urgency. Low back and suprapubic pain, hematuria, and cloudy/foul-smelling urine are also common symptoms. Fever and systemic symptoms are rare. Typically, urinalysis demonstrates white blood cells in the urine, and hematuria may be present. Urine culture is required to confirm the diagnosis and identify the causative organism. However, when the clinical picture and urinalysis are highly suggestive of the diagnosis of acute cystitis, urine culture may not be needed. E. coli. causes most of the acute cystitis.

3.1.2 Radiographic imaging

In uncomplicated infection of the bladder, radiologic evaluation is often not necessary.

3.1.3 Management

Management for acute cystitis consists of a short course of oral antibiotics. Trimethoprim-sulfamethoxazole, nitrofurantoin, and fluoroquinolones have excellent activity against most pathogens that cause cystitis. Trimethoprim-sulfamethoxazole and nitrofurantoin are less expensive and thus are recommended for the treatment of uncomplicated cystitis. In adults and children, the duration of treatment is usually limited to 3-5 days. Longer therapy is not indicated. Single-dose therapy for the treatment of recurrent cystitis/UTI appears to be less effective; however, fluoroquinolones with long half-lives may be suitable for single-dose therapy.

3.2 Urethritis

Infection of the urethra can be categorized into those types caused by Neisseria gonorrhoeae and by other organisms(Chlamydia trachomatis, Ureaplasma urealyticum, Trichomonas vaginalis, and herpes simplex virus). Most cases are acquired during sexual intercourse.

3.2.1 Presentation and findings

Patients with urethritis may present with urethral discharge and dysuria. The amount of discharge may vary significantly, from profuse to scant amounts. Obstructive voiding symptoms are primarily present in patients with recurrent infection, in whom urethral strictures subsequently develop. It is important to note that approximately 40% of patients with gonococcal urethritis are asymptomatic. The diagnosis is made from examination and culture of the urethra. It is important to obtain the specimen from within the urethra, rather than from just the discharge.

3.2.2 Radiologic imaging

Retrograde urethrogram is only indicated in patients with recurrent infection and obstructive voiding symptoms. Most patients with uncomplicated urethritis do not require any radiologic imaging.

3.2.3 Management

Pathogen-direct antibiotic therapy is required. In patients with gonococcal urethritis, ceftriaxone (250 mg intramuscularly) or fluoroquinolones(ciprofloxacin 250 mg) or norfloxacin 800 mg may be used. For patients with nongonococcal urethritis, treatment is with tetracycline or erythromycin (500 mg 4 times daily) or doxycycline(100 mg twice daily) for 7-14 days. However, the most essential component of treatment is prevention. Sexual partners of the affected patients should be treated, and protective sexual practices are recommended.

Chapter 4

Male Genital Infection

4.1 Chronic Bacterial Prostatitis

In contrast to the acute form, chronic bacterial prostatitis has a more insidious onset, characterized by relapsing, recurrent UTI caused by the persistence of pathogen in the prostatic fluid despite antibiotic therapy.

4.1.1 Clinical presentation

Most patients with chronic bacterial prostatitis typically present with dysuria, urgency, frequency, nocturia, and low back/perineal pain. Others are asymptomatic, but the diagnosis is made after investigation for bacteriuria. In patients with chronic bacterial prostatitis, digital rectal examination of the prostate is often normal; occasionally, tenderness, firmness, or prostatic calculi may be found on examination. Urinalysis demonstrates a variable degree of white blood cells and bacteria in the urine, depending on the extent of the disease. Serum blood analysis normally does not show any evidence of leukocytosis. Prostate-specific antigen levels may be elevated. Diagnosis is made after identification of bacteria from prostate expressate or urine specimen after a prostatic massage. The causative organisms are similar to those of acute bacterial prostatitis. It is currently believed that other gram-positive bacteria, Mycoplasma, Ureaplasma, and Chlamydia spp. are not causative pathogens in chronic bacterial prostatitis.

4.1.2 Radiologic imaging

Radiologic imaging is rarely indicated in patients with chronic prostatitis. Transrectal ultrasonography is only indicated if a prostatic abscess is suspected.

4.1.3 Management

Antibiotic therapy is similar to that for acute bacterial prostatitis. Interestingly, the presence of leukocytes or bacteria in the urine and prostatic massage does not predict antibiotic response in patients with chronic prostatitis. In patients with chronic bacterial prostatitis, the duration of antibiotic therapy may be 3-4 months. Using fluoroquinolones, some patients may respond after 4-6 weeks of treatment. The addition of an alpha blocker to antibiotic therapy has been shown to reduce symptom recurrences. Despite maximal therapy, cure is not often achieved due to poor penetration of antibiotic into prostatic tissue and relative isolation of the bacterial foci within the prostate. When recurrent episodes of infection occur despite antibiotic therapy, suppressive antibiotic may be used. Transurethral resection of the prostate has been used to treat patients with refractory disease; however, the success rate has been variable and this approach is not generally recommended.

4.2 Prostate Abscess

Most cases of prostatic abscess result from complications of acute bacterial prostatitis that were inadequately or inappropriately treated. Prostatic abscesses are often seen in patients with diabetes; those receiving chronic dialysis; or patients who are immunocompromised, undergoing urethral instrumentation, or who have chronic indwelling catheters.

4.2.1 Clinical presentation

Patients with prostatic abscess present with similar symptoms to those with acute bacterial prostatitis. Typically, these patients were treated for acute bacterial prostatitis previously and had a good initial response to treatment with antibiotics. However, their symptoms recurred during treatment, suggesting development of prostatic abscesses. On digital rectal examination, the prostate is usually tender and swollen. Fluctuance is only seen in 16% of patients with prostatic abscess.

4.2.2 Radiologic imaging

Imaging with transrectal ultrasonography or pelvic CT scan is crucial for diagnosis and treatment.

4.2.3 Management

Antibiotic therapy in conjunction with drainage of the abscess is required. Transrectal ultrasonography or CT scan can be used to direct transrectal drainage of the abscess. Transurethral resection and drainage may be required if transrectal drainage is inadequate. When properly diagnosed and treated, most cases of prostatic abscess resolve without significant sequelae.

4.3 Epididymitis

Infection and inflammation of the epididymis most often result from an ascending infection from the lower urinary tract. Most cases of epididymitis in men younger than 35 years are due to sexually transmitted organisms; those in children and older men are due to urinary pathogens such as E. coli. The infection in the epididymis may spread to involve the testis.

4.3.1 Clinical presentation

Patients with epididymitis present with severe scrotal pain that may radiate to the groin or flank. Scrotal enlargement due to the inflammation of the epididymis/ testis or a reactive hydrocele may develop rapidly. Other symptoms of urethritis, cystitis, or prostatitis may be present before or concurrent with the onset of scrotal pain. On physical examination, an enlarged and red scrotum is present, and it is often difficult to distinguish the epididymis from the testis during the acute infection. A thickened spermatic cord can occasionally be palpated. Urinalysis typically demonstrates white blood cells and bacteria in the urine or urethral discharge. Serum blood analysis often reveals leukocytosis.

4.3.2 Radiologic imaging

Frequently, it is difficult to distinguish epididymitis from acute testicular torsion based on the history and physical examination alone. Scrotal Doppler ultrasonography or radionuclide scanning can be used to confirm the diagnosis. The presence of blood flow in the testis on ultrasonography or uptake of the tracers into the center of the testis on radionuclide scanning rule out torsion. On scrotal ultrasonography, patients with epididymitis commonly have an enlarged epididymis with increased blood flow. A reactive hydrocele or testicular involvement may also be seen.

4.3.3 Management

Oral antibiotic treatment is directed against specific causative organisms. In addition, bed rest, scrotal elevation, and the use of nonsteroidal anti-inflammatory agents are helpful in reducing the duration of the symptoms. In patients with epididymitis caused by sexually transmitted organisms, treatment of their sexual partners is recommended to prevent reinfection. For patients with sepsis or severe infection, hospitalization and parenteral antibiotic therapy may be needed. Open drainage is indicated in cases in which an abscess develops. Occasionally, patients with chronic, relapsing epididymitis and scrotal pain may require epididymectomy for relief of their symptoms.

Part 43

Genitourinary Tuberculosis

Genitourinary tuberculosis is commonly missed in the clinic, and it should be considered in any case of pyuria without bacteriuria or in any cause of urinary tract infection that does not respond to the common treatment. The kidneys and the prostate are the principal sites of urinary tract involvement.

Chapter 1

Urinary Tuberculosis

Tubercle bacilli may invade one or more of the organs of the genitourinary tract and cause a chronic granulomatous infection that shows the same characteristics as tuberculosis in other organs. Urinary tuberculosis is a disease of young adults. The infected organism is Mycobacterium tuberculosis, which reaches the genitourinary organs by the hematogenous route from the lungs. The primary site is often not symptomatic or apparent.

The kidney and possibly the prostate are the primary sites of tuberculous infection in the genitourinary tract. All other genitourinary organs become involved by either ascent (prostate to bladder) or descent (kidney to bladder, prostate to epididymis). The testis may become involved by direct extension from epididymal infection.

1.1 Clinical Findings

1.1.1 Symptoms

There is no classic clinical manifestation of renal tuberculosis. Most symptoms of this disease, even in the most advanced stage, are vesical in origin (cystitis). Vague generalized malaise, fatigability, low-grade but persistent fever, and night sweats are some of the nonspecific complaints. Even vesical irritability may be absent, in which case only proper collection and examination of the urine will afford the clue.

Because of the slow progression of the disease, the affected kidney is usually completely asymptomatic. On occasion, however, there may be a dull ache in the flank. The passage of a blood clot, secondary calculi, or a mass of debris may cause renal and ureteral colic. The earliest symptoms of renal tuberculosis may arise from secondary vesical involvement. These include burning, frequency, and nocturia. Hematuria is occasionally found and is of either renal or vesical origin. At times, particularly in a late stage of the disease, the vesical irritability may become extreme. If ulceration occurs, suprapubic pain may be noted when the bladder becomes full.

1.1.2 Signs

There is usually no enlargement or tenderness of the involved kidney. Evidence of extragenital tuberculosis may be found(lungs, bone, lymph nodes, tonsils, intestines).

1.1.3 Laboratory findings

Proper urinalysis affords the most important clue to the diagnosis of genitourinary tuberculosis. Persistent pyuria without organisms on culture or on the smear stained with methylene blue means tuberculosis until proved otherwise. Acid-fast stains done on the concentrated sediment from a 24 h specimen are positive in at least 60% of cases. However, this must be corroborated by a positive culture. If clinical response to adequate treatment fails and pyuria persists, tuberculosis must be ruled out by bacteriologic and roentgenologic means.

Cultures for tubercle bacilli from the first morning urine are positive in a very high percentage of cases of tuberculous infection. If positive, sensitivity tests should be ordered. In the face of strong presumptive evidence of tuberculosis, negative cultures should be repeated. The bloodcells count may be normal or may show anemia in advanced disease. The sedimentation rate is usually accelerated. Renal function is normal unless there is bilateral damage; as one kidney is slowly injured, compensatory hypertrophy of the normal kidney develops. It can also be infected with tubercle bacilli, or it may become hydronephrotic from fibrosis of the bladder wall(ureterovesical stenosis) or vesicoureteral reflux.

If tuberculosis is suspected, the tuberculin test should be performed. A positive test, particularly in an adult, is hardly diagnostic, but a negative test in an otherwise healthy patient speaks against a diagnosis of tuberculosis.

1.1.4 X-ray findings

A chest film that shows evidence of tuberculosis should cause the physician to suspect tuberculosis of the urogenital tract in the presence of urinary signs and symptoms. A plain film of the abdomen may show enlargement of one kidney or obliteration of the renal and psoas shadows due to perinephric abscess. Punctate calcification in the renal parenchyma may be due to tuberculosis.

Excretory urograms can be diagnostic if the lesion is moderately advanced. The typical changes include the following: ①A "moth-eaten" appearance of the involved ulcerated calyces. ②Obliteration of one or more calyces. ③Dilatation of the calyces due to ureteral stenosis from fibrosis. ④Abscess cavities that connect with calyces. ⑤Single or multiple ureteral strictures, with secondary dilatation, with shortening and therefore straightening of the ureter. ⑥Absence of function of the kidney due to complete ureteral occlusion and renal destruction(autonephrectomy).

If the excretory urograms demonstrate gross tuberculosis in one kidney, there is no need to do a retrograde urogram on that side. In fact, there is at least a theoretic danger of hematogenous or lymphogenous dissemination resulted from the increased intrapelvic pressure. Retrograde urography may be carried out on the unsuspected side, however, as a verification of its normality. This is further substantiated if the urine from that side is free of both pus cells and tubercle bacilli.

1.1.5 Instrumental examination

Thorough cystoscopic study is indicated even when the offending organism has been found in the urine and excretory urograms show the typical renal lesion. This study clearly demonstrates the extent of the disease. Cystoscopy may reveal the typical tubercles or ulcers of tuberculosis. Biopsy can be done if necessary. Severe contracture of the bladder may be noted. A cystogram may reveal ureteral reflux. A clean specimen of urine should also be obtained for further study.

1.2 Complications

Perinephric abscess may cause an enlarging mass in the flank. Scarring with stricture formation is one of the typical lesions of tuberculosis and most commonly affects the juxtavesical portion of the ureter. This may cause progressive hydronephrosis. Complete ureteral obstruction may cause complete nonfunction of the kidney(autonephrectomy). When severely damaged, the bladder wall becomes fibrosed and contracted. Stenosis of the ureters or reflux occurs, causing hydronephrotic atrophy.

1.3 Treatment

Tuberculosis must be treated as a generalized disease. Even when it can be demonstrated only in the urogenital tract, one must assume activity elsewhere. This means that the basic treatment is medical. Surgical excision of an infected organ, when indicated, is merely an adjunct to overall therapy. Optimal nutrition is no less important in treating tuberculosis of the genitourinary tract than in the treatment of tuberculosis elsewhere.

1.3.1 Renal tuberculosis

A strict medical regimen should be instituted. A combination of drugs is usually desirable. The following drugs are effective in combination, which include isoniazid, rifampin, ethambutol, streptomycin and pyrazinamide. It is preferable to begin treatment with a combination of isoniazid, rifampin, and ethambutol.

1.3.2 Vesical tuberculosis

Tuberculosis of the bladder is always secondary to renal or prostatic tuberculosis. It tends to heal promptly when definitive treatment for the "primary" genitourinary infection is given. Vesical ulcers that fail to respond to this regimen may require transurethral electrocoagulation. If extreme contracture of the bladder develop, it may be necessary to divert the urine from the bladder or perform augmentation cystoplasty after subtotal cystectomy to increase bladder capacity.

1.3.3 Treatment of other complications

Perinephric abscess must be drained, and nephrectomy should be done either then or later to prevent development of a chronic draining sinus. Prolonged antimicrobial therapy is indicated. If ureteral stricture develops on the involved side, ureteral dilatations offer a better than 50% chance of cure.

Chapter 2

Male Genital Tuberculosis

The passage of infected urine through the prostatic urethra ultimately leads to invasion of the prostate and one or both seminal vesicles. Prostatic infection can ascend to the bladder and descend to the epididymis. Tuberculosis of the prostate can extend along the vas or through the perivasal lymphatics and affect the epididymis. If the epididymal infection is extensive and an abscess forms, it may rupture through the scrotal skin, thus establish a permanent sinus, or it may extend into the testicle.

2.1 Symptoms

Tuberculosis of the prostate and seminal vesicles usually causes no symptoms. Tuberculosis of the epididymis usually presents as a painless or only mildly painful swelling. An abscess may drain spontaneously through the scrotal wall. A chronic draining sinus should be regarded as tuberculous until proved otherwise.

2.2 Signs

A thickened, nontender, or only slightly tender epididymis may be discovered. The vas deferens often is thickened and beaded. A chronic draining sinus through the scrotal skin is almost pathognomonic of tuberculous epididymitis. Hydrocele occasionally accompanies tuberculous epididymitis. Involvement of the penis and urethra is rare. Prostate and seminal vesicles may be normal to palpation. Ordinarily, however, the tuberculous prostate shows areas of induration, even nodulation. The involved seminal vesicle is usually indurated, enlarged, and fixed. If epididymitis is present, the ipsilateral seminal vesicle usually shows changes as well.

2.3 Treatment

Tuberculosis of the epididymis never produces an isolated lesion. The prostate is always involved and usually the kidney as well. Only rarely does the epididymal infection break through into the testis. Treatment is medical. If an abscess or a draining sinus exists after months of treatment, epididymectomy is indicated. The removal of the entire prostate and the vesicles when they become involved by tuberculosis is not necessary, and the majority opinion is that only medical therapy. Control can be checked by culture of the semen for tubercle bacilli.

Part 44

Urinary Tract Obstruction

Chapter 1

Introduction

Obstruction is one of the most important abnormalities of the urinary tract. It eventually leads to decompensation of the muscular conduits and reservoirs, back pressure, and atrophy of renal parenchyma. It also invites infection and stone formation, which cause further damage and can ultimately end in complete unilateral or bilateral destruction of the kidney.

4.1 Etiology

Obstruction may be classified according to cause (congenital or acquired).

4.1.1 Congenital

The common sites of congenital narrowing are the external meatus in boys (meatal stenosis) or just inside the external urinary meatus in girls, the distal urethra (stenosis), posterior urethral valves, ectopic ureters, ureteroceles, and the ureterovesical and ureteropelvic junctions. Another congenital cause of urinary stasis is the damage to sacral roots 2–4 as seen in spina bifida and myelomeningocele. Vesicoureteral reflux causes both vesical and renal stasis.

4.1.2 Acquired

Acquired obstructions are numerous and may be primary in the urinary tract or secondary to retroperitoneal lesions that invade or compress the urinary passages. Among the common causes are as follows:

(1) Urethral stricture secondary to infection or injury.

(2) Benign prostatic hyperplasia or cancer of the prostate.

(3) Vesical tumor involving the bladder neck or one or both ureteral orifices.

(4) Local extension of cancer of the prostate or cervix into the base of the bladder, occluding the ureters.

(5) Compression of the ureters at the pelvic brim by metastatic nodes from cancer of the prostate or cervix.

(6) Ureteral stone.

(7) Retroperitoneal fibrosis or malignant tumor.

(8) Pregnancy.

4.2 Pathogenesis

These changes induced by obstruction can be well understood by considering the effects of a severe meatal stricture on the lower tract(distal to the bladder neck), a large obstructing prostate on the midtract (bladder), and an impacted stone in the ureter on the upper tract(ureter and kidney).

4.2.1 Lower tract

Hydrostatic pressure proximal to the obstruction causes dilation of the urethra. The wall of the urethra may become thinner, and a diverticulum may form. If the urine becomes infected, urinary extravasation may occur, which can result in periurethral abscess. The prostatic ducts may become widely dilated.

4.2.2 Midtract

In the earlier stages(compensatory phase), to balance the increasing outlet resistance, the muscle wall of the bladder hypertrophied and thickened. Its thickness may double or triple. Complete emptying of the bladder becomes possible. The hypertrophied muscle may be seen endoscopically. With secondary infection, the effects of infection are often superimposed. There may be edema of the submucosa, which may be infiltrated with plasma cells, lymphocytes, and polymorphonuclear cells. With decompensation, it becomes less contractile and, therefore, weakened, resulting in the presence of a large amount of residual urine after voiding.

4.2.3 Upper tract(ureter)

In the early stages of obstruction, intravesical pressure is normal while the bladder fills and is increased only during voiding. The pressure is not transmitted to the ureters and renal pelves because of the competence of the ureterovesical "valves" (A true valve is not present; the ureterotrigonal unit, by virtue of its intrinsic structure, resists the retrograde flow of urine). However, owing to trigonal hypertrophy and to the resultant increase in resistance to urine flow across the terminal ureter, there is progressive back pressure on the ureter and kidney, resulting in ureteral dilatation and hydronephrosis. Later, with the phase of decompensation accompanied by residual urine, there is an added stretch effect on the already hypertrophied trigone that increases appreciably the resistance to flow at the lower end of the ureter and induces further hydroureteronephrosis. With decompensation of the ureterotrigonal complex, the valve-like action may be lost, vesicoureteral reflux occurs, and the increased intravesical pressure is transmitted directly to the renal pelvis, aggravating the degree of hydroureteronephrosis. Secondary to the back pressure resulting from reflux or from obstruction by the hypertrophied and stretched trigone or by a ureteral stone, the ureteral musculature thickens in its attempt to push the urine downward by increased peristaltic activity(stage of compensation). This causes elongation and some tortuosity of the ureter. At times, this change becomes marked, and bands of fibrous tissue develop. On contraction, the bands further angulate the ureter, causing a secondary ureteral obstruction. Finally, because of increasing pressure, the ureteral wall becomes attenuated and therefore loses its contractile power(stage of decompensation).

4.2.4 Upper tract(kidney)

The pressure within the renal pelvis is normally close to zero. If the intrapelvic pressure in the hydronephrotic kidney rapidly increases to a level approaching filtration pressure (resulting in cessation of filtration), a safety mechanism is activated that produces a break in the surface lining of the collecting structure at the weakest point—the fornices. This leads to escape and extravasation of urine from the renal pelvis into the parenchymal interstitium (pyelointerstitial backflow). The extravasated fluid is absorbed by the renal lymphatics, and the pressure in the renal pelvis drops, allowing further filtration of urine. With the persistence of increased intrapelvic pressure, compression from the increase in intrapelvic pressure causes an ischemic effect, thus impairing the renal function. The degree of hydronephrosis that develops depends on the duration, degree, and site of the obstruction. The higher the obstruction, the greater the effect on the kidney. In the earlier stages, the renal pelvic musculature undergoes compensatory hypertrophy in its effort to force urine past the obstruction. Later, however, the muscle becomes stretched and atonic (and decompensated). Eventually, the kidney is completely destroyed and appears as a thin-walled sac filled with clear fluid (water and electrolytes) or pus.

Chapter 2

Hydronephrosis

Hydronephrosis is an aseptic dilatation of the kidney caused by obstruction.

2.1 Etiology

Hydronephrosis shares the same etiology with urinary tract obstruction, but causes of upper urinary tract obstruction are more relevant to hydronephrosis.

2.2 Epidemiology

Hydronephrosis is found to be more prevalent in women from the ages of 20–60 years, which is attributed to pregnancy and the development of gynecologic malignancies. In contrast, hydronephrosis is more prevalent in men after age 60 because of the presence of prostatic disease. Among children, hydronephrosis appears to be somewhat more prevalent in boys and the majority of cases occur in subjects younger than 1 year.

2.3 Clinical Manifestations

2.3.1 Unilateral hydronephrosis

Unilateral hydronephrosis (commonly caused by idiopathic pelviureteric junction obstruction or calculus) is more common in women and on the right. Presenting features include the following:

(1) Mild pain or dull aching in the loin, often a dragging heaviness worsened by excessive fluid intake. The kidney may be palpable.

(2) Intermittent hydronephrosis (Dietl's crisis). Loin swelling is associated with acute renal pain. The pain goes and the swelling disappears when a large volume of urine is passed.

(3) Antenatal detection in the fetus by ultrasound scan. Many of these cases are benign, but postnatal

investigation is required to detect those with significant pelviureteric junction obstruction

2.3.2 Bilateral hydronephrosis

(1) From lower urinary obstruction: Symptoms of bladder outflow obstruction predominate. The kidneys are usually impalpable because renal failure intervenes before they enlarge.

(2) From bilateral upper urinary tract obstruction: Idiopathic retroperitoneal fibrosis affects both ureters and idiopathic pelviureteric junction obstruction can be bilateral. Symptoms may be referred to one side.

(3) From pregnancy: Dilatation of the ureters and renal pelves occurs early in pregnancy up to the 20th week. It results from the effects on the ureteric smooth muscle of high levels of circulating progesterone and is part of normal pregnancy. The ureters return to their normal size within 12 weeks of delivery. This physiological condition is associated with an increased liability to infection and there is a possibility that abdominal pain during pregnancy may be erroneously ascribed to ureteric obstruction.

2.4 Laboratory Examination

Anemia may be found in advanced bilateral hydronephrosis. Leukocytosis is to be expected in the acute stage of infection. Little, if any, the elevation of the white blood count accompanies the chronic process. In the presence of significant bilateral hydronephrosis, both urea and creatinine are elevated. The urinalysis and microscopic analysis are necessary in the complete evaluation of a patient suspected of having urinary tract obstruction and/or renal failure. The urinalysis can provide an estimation of osmolality, evidence of UTI, insight into stone formation based on crystals that may be present in the urine, and the possible presence of medical renal disease with the presence of protein and/or cellular casts. Microscopic hematuria may indicate renal or vesical infection, tumor, or stone. Pus cells and bacteria may or may not be present.

2.5 Imaging Examination

2.5.1 Ultrasonography

Renal ultrasonography remains a first-line imaging modality in the evaluation of a patient suspected of having urinary tract obstruction. The renal ultrasound primarily provides anatomic information about the kidney, including renal size, cortical thickness, corticomedullary differentiation, and grade of collecting system dilation. Parenchymal thinning and small renal size can be the evidence of chronic renal obstruction

2.5.2 InIntraudio videoenous urography (IVU)

IVU helps only if there is a significant function in the obstructed kidney. The extrarenal pelvis is dilated and the minor calyces lose their normal cupping and become "clubbed". If the level of obstruction is in doubt, it can help to take follow-up films 36 hours after the contrast has been injected. Contrast slowly diffuses to fill the obstructed system down to the blockage.

2.5.3 Nuclear renography

Isotope renography is the best test to confirm obstructive dilatation of the collecting system. A substance[usually diethylenetriaminepenta-acetic acid(DTPA) or MAG-3] is injected intravenously. The DTPA is labelled with technetium-99m, a gamma-ray emitter, so that the passage of ^{99m}Tc-labeled DTPA through the kidneys can be tracked using a gamma camera. ^{99m}Tc-DTPA is cleared from a normal kidney but stays in the renal pelvis on the obstructed side and is retained even if urine flow is increased by administering frusemide.

2.5.4 Computed tomography

CT has a reported sensitivity of 96% for stone detection with a specificity and positive predictive value of 100% and can detect most radiolucent stones with the exception of protease inhibitor stones(i. e. , indinavir sulfate) and mucoid matrix stones.

2.5.5 Magnetic resonance urography

With the exception of pregnant women due to the irradiation, MRI is the preferred test. However, the test has limited value in delineating ureteral anatomy if it is not dilated.

2.5.6 Whitaker test

Very occasionally, a Whitaker test is indicated. The Whitaker test involves placement of a percutaneous needle in the collecting system of the kidney and the infusion of contrast at a rate of 10 mL/min. A urodynamic catheter is also placed in the bladder, and intravesical pressures are monitored and subtracted from measured intrapelvic pressures during the infusion. Intrapelvic pressures are noted at the time that contrast is first seen extending past the ureteropelvic junction and past the ureterovesical junction. Pressures less than 15 cmH_2O are considered normal, greater than 22 cmH_2O are indicative of obstruction, and between 15 and 22 cmH_2O are considered indeterminate.

2.5.7 Retrograde pyelography

Retrograde pyelography is rarely indicated but will confirm the site of obstruction immediately before corrective surgery.

2.6 Complications

Stagnation of urine leads to infection, which then may spread throughout the entire urinary system. Once established, infection is difficult and at times impossible to be eradicated even after the obstruction has been relieved.

Often, the invading organisms are urea splitting(Proteus, staphylococci), which causes the urine to become alkaline. Calcium salts precipitate and form bladder or kidney stones more easily in alkaline urine. If both kidneys are affected, the result may be renal insufficiency. Secondary infection increases renal damage.

Pyonephrosis is the end stage of a severely infected and obstructed kidney. The kidney is functionless and filled with thick pus. At times, a plain film of the abdomen may show an air urogram caused by gas liberated by infecting organisms.

2.7 Treatment

The indications for operation are bouts of renal pain, increasing hydronephrosis, evidence of parenchymal damage and infection. Nephrectomy should be considered only when the kidney has been largely destroyed. Mild cases should be followed by serial ultrasound scans and operated upon if dilatation is increasing.

2.7.1 Pyeloplasty

In the Anderson–Hynes operation, the upper third of the ureter and the renal pelvis are mobilised. A renal vein overlying the distended pelvis can be divided, but an artery in this situation should be preserved to avoid infarction of the territory that it supplies. The anastomosis is made in front of such an artery. A nephrostomy tube or a ureteric stent protects the anastomosis. Laparoscopic pyeloplasty is becoming increasingly popular.

2.7.2 Endoscopic pyelolysis

Disruption of the pelviureteric junction by a balloon passed up the ureter and distended under radiographic control has been used to treat idiopathic pelviureteric junction obstruction. The long–term efficacy and various forms of endoscopic pyelotomy have still to be proved. The alternative minimal access procedure, laparoscopic pyeloplasty, is increasingly popular.

Chapter 3

Benign Prostatic Hyperplasia

Benign prostatic hyperplasia(BPH) is a histologic diagnosis that refers to the proliferation of smooth muscle and epithelial cells within the prostatic transition zone.

3.1 Etiology

The precise molecular etiology of this hyperplastic process is uncertain. Androgens, estrogens, stromal-epithelial interactions, growth factors, and neurotransmitters may play a role, either singly or in combination, in the etiology of the hyperplastic process.

3.2 Epidemiology

BPH is prevalent, affecting approximately 70% of men between the ages of 60 and 69 years, making it one of the most common conditions treated by urologists.

3.3 Pathology

BPH affects both glandular epithelium and connective tissue stroma to variable degrees. These changes are similar to those occurring in breast dysplasia, in which adenosis, epitheliosis and stromal proliferation are seen in differing proportions. BPH typically affects the submucous group of glands in the transitional zone, forming a nodular enlargement. Eventually, this overgrowth compresses the peripheral zone(PZ) glands into a false capsule and causes the appearance of the typical "ateral" lobes. When BPH affects the subcervical central zone(CZ) glands, a "middle" lobe develops that projects up into the bladder within the internal sphincter. Sometimes, both lateral lobes also project into the bladder, so that, when viewed from within, the sides and back of the internal urinary meatus are surrounded by an intravesical prostatic collar.

3.4 Pathophysiology

By upsetting the mechanism for opening and funneling the vesical neck at the time of voiding, hyperplasia of the prostate causes increased outflow resistance. Consequently, a higher intravesical pressure is required to accomplish voiding, causing hypertrophy of the vesical and trigonal muscles. Hypertrophy of the trigone causes excessive stress on the intravesical ureter, producing functional obstruction and resulting in hydroureteronephrosis in late cases. Stagnation of urine can lead to infection; the onset of cystitis will exacerbate the obstructive symptoms.

3.5 Clinical Manifestations

It is important to realize that the relationship between anatomical prostatic enlargement, lower urinary tract symptoms (LUTS) and urodynamic evidence of bladder outflow obstruction (BOO) is complex (Figure 44-3-1).

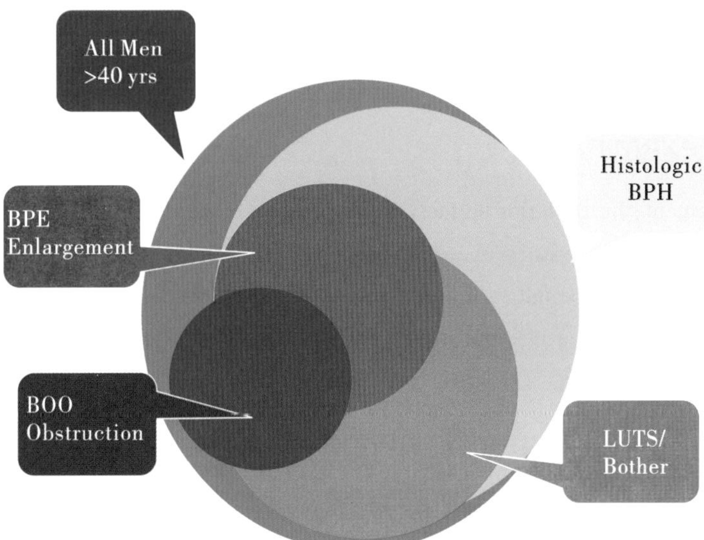

Figure 44-3-1 The relationship between histologic hyperplasia of the prostate (BPH), lower urinary tract symptoms, benign prostate enlargement (BPE), and bladder outlet obstruction

The enlarged gland has been proposed to contribute to the LUTS complex via at least two routes: ①Direct bladder outlet obstruction from enlarged tissue (static component). ② from increased smooth muscle tone and resistance within the enlarged gland (dynamic component). But BPH is certainly not the only cause of LUTS in aging men. LUTS can be divided into storage, voiding and post-micturition symptoms.

3.5.1 Storage symptoms

Storage symptoms are experienced during the storage phase of the bladder, including increased daytime frequency(the complaint of voiding too often by day),nocturia,urgency,and urinary incontinence(the complaint of any involuntary leakage of urine).

3.5.2 Voiding symptoms

Voiding symptoms are experienced during the voiding phase, including slow stream, splitting or spraying of the urine stream, intermittent stream, hesitancy(difficulty in initiating micturition, resulting in a delay in the onset of voiding after the individual is ready to pass urine), straining to void, and terminal dribble (a prolonged final part of micturition, when the flow has slowed to a trickle/dribble).

3.5.3 Post micturition symptoms

Post micturition symptoms are experienced immediately after micturition, including the feeling of incomplete emptying and post micturition dribble(the involuntary loss of urine immediately after one has finished passing urine).

LUTS are usually assessed by means of scoring systems, including the International Prostate Symptom Score(IPSS), the International Consultation on Incontinence Questionnaire(ICIQ-MLUTS), and Danish Prostate Symptom Score(DAN-PSS).

3.6 Laboratory Examination

3.6.1 Rectal examination

In benign enlargement, the posterior surface of the prostate is smooth, convex and typically elastic, but the fibrous element may give the prostate a firm consistency. The rectal mucosa can be made to move over the prostate. Residual urine may be felt as a fluctuating swelling above the prostate. It should be noted that, if there is a considerable amount of residual urine present, it pushes the prostate downwards, making it appear larger than it is.

3.6.2 Serum prostate-specific antigen(PSA)

PSA should be measured if a suspected diagnosis of prostate cancer is established or if it assists in the treatment and/or decision making process.

3.6.3 Flow rate measurement

For this to be meaningful, two or three voids should be recorded, and the voided volume should be in excess of 150-200 mL. This usually means the patient attending a special flow rate clinic. A typical history and a flow rate <10 mL/s(for a voided volume of >200 mL) will be sufficient for most urologists to recommend treatment. Usually, a flow rate measurement will be coupled with ultrasound measurement of post-void residual urine.

3.6.4 Pressure-flow urodynamic studies

Pressure-flow urodynamic studies should be performed on the following patients: men with a doubtful history and those with flow rates in the near-normal range(~ or >15 mL/s); men with invalid flow rate measurements(because of low voided volumes); men with a dominant history of irritative symptoms and men with lifelong urgency and frequency. The value of pressure–flow studies is debatable, especially in men who elect watchful waiting or medical therapy as their management option.

3.6.5 Urinalysis

Urinalysis (dipstick or sediment) must be included in the primary evaluation of any patient presenting with LUTS to identify conditions, such as urinary tract infections.

3.7 Imaging Examination

Transrectal ultrasound scanning (TRUS): TRUS is the method of choice to accurately evaluate the prostate (including prostate shape, size, configuration and protrusion into the bladder) and to guide a needle biopsy of suspicious areas, or to perform systematic biopsies to rule out prostate cancer.

3.8 Treatment

3.8.1 Conservative treatment

Conservative measures include watchful waiting in conjunction with behavioural and dietary modifications. Watchful waiting is a viable option for many men with non–bothersome LUTS as few will progress to acute urine retention and complications (e. g., renal insufficiency or stones), whilst others can remain stable for years. It is customary to give education about the patient's condition, reassurance, periodic monitoring, and lifestyle advice, including fluid restriction, reduction in caffeine intake, use of relaxed and double–voiding techniques, urethral milking to prevent post–micturition dribble, distraction techniques, etc.

3.8.2 Pharmacological treatment

(1) α_1–adrenoceptor antagonists (α_1–blockers)

α_1–blockers aim to inhibit the effect of endogenously released noradrenaline on smooth muscle cells in the prostate and thereby reduce prostate tone and BOO. α_1–blockers are often considered the first–line drug treatment of male LUTS. However, α_1–blockers do not prevent the occurrence of urinary retention or the need for surgery.

(2) 5α–reductase inhibitors

Androgen effects on the prostate are mediated by dihydrotestosterone (DHT), which is converted from testosterone by the enzyme 5 α–reductase, a nuclear–bound steroid enzyme. Two isoforms of this enzyme exist: 5 α–reductase type 1, with minor expression and activity in the prostate but predominant activity in extraprostatic tissues, such as skin and liver; 5 α–reductase type 2, with predominant expression and activity in the prostate. Two 5α–reductase inhibitors (5–ARIs) are available for clinical use: dutasteride and finasteride. Finasteride inhibits only 5α–reductase type 2, whereas dutasteride inhibits 5α–reductase type 1 and 2 with similar potency (dual 5–ARI). Treatment with 5–ARIs should be considered in men with moderate–to–severe LUTS and an enlarged prostate (> 40 mL) and/or elevated PSA concentration (> 1.4–1.6 ng/mL). 5α–reductase inhibitors can prevent disease progression with regard to acute urinary retention and the need for surgery. Due to the slow onset of action. They are suitable only for long–term treatment (years).

(3) Phosphodiesterase 5 inhibitors

Phosphodiesterase 5 inhibitors (PDE5Is) increase intracellular cyclic guanosine monophosphate, thus reducing smooth muscle tone of the detrusor, prostate and urethra. Nitric oxide and PDEs might also alter reflex pathways in the spinal cord and neurotransmission in the urethra, prostate, or bladder. Moreover, chronic treatment with PDE5Is seems to increase blood perfusion and oxygenation in the LUT. Finally, PDE5Is could reduce chronic inflammation in the prostate and bladder. The exact mechanism of PDE5Is on LUTS remains unclear.

(4) Plant extracts-phytotherapy

Phytotherapeutic agents are a heterogeneous group and may contain different concentrations of active ingredients. Hence, meta-analyses may not be justified and results of any analyses have to be interpreted with caution.

3.8.3 Surgical treatments

(1) Transurethral resection of the prostate and transurethral incision of the prostate

Transurethral resection of the prostate (TURP) removes tissue from the transition zone of the gland. Transurethral incision of the prostate (TUIP) involves incising the bladder outlet without tissue removal. TURP and TUIP are effective treatments for moderate-to-severe LUTS secondary to BPH. The choice should be based primarily on prostate volume (< 30 mL and 30-80 mL suitable for TUIP and TURP, respectively). The upper limit for TURP is suggested at 80 mL (based on Panel expert opinion, under the assumption that this limit depends on the surgeon's experience, resection speed, and choice of resectoscope size).

(2) Open prostatectomy

Open prostatectomy is the most invasively surgical method but it is an effective and durable procedure for the treatment of LUTS secondary to BPH. In the absence of an endourological armamentarium, open prostatectomy is the surgical treatment of choice for men with prostates > 80 mL.

3.8.4 Other treatment modalities

Other treatment modalities include transurethral microwave therapy (TUMT), transurethral needle ablation of the prostate, laser enucleation and holmium laser resection of the prostate, prostatic stents, prostatic urethral lift, intra-prostatic injections, minimal invasive simple prostatectomy, etc.

Chapter 4

Acute Urinary Retention

4.1 Etiology

Acute urinary retention(AUR)can happen in men or women and results from a variety of causes, although it most commonly occurs in men with BPH. Other chronic causes of poor bladder emptying, such as diabetic neuropathy, urethral stricture, multiple sclerosis, or Parkinson's disease, can result in episodes of complete urinary retention, often when the bladder becomes overdistended. This frequently occurs in the hospital setting when patients have limited mobility and is receiving medications that decrease bladder contractility, including opiates or anticholinergics. Constipation, a common side effect of those medications, can itself worsen urinary retention. Significant hematuria can result in the formation of blood clots, which may block the urethra and cause retention.

4.2 Clinical Manifestations

Clinical features include the following: no urine is passed for several hours; although some patients receiving large doses of narcotics or those with chronically decompensated bladders may not experience discomfort, most patients with AUR have significant pain; the bladder is visible, palpable, tender and dull to percussion; if the urinary retention has lasted several days(often accompanied by overflow incontinence), patients may develop acute renal failure; potential neurological causes should be excluded by checking reflexes in the lower limbs and perianal sensation.

4.3 Treatment

Treatment should include placement of a urethral catheter as quickly as possible. However, BPH or urethral strictures often make the placement of a catheter difficult. For men with BPH, a coude(French for-curved)catheter is helpful in negotiating past the angulation in the prostatic urethra. A urethral stricture should be suspected when the catheter meets resistance closer to the meatus, as many strictures occur in the distal urethra, which is narrower than the proximal portion. Using a 12F or 14F catheter often will allow the passage of the catheter into the bladder. If catheter placement is not successful, it is recommended to use a cystoscope, guidewire, and urethral dilators to dilate the stricture and place a Counseltip catheter via Seldinger technique; or place a suprapubic tube approximately two fingerbreadths above the pubic symphysis. If hematuria is the cause of retention, continuous bladder irrigation often is necessary to prevent clot formation.

A urinalysis should be checked because a poorly emptying bladder is prone to infection. Renal function also should be assessed for those in AUR by checking the creatinine level. An elevated creatinine level suggests that AUR has resulted in renal dysfunction, and these patients are at risk for postobstructive diuresis. These patients must be closely watched for excessive urine output. Fluid and electrolytes must be replaced if the urine output exceeds 200 mL/h, especially if hemodynamic instability or electrolyte imbalances is seen.

Once the bladder is adequately drained, the cause of AUR should be addressed. Narcotics should be tapered as tolerated. Postvoid residuals should be checked with a portable ultrasound device (bladder scanner) or by "straight" catheterization to determine the residual amount of urine left after the patient tries to empty his or her bladder. The inability to void or the presence of a postvoid residual over 200 mL is concerning for development of another episode of AUR. Patients may be given the option of an indwelling catheter for another few days with a subsequent voiding trial, or learning to clean intermittent catheterization (CIC), whereby, after predetermined intervals (4–6 hours) or after voiding attempts, the patient passes a catheter into the bladder and empties it.

Part 45

Urolithiasis

Chapter 1

Introduction

Stone disease is one of the most common afflictions of modern society, and urinary tract stones are a common cause of visits to the emergency department. Revolutionary advances in the minimally invasive and noninvasive management of stone disease over the past two decades have greatly facilitated the ease with which stones are removed. However, the overall estimated annual expenditure for patients with nephrolithiasis was nearly $ 2.1 billion in 2000. A thorough understanding of the etiology, epidemiology, and pathogenesis of urinary tract stone disease is necessary.

1.1 Epidemiology

The lifetime prevalence of kidney stone disease is estimated at 1% –15%, varying according to age, gender, race, and geographic location. The incidence of stone disease peaks in the fourth to sixth decades of life and is more common to men than women by ratio of 2 : 1. The geographic distribution of stone disease tends to roughly follow environmental risk factors. A higher prevalence of stone disease is found in hot, arid, or dry climates such as the mountains, desert, or tropical areas. However, genetic factors and dietary influences may outweigh the effects of geography.

Stones consist of both crystalline and noncrystalline components. The noncrystalline component is termed matrix, which typically accounts for about 2.5% of the weight of the stone. In some cases, matrix comprises the majority of the stone (up to 65%), usually in association with chronic urinary tract infection. Table 45–1–1 lists the clinically most relevant substances and their mineral components.

Table 45-1-1 Stone composition

Chemical name	Mineral name	Chemical formula
Calcium oxalate monohydrate	Whewellite	$CaC_2O_4 \cdot H_2O$
Calcium oxalate dihydrate	Wheddelite	$CaC_2O_4 \cdot 2H_2O$
Basic calcium phosphate	Apatite	$Ca_{10}(PO_4)_6 \cdot (OH)_2$
Calcium hydroxyl phosphate	Carbonite apatite	$Ca_5(PO_3)_3(OH)$
b-tricalcium phosphate	Whitiockite	$Ca_3(PO_4)_2$
Carbonate apatite phosphate	Dahllite	$Ca_5(PO_4)_3OH$
Calcium hydrogen phosphate	Brushite	$PO_4 \cdot 2H_2O$
Calcium carbonate	Aragonite	$CaCO_3$
Octacalcium phosphate		$Ca_8H_2(PO_4)_6 \cdot 5H_2O$
Uric acid	Uricite	$C_5H_4N_4O_3$
Uric acid dihydrate	Uricite	$C_5H_4O_3-2H_2O$
Ammonium urate		$NH_4C_5H_3N_4O_3$
Sodium acid urate monohydrate		$NaC_5H_3N_4O_3 \cdot H_2O$
Magnesium ammonium phosphate	Struvite	$MgNH_4PO_4 \cdot 6H_2O$
Magnesium acid phosphate trihydrate	Newberyite	$MgNH_4(PO_4) \cdot 1H_2O$
Magnesium ammonium phosphate monohydratet	Dittmarite	$[SCH_2CH(NH_2)COOH]_2$
Cystine		
Xanthine		
2,8-Dihydroxyadenine		
Proteins		
Cholosterol		
Calcite		
Potassium urate		
Trimagnesium phosphate		
Melamine		
Matrix		
Drug stones	· Active compounds crystallising in urine · Substances impairing urine composition (Section 4.11)	
Foreign body calculi		

1.2 Pathogenesis

The development of stones in the urinary tract is a complex, poorly understood, multifactorial process. It begins with urine that becomes supersaturated with respect to stone-forming salts, such that dissolved ions or molecules precipitate out of solution and form crystals or nuclei. Once formed, crystals may flow out with the urine or become retained at anchoring sites that promote growth and aggregation, ultimately leading to stone formation. A number of chemical and physical factors engaged in this process are known for playing a role.

1.2.1 Supersaturation

When there is an overabundance of solute in solution, supersaturation is said to be present. This state depends not only on the amount of solute presented to the kidney but also on urine pH and temperature. In the supersaturated state, nucleation and aggregation of solute crystals may occur, leading to stone formation. Supersaturation and crystallization account fairly well for uric acid and cystine stone formation but do not completely explain calcium stone formation. In the presence of urinary inhibitors and other substances, calcium oxalate precipitation occurs only when supersaturation exceeds solubility by 7-11 times.

1.2.2 Inhibitors

Inhibitors are substances in the urine that can block crystallization. One theory of stone formation holds that persons who form stones differ from those who do not in their lack of sufficient urinary inhibitors. Substances that are known to act as urinary inhibitors include pyrophosphate, citrate, magnesium, zinc, and macromolecules.

1.2.3 Matrix

Matrix is a noncrystalline mucoprotein often associated with urinary calculi. In persons who do not form stones, urinary matrix may act as an inhibitor. However, matrix may act as an initiator in some stone formers and may even provide the framework on which crystal deposition occurs. Pure matrix calculi may be seen in association with proteus infection.

1.2.4 Exogenous substances

Exogenous substances may be ingested and become stone components.

1.3 Etiology

Most classification systems for urolithiasis differentiate stones on the basis of the underlying metabolic or environmental abnormalities with which they are associated.

1.3.1 Calcium stones

(1) Hypercalciuria

Hypercalciuria is the most common abnormality identified in calcium stone formers. High urinary calcium concentrations lead to increase urinary saturation of calcium salts and reduced urinary inhibitory activity by way of complexation with negatively charged inhibitors such as citrate and chondroitin sulfate. Causes of hypercalciuria include the increased intestinal calcium absorption, renal calcium leak, primary hyperparathyroidism, sarcoid and granulomatous disease, malignancy.

(2) Hyperoxaluria

Hyperoxaluria eads to increase urinary saturation of calcium oxalate and subsequent promotion of calcium oxalate stones. Causes of hyperoxaluria include disorders in biosynthetic pathways (primary hyperoxaluria); intestinal malabsorptive states associated with inflammatory bowel disease, celiac sprue, or intestinal resection (enteric hyperoxaluria); and excessive dietary intake or high substrate levels (vitamin C) (dietary hyperoxaluria).

(3) Hyperuricosuria

The mechanism by which hyperuricosuria induces calcium oxalate stones is not completely elucidated. Not all evidence supports a role of uric acid in calcium oxalate stone formation. The most common cause of hyperuricosuria is increased dietary purine intake.

(4) Hypocitraturia

Citrate is an important inhibitor that can reduce calcium stone formation. Urinary citrate results from a variety of pathologic states associated with acidosis.

(5) Low urine pH

At low urine pH (<5.5), the undissociated form of uric acid predominates, leading to uric acid and/or calcium stone formation.

(6) Renal tubular acidosis (RTA)

Distal and proximal RTA occur as a result of impairment of net excretion of acid into the urine (distal or type 1) or of reabsorption of bicarbonate (proximal or type 2). Distinction between these abnormalities provides the basis for classification of RTA into proximal or distal, although both share the characteristic findings of hyperchloremic metabolic acidosis associated with inappropriately high urinary pH.

(7) Hypomagnesiuria

Hypomagnesiuria is a rare cause. Magnesium complexes with oxalate and calcium salt, and therefore low magnesium levels result in reduced inhibitory activity. Low urinary magnesium is also associated with decreased urinary citrate levels, which may further contribute to stone formation.

1.3.2 Uric acid stones

The three main determinants of uric acid stone formation are low pH, low urine volume, and hyperuricosuria. The most important pathogenetic factor is low urine pH because most patients with uric acid stones have normal uric acid excretion but invariably demonstrate persistent low urine pH. Hyperuricosuria predisposes to uric acid stone formation by causing supersaturation of the urine with respect to sparingly soluble undissociated uric acid. All conditions that contribute to low urinary volume increase the risk of uric acid supersaturation.

1.3.3 Cystine stones

In cystinuria, the defect in cystine transport results in high urinary levels. Several factors determine the solubility of cystine, including cystine concentration, pH, ionic strength, and urinary macromolecules. The main contributor to cystine crystallization is supersaturation because there is no specific inhibitor of cystine crystallization in the urine. Because of the poor solubility of cystine in urine, precipitation of cystine and subsequent stone formation occurs at physiologic urine conditions. The genetics of cystinuria has been studied extensively. Two genes involved in the disease have been identified: SLC3A1, which resides on the short arm of chromosome 2 and codes for a 663-amino acid heavy subunit (rBAT) of the cystine transporter, and SLC7A9, which is located on the long arm of chromosome 19 and codes for a 487-amino acid light subunit (b°, +AT) of the cystine transporter. The two subunits form a heterodimer that resides in the apical membrane of the proximal tubule cells. It has been revised by the International Cystinuria Consortium (ICC) to take into account the chromosomal localization of the mutation: type A (chromosome 2), type B (chromosome 19), and type AB (both chromosomes).

1.3.4 Infection stones

Infection stones are composed primarily of magnesium ammonium phosphate hexahydrate ($MgNH_4PO_4 \cdot 6H_2O$) but may in addition contain calcium phosphate in the form of carbonate apatite [$Ca_{10}(PO_4)_6 \cdot CO_3$]. Struvite stones (magnesium ammonium phosphate) occur only in association with urinary infection by urea-splitting bacteria. The most common urease-producing pathogens are Proteus, Klebsiella, Pseudomonas, and Staphylococcus species, with Proteus mirabilis the most common organism associated with infection stones.

1.3.5 Miscellaneous stones

(1) Xanthine and dihydroxyadenine stones

They form as a result of an inherited disorder in the catabolic enzyme xanthine dehydrogenase or xanthine oxidase, which catalyzes the conversion of xanthine to uric acid.

(2) Ammonium acid urate stones

The underlying pathophysiologic mechanism of ammonium acid urate stone formation attributable to laxative abuse has been postulated to be dehydration resulting from gastrointestinal fluid loss, causing intracellular acidosis and enhanced ammonia excretion. Because urinary sodium is low in the setting of laxative use, urate complexes with abundant ammonia, thereby leading to urinary supersaturation of ammonium acid urate.

(3) Matrix stones

The association between urinary proteins and stone formation has long been recognized. But the mechanism remains unclear.

(4) Medication-related stones

Drug-induced stones form either directly as a result of precipitation and crystallization of a drug or its metabolite or indirectly by altering the urinary environment, making it favorable for metabolic stone formation. Medications that directly promote stone formation include antiretroviral agents, triamterene, guaifenesin and ephedrine, silicate stones. Medications that indirectly promote stone formation include corticosteroids, vitamin D, and phosphate binding antacids, thiazides.

(5) Anatomic predisposition to stones

Patients with anatomic anomalies associated with urinary obstruction and/or stasis have been noted to have a high incidence of associated stones. Anatomic anomalies include ureteropelvic junction obstruction, horseshoe kidney, calyceal diverticula, medullary sponge kidney.

(6) Stones in pregnancy

Important physiologic changes in the kidney occur during pregnancy and modulate urinary stone risk factors. Renal blood flow increases, leading to a 30%-50% rise in glomerular filtration rate, which subsequently increases the filtered loads of calcium, sodium, and uric acid. Despite increases in a number of stone-inducing analytes, pregnant women have been shown to excrete increased amounts of inhibitors such as citrate, magnesium, and glycoproteins.

Chapter 2

Renal and Ureteral Calculi

2.1 Clinical Manifestation

2.1.1 Pain

Renal colic and noncolicky renal pain are the two types of pain originating from the kidney. Renal colic usually is caused by stretching of the collecting system or ureter, whereas noncolicky renal pain is caused by distention of the renal capsule. In the ureter, local pain is referred to the distribution of the ilioinguinal nerve and the genital branch of the genitofemoral nerve, whereas pain from obstruction is referred to the same areas as for collecting system calculi (flank and costovertebral angle). The stone burden does not correlate with the severity of the symptoms.

(1) Renal calyx

Stones or other objects in calyces or calyceal diverticula may cause obstruction and renal colic. In general, unobstructed stones cause pain only periodically, owing to intermittent obstruction. The pain is a deep, dull ache in the flank or back that can vary in intensity from severe to mild. The pain may be exacerbated after consumption of large amounts of fluid. The presence of infection or inflammation in the calyx or diverticulum (e. g., milk of calcium) in addition to obstruction may contribute to pain perception.

(2) Renal pelvis

Stones in the renal pelvis 1 cm in diameter commonly obstruct the ureteropelvic junction, generally causing severe pain in the costovertebral angle, just lateral to the sacrospinalis muscle and just below the 12th rib. This pain may vary from dull to excruciatingly sharp and is usually constant, boring, and difficult to ignore. It often radiates to the flank and also anteriorly to the upper ipsilateral abdominal quadrant. Acquired or congenital ureteropelvic junction obstruction may cause a similar constellation of symptoms. Symptoms frequently occur on an intermittent basis following a drinking binge or consumption of large quantities of fluid.

Partial or complete staghorn configured calculi that are present in the renal pelvis is not necessarily obstructive. In the absence of obstruction, these patients often have surprisingly few symptoms such as flank or back pain. Recurrent urinary tract infections frequently culminate in radiographic evaluation with the discovery of a large calculus. If untreated, these "silent" staghorn calculi can often lead to significant.

(3) Upper and mid-ureter

Stones or other objects in the upper or mid ureter often cause severe, sharp back (costovertebral angle) or flank pain. The pain may be more severe and intermittent if the stone is progressing down the ureter and causing intermittent obstruction. A stone that becomes lodged at a particular site may cause less pain, especially if it is only partially obstructive. Stationary calculi that result in high-grade but constant obstruction may allow autoregulatory reflexes and pyelovenous and pyelolymphatic backflow to decompress the upper tract, with diminution in intraluminal pressure gradually easing the pain. Pain associated with ureteral calculi often projects to corresponding dermatomal and spinal nerve root innervation regions. The pain of upper ureteral stones thus radiates to the lumbar region and flank. Mid ureteral calculi tends to cause pain that radiates caudally and anteriorly toward the mid and lower abdomen in a curved, band-like fashion. This band initially parallels the lower costal margin but deviates caudad toward the bony pelvis and inguinal ligament. The pain may mimic acute appendicitis if on the right or acute diverticulitis if on the left side, especially if concurrent gastrointestinal symptoms are present.

(4) Distal ureter

Calculi in the lower ureter often causes pain that radiates to the groin or testicle in males and the labia majors in females. This referred pain is often generated from the ilioinguinal or genital branch of the genitofemoral nerves. Diagnosis may be confused with testicular torsion or epididymitis. Stones in the intramural ureter may mimic cystitis, urethritis, or prostatitis by causing suprapubic pain, urinary frequency and urgency, dysuria, stranguria, or gross hematuria. Bowel symptoms are not uncommon. In women, the diagnosis may be confused with menstrual pain, pelvic inflammatory disease, and ruptured or twisted ovarian cysts. Strictures of the distal ureter from radiation, operative injury, or previous endoscopic procedures can present with similar symptoms. This pain pattern is likely due to the similar innervation of the intramural ureter and bladder.

2.1.2 Hematuria

Patients frequently admit to intermittent gross hematuria or occasional tea-colored urine (old blood). Most patients will have at least microhematuria. Rarely (10-15% of cases), complete ureteral obstruction presents without microhematuria.

2.1.3 Infection

Infection may be a contributing factor to pain perception. Uropathogenic bacteria may alter ureteral peristalsis by the production of exotoxins and endotoxins. Local inflammation from infection can lead to chemoreceptor activation and perception of local pain with its corresponding referral pattern.

2.1.4 Associated fever

The association of urinary stones with fever is a relative medical emergency. Signs of clinical sepsis are variable and include fever, tachycardia, hypotension, and cutaneous vasodilation. Costovertebral angle tenderness may be marked with acute upper-tract obstruction; however, it can not be relied upon to be present in instances of long-term obstruction. In such instances, a mass may be palpable resulting from a grossly hydronephrotic kidney.

2.1.5 Nausea and vomiting

Upper-tract obstruction is frequently associated with nausea and vomiting.

2.2 Laboratory examinations

2.2.1 Blood test

A multichannel blood screen is helpful in identifying certain systemic problems. These include primary hyperparathyroidism(high serum calcium and low serum phosphorus), renal phosphate leak (hypophosphatemia), uric acid lithiasis(hyperuricemia), and distal RTA(hypokalemia, decreased serum carbon dioxide).

2.2.2 Urine test

Voided urine specimens should be obtained for comprehensive urinalysis and culture. The urinalysis should include pH determination(preferably with an electrode), because a pH greater than 7.0 is suggestive of infection lithiasis or RTA, whereas a pH less than 5.5 suggests uric acid lithiasis secondary to gouty diathesis.

The urine sediment should be examined for crystalluria, because particular crystal types may give a clue as to the composition of stones the patient is forming. Tetrahedral "envelopes" are seen in calcium oxalate lithiasis, and rectangular, "coffinlid" crystals are often seen in patients with struvite calculi. Hexagonal crystals confirm cystinuria; uric acid crystals may be seen as amorphous fibers or as irregular plates.

Urine cultures are performed if there is a suspicion of infection-related calculi or if there are signs or symptoms of a UTI.

2.2.3 Crystalline composition test

Available stones should be analyzed to determine their crystalline composition. The presence of uric acid or cystine would suggest the presence of a gouty diathesis or cystinuria, respectively. The finding of struvite, carbonate apatite, and magnesium ammonium phosphate would suggest infection lithiasis. A predominance of a hydroxyapatite component suggests the presence of RTA or primary hyperparathyroidism and warrants an assessment of basic electrolytes. Stones composed of pure calcium oxalate or mixed calcium oxalate and hydroxyapatite are less useful diagnostically because they may occur in several entities, including absorptive and renal hypercalciuria, hyperuricosuric calcium nephrolithiasis, enteric hyperoxaluria, hypocitraturic calcium nephrolithiasis, and low urine volume.

2.3 Imaging Examinations

2.3.1 Ultrasonography

Ultrasound should be used as the primary diagnostic imaging tool, although pain relief, or any other emergency measures should not be delayed by imaging assessments. It can identify stones located in the calices, pelvis, and pyeloureteric and vesicoureteric junctions(ultrasound with filled bladder), as well as in patients with upper urinary tract dilatation. Ultrasound has a sensitivity of 45% and specificity of 94% for ureteric stones and a sensitivity of 45% and specificity of 88% for renal stones.

2.3.2 Kidney-ureter-bladder (KUB) radiography films

The sensitivity and specificity of KUB is 44% -77% and 80% -87%, respectively. Kidney-ureter-bladder radiography should not be performed if non-contrast-enhanced computed tomography (NCCT) is considered. However, KUB is helpful in differentiating between radiolucent and radiopaque stones and be used for comparison during follow-up. Table 45-2-1 lists different types of stones with different radiation properties.

Table 45-2-1 Different types of stones with different radiation properties

Radiopaque	Poor radiopacity	Radiolucent
Calcium oxalate dihydrate	Magnesium ammonium phosphate	Uric acid
Calcium oxalate monohydrate	Apatite	Ammonium urate
Calcium phosphates	Cystine	Xanthine
		2,8-Dihydroxyadenine
		Drug-stones (Section 4.11)

2.3.3 NCCT

NCCT has become the standard for diagnosing acute flank pain, and has replaced IVU. NCCT can determine stone diameter and density. When stones are absent, the cause of abdominal pain should be identified. In evaluating patients with suspected acute urolithiasis, NCCT is significantly more accurate than IVU. NCCT can detect uric acid and xanthine stones, which are radiolucent on plain films, but not indinavir stones. NCCT can determine stone density, inner structure of the stone and skin-to-stone distance and surrounding anatomy; all of which affect selection of treatment modality.

2.3.4 IVU

Intravenous urography can provide information about renal function, the anatomy of the collecting system as well as the level of an obstruction.

2.3.5 Magnetic resonance urography

Magnetic resonance urography (MRU) can not be used to detect urinary stones. However, it might provide detailed anatomical information about the urinary collecting system, the location of an obstruction or stenosis in the ureter, and renal parenchymal morphology.

2.4 Differential Diagnosis

Urinary stones can mimic other retroperitoneal and peritoneal pathologic states. A full differential diagnosis of the acute abdomen should be made, including acute appendicitis, ectopic and unrecognized pregnancies, ovarian pathologic conditions including twisted ovarian cysts, diverticular disease, bowel obstruction, biliary stones with and without obstruction, peptic ulcer disease, acute renal artery embolism, and abdominal aortic aneurysm—to mention a few. Peritoneal signs should be sought during physical examination.

2.5 Treatment

Basic treatment algorithms for renal calculi and ureteral calculi are presented in Figure 45-2-1 and Figure 45-2-2, respectively.

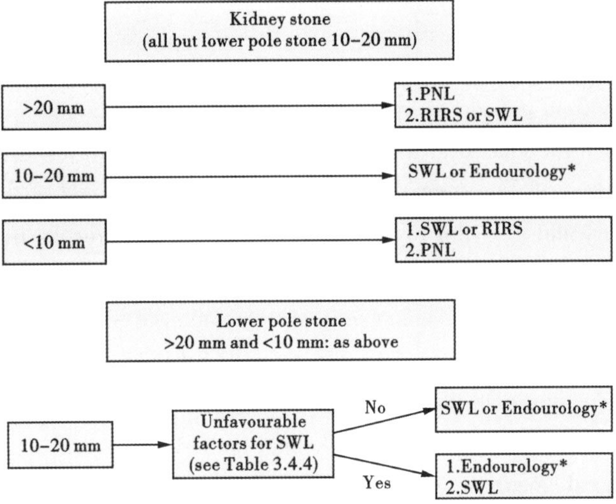

Figure 45-2-1 Treatment algorithm for renal calculi

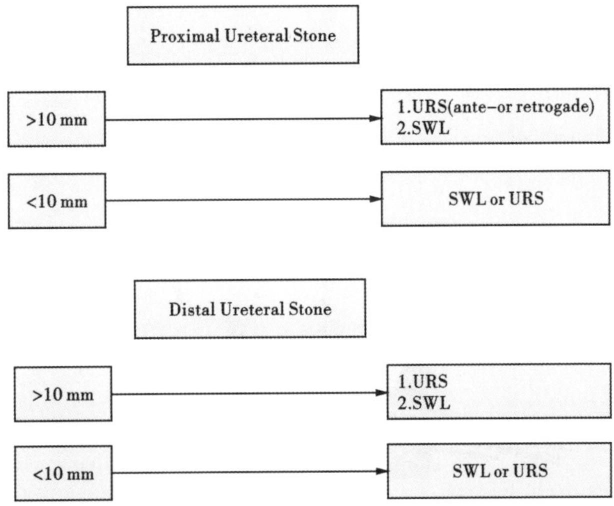

Figure 45-2-2 Treatment algorithm for ureteral calculi

2.5.1 Management of emergency (relief of renal colic)

Renal colic may be relieved with medications and fluid infusion, such as atropine, prosgesterone, calcium channel blocker, indomethacin, or dolantin.

2.5.2 Conservative measures

Intervention is not required for small, nonobstructive, asymptomatic caliceal stones. Hydration and dietary management may be sufficient to prevent growth of existing or new calcium stones in patients without metabolic abnormalities. Most ureteral calculi pass and do not require intervention. Spontaneous passage depends on stone size, shape, location, and associated ureteral edema. Ureteral calculi with 5 mm in size have a 40% –50% chance of spontaneous passage.

The effectiveness of dissolution agents depends on stone surface area, stone type, volume of irrigant, and mode of delivery. Oral alkallsing agents include sodium or potassium bicarbonate and potassium citrate.

2.5.3 Shock wave lithotripsy

Shock wave lithotripsy(SWL) requires an energy source to create the shock wave, a coupling mechanism to transfer the energy from outside to inside the body, and either fluoroscopic or ultrasonic modes, or both, to identify and position the calculi at a focus of converging shock waves. Shock waves are capable of fragmenting stones when focused. Fragmentation is achieved by erosion and shattering. Cavitational forces result in erosion at the entry and exit sites of the shock wave. Shattering results from energy absorption with stress, strain, and shear forces. Surrounding biologic tissues are resilient because they are neither brittle nor are the shock waves focused on them. A diagrammatic representation of SWL is presented in Figure 45-2-3. There are several contraindications to the use of extracorporeal SWL, including pregnancy, due to the potential effects on the foetus; bleeding diatheses, which should be compensated for at least 24 hours before and 48 hours after treatment; uncontrolled UTIs; severe skeletal malformations and severe obesity, which prevent targeting of the stone; arterial aneurysm in the vicinity of the stone; anatomical obstruction distal to the stone.

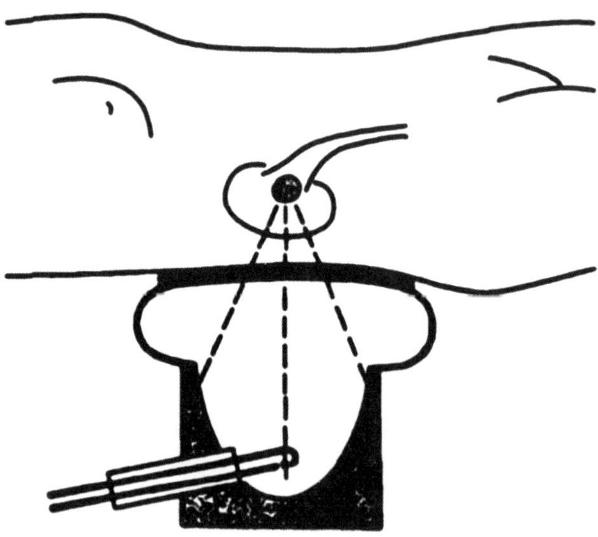

Figure 45-2-3 Diagrammatic representation of SWL

2.5.4 Percutaneous nephrolithotomy

Percutaneous nephrolithotripsy(PNL) remains the standard procedure for large renal calculi. Needle puncture is directed by fluoroscopy, ultrasound, or both, and is routinely placed from the posterior axillary line into a calyx or a caliceal. Tract dilation is performed and tracts placed during open renal procedures are frequently tortuous and suboptimal for subsequent endourologic extraction of calculi (Figure 45-2-4). Patients receiving anticoagulant therapy must be monitored carefully pre-and post-operatively. Anticoagulant therapy must be discontinued before PNL. Other important contraindications include tumour in the presumptive access tract area; potential malignant kidney tumour; pregnancy; untreated UTI.

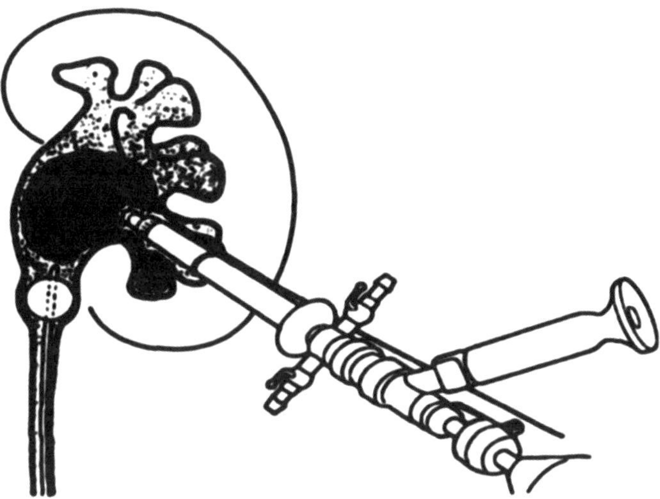

Figure 45-2-4 Diagrammatic representation of PNL

2.5.5 Ureterorenoscopy

Use flexible Ureterorenoscopy (URS) in case percutaneous nephrolithotomy or shock wave lithotripsy is not an option (even for stones > 2 cm). The ureteral access can be established and a variety of lithotrites can be placed through an ureteroscope, including electrohydraulic, solid and hollow-core ultrasonic probes, a variety of laser systems, and pneumatic systems for stone extraction. Apart from general problems, for example, with general anaesthesia or untreated UTIs, URS can be performed in all patients without any specific contraindications.

2.5.6 Retrograde renal surgery

Retrograde renal surgery (RIRS) can not be recommended as first-line treatment for stones > 20 mm in uncomplicated cases as SFRs decrease, and staged procedures will be required. However, it may be a first-line option in patients where PNL is not an option or contraindicated.

2.5.7 Open stone surgery

Open stone surgery is the historic way to remove calculi, yet it is rarely used today. The morbidity of the incision, the possibility of retained stone fragments, and the ease and success of less invasive techniques have made these procedures rare.

2.5.8 Other renal procedures

Partial nephrectomy is appropriate with a large stone burden in a renal pole with marked parenchymal thinning. Caution should be taken with a simple nephrectomy even with a normal contralateral kidney, as stones are frequently associated with a systemic metabolic defect that may recur in the contralateral kidney.

2.5.9 Ureterolithotomy

Long-standing ureteral calculi—those inaccessible with endoscopy and those resistant to SWL—can be extracted with an ureterolithotomy.

2.6 Prophylaxis

In general, 50% of patients experience recurrent urinary stones within 5 years without prophylactic intervention. Appropriate education and preventive measures are best instituted with a motivated patient after spontaneous stone passage or surgical stone removal. Risk factors as described previously should be identified and modified, if possible. Irrespective of the final metabolic evaluation and stone analysis, the patient's fluid intake should be 1.5–2.0 L/2 hour. Fluids should be encouraged during mealtime. In addition, liquids should be increased approximately 2 hours after meals. Water produced as a metabolic by-product reaches its nadir at this time, and thus the body is relatively dehydrated. Fluid ingestion also should be encouraged to force a nighttime diuresis adequate to awaken the patient to void. Awakening and ambulating to void limits urinary stasis and offers an opportunity to ingest additional fluids. These lifestyle changes are difficult to maintain and should be encouraged during subsequent office visits. Motivated patients who regularly return to the urinary stone clinic have a reduced stone recurrence rate that is probably due to increased compliance.

Chapter 3

Bladder Stones

Bladder calculi usually is a manifestation of an underlying pathologic condition, including voiding dysfunction or a foreign body. Voiding dysfunction may be due to an urethral stricture, BPH, bladder neck contracture, or flaccid or spastic neurogenic bladder, all of which result in static urine. Foreign bodies such as Foley catheters and forgotten double-J ureteral catheters can serve as nidi for stones. Most bladder calculi are seen in men. In developing countries, they are frequently found in prepubescent boys. Stone analysis frequently reveals ammonium urate, uric acid, or calcium oxalate stones. Bladder stones can be solitary or numerous. Patients present with irritative voiding symptoms, intermittent urinary stream, urinary tract infections, hematuria, or pelvic pain. Physical examination is unrevealing. A large percentage of bladder stones are radiolucent (uric acid). Ultrasound of the bladder identifies the stone with its characteristic postacoustic shadowing. The stone moves with changing body position. Stones within an ureterocele do not move with body position as seen on ultrasound examination. They frequently are nonobstructive. Endoscopic incision and stone removal rarely results in vesicoureteral reflux. The mode of stone removal for other bladder stones should be directed by the underlying cause. Early instruments used to remove bladder calculi were both clever and bizarre. Simple mechanical crushing devices are still used today. Mechanical lithotrites should be used with caution to prevent bladder injury when the jaws are closed. Ensuring a partially full bladder and endoscopic visualization of unrestricted lateral movement before forceful crushing of the stones helps reduce this troublesome complication. Cystolitholapaxy allows most stones to be broken and subsequently removed through a cystoscope. Electrohydraulic, ultrasonic, laser, and pneumatic lithotrites similar to those used through a nephroscope are effective. Cystolithotomy can be performed through a small abdominal incision.

Chapter 4

Urethral Stones

Urethral calculi usually originates from the bladder and rarely from the upper tracts. Most ureteral stones that pass spontaneously into the bladder can pass through the urethra unimpeded. Urethral stones may develop secondary to urinary stasis, secondary to a urethral diverticulum, near urethral strictures, or at sites of previous surgery. Most urethral stones in men present in the prostatic or bulbar regions and are solitary. Patients with recurrent pendulous urethral calculi without evidence of other pathologic conditions should be suspected of self-introduction of such stones in an attempt to obtain pain medications or for attention, as seen in Munchausen syndrome. Females rarely develop urethral calculi owing to their short urethra and a lower incidence of bladder calculi. Most urethral stones found in women are associated with urethral diverticula. Symptoms are similar to bladder calculi—intermittent urinary stream, terminal hematuria, and infection. The stones may present with dribbling or during acute urinary retention. Pain may be severe and, in men, may radiate to the tip of the penis. The diagnosis may be confirmed by palpation, endoscopic visualization, or radiographic study. Treatment should be directed by the underlying cause. Stones associated with a dense urethral stricture or complex diverticula can be removed during definitive open surgical repair. Small stones may be grasped successfully and removed intact. More frequently, they need to be fragmented and removed. Long-standing, large impacted stones are best removed through a urethrotomy.

Part 46

Urologic and Male Genital Tumors

Chapter 1

Renal Neoplasm

Renal neoplasms can be malignant or benign. Malignant renal tumors include renal cell carcinoma (RCC), urothelium-based malignancies, sarcomas, embryonic or pediatric tumors, lymphomas, and metastases. Benign renal tumors are diverse and present unique diagnostic challenges, including adenoma, aangioma, aangiomyolipoma.

Renal Cell Carcinoma(RCC) is the most lethal cancer of the common urologic cancers.

1.1 Etiology

RCCs were traditionally thought to arise primarily from the proximal convoluted tubules, and this is probably true for the clear cell and papillary variants. However, we now know that other histologic subtypes of RCC, such as chromophobe RCC and collecting duct carcinoma, are derived from the more distal components of the nephron.

The most generally accepted environmental risk factor for RCC is tobacco exposure, although the relative associated risks have been modest. Tobacco user for 20%–30% of cases of RCC in men and 10%–20% in women. Obesity is now accepted as another major risk factor for RCC. Hypertension appears to be the third major etiologic factor for RCC. Novel familial syndromes of RCC have been identified, and the tumor suppressor genes and oncogenes contributing to the development of both sporadic and familial forms of this malignancy have been characterized. Eliminating cigarette smoking and reducing weight are the most important primary prevention of RCC.

1.2 Epidemiology

Renal cell cancer represents 2%–3% of all cancers and there is a 1.5 : 1 male predominance, with a peak incidence between 60 and 70 years old.

1.3 Pathology

Renal cell carcinomas comprise a broad spectrum of histopathological entities described in the 2016 World Health Organization classification. There are three main RCC types: clear cell(70%–80%), papillary(10%–15%) and chromophobe(5%).

Overall, clear-cell RCC(ccRCC) is well circumscribed and a capsule is usually absent. The cut surface is golden-yellow, often with haemorrhage and necrosis.

Macroscopically, papillary RCC(pRCC) is well circumscribed with pseudocapsule, yellow or brown in colour, and a soft structure. pRCC has traditionally been subdivided into two types. Exophytic spherical growth, pseudo-necrotic changes and pseudo-capsule are typical signs of pRCC type 1. Tumours are usually fragile.

Chromophobe(chRCC) is a pale tan, relatively homogenous and tough, well-demarcated mass without a capsule.

RCCs are vascular tumors that tend to spread either by direct invasion through the renal capsule into perinephric fat and adjacent visceral structures or by direct extension into the renal vein. 25%–30% of patients have evidence of metastatic disease at presentation. The most common site of distant metastases is the lung. However, liver, bone(osteolytic), ipsilateral adjacent lymph nodes and adrenal gland, brain, the opposite kidney, and subcutaneous tissue are frequent sites of disease spread.

The tumour node metastasis(TNM) classification system is recommended for clinical use(Table 46-1-1). Tumour size, venous invasion, renal capsular invasion, adrenal involvement, and lymph node and distant metastasis are included in the TNM classification system.

Table 46-1-1 The TNM classification system for RCC

T-Primary Tumour	
TX	Primary tumour cannot be assessed
T0	No evidence of primary tumour
T1	Clinically inapparent tumour that is not palpable
	T1a Tumour incidental histological finding in 5% or less of tissue ressected
	T1b Tumour incidental histological finding in more than 5% of tissue resected
	T1c Tumour identified by needle biopsy (e. g. because of elevated prostate-specific antigen(PSA) level)
T2	Tumour that is palpable and confined within the prostate
	T2a Tumour involves one half of one bobe or less
	T2b Tumour involves more than half of one lobe, but not both lobes
	T2c Tumour involves both lobes
T3	Tumour extends through the prostatic capsule[1]
	T3a Extracapsular extension (unilateral or bilateral) including microscopic bladder neck involvement
	T3b Tumour invades seminal veslcle(s)
T4	Tumour is fixed or invades adjacent structures other than seminal vesicles: extemal sphincter, rectum, levator muscles, and/or pelvic wall

Continue to Table 46-1-1

N-Regional Lymph Nodes[2]		
NX	Regional lymph nodes cannot be assessed	
N0	No regional lymph node metastasis	
N1	Regional lymph node metastasis	
M-Distant Metastasis[3]		
M0	No distant metastasis	
M1	Distant metastasis	
	M1a	Non-regional lymph node(s)
	M1b	Bone(s)
	M1c	Other site(s)

[1] Invasion into the prostate apex or into (but not beyond) the prostate capsule is not classified as T3, but as T2.

[2] Metastasis no larger than 0.2 cm can be designated pNmi.

[2] T2a to c only exist for clinical T2(cT2). For pathological T2 they are no longer present in the 2017 TNM. Only pT2 exists.

[3] When more than one site of metastasis is present, the most advanced category is used. (p)M1c is the most advanced category.

1.4 Clinical manifestation

The classically described triad of gross hematuria, flank pain, and a palpable mass occurs in only 7% - 10% of patients and is frequently a manifestation of advanced disease. Patients may also present with hematuria, dyspnea, cough, and bone pain that are typically symptoms secondary to metastases. With the routine use of CT scanning for evaluation of nonspecific findings, asymptomatic renal tumors are increasingly detected incidentally.

RCC is associated with a wide spectrum of paraneoplastic syndromes including erythrocytosis, hypercalcemia, hypertension, and nonmetastatic hepatic dysfunction. Paraneoplastic syndromes are listed as followings:

(1) Erythrocytosis

RCC is the most common causes of paraneoplastic erythrocytosis, reported to occur in 3% - 10% of patients with this tumor.

(2) Hypercalcemia

Hypercalcemia has been reported to occur in up to 20% of patients with RCC. Hypercalcemia may be due to production of a parathyroid hormone-related peptide that mimics the function of parathyroid hormone or other.

(3) Hypertension

Hypertension associated with RCC has been reported in up to 40% of patients and renin production by the neoplasm has been documented in 37%.

(4) Stauffer's syndrome

Stauffer's syndrome was described as a reversible syndrome of hepatic dysfunction in the absence of hepatic metastases associated with RCC. Hepatic function abnormalities include elevation of alkaline phosphatase and bilirubin, hypoalbuminemia, prolonged prothrombin time, and hypergammaglobulinemia. Stauffer's syndrome tends to occur in association with fever, fatigue, and weight loss and typically resolves after nephrectomy. The reported incidence of Stauffer's syndrome varies from 3% to 20%. It may be due to overproduction of granulocytemacrophage colony stimulating factor by the tumor.

(5) Other syndromes

RCC is known to produce a multitude of other biologically active products that result in clinically significant syndromes, including adrenocorticotropic hormone (Cushing's syndrome), enteroglucagon (protein enteropathy), prolactin (galactorrhea), insulin (hypoglycemia), and gonadotropins (gynecomastia and decreased libido; or hirsutism, amenorrhea, and male pattern balding) (A paraneoplastic syndrome present at the time of disease).

1.5 Laboratory examination

Commonly assessed laboratory parameters are serum creatinine, glomerular filtration rate (GFR), complete cell blood count, erythrocyte sedimentation rate, liver function study, alkaline phosphatase, lactate dehydrogenase (LDH), serum corrected calcium, coagulation study, and urinalysis. For central renal masses abutting or invading the collecting system, urinary cytology and possibly endoscopic assessment should be considered in order to exclude urothelial cancer. Split renal function should be estimated using renal scintigraphy in the following situations: when renal function is compromised, as indicated by increased serum creatinine or significantly decreased GFR or when renal function is clinically important, e. g., in patients with a solitary kidney or multiple or bilateral tumours.

Fine-needle aspiration of renal lesions is the diagnostic approach of choice in those patients with clinically apparent metastatic disease who may be candidates for nonsurgical therapy. Other settings in which fine-needle aspiration may be appropriate include establishing a diagnosis in patients who are not surgical candidates, differentiating a primary RCC from a renal metastasis in patients with known primary cancers of nonrenal origin, and evaluating some radiographically indeterminate lesions. Fine needle aspiration is being increasingly used to confirm the diagnosis of a neoplasm particularly in patients who may undergo observation or percutaneous ablative therapy.

1.6 Imaging examination

(1) Ultrasonography

Ultrasonography (US) examination is a noninvasive, relatively inexpensive technique able to further delineate a renal mass. It is approximately 98% accurate in distinguishing simple cysts from solid lesions.

(2) CT Scanning

CT scanning is more sensitive than US for detection of renal masses. A typical finding of RCC on CT is a mass that becomes enhanced with the use of intravenous contrast media. In general, RCC exhibits an overall decreased density in Hounsfield units compared with normal renal parenchyma but shows either a homogeneous or heterogeneous pattern of enhancement (increase in density of 10 Hounsfield units) following contrast administration. In addition to defining the primary lesion, CT scanning is also the method of choice in staging the patient by visualizing the renal hilum, perinephric space, renal vein and vena cava, adrenals, regional lymphatics, and adjacent organs. In patients with equivocal chest X-ray findings, a CT scan of the chest is indicated. Patients who present with symptoms consistent with brain metastases should be evaluated with either head CT or MRI.

(3) MRI

MRI is indicated in patients who are allergic to intravenous CT contrast medium and in pregnancy without renal failure. Its primary advantage is in the evaluation of patients with suspected vascular extension.

(4) Renal angiography

With the widespread availability of CT scanners, the role of renal angiography in the diagnostic evaluation of RCC has markedly diminished and is now very limited.

(5) Radiographic investigations to evaluate RCC metastases

Chest CT is accurate for chest staging. Bone scan, brain CT, or MRI may be used in the presence of specific clinical or laboratory signs and symptoms.

1.7 Differential diagnosis

When a patient presents with clinical findings consistent with metastatic disease and is found to have a renal mass, a diagnosis of RCC can be straightforward. The differential diagnosis of RCC includes other solid renal lesions. The great majority of renal masses are simple cysts. Once the diagnosis of a cyst is confirmed by US, no additional evaluation is required if the patient is asymptomatic. Differentiation of benign from malignant lesions is frequently difficult. Findings on CT scan that suggest malignancy include amputation of a portion of the collecting system, presence of calcification, a poorly defined interface between the renal parenchyma and the lesion, invasion into perinephric fat or adjacent structures, and the presence of abnormal periaortic adenopathy or distant metastatic disease. The frequency of benign lesions among renal masses < 7 cm in size is as high as 16% – 20%. Masses > 7 cm are rarely benign. Some characteristic lesions can be defined using CT criteria in combination with clinical findings. Angiomyolipomas (with large fat components) can be easily identified by the low-attenuation areas classically produced by substantial fat content. A renal abscess may be strongly suspected in a patient presenting with fever, flank pain, pyuria, and leukocytosis, and an early needle aspiration and culture should be performed. Other benign renal masses (in addition to those previously described) include granulomas and arteriovenous malformations. Renal lymphoma (both Hodgkin's disease and non-Hodgkin's disease), transitional cell carcinoma of the renal pelvis, adrenal cancer, and metastatic disease (most commonly from a lung or breast cancer primary) are additional diagnostic possibilities that may be suspected based on CT and clinical findings.

1.8 Treatment

(1) T1 tumours (< 7 cm)

1) Partial nephrectomy (PN)

PN is recommended as the preferred option in organ-confined tumors measuring up to 7 cm since it preserves kidney function better and in the long term limits development of metabolic as well as cardiovascular disorders. In patients with compromised renal function, solitary kidney or bilateral tumours, PN is also the standard of care, with no tumour size limitation. PN can be carried out via open, laparoscopic or laparoscopic robot-assisted approaches. PN is unsuitable for some patients with localised RCC due to insufficient volume of remaining parenchyma to maintain proper organ function; renal vein thrombosis; unfavourable tumour location, e. g. , adherence to the renal vessels; use of anticoagulants. In these situations the curative therapy is RN including removal of the tumour-bearing kidney.

2) Ablative therapies

Radio frequency ablation (RFA) or cryoablation (CA) treatments are options in patients with small cortical tumors ($\leqslant$ 3 cm), especially for patients who are frail, present a high surgical risk and those with a solitary kidney, compromised renal function, hereditary RCC or multiple bilateral tumours. Renal biopsy is recommended to confirm malignancy and subtype in this setting.

3) Active surveillance

Active surveillance is an option in elderly patients with significant co-morbidities or those with a short-life expectancy and solid renal tumours measuring < 40 mm. Renal biopsy is recommended to select patients with small masses for active surveillance with high accuracy.

(2) T_2 tumours (> 7 cm)

Laparoscopic radical nephrectomy (RN) is the preferred option.

(3) Locally advanced RCC (T_3 and T_4)

Open RN remains the standard of care. Systematic adrenalectomy is not recommended when abdominal CT shows no evidence of adrenal invasion. In patients with clinically enlarged lymph nodes, lymph node dissection should be performed for staging purposes or local control. All patients with nonmetastatic disease and venous tumour thrombus, should be considered for surgical intervention, irrespective of the extent of tumour thrombus at presentation.

Currently, there is no evidence that adjuvant therapy is of survival benefit or prolongs.

(4) Metastatic disease

1) Cytoreductive nephrectomy

For most patients with metastatic disease, cytoreductive nephrectomy (CN) is palliative and systemic treatments are necessary. Cytoreductive nephrectomy is currently recommended in metastatic (mRCC) patients with a good performance status, large primary tumours and low metastatic volume. In patients with poor performance status or Metastatic Renal Cancer Database Consortium (IMDC) risk, small primaries and high metastatic volume and/or a sarcomatoid tumour, CN is not recommended.

2) Metastasectomy and other local treatment strategies

Local therapy for metastatic disease (including metastasectomy) should be considered in patients with a favourable risk profile in whom complete resection is achievable or when local symptoms need to be controlled.

3) Systemic treatment

An algorithm for systemic treatment in mRCC is presented in Figure 46-1-1.

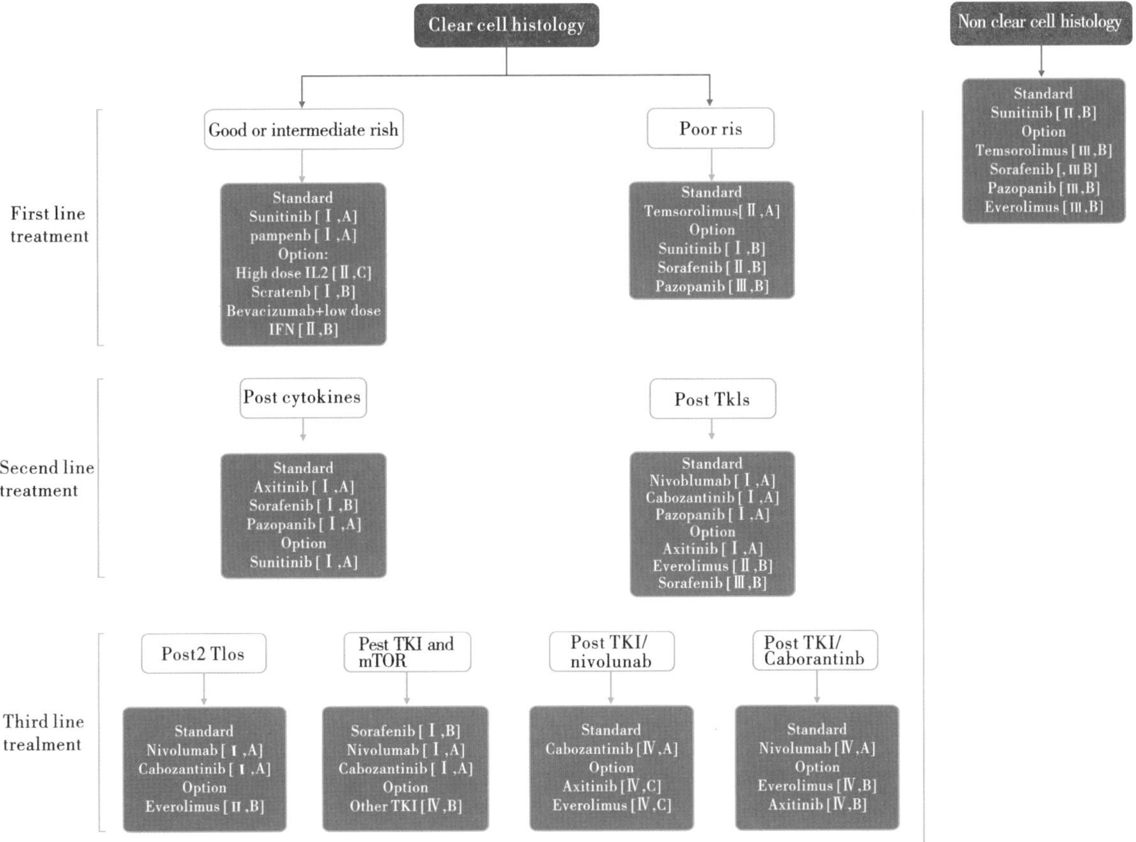

Figure 46-1-1 An algorithm for systemic treatment in mRCC

1.9 Prognosis

Prognostic factors can be classified into anatomical, histological, clinical, and molecular. In RCC patients, TNM stage, tumour nuclear grade, and RCC subtype provide important prognostic information.

Chapter 2

Nephroblastoma (Wilms Tumor)

Nephroblastoma, also known as Wilms tumor, is the most common solid renal tumor of childhood.

2.1 Etiology

A two-hit hypothesis was proposed to explain the earlier age of onset and bilateral presentation in children with a familial history of Wilms tumor. In this hypothesis, the pathogenesis of the sporadic form of Wilms tumor results from two postzygotic mutations in a single cell. In contrast, the familial form of the disease arises after one prezygotic mutation and a subsequent postzygotic event.

Karyotypic analyses of Wilms tumor patients with various congenital malformations and loss of heterozygosity studies helped identify a region on the short arm of chromosome 11. This work ultimately led to the identification of a gene associated with Wilms tumor development (WT1), which maps to chromosome 11p13. Although alterations in this gene have been associated with Wilms tumor and genitourinary abnormalities, only 5%–10% of sporadic Wilms tumors have been demonstrated to have WT1 mutations.

2.2 Epidemiology

Nephroblastoma accounts for roughly 5% of childhood cancers. The peak age for presentation is during the third year of life, and there is no sex predilection. The disease is seen worldwide with a similar age of onset and sex distribution. Tumors are commonly unicentric, but they occur in either kidney with equal frequency. In 5% of cases the tumors are bilateral.

2.3 Pathology

The typical Wilms tumor consists of blastemal, epithelial, and stromal elements in varying proportions. Grossly, Wilms tumors are generally large, multilobulated, and gray or tan in color with focal areas of hemorrhage and necrosis. A fibrous pseudocapsule is occasionally seen. Tumor dissemination can occur by direct extension through the renal capsule, hematogenously via the renal vein and vena cava, or via lymphatic spread. Metastatic disease is present at diagnosis in 10% –15% of patients, with the lungs(85% –95%) and liver(10% –15%) the most common sites of involvement. Regional lymphatics are involved in as many as 25% of patients. Metastases to liver, bone, and brain are uncommon.

The NWTS staging system is most widely used and is based on surgical and pathologic findings.

Stage Ⅰ—Tumor limited to kidney and completely excised. No penetration of renal capsule or involvement of renal sinus vessels. Tumor is not ruptured before or during removal. There is no residual tumor apparent beyond the margins of resection.

Stage Ⅱ—Tumor extends beyond the kidney but is completely removed. There is either penetration through the outer surface of the renal capsule, invasion of renal sinus vessels, biopsy of tumor before removal, or spillage of tumor locally during removal. There is no residual tumor apparent at or beyond the margins of excision and no lymph node involvement.

Stage Ⅲ—Residual nonhematogenous tumor confined to abdomen. Any one or more of the following occur: ①Regional lymph node involvement. ②Diffuse peritoneal contamination by tumor, such as spillage of tumor beyond the flank before or during surgery, or by tumor growth that has penetrated through the peritoneal surface. ③Implants are found on the peritoneal surfaces. ④The tumor extends beyond the surgical margins either microscopically or grossly. ⑤The tumor is not completely resectable because of local infiltration into vital structures. ⑥Tumor spills not confined to the flank occurred either before or during surgery. ⑦Transected tumor thrombus.

Stage Ⅳ—Hematogenous metastases to lung, liver, bone, and brain.

Stage Ⅴ—Bilateral renal involvement at diagnosis. An attempt should be made to stage each side according to the previously given criteria on the basis of extent of disease before biopsy.

2.4 Clinical Manifestation

The diagnosis of Wilms tumor is most commonly made after the discovery of an asymptomatic mass by a family member or a physician during a routine physical examination. Common symptoms of presentation include abdominal pain and distention, anorexia, nausea and vomiting, fever, and hematuria. The most common sign is an abdominal mass. Hypertension is seen in 25% –60% of cases and is caused by elevated renin levels. Up to 30% of patients demonstrate hematuria and coagulopathy can occur in 10%.

2.5 Laboratory and Imaging Examination

Urinalysis may show evidence of hematuria, and anemia may be present, particularly in patients with evidence of subcapsular hemorrhage. Patients with liver metastases may have abnormal serum chemistries.

Abdominal US and CT scanning are performed initially to evaluate the mass. Abdominal MRI can sometimes be used to distinguish between nephrogenic rests and Wilms tumor but is otherwise not routinely indicated. MRI can also provide important information in defining the extent of tumor into the inferior vena cava, Chest X–ray remains the initial examination of choice to evaluate for the presence of lung metastases. The role of a chest CT scan is controversial, and it is probably not indicated for routine use in low–risk patients.

The preoperative biopsy is indicated routinely only in tumors deemed too large for safe primary surgical resection and for which preoperative chemotherapy or radiation therapy is planned.

2.6 Differential Diagnosis

The differential diagnosis of a flank mass in a child includes hydronephrosis, cystic kidneys, intrarenal neuroblastoma, mesoblastic nephroma, and various very rare sarcomas.

2.7 Treatment

Significant improvements in survival rates for children with Wilms tumor have been achieved by an improved understanding of the disease and a multimodality approach to therapy, which incorporates surgery, radiation therapy, and chemotherapy.

For patients with unilateral kidney involvement whose tumors are deemed surgically resectable (tumors not crossing the midline or involving adjacent visceral organs), radical nephrectomy via a transabdominal incision is the procedure of choice. A child with bilateral Wilms tumor requires renal-sparing surgery.

Chemotherapy regimens include agents such as cyclophosphamide, ifosfamide, carboplatin, etoposide, vincristine and dactinomycin.

Postoperative radiation is recommended for patients with stage Ⅲ or Ⅳ disease with favorable histology, stages Ⅱ-Ⅳ with focal anaplasia and clear cell sarcoma, and all stages of rhabdoid tumor of the kidney.

2.8 Prognosis

The multimodality approach to the treatment of children with Wilms tumors has significantly improved outcomes. The 4-year survival of patients with favorable histology Wilms tumor now approaches 90%. The most important negative prognostic factors remain the unfavorable histologic subtypes (clear cell sarcoma, rhabdoid, and anaplastic tumors).

Chapter 3

Tumor of the Ureter

Carcinomas of the renal pelvis and ureter are rare, accounting for only 4% of all urothelial cancers.

3.1 Etiology

An increased risk of upper urinary tract TCCs is associated with smoking, exposure to certain industrial dyes or, a contrast agent termed Thorotrast, increased frequency in patients with a long history of excessive analgesic or coffee intake, Balkan nephropathy, aristolochic acid nephropathy, chronic inflammation, infection, or iatrogenesis.

3.2 Epidemiology

Carcinomas of the renal pelvis and ureter are rare, accounting for only 4% of all urothelial cancers. The ratio of bladder–renal pelvic–ureteral carcinomas is approximately 51 ∶ 3 ∶ 1. The mean age at diagnosis is 65 years, and the male–female ratio is (2–4) ∶ 1.

3.3 Pathology

The mucosal lining of the renal pelvis and ureter is similar to that of the urinary bladder, being composed of transitional cell epithelium. Thus, most ureteral cancers (97%) are TCCs. Ureteral cancers with pure nonurothelial histologyare rare, these variants correspond to high–grade tumours with worse prognosis compared with pure UC. Squamous cell carcinoma is rare within the ureter. Squamous cell carcinoma of the urinary tract is assumed to be associated with chronic inflammatory diseases and infections arising from urolithiasis. Other variants include micropapillary and sarcomatoid carcinomas, and lymphoepithelioma. The TNM classification is shown in Table 46–3–1.

Table 46-3-1 TNM classification 2017 for upper tract urothelial carcinoma

T-primoary tumour	
Tx	Primary tumour can not be assessee
	Ta:Noninvasive papillary carcinoma
	Tis:Carcinoma in situ
T1	Tumour invades subepithelial connective tissue
T2	Tumour invades muscularis
T3	Tumour invades beyond muscularis into peripelvic fat or renal parenchyma(renal pelvis) Tumour invades beyond muscularis into periureteric fat(ureter)
T4	Tumour invades adjacent organs or through the kidney into perinephric fat
N-regional lymph nodes	
Nx	Regional lymph nodes can not be assessed
N0	No regional lymph node metastasis
N1	Metastasis in a single lymph node≤2 cm in the greatest dimension
N2	Metastasis in a single lymph node>2 cm, or multiple lymph nodes
M-distant metastasis	
M0	No distant metastasis
M1	Distant metastasis
TNM = tumour, node, metastasis(classfication)	

3.4 Clinical Manifestation

The most common symptom is visible or nonvisible haematuria(70% -80%). Flank pain occurs in approximately 20% of cases, and a lumbar mass is present in approximately 10%. Systemic symptoms(including anorexia, weight loss, malaise, fatigue, fever, night sweats, or cough) associated with UTUC should prompt more rigorous metastatic evaluationwhich confers a worse prognosis.

3.5 Laboratory Examination

Hematuria is identified in most patients but may be intermittent. Elevated liver function levels due to liver metastases are noted in a few patients. Pyuria and bacteriuria may be identified in patients with concomitant urinary tract infection from obstruction and urinary stasis. Upper urinary tract cancers may be identified by examining exfoliated cells in the urinary sediment. The utility of the newer voided markers, such as the UroVysion has been found to have better sensitivity and specificity relative to cytology of upper-tract washings for the diagnosis of ureteric tumors.

3.6 Imaging Examination

3.6.1 Computed tomography urography and magnetic resonance urography

Computed tomography urography(CTU) has the highest diagnostic accuracy of the available imaging techniques. CTU is generally preferred to MR urography for diagnosing and staging ureteral cancer. Magnetic resonance urography(MRU) is indicated in patients who can not undergo CTU, usually when radiation or i-odinated contrast media are contraindicated.

3.6.2 Diagnostic ureteroscopy

Flexible ureteroscopy is used to visualise the ureter, renal pelvis, and collect system and biopsy suspicious lesions.

3.7 Treatment

Surgical treatment decision is based on the location and risk status(Figure 46-3-1).

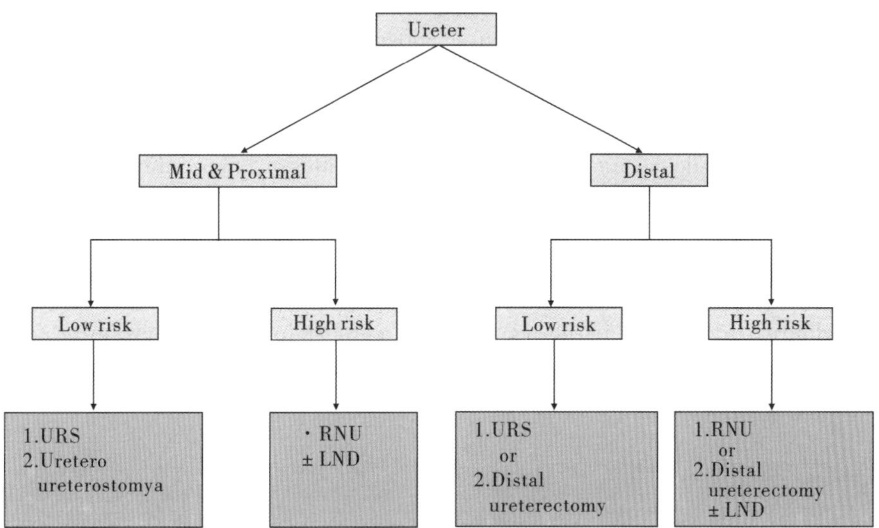

Figure 46-3-1 Treatment algorithm for ureter cancer

1 = first treatment option; 2 = secondary treatment option. LND = lymph node. dissection; RNU = radical nephroureterectomy; URS = ureteroscopy.

3.7.1 Risk stratification of ureter cancer

(1) Low-risk

Low-risk ureter cancer is considered in the following situations: unifocal disease, tumor size < 2 cm, low-grade cytology, low-grade URS biopsy, no invasive aspect on CTU.

(2) High-risk

High-risk ureter cancer is considered in the following situations: hydronephrosis, tumor size > 2 cm, high-grade cytology, high-grade URS biopsy, multifocal disease, previous radical cystectomy for bladder cancer, variant histology.

3.7.2 Localised disease

(1) Ureteroscopy

Endoscopic ablation can be considered in patients with clinically low-risk cancer in the following situations: ①Laser generator and pliers available for biopsies. ②In case a flexible (rather than a rigid) ureteroscope is available. ③The patient is informed of the need for early (second look), closer, more stringent, surveillance④Complete tumour resection or destruction can be achieved.

(2) Segmental ureteral resection

Segmental ureteral resection with wide margins provides adequate pathological specimens for staging and grading while preserving the ipsilateral kidney. Lymphadenectomy can also be performed during segmental ureteral resection. Complete distal ureterectomy with neocystostomy is indicated for low-risk tumours in the distal ureter that can not be removed completely endoscopically and for high risk tumours when renal function preservation is necessary.

(3) Adjuvant topical agents

The antegrade instillation of bacillus Calmette-Guérin (BCG) vaccine or mitomycin C (MMC) in the upper urinary tract by percutaneous nephrostomy is feasible after kidney-sparing management or for treatment of CIS. Retrograde instillation through a ureteric stent is also used, but it can be dangerous due to possible ureteric obstruction and consecutive pyelovenous influx during instillation/perfusion.

(4) Radical nephroureterectomy

Open radical nephroureterectomy with bladder cuff excision is the standard for high-risk ureter cancer, regardless of tumour location. Laparoscopic approaches have equivalent efficacy and safety in T1-2/N0 upper tract urothelial carcinoma.

3.7.3 Advanced disease

In patients with metastatic ureter cancer, radical nephroureterectomy is applied for palliative considerations. There are several platinum-based regimens, but not all patients can receive adjuvant chemotherapy because of comorbidities and impaired renal function after radical surgery. Chemotherapy-related toxicity, particularly nephrotoxicity due to platinum derivatives, may significantly reduce survival in patients with postoperative renal dysfunction.

3.7.4 Prognosis

Ureter cancers that invade the muscle wall usually have a very poor prognosis. The 5-year specific survival is $<50\%$ for pT2/pT3 and $<10\%$ for pT4.

Chapter 4

Tumor of the Bladder

4.1 Etiology

(1) Tobacco smoking

Tobacco smoking accounts for 65% of cases in men and 20%–30% in women. In general, smokers have Two to three fold increase risk of bladder cancer (BC) than nonsmokers, and the association appears to be dose related.

(2) Occupational exposure to chemicals

Occupational exposure accounts for 15%–35% of cases in men and 1%–6% in women. Workers in the chemical, dye, rubber, petroleum, leather, and printing industries are at increased risk. Specific occupational carcinogens include benzidine, beta-naphthylamine, and 4-aminobiphenyl, and the latency period between exposure and tumor development may be prolonged.

(3) Radiotherapy

Increased rates of secondary bladder malignancies have been reported after external-beam radiotherapy (EBRT) for gynaecological malignancies, with relative risks of 2–4.

(4) Bladder schistosomiasis and chronic urinary tract infection

There is a well-established relationship between schistosomiasis and urothelial carcinoma of the bladder, which can progress to squamous cell carcinoma (SCC). Invasive SCC has been linked to the presence of chronic UTI distinct from schistosomiasis.

(5) Genetic factors

There is growing evidence that genetic susceptibility factors and family association may influence the incidence of bladder cancer (BC).

4.2 Epidemiology

BC is the seventh most commonly diagnosed cancer in the male population worldwide, while it drops to eleventh when both genders are considered. The worldwide age-standardised incidence rate (per 100,000 person/years) is 9.0 for men and 2.2 for women. In the European Union the age-standardised incidence rate is 19.1 for men and 4.0 for women. Approximately 75% of patients with BC present with a disease confined to the mucosa (stage Ta, CIS) or submucosa (stage T1); in younger patients (< 40) this percentage is even higher. Patients with TaT1 and CIS have a high prevalence due to long-term survival in many cases and lower risk of cancer-specific mortality compared to T2-4 tumours.

4.3 Pathology

98% of all bladder cancers are epithelial malignancies, with the predominant majority being transitional cell carcinomas (TCCs). About 5% are adenocarcinomas or squamous cell carcinomas. lymphoepithelioma, small-cell carcinomas, micropapillary and microcystic urothelial carcinoma, sarcomatoid carcinomas are rare.

4.3.1 TNM classification

See Table 46-4-1.

Table 46-4-1 TNM classification of urinary bladder cancer

T-primoary tumour	
Tx	Primary tumour cannot be assessed
T0	No evidence of primary tumour
Ta	Non-invasive papillary carcinoma
Tis	Carcinoma in situ: "flat tumour"
T1	Tumour invades subepithelial connective tissue
T2	Tumour invades muscle
	T2a Tumour invades superlicial muscle (inner half)
	T2b Tumour invades deep muscle (outer half)
T3	Tumour invades perivesical tissue:
	T3a microscopically
	T3b macroscopically (extravesical mass)
T4	Tumour invade any of the following: prostate stroma, seminal vesicles, uterus, vagina, pelvic wall, abdominal wall
	T4a Tumour invades prostate stroma, seminal vesicles, uterus, or vagina
	T4b Tumour invades pelvic wall or abdominal wall
N-regional lymph nodes	
Nx	Regional lymph nodes cannot be assessed
N0	No regional lymph node metastasis
N1	Metastasis in a single lymph node in the true pelvis (hypogastric, obturator, external iliac, or presacral)
N2	Metastasis in multiple regional lymph nodes in the true pelvis (hypogastric, obturator, extrnal illac, or presacral)
N3	Metastasis in a common iliac lymph node(s)

Continue to Table 46-4-1

M-distant metastasis	
M0	No distant metastasis
	M1a Non-regional lymph nodes
	M1b Other distant metastasis

4.3.2 WHO grading

2004 WHO grading system(papillary lesions):①2004 WHO grading system(papillary lesions). ②Papillary urothelial neoplasm of low malignant potential (PUNLMP). ③Low-grade(LG) papillary urothelial carcinoma. ④High-grade(HG) papillary urothelial carcinoma.

4.3.3 Non-muscle invasive bladder cancer and muscle-invasive bladder cancer

Tumours(Tis, Ta, T1) can be treated by transurethral resection of the bladder(TURB), eventually in combination with intravesical instillations and are therefore grouped under the heading of non-muscle invasive bladder cancer(NMIBC) for therapeutic purposes. Muscle invasive bladder cancer(MIBC) includes stage T2 or greater bladder cancer at diagnosis. In MIBC all cases are high-grade urothelial carcinomas.

NMIBC are usually papillary tumours that grow in an exophytic fashion into the bladder lumen. They may be single or multiple and may appear pedunculated, arising on a stalk with a narrow base, but if the tumours are less well differentiated they are more solid with a wider base. The mucosa round the tumour is often rather oedematous, with angry-looking, dilated blood vessels. These areas may contain situ changes.

The histological appearance of irregularly arranged cells with large nuclei and a high mitotic index replacing the normally well-ordered urothelium is known as TIS. It may occur alone(primary CIS) or in association with a new tumour(concomitant Tis) or it may occur later in a patient who has previously had a tumour(secondary Tis).

Muscle-invasive tumors are nearly always solid, although there may be a low tufted surface. These tumors are often large and broad-based, having an irregular, ulcerated, appearance within the bladder. The incidence of metastases, whether from lymphatic invasion in the pelvis or blood-borne to the lung, liver or bones, is much more common and will cause the death of 30%-50% per cent of patients.

4.4 Clinical Manifestation

Hematuria is the presenting symptom in 85%-90% of patients with bladder cancer. It may be gross or microscopic, intermittent rather than constant. In a smaller percentage of patients, it is accompanied by symptoms of vesical irritability: frequency, urgency, and dysuria. Irritative voiding symptoms seem to be more common in patients with diffuse CIS. Symptoms of advanced disease include bone pain from bone metastases or flank pain from retroperitoneal metastases or ureteral obstruction.

Patients with large-volume or invasive tumors may be found to have bladder wall thickening or a palpable mass-findings that may be detected on a careful bimanual examination under anesthesia. If the bladder is not mobile, fixation of tumor to adjacent structures by direct invasion is suggested. Hepatomegaly and supraclavicular lymphadenopathy are signs of metastatic disease. Lymphedema from occlusive pelvic lymphadenopathy may be seen occasionally. Patients may also present with back pain or pathologic fracture from bony metastases. On rare occasions, metastases can occur in unusual sites such as the skin presenting as painful nodules with ulceration.

4.5 Laboratory Examination

4.5.1 Routine testing

The most common laboratory abnormality is hematuria. It may be accompanied by pyuria, which on occasion may result from concomitant urinary tract infection. Azotemia may be noted in patients with ureteral occlusion owing to the primary bladder tumor or lymphadenopathy. Anemia may be a presenting symptom owing to chronic blood loss, or replacement of the bone marrow with metastatic disease.

4.5.2 Urinary cytology

Exfoliated cells from both normal and neoplastic urothelium can be readily identified in voided urine. Larger quantities of cells can be obtained by gently irrigating the bladder with isotonic saline solution through a catheter or cystoscope (barbotage). Cytologic examination of exfoliated cells may be especially useful in detecting cancer in symptomatic patients and assessing response to treatment. Detection rates are high for tumors of high grade and stage as well as CIS but not as impressive for low-grade superficial tumors.

4.5.3 Other markers testing

Several new tests have been developed in order to overcome the shortcomings of urinary cytology such as the low sensitivity for low-grade superficial tumors and inter-observer variability. Commercially available tests include, the bladder tumor antigen (BTA) stat test, the BTA TRAK assay, the NMP22 assay, and the NMP22 BladderChek test, ImmunoCyt and UroVysion. These tests can detect cancer specific proteins in urine (BTA/NMP22) or augment cytology by identifying cell surface or cytogenetic markers in the nucleus (UroVysion and Immuno Cyt).

4.6 Imaging Examination

4.6.1 Computed tomography urography and intravenous urography

CTU is used to detect papillary tumours in the urinary tract. Bladder tumors may be recognized as pedunculated, radiolucent filling defects projecting into the lumen; nonpapillary, infiltrating tumors may result in fixation or flattening of the bladder wall. Hydronephrosis from ureteral obstruction is usually associated with deeply infiltrating lesions and poor outcome after treatment. IVU is an alternative if CT is not available, but particularly in muscle-invasive tumours of the bladder and in UTUCs, CTU gives more information than IVU (including status of lymph nodes and neighbouring organs).

4.6.2 Ultrasound

Renal and bladder ultrasound may be used during the initial work-up in patients with haematuria, and it permits characterisation of renal masses, detection of hydronephrosis, and visualisation of intraluminal masses in the bladder. However, it can not exclude the presence of UTUC and can not replace CTU.

4.6.3 Cystoscopy

The diagnosis of papillary BC ultimately depends on cystoscopic examination of the bladder and histological evaluation of sampled tissue by either cold-cup biopsy or resection. Cystoscopy should be performed in all patients with symptoms suggestive of bladder cancer. Superficial, low-grade tumors usually appear as single or multiple papillary lesions. Higher grade lesions are larger and sessile. CIS may appear as flat areas of erythema and mucosal irregularity. As a standard procedure, cystoscopy is performed using white light. However, the use of white light can lead to missing lesions that are present but not visible.

Photodynamic diagnosis (PDD) is performed using violet light after intravesical instillation of 5-aminolaevulinic acid (ALA) or hexaminolaevulinic acid (HAL). It has been confirmed that fluorescence-guided biopsy and resection are more sensitive than conventional procedures for the detection of malignant tumours, particularly for CIS.

Narrow-band imaging (NBI) can enhance the contrast between normal urothelium and hyper-vascular cancer tissue. Initial studies have demonstrated improved cancer detection by NBI-guided biopsies and resection.

4.6.4 Imaging for staging of MIBC

The treatment and prognosis of MIBC is determined by tumour stage and grade. In clinical practice, CT and MRI are the imaging techniques used. The purpose of using imaging for staging MIBC is to determine prognosis and provide information to assist treatment selection. Imaging parameters required for staging MIBC are extent of local tumour invasion; tumour spread to lymph nodes; tumour spread to the upper urinary tract (UUT) and other distant organs (e.g., liver, lungs, bones, peritoneum, pleura, and adrenal glands).

4.7 Treatment

4.7.1 NMIBC

Treatment decision for NMIBC is based on the risk stratification (Table 46-4-2).

Table 46-4-2 Treatment recommendations in TaT1 tumors and carcinoma in situ according to risk stratification

Risk category	Definition	Treatment recommendation
Low-risk tumours	Primary, solitary, TaG1 (PUNLMP, LG). <3 cm, no CIS	One im mediate instillation of intravesical chemotherapy after TURB.
Intermediate-risk tumours	All tumours not defined in the two adjacent categories (between the category of low-and high-risk).	In patients with previous low recurrence rate (less than or equal to one recurrence per year) and expected EORTC recurrence score < 5, one immediate instillation of intravesical chemotherapy after TURB. In all patients either one-year ful-dose BCG treatment (induction plus three-weekly instillations at three, six and twelve months), or instilations of chemotherapy (the optimal schedule is not known) for a maximum of one year.
High-risk tumours	Any of the following: · T1 tumours; · G3 (HG) tumour: · Multiple, recurrent and large (> 3 cm) TaG1G2/LG tumours (all features must be present).	Intravesical full-dose BC G instilations for one-three years or radical cystectomy (in highest-risk turnours -see below).
	Subgroup of highest-risk tumours	
	T1G3/HG associated with concurrent bladder CIS, multiple and/or largeT1G3/HG and/or recurrent T1G3/HG, T1G3/HG with CIS in the prostatic urethra, some forms of variant histology of urothelial carcinoma, LVI (see Sections 4.7 and 6.4).	Radical cystectomy should be considered. In those who refuse or are unfit for RC intravesical full-dose BCG instillations for one-three years.
	BCG failures.	Radical cystectomy is recommended.

(1) TURB

The goal of TURB in TaT_1 BC is to make the correct diagnosis and completely remove all visible lesions. It is a crucial procedure in the diagnosis and treatment of BC. The presence of detrusor muscle in the specimen is considered as the surrogate criterion of the resection quality and is required, because the absence of detrusor muscle in the specimen is associated with a significantly higher risk of residual disease, early recurrence and tumour understaging. Carcinoma in situ can present as a velvet-like, reddish, area indistinguishable from inflammation, or it may not be visible at all. For this reason, the strategy of taking biopsies from abnormal urothelium and biopsies from normal-looking mucosa (random/mapping biopsies) is recommended. The significant risk of residual tumour after initial TURB of TaT_1 lesions leads to a second TURB in the following situations: after (suspicion of) incomplete initial TURB (in the case of any doubt aboutthe completeness of a TURB); if there is no muscle in the specimen after initial resection, with the exception of $TaLG/G_1$ tumours and primary CIS; in T1 tumours. If indicated, perform a second TURB within 2-6 weeks after initial resection.

(2) Intravesical therapy

BCG is an attenuated strain of Mycobacterium bovis. The exact mechanism by which BCG exerts its antitumor effect is unknown, but it seems to be immunologically mediated. Activated helper T lymphocytes can be identified in the granulomas, and interleukin-2 reportedly can be detected in the urine of treated patients. BCG has been shown to be very effective both therapeutically and prophylactically. It appears to be the most efficacious intravesical agent for the management of CIS. BCG has been shown to be superior to intravesical chemotherapy in preventing recurrence in patients with high-risk superficial bladder cancer, but BCG intravesical treatment is associated with more side effects: symptoms of cystitis, haematuria, symptomatic granulomatous prostatitis, epididymo-orchitis, general malaise, fever, arthralgia and/or arthritis, BCG sepsis, allergic reactions. Absolute contraindications of BCG intravesical instillation are as follows: during the first two weeks after TURB; in patients with visible haematuria; after traumatic catheterisation; in patients with symptomatic urinary tract infection.

Immediate single instillation (SI) of chemotherapy has been shown to act by destroying circulating tumour cells after TURB, and by an ablative effect (chemo resection) on residual tumour cells at the resection site and on small overlooked tumours. Mitomycin C, epirubicin, and pirarubicin have all shown a beneficial effect. To maximize the efficacy of SI, flexible practices should be devised that allow the instillation to be given as soon as possible after TURB, preferably within the first two hours in the recovery room or even in the operating theatre. The need for further adjuvant intravesical therapy depends on prognosis. In low-risk patients, a SI reduces the risk of recurrence and is considered to be the standard and complete treatment. For other patients, however, a SI remains an incomplete treatment because of the considerable likelihood of recurrence and/or progression.

(3) Cystectomy

There are several reasons to consider immediateradical cystectomy for selected patients with NMIBC: The staging accuracy for T1 tumours by TURB is low with 27%-51% of patients being upstaged to muscle-invasive tumour at radical cystectomy; Some patients with NMIBC experience disease progression to muscle-invasive disease. The potential benefit of RC must be weighed against its risks, morbidity, and impact on the quality of life. It is reasonable to propose immediate RC in those patients with NMIBC who are at the highest risk of disease progression.

4.7.2 MIBC

(1) Neoadjuvant chemotherapy

Neoadjuvant chemotherapy (NAC) is recommended for T2-T4a, cN0M0 bladder cancer. In this case, cisplatin-based combination therapy is always used. NAC is not offered to patients who are ineligible for cisplatin-based combination chemotherapy. Toxicities of cisplatin, including nephrotoxicity, diminished cardiac function, neurotoxicity and hearing loss, preclude 30%-50% of MIBC patients from safe receipt of cisplatin-based chemotherapy.

(2) Radical cystectomy and urinary diversion

Radical cystectomy is the standard treatment for localised MIBC. In men, standard RC includes removal of the bladder, prostate, seminal vesicles, distal ureters, and regional LNs. In women, standard RC includes removal of the bladder, entire urethra and adjacent vagina, uterus, distal ureters, and regional LNs. Different approaches have been described to improve voiding and sexual function in patients undergoing RC for BC. Four main types of sexual-preserving techniques in men have been described:

1) Prostate sparing cystectomy, part or the whole prostate is preserved including seminal vesicles, vas deferens and neurovascular bundles.

2) Capsule sparing cystectomy: the capsule or peripheral part of the prostate is preserved with adenoma (including prostatic urethra) removed by TURP or en bloc with the bladder. Seminal vesicles, vas deferens and neurovascular bundles are also preserved.

3) Seminal sparing cystectomy: seminal vesicles, vas deferens and neurovascular bundles are preserved.

4) Nerve sparing cystectomy: the neurovascular bundles are the only tissue left in place.

Sexual-preserving techniques are offered to those motivated to preserve their sexual function since the majority will benefit. Patients are selected based on: organ-confined disease; absence of any kind of tumour at the level of the prostate, prostatic urethra or bladder neck in men; absence of tumour in bladder neck or urethra in women.

Urinary diversion may be accomplished. The choice of urinary diversion has a significant impact on long-term quality of life for patients who undergo radical cystectomy, and each type of diversion is associated with its own unique potential complications. From an anatomical standpoint, three alternatives are currently used after cystectomy: ①Abdominal diversion, such as an ureterocutaneostomy, ileal or colonic conduit, and various forms of a continent pouch. ②Urethral diversion, which includes various forms of gastrointestinal pouches attached to the urethra as a continent, orthotopic urinary diversion (neobladder, orthotopic bladder substitution). ③Rectosigmoid diversions, such as uretero-(ileo-) rectostomy.

(3) Multi-modal bladder preserving therapy

Multimodality treatment (MMT) or trimodality treatment combines TURB, chemotherapy and radiation. The rationale for performing TURB and radiation is to achieve local tumour control. The addition of systemic chemotherapy or other radiosensitisers (mentioned below) aims at the potentiation of RT. Micrometastases are targeted by platinum-based combination chemotherapy. The aim of multimodality therapy is to preserve the bladder and QoL, without compromising outcome. Following TURB and staging, treatment comprises EBRT with concurrent radiosensitising drugs. Two schedules are in common use worldwide: a split dose format with interim cystoscopy or single-phase treatment. For radiosensitising chemotherapy, cisplatin or mitomycin C plus 5-fluorouracil (5-FU) can be used, but also other schedules have been used. Multimodality treatment is recommended as an alternative in selected, well-informed and compliant patients, especially for whom cystectomy is not an option.

4.7.3 Metastatic disease

Cisplatin-containing combination chemotherapy has been the standard of care. Cisplatin-containing combination chemotherapy with GC, MVAC, preferably with G-CSF, HD-MVAC with G-CSF or PCG is recommended as first-line treatment.

4.8 Prognosis

For patients undergoing RC for BC, the 5-year recurrence-free survival was 58% and the CSS was 66%. Recurrence-free survival and OS in a large single-center study of 1,054 patients was 68% and 66% at 5 years and 60% and 43%, at 10 years, respectively. However, the 5-year recurrence-free survival in node-positive patients who underwent cystectomy was considerably less at 34%-43%. In a surgery-only study, the 5-year recurrence-free survival was 76% in patients with pT1 tumours, 74% for pT2, 52% for pT3, and 36% for pT4.

Chapter 5

Tumor of the Penis

Cancers of the penis are uncommon tumors that are often devastating for the patient and frequently diagnostically and therapeutically challenging for the urologist.

5.1 Etiology

The one etiologic factor most commonly associated with penile carcinoma is poor hygiene. The disease is virtually unheard of in males circumcised near birth. One theory postulates that smegma accumulation under the phimosis foreskin results in chronic inflammation leading to carcinoma. HPV viral cause has also been suggested as a result of the association of this tumor with cervical carcinoma. Other factors include circumcision practice, phimosis, number of sexual partners, infection, exposure to tobacco products, etc.

5.2 Epidemiology

There is marked variation in incidence with geographic location. Penile malignant neoplasms constitute a substantial health concern in many African, South American, and Asian countries. Penile carcinoma occurs most commonly in the sixth decade of life, although rare case reports have included children.

5.3 Pathology

Squamous cell carcinoma composes most penile cancers. It most commonly originates on the glans, with the next most common sites, in order, being the prepuce and shaft. The appearance may be papillary or ulcerative. Verrucous carcinoma is a variant of squamous cell carcinoma composing 5%–16% of penile carcinomas. This lesion is papillary in appearance, and on histologic examination it is noted to have a well-demarcated deep margin unlike the infiltrating margin of the typical squamous cell carcinoma.

Bowen disease is a squamous cell carcinoma in situ typically involving the penile shaft. The lesion appears as a red plaque with encrustation. Erythroplasia of Queyrat is also characterized by the noninvasive changes of carcinoma in situ. It is a velvety, red lesion with ulcerations that usually involve the glans. Microscopic examination shows typical, hyperplastic cells in a disordered array with vacuolated cytoplasm and mitotic figures.

Invasive carcinoma of the penis begins as an ulcerative or papillary lesion, which may gradually grow to involve the entire glans or shaft of the penis. Buck's fascia represents a barrier to corporal invasion and hematogenous spread. Primary dissemination is via lymphatic channels to the femoral and iliac nodes. The prepuce and shaft skin drain into the superficial inguinal nodes (superficial to fascia lata), while the glans and corporal bodies drain to both superficial and deep inguinal nodes (deep to fascia lata). There are many cross communications so that penile lymphatic drainage is bilateral to both inguinal areas. Drainage from the inguinal nodes is to the pelvic nodes. Involvement of the femoral nodes may result in skin necrosis and infection or femoral vessel erosion and hemorrhage. Distant metastases are clinically apparent in < 10% of cases and may involve lung, liver, bone, or brain.

5.4 Staging

The TNM staging system (Table 46-5-1) is proposed for clinical use.

Table 46-5-1 2009 TNM clinical and pathological classification of penile cancer

Clinical classification	
T: primary tumour	
TX	Primary tumour cannot be assessed
TO	No evidence or primary cumour
Tis	Carcinoma in sicu
Ta	Non-invasive carcinoma
T1	Tumour invades subepithelial connective tissue
	T1a Tumour invades subepithelial connective tissue without lymphovascular invasion and is not poorly differentiated or undifferentiated (T1G1-2) T1b Tumour invades subepithelial connective tissue with lymphovascular invasion or is poorly differentiated or undifferentiated (T1G3-4)
T2	Tummour invades corpus spongiosum and /or corpora cavernosa
T3	Tumour invades urethra
T4	Tumour invades other adjacent structures
N: Regional lymph nodes	
NX	Regional lymph nodes cannot be assessed
NO	No palpable or visibly enlarged inguinal lymph node
N1	Palpable mobile unilateral inguinal lymph node
N2	Palpable mobile mulciple unilateral or bilateral inguinal lymph nodes
N3	Fixed inguinal nodal mass or pelvic lymphadenopathy. unilateral or bilateral

Continue to Table 46-5-1

Clinical classification	
M: Distant metastasis	
MO	No distanc metastasis
M1	Distanc metastasis
Pathologic classification	
The pT categories correspong to the clinical T categories. THe pN categories are based upon biopsy or surgical excision.	
pN: Regional lymph nodes	
pNX	Regional lymph nodes cannot be assessed
pN0	No regional lymph node metastasis
pN1	Intranodal metastasis in a singte inguinal lymph node
pN2	Metastasis in multiple or bilateral inguinal lymph nodes
pN3	Metastasis in pelvie lymph node(s). unilateral or bilateral or extrampda; extension of any regional lymph node metastasis
pM: Distant metasis	
pM0	No distant metastasis
PM1	Distant metastasis
G: Histopathologie grading	
GX	Grade or differentiation cannot be assessed
G1	Well differentiated
G2	Moderately differentiated
G3-4	Poorly differentiated/undifferentiated

5.5 Clinical Manifestation

The most common complaint at presentation is the lesion itself. It may appear as an area of induration or erythema, an ulceration, a small nodule, or an exophytic growth. Phimosis may obscure the lesion and result in a delay in seeking medical attention. Other symptoms include pain, discharge, irritative voiding symptoms, and bleeding. Lesions are typically confined to the penis at presentation.

The primary lesion should be characterized with respect to size, location, and potential corporal body involvement. Careful palpation of the inguinal area is mandatory because >50% of patients present with enlarged inguinal nodes. This enlargement may be secondary to inflammation or metastatic spread.

5.6 Examination

Laboratory evaluation is typically normal. Anemia and leukocytosis may be present in patients with a long-standing disease or extensive local infection. Hypercalcemia in the absence of osseous metastases may be seen in 20% of patients and appears to correlate with the volume of disease.

Ultrasound or magnetic resonance(MR) with an artificial erection can give information about infiltration of the corpora. Penile carcinoma is often clinically obvious but can be hidden under a phimosis.

Metastatic workup should include CXR, bone scan, and CT scan of the abdomen and pelvis. Disseminated disease is present in < 10% of patients at presentation.

The diagnosis of penile cancer is often without doubt, but in doubtful cases and if nonablative treatment is planned, histological verification is mandatory.

5.7 Differential Diagnosis

In addition to the dermatologic lesions discussed previously, carcinoma of the penis must be differentiated from several infectious lesions. The Syphilitic chancre may present as painless ulceration. Serologic and dark field examination should establish the diagnosis. Chancroid typically appears as a painful ulceration of the penis. Selective cultures for Haemophilus ducreyi should identify the cause. Condylomata acuminata appear as exophytic, soft, "grape cluster" lesions anywhere on the penile shaft or glans. The Biopsy can distinguish this lesion from carcinoma if any doubt exists.

5.8 Treatment

5.8.1 Primary tumour

The aims of treatment are radical tumour removal with as much organ preservation as possible. Treatment varies depending on the pathology as well as the location of the lesion. For CIS, topical chemotherapy with imiquimod or 5-fluorouracil(5-FU) is a first-line treatment. Patients must come for frequent follow-up examinations to monitor response. The goal of treatment in invasive penile carcinoma is complete excision with adequate margins. For lesions involving the prepuce, this may be accomplished by simple circumcision. For lesions involving the glans or distal shaft, partial penectomy with a 2 cm margin to decrease local recurrence has traditionally been suggested. Less aggressive surgical resections such as Mohs micrographic surgery and local excisions directed at penile preservation yet attaining a negative surgical margin have gained popularity. For lesions involving the proximal shaft or when partial penectomy results in a penile stump of insufficient length for sexual function or directing the urinary stream, total penectomy with perineal urethrostomy has been recommended.

5.8.2 Regional lymph nodes

Penile carcinoma spreads primarily to the inguinal lymph nodes. However, enlargement of inguinal nodes at presentation does not necessarily imply metastatic disease. In fact, up to 50% of the time this enlargement is caused by inflammation. Thus, patients who present with enlarged inguinal nodes should undergo treatment of the primary lesion followed by a 4-to 6-week course of oral broad-spectrum antibiotics. Persistent adenopathy following antibiotic treatment should be considered to be the metastatic disease, and sequential bilateral ilioinguinal node dissections should be performed. If lymphadenopathy resolves with antibiotics, observation in low-stage primary tumors(Tis, T1) is warranted. However, if lymphadenopathy resolves in higher-stage tumors, more limited lymph node samplings should be considered, such as the sentinel node biopsy. If positive nodes are encountered, bilateral ilioinguinal node dissection should be performed. Patients who initially have clinically negative nodes but in whom clinically palpable nodes later develop should undergo a unilateral ilioinguinal node dissection. Patients who have inoperable disease and bulky inguinal metastases are treated with chemotherapy (cisplatin and 5-fluorouracil). In some cases, regional radiotherapy can provide significant palliation by delaying ulceration and infectious complications and alleviating pain.

5.8.3 Systemic disease

Four chemotherapeutic agents demonstrate activity against penile carcinoma: bleomycin, methotrexate, cisplatin, and 5-fluorouracil.

5.9 Prognosis

Survival in penile carcinoma correlates with the presence or absence of nodal disease. 5-year survival rates for patients with node-negative disease range from 65% to 90%. For patients with positive inguinal nodes, this rate decreases to 30%-50% and with positive iliac nodes decreases to 20%. In the presence of soft tissue or bony metastases, no 5-year survivors have been reported.

Chapter 6

Tumors of the Testis

6.1 Etiology

The cause of testicular cancer is unknown, both congenital and acquired factors have been associated with tumor development. The strongest association has been with the cryptorchid testis. 7%–10% of testicular tumors develop in patients who have a history of cryptorchidism; seminoma is the most common form of tumor these patients have. The relative risk of malignancy is highest for the intra-abdominal testis (1 in 20) and is significantly lower for the inguinal testis (1 in 80). Placement of the cryptorchid testis into the scrotum (orchiopexy) lowers the risk of malignancy if it is performed prior to the age of 13.

Exogenous estrogen administration to the mother during pregnancy has been associated with an increased relative risk for testicular tumors in the fetus, ranging from 2.8 to 5.3 over the expected incidence. Other acquired factors such as trauma and infection-related testicular atrophy have been associated with testicular tumors; however, a causal relationship has not been established.

6.2 Epidemiology

Testicular cancer represents 1% of male neoplasms and 5% of urological tumors. At diagnosis, 1%–2% of cases are bilateral and the predominant histology is germ cell tumour (90%–95% of cases). Peak incidence is in the third decade of life for non-seminoma, and in the fourth decade for pure seminoma.

6.3 Pathology

Testicular cancers constitute a morphologically and clinically diverse group of tumors, of which more than 95% are germ cell tumors (GCTs). GCTs are broadly classified as seminoma and nonseminoma germ cell tumors (NSGCT), and the relative distribution is 52%–56% and 44%–48%, respectively. NSGCTs include embryonal carcinoma (EC), yolk sac tumor, teratoma, and choriocarcinoma subtypes, occurring either alone as pure forms or in combination as mixed GCT with or without seminoma. Most NSGCTs are mixed tumors that are composed of two or more GCT subtypes. GCTs that contain both NSGCT subtypes and seminoma are classified as NSGCTs.

6.4 Staging

The staging system recommended is the 2017 Tumour, Node, Metastasis of the International Union Against Cancer(Table 46-6-1). This includes determination of the anatomical extent of disease; assessment of serum tumour markers, including nadir values of hCG, AFP and LDH after orchiectomy(S category); definition of regional nodes; N-category modifications related to node size.

Table 46-6-1 TNM classification for testicular cancer

pT	Primary Tumour[1]	
	pTX	Primary tumour canrnot be assessed (see note t)
	pT0	No evidence of primary turmour (e. g. hiatological scar in testin)
	pTis	intratubular ger m cel neoptasia (carcino ma in situ)
	pT1	Tumour limited to testis and epididymis without vascular/lymphatic invasior; tumour may invade tunica albuginea but not turnica vaginalis
	pT2	Tumour limited to testis and epididyrnis with vascularflymphatic arvasion, or tumour extending trhvough tunica albuginea win invotvement of tunica vaginais
	pT3	Tumour invades spermatic cord with or without vascular/lymphatic irvasion
	pT4	Tumour invades scrotum with or without vascutar/lymphatic invasion
N	Regional Lymph Nodes -Clinical	
	Nx	Regional lymph nodes cannot be assessed
	N0	No regional lymph node metastasis
	N1	Metastasis wih a lyrmph node mass 2 om or less in greatest dimension or multiple bymph nodes, none more than 2 c m in greatest dirmension
	N2	Metastasis with a lymph node mass more than 2 cm but not more than 5 cm in greatest dimension. or multiple lymph nodes, any one mass more than 2 cm but not more than s cm in greatest dimension.
	N3	Metastasis with a lymph node mass more than 5 cm in greatest dimension dimension
Pn	Regional Lymph Nodes - Pathological	
	pNX	Regional lyrmph nodes cannot be assessed
	pN0	No rogional lymph node motastasis
	pN1	Metastasis with a tyrmph node mass 2 cm or ies in greatest dinersion and 5 or fewer positive nodes, none more than 2 cm in greatest dimension
	pN2	Metastasis with a iymph node mass more than 2 c m but not more than 5 cm in greatest dimension; or more than 5 nodes positive, none more than 5 cm; or evidence or extranodal extension of tumour
	pN3	Metastasis with a lymph nodc mass morc than 5 cm in greatest dimension

Continue to Table 46-6-1

M	Distant Metastasis			
	MX	Distant metastasis cannot be assessed		
	N1	No distant metastasis		
	M1	Dintant metastasin		
		M1a Non-rogional lymph nodeísj or lung motastanis		
		M1b Distant metastasis other than non-regional lymph nodes and lung		
S	Serum Tumour Markers			
	SX	Serum marker studies not avallable or not performed		
	S0	Serum marker study levels within normat timits		
		LDH (U/I)	hCG (mlU/mL)	AFP (ng/mL)
	S1	<1.5×N and	< 5,000 and	< 1.000
	S2	1.5-10×N or	5,000-50,000 or	1,000-10,000
	S3	>10×N or	>50.000 or	>10,000

N indicates the upper limit of normal for the LD H assay.

L. DH=lactate cforydrogonuse:hCG = human chnionic gonadotropthirn: AFP = aipha-tetoproteirt.

* AJCC subdivides T1 by T1a and T1b depending on sire no greater than 3 cm or greater than 3 cm in greatest dimension.

[1] Ercept for p Tis and pT4, where radical orchidectomy is not ahways necessary for classification purposes, the extent of the primary tumour is classified after radical orchcectomy, see pT. In other crcumstanoes. TX s uaed if no radical orchidectomy has been performed.

Stage grouping				
Stage 0	pTis	N0	M0	S0
Stage 1	pT1-T4	N0	M0	SX
Stage IA	pT1	N0	M0	S0
Stage IB	pT2-pT4	N0	M0	S0
Stage IS	Any patient/TX	N0	M0	S1-3
StageII	Any paticnt/TX	N1-N3	M0	SX
Stage IIA	Any patient/TX	N1	M0	S0
	Any patient/TX	N1	M0	S1
Stage IIB	Any patient/TX	N2	M0	S0
	Any patient/TX	N2	M0	S1
Stage II	Any patient/TX	N3	M0	S0
	Any patient/TX	N3	M0	S1
Stage III	Any patient/TX	Any N	M1a	SX
Stage IIIA	Any patient/TX	Any N	M1a	SX
	Any patient/TX	Any N	M1a	S1
Stage IIIB	Any patient/TX	N1-N3	M0	S2
	Any patient/TX	Any N	M1a	S2
Stage IIIC	Any patient/TX	N1-N3	M0	S3
	Any patient/TX	Any N	M1a	S3
	Any patient/TX	Any N	M1b	Any S

6.5 Clinical Manifestation

The most common symptom of testicular cancer is a painless enlargement of the testis. Enlargement is usually gradual, and a sensation of testicular heaviness is not unusual. Acute testicular pain is seen in approximately 10% of cases and may be the result of intratesticular hemorrhage or infarction. Approximately 10% of patients present with symptoms related to metastatic disease. Back pain (retroperitoneal metastases involving nerve roots) is the most common symptom. Other symptoms include cough or dyspnea (pulmonary metastases); anorexia, nausea, or vomiting (retroduodenal metastases); bone pain (skeletal metastases); and lower extremity swelling (vena caval obstruction). Approximately 10% of patients are asymptomatic at presentation, and the tumor may be detected incidentally following trauma.

A testicular mass or diffuse enlargement is found in most cases. The mass is typically firm and nontender and the epididymis should be easily separable from it. A hydrocele may accompany the testicular tumor and help to camouflage it. Transillumination of the scrotum can help to distinguish between these entities. Palpation of the abdomen may reveal bulky retroperitoneal disease; assessment of supraclavicular, scalene, and inguinal nodes should be performed. Gynecomastia is present in 5% of all germ cell tumors but may be present in 30%–50% of Sertoli and Leydig cell tumors. Its cause seems to be related to multiple complex hormonal interactions involving testosterone, estrone, estradiol, prolactin, and hCG. Hemoptysis may be seen in advanced pulmonary disease.

6.6 Laboratory Examination

Anemia may be detected in advanced disease. Liver function tests may be elevated in the presence of hepatic metastases. Renal function may be diminished (elevated serum creatinine) if ureteral obstruction secondary to bulky retroperitoneal disease is present. The assessment of renal function (creatinine clearance) is mandatory in patients with advanced disease who require chemotherapy.

Several biochemical markers are of importance in the diagnosis and management of testicular carcinoma, including AFP, hCG, and lactic acid dehydrogenase (LDH). Other markers have been described for testis cancer, including placental alkaline phosphatase (PLAP) and gamma-glutamyl transpeptidase (GGT).

6.7 Imaging Examination

The primary testicular tumor can be rapidly and accurately assessed by scrotal ultrasonography. This technique can determine whether the mass is truly intratesticular, can be used to distinguish the tumor from epididymal pathology, facilitate testicular examination in the presence of a hydrocele, and may also explore the contralateral testis.

Once the diagnosis of testicular cancer has been established by inguinal orchiectomy, careful clinical staging of the disease is mandatory. If the diagnosis is not clear, a testicular biopsy (and enucleation of the intraparenchymal tumour) is taken for frozen (fresh tissue) section histological examination. In cases of life-threatening disseminated disease, lifesaving chemotherapy should be given up-front, especially when the clinical picture is very likely TC and/or tumour markers are increased. Orchiectomy may be delayed until clinical stabilisation occurs or in combination with resection of residual lesions.

Chest radiographs (posteroanterior and lateral) and CT scans of the abdomen and pelvis are used to assess the two most common sites of metastatic spread, namely, the lungs and retroperitoneum. The role of CT scanning of the chest remains controversial because of its decreased specificity. Of note is the fact that routine chest X-rays (CXR) detect 85% -90% of pulmonary metastases. Pedal lymphangiography (LAG) is rarely used owing to its invasiveness as well as low specificity, although it may be warranted in patients undergoing a surveillance protocol.

6.8 Differential Diagnosis

The differential diagnosis of a testis mass includes epididymoorchitis, torsion, hematoma, or paratesticular neoplasm (benign or malignant). Other diagnostic possibilities include hernia, varicocele, or spermatocele, although these usually can be distinguished from a testis mass by physical examination. A firm intratesticular mass should be considered cancer until proved otherwise and should be evaluated further with a scrotal ultrasound scan. Patients with a presumptive diagnosis of epididymo-orchitis should be re-evaluated within 2-4 weeks of completion of an appropriate course of oral antibiotics. A persistent mass or pain should be evaluated further with scrotal ultrasonography.

6.9 Treatment

The management of GCTs is governed by the potential for rapid growth and for the cure in essentially all patients, which translates into a need for rapid diagnosis and staging and expeditious application of appropriate treatment so as not to have patients die unnecessarily or experience side effects from treatment that would not have been required with earlier diagnosis and proper management. The probability of cure even in the presence of metastatic disease has led to an aggressive approach with regard to the administration of chemotherapy and the performance of surgery after chemotherapy to resect residual masses. Chemotherapy is generally administered regardless of low white blood cell counts or thrombocytopenia, and nephrotoxic chemotherapy (cisplatin) is often administered even in the presence of moderate to severe renal insufficiency. Similarly, an aggressive surgical approach is taken to resect all sites of residual disease after chemotherapy for NSGCT even if this involves multiple anatomic sites. The young age and general good health of patients with GCTs permit an aggressive treatment approach if needed.

Serum tumor markers strongly influence the management of GCTs, particularly NSGCTs. As discussed, elevated serum AFP or hCG after orchiectomy indicates the presence of metastatic disease, and these patients are preferentially given chemotherapy. For patients receiving chemotherapy, increasing serum tumor marker levels during or after therapy generally indicate refractory or relapsed disease, respectively. Serum AFP, hCG, and LDH levels in the initiation of chemotherapy are important prognostic factors and influence the selection and duration of chemotherapy regimens.

Testis cancer is a relatively rare disease, and the treatment algorithms are complex and nuanced. Whenever possible, patients with GCTs should be treated at high-volume centers, and RPLND should be performed by surgeons who are experienced with this operation.

6.10 Prognosis

The vast majority of patients will be cured and 5-year relative survival rates approximate 95%. Furthermore, TC patients are usually between 18 and 40 years at diagnosis such that life expectancy after cure extends over several decades.

Chapter 7

Carcinoma of the Prostate

7.1 Etiology

Family history and racial/ethnic background are associated with an increased cancer of prostate(CaP) incidence suggesting a genetic predisposition. A wide variety of exogenous/environmental factors have been discussed as being aetiologically important for the risk of progression from latent to clinical CaP, including metabolic syndrome, dietary factors, hormonally active medication, balding, gonorrhoea, occupational exposure, etc.

7.2 Epidemiology

Prostate cancer remains the second most commonly diagnosed cancer in men, with an estimated 1.1 million diagnoses worldwide in 2012, accounting for 15% of all cancers diagnosed. Autopsy studies showed a prevalence of CaP at age < 30 years of 5% (95% CI: 3% – 8%), increasing by an odds ratio of 1.7 (1.6 – 1.8) per decade, to a prevalence of 59% (48% – 71%) by age > 79 years. There is relatively less variation in mortality rates worldwide, although rates are generally high in populations of African descent.

7.3 Pathology

More than 95% of prostate cancers are adenocarcinomas. The histology of the remaining 5% of prostate cancer is heterogeneous, arising from stromal, epithelial, or ectopic cells. Nonadenocarcinoma variants can be categorized into two groups based on the cellular origin: epithelial and nonepithelial. Epithelial variants consist of endometrioid, mucinous, signet-ring, adenoid cystic, adenosquamous, squamous cell, transitional cell, neuroendocrine, and comedocarcinoma. Nonepithelial variants include rhabdomyosarcoma, leiomyosarcoma, osteosarcoma, angiosarcoma, carcinosarcoma, malignant lymphoma, and metastatic neoplasms among others.

The cytologic characteristics of CaP include hyperchromatic, enlarged nuclei with prominent nucleoli. The Cytoplasm is often abundant and often slightly blue-tinged or basophilic. The basal cell layer is absent in CaP, whereas it is present in normal glands, BPH glands, and the precursor lesions of CaP. If the diagnosis of CaP is in question, high molecular-weight keratin immunohistochemical staining is useful, as it preferentially stains basal cells. Absence of staining is thus consistent with CaP.

60%-70% of cases of CaP originate in the peripheral zone, 10%-20% originate in the transition zone, and 5%-10% in the central zone. Prostate cancer is frequently multifocal. Penetration of the prostatic capsule by cancer is a common event and often occurs along perineural spaces. Lymphatic metastases are most often identified in the obturator, external iliac, and internal lymph node chains. The axial skeleton is the most usual site of distant metastases, with the lumbar spine being most frequently implicated. The bone lesions of metastatic CaP are typically osteoblastic. Visceral metastases most commonly involve the lung, liver, and adrenal gland. Central nervous system involvement is usually a result of direct extension from skull metastasis.

The 2017 Tumor, Node, Metastasis classification for the staging of CaP and the EAU risk group classification are used to combine patients with a similar clinical outcome.

7.3.1 TNM classification

The TNM classification of Cap is shown in Table 46-7-1.

Table 46-7-1 TNM classification of CaP

T-Primary Tumour		
TX	Primary tumour cannot be assessed	
T0	No evdence of primary turmour	
T1	Cinicaly irnapparert turmour that is not palpable	
	T1a	Tumour incidentai histological finding in 59% or iess of tissue resected
	T1b	Tumour incidental histological finding in more than 5% of tissue resected
	T1c	Tumour identified by needle biopey (e g. because of elevated prostate -specific antigon (PSA) leve)
T2	Turnour that is palpabie and confined within the prostate	
	T2a	Tumour involves one halt of one lobe or less
	T2b	Tumour involves more thar half of one lobe, but not both lobes
	T2c	Tumour involves both iobes
T3	Tumour extends through the prostatic capsule!	
	T3a	Extracapsular extension (unilateral or bilateral) including microscopic biadder neck involverment
	T3b	Turmour irvades serminal vesicle(s)
T4	Tumour is fixed or invaden adjacent structures other than saminaf vesicles: externai sphincter, rectum, levator tmuscles, and/or pelvic wall	
N-Regional Lymph Nodes?		
NX	Regional lymph nodes cannot be assessed	
N0	No regional tymph node metastasig	
N1	Ragional lymph node metastasis	
M- Distant Metastasis?		
M0	No distarnt metastasis	
M1	Distant metastasis	
	M1a	Mta Non-regionat lymph node(s)
	M1b	M1b Bonet(s)
	M1c	M1c Other sitei(s)

[1] trvasion into the prostate aper or into (but not beyond) the prostate capsufe is not ciassibed as T3, but as T2

[2] PMetastasis no larger tman 0.2 c m can be dasigrated phNmi.

[2] aT2a to c onty eust for cinical T2 (cT2) For pathological T2 they are no longer present in the 2017 TNM. Only pT2 cxisis.

[3] When more than one site of metastasis s presont, tme most acvanced category is used. (p) hftc s the mest acvanced citegory.

7.3.2 EAU risk group classification

The EAU risk group classification is shown in Table 46-7-2.

Table 46-7-2 EAU risk gruops for biochemical recurrence of localized and locally advanced CaP

Definition			
Low-risk	intermediate-risk	High-risk	
PSA<10 ng/mL and GS<7(ISUP grade 1) and cT1-T2a	PSA 10-20 ng/mL or GS 7(ISUP grade 2/3) or cT2b	PSA>20 ng/mL or GS>7(ISUP grade 4/5) or cT2c	any PSA and GS cT3-T4 or cN + Any ISUP grade
Localised			Locally advanced

7.3.3 Gleason score and international society of urological pathology 2014 grade groups

The Gleason system relies on the low-power appearance of the glandular architecture under the microscope. In assigning a grade to a given tumor, pathologists assign a primary grade to the pattern of cancer that is most commonly observed and a secondary grade to the second most commonly observed pattern in the specimen. Grades range from 1 to 5. The Gleason system is the most commonly employed grading system. The system relies on the low-power appearance of the glandular architecture under the microscope. In assigning a grade to a given tumor, pathologists assign a primary grade to the pattern of cancer that is most commonly observed and a secondary grade to the second most commonly observed pattern in the specimen. Grades range from 1 to 5 are obtained by adding the primary and secondary grades together. Traditionally, Gleason grades ranged from 1 to 5, and Gleason scores thus ranged from 2 to 10.

The ISUP 2014 Gleason grading (Table 46-7-3) represents a compression of Gleason scores < 6 to ISUP grade 1, and Gleason scores 9-10 to ISUP grade 5, whereas Gleason score 7 is expanded to ISUP grade 2, i. e., 7(3 + 4) and ISUP grade 3, i. e., 7(4 + 3).

Table 46-7-3 Internatianal society of urological pathology 2014 grades

Gleason score	ISUP grade
2-6	1
7(3+4)	2
7(4+3)	3
8(4+4 or 3+5 or 5+3)	4
9-10	5

7.4 Clinical Manifestation

The large majority of patients with early-stage CaP are asymptomatic. The presence of symptoms often suggests locally advanced or metastatic disease. Obstructive or irritative voiding complaints can result from local growth of the tumor into the urethra or bladder neck or from its direct extension into the trigone of the bladder. Much more commonly, however, such symptoms are attributable to coexisting BPH. Metastatic disease to the bones may cause bone pain. Metastatic disease to the vertebral column with impingement on the spinal cord may be associated with symptoms of cord compression, including paresthesias and weakness of the lower extremities and urinary or fecal incontinence.

A physical examination, including a digital rectal exam, is needed. Induration or nodularity, if detected, must alert the physician to the possibility of cancer and the need for further evaluation. Most CaPs are located in the peripheral zone and can be detected by DRE when the volume is greater than 0.2 mL. Locally advanced disease with bulky regional lymphadenopathy may lead to lymphedema of the lower extremities. Specific signs of cord compression relate to the level of the compression and may include weakness or spasticity of the lower extremities and a hyper-reflexive bulbocavernosus reflex.

7.5 Laboratory Examination

7.5.1 Prostate-specific antigen

PSA is a serine protease in the human kallikrein(hK) family produced by benign and malignant prostate tissues. It circulates in the serum as uncomplexed(free or unbound) or complexed(bound) forms. PSA is used both as a diagnostic(screening) tool and as a means of risk-stratifying known prostate cancers. Its use is complicated by the fact that PSA is prostate specific, not prostate cancer specific. There are no agreed standards defined for measuring PSA. PSA is a continuous parameter, with higher levels indicating a greater likelihood of CaP.

A "normal" PSA has traditionally been defined as < 4 ng/mL, and the positive predictive value of a serum PSA between 4 and 10 ng/mL is 20%-30%. For levels in excess of 10 ng/mL, the positive predictive value increases from 42% to 71.4%.

7.5.2 Prostate biopsy

The need for prostate biopsy is based on PSA level and/or suspicious DRE. Age, potential comorbidity, and therapeutic consequences should also be considered and discussed beforehand. Risk stratification is a potential tool for reducing unnecessary biopsies. Ultrasound-guided biopsy is now the standard of care. A transrectal approach is used for most prostate biopsies, although some urologists prefer a perineal approach.

7.6 Imaging Laboratory

7.6.1 Multiparametric magnetic resonance imaging

Multiparametric magnetic resonance imaging(mpMRI) can reliably detect aggressive tumours in candidates for prostate biopsy with a negative(NPV) and positive predictive value(PPV) ranging from 63 to 98% and from 34 to 68%, respectively. mpMRI is increasingly performed before prostate biopsy. Before biopsy is repeated, mpMRI should be performed when clinical suspicion of CaP persists in spite of negative biopsies.

7.6.2 Bone scan

Bone scan(BS) has been the most widely used method for evaluating bone metastases of CaP. When prostate cancer metastasizes, it most commonly does so to the bone. Soft tissue metastases(e. g. , lung and liver) are rare at the time of initial presentation. Bone scanning should be performed in symptomatic patients, independent of PSA level, Gleason score or clinical stage.

7.6.3 Transrectal ultrasound and computed tomography

Grey-scale transrectal ultrasound(TRUS) is not reliable at detecting CaP. Currently there is not enough evidence for their routine use.

Because of the low sensitivity, CT should not be used for nodal staging in low-risk patients and be reserved for high-risk cancer patients.

7.7 Treatment

7.7.1 For localized CaP

Different treatment strategies is listed in Table 46-7-4.

Table 46-7-4 Treatment strategies correlating with the different-risk CaP

Treatment	Low-risk CaP	Intermediate-risk CaP	Low-risk Cap
Active surveillance	(1) Offer active survelance (AS) to patients with the lowest risk of caner progreslor. > 10 years lfe espectancy, cT1/2, prostate-specifitc antgen (PSA) ≤ 10 ng/mL, biopsy Gleaston scores ≤ 6, ≤ 2 positive biopsies, minimal biopsy core involvement (≤ 50% cancer per biopsy}. (2) Base follow up on digital rectal examination (DRE), PSA and rectal examination (DRE), PSA and repeated biopsie. (3) Counsel patients about the posibllty of needing further treatment in the future.	Not an option.	Not appropriate.

Continue to Table 46-7-4

Treatment	Low-risk CaP	Intermediate-risk CaP	Low-risk Cap
Watchful waiting	Offer watchful waiting (WW) to patients not eligible for local curative treatment and with a short life espectancy.	Offer WW to patients not eligible for local curative treatment and with a short lfe expectancy.	(1) High risk locelised: Offer W W to patients not eligible for local curative treatment and with a short ife erpectancy. (2) High rtak localy advanced: n locoly advanced MO patients unwilling or unable to receive any for m of local treattnent. offer a deferred treatment polley to asymptomatik patients wth a pSA DT>12 months and a PSAc S0ng/mL and non- poorhy diterentiated tumor.
Radical prostatectomy	(1) Offer both radical prostectormy (RP) and radiotherapy (RT) in patients with low-risk CaP and a life expectaney>10 years. (2) Do not perform lymph node dlissection (LND) in low-risk CaP.	(1) Offer both RP and RT in patients with inter mediate-risk disease and a life expectancy>10 years. (2) Offer nerve sparing surgery in patients with a low risk of extracapsular disease. Offter nerve-sparing surgery in patients with a lo w risk of estracapsular disease (3) Perform an extended (ND (eL ND) if the estirmated risk for postve lymph nodes (LNs) esceeds 5%. Do not perform a limited LND. (4) In patients with pT3, NOMO PC and an undetectable PSA folliowing RP. discuss adjuvant EBRT because t at least improves biochemical-free survival. inform patients with pT3. NOMO PCa and an undetectabie PSA folowing RP about saltvage irradiation as an alternative to adjuevant irradiation when PSA increases. (5) Do not offer adjuvant hormonal therapy (HT) after RP for pN0 disease.	(1) Do not offer neoadjuvant hormonal therapy before RP. (2) Offer RP in selected patients withs locally advanced (cT3a) disease and life erpectancy > 10 years onhy s part of muti-rmodaltherapy (3) Offer RP in selected patients with localy advanced (cT3a) disese and a life expectancy > 10years only as part of muti modal therapy. (4) Perform an elND in high-risk PCa. (5) High risk localised: Offer RP in patients with hightisk localised PCa and alfe espectancy of > 10 years only as part of multi-modal therapy. in high risk discasc. usc mpMit as a decisicn-making tool to select patents for nerve sparing procedures. (6) High risk localy advanced: Offer RP in higbiy selected patients with (cT3b-T4 NO or any T N1) only as partoef mut modia therapy. In patients with pT3, NOMO PCa and an undetectable PSA following RP, discus adiuvant EBRT because it astleast improres biochemical-free survival. ihform patients with pT3. A0ttO PCa and an undetectable PSA following RP about salveag radiatien as an alternative to adjuvan adjuvant irradiation when PSA increases.

Continue to Table 46-7-4

Treatment	Low-risk CaP	Intermediate-risk CaP	Low-risk Cap
Radiotherapy	(1) In low-risk PCa, use a total dose of 74 to 78 Gy for external beam radiotherapy(EBRT). (2) in low-risk PCa, use a total dose of 74 to 78 Gy for eaternal beam radiotherapy (EBRT)	(1) In intermedlate - risk PCa use a total dose of 76-78Gy. in combinstion with short-term androgen deprivation therapy (ADT) (four to stx months). (2) in selected intermediate-risk patients. without a previous TURP and with a good IPSS and a prostate volume < 50 mL, offer LDR brachytherapy.	(1) inform patients with an undetectable PSA following RP about salvage irradiation as an alternative to adjuvant irradiation when PSA increases. (2) Inform patients with an undetectable PSA following RP about salvage irradiation as an alternative to adjuvant irradiation when PSA increases. (3) in patients with focally advanced cNo pCa. offer RT in combination with long term ADT (two to three years is recommended).
Androgen suppression	Unsuitable.	No place in asymptomatic patients.	(1) In patients with localy advanced cNO PCa, offer RT in conbination with long term ADT (two to three years is recom mended). (2) Do not ofler ADT to patlents with a PSA-DT > 12 months.

(1) Active surveillance

Active surveillance(Table 46-7-5) aims to achieve correct timing for curative treatment in patients with clinically localized CaP, rather than delay palliative treatment. Patients remain under close surveillance, and treatment is prompted by predefined thresholds indicative of potentially life-threatening disease, still potentially curable, while considering individual life expectancy.

(2) Watchful waiting

Watchful waiting(Table 46-7-5) is also known as deferred or symptom-guided treatment. It refers to conscrvativc managcmcnt, until thc dcvclopmcnt of local or systcmic progrcssion with (immincnt) discasc-related complaints. Patients are then treated according to their symptoms, in order to maintain QoL.

Table 46-7-5 Definitions of active surveillance ans watchful waiting

	Active surveillance	Watchful waiting
Treatment intent	Curative	Palliative
Follow-up	Predefined schedule	Patient-specitic
Assessment/markers used	DRE, PSA, re-biopsy, mpMRI	Not predefined
Life expectancy	>10 years	<10 years
Aim	Minimise treatment - related toxicity without compromising survival	Minimise treatment-related toxicity
Comments	Low-risk patients	Can apply to patients with all stages

DRE = digital rectal examination; PSA = prostate-specific antigen; mpMRI = multiparametric magnetic resonance imaging.

(3) Radical prostatectomy

The goal of RP by any approach must be eradication of disease, while preserving continence and, whenever possible, potency. estimation of life expectancy is paramount in counseling a patient about surgery. Radical prostatectomy can be performed by open, laparoscopic or robot-assisted (RARP) approach. Laparoscopy reduces blood loss substantially, shortens the overall recovery time, and in some series reduces hospitalization time. Whether robot-assisted or unassisted laparoscopic surgery results in better or worse results in terms of the critical outcomes of cancer control, however, remains unclear.

(4) Radiotherapy

1) External beam therapy

Traditional external beam radiotherapy (XRT) techniques allow the safe delivery of 6500-7000 cGy to the prostate. Standard XRT techniques depend upon bony landmarks to define treatment borders or a single CT slice to define the target volume. Often, these XRT techniques fail to provide adequate coverage of the target volume in as many as 20-41% of patients with CaP irradiated. Improved imaging and use of novel treatment planning [three-dimensional, conformal radiation therapy (3DCRT) and intensity-modulated radiation therapy (IMRT)] allow for better targeting, conforming, or shaping radiation volume more closely around the prostate, and the use of higher doses without exceeding tolerance of surrounding normal tissues. Such radiotherapy has resulted in dramatic reductions in acute and late toxicity of radiation treatment and improved tumor control compared with conventional-dose radiotherapy. IMRT, with or without image-guided radiotherapy (IGRT), is the accepted best standard for EBRT.

2) Brachytherapy

A resurgence in the interest in brachytherapy has occurred because of the technologic developments making it possible to place radioactive seeds under TRUS guidance. Implants can be permanent (iodine 125 or palladium 103) in that the seeds are placed in the prostate, and the radiation dose is delivered over time or temporary in that the seeds are loaded into hollow-core catheters and both the seeds (iridium 192) and catheters are removed after a short period of hospitalization and radiation exposure.

(5) Hormonal therapy

Androgen deprivation treatment (ADT) can be achieved by either suppressing the secretion of testicular androgens or inhibiting the action of circulating androgens at the level of their receptor. These two methods can be combined to achieve what is known as complete (or maximal or total) androgen blockade (CAB).

1) Surgical castration is still considered for the primary treatment modality as ADT.

2) Treatment with oestrogen results in testosterone suppression. Due to severe side effects, especially thromboembolic complications, even at lower doses, these drugs are not considered as standard first-line treatment.

3) Long-acting LHRH agonists are currently the main forms of ADT. After the first injection, they induce a transient rise in luteinizing hormone (LH) and follicle-stimulating hormone (FSH) leading to the "testosterone surge" or "flare-up" phenomenon, which starts 2-3 days after administration and lasts for about 1 week.

4) Luteinizing-hormone releasing hormone antagonists immediately bind to LHRH receptors, leading to a rapid decrease in LH, FSH and testosterone levels without any flare.

5) Anti-androgens compete with androgens at the receptor level. This is the sole action of non-steroidal antiandrogens and leads to an unchanged or slightly elevated testosterone level. Conversely, steroidal anti-androgens have progesterone properties leading to central inhibition by crossing the blood-brain barrier.

6) Abiraterone acetate and enzalutamide, both are currently approved for mCRPC only. Abiraterone ac-

etate(AA) is a CYP17 inhibitor(a combination of 17-hydrolase and 17,20-lyase inhibition). By blocking CYP17, AA significantly decreases the intracellular testosterone level by suppressing its synthesis at the adrenal level and inside the cancer cells(intracrine mechanism). Enzalutamide is a novel anti-androgen with a higher affinity than bicalutamide for the AR receptor. While nonsteroidal anti-androgens still allow the transfer of ARs to the nucleus, enzalutamide also blocks AR transfer and therefore suppresses any possible agonist-like activity.

7.7.2 For metastatic CaP

Primary ADT has been the standard of care for over 50 years. Castration combined with chemotherapy (docetaxel) is recommended for all patients whose first presentation is M1 disease and who fit enough for chemotherapy. Offer castration alone with or without an anti-androgen, to patients unfit for, or unwilling to consider, castration combined with chemotherapy.

7.8 Prognosis

The Gleason score at radical prostatectomy correlates well with prognosis. The 5-year postoperative biochemical risk, free of disease, is 96.6%, 88.1%, 69.7%, 63.7%, and 34.5% for Gleason scores less than or equal to 6; 3+4=7; 4+3=7; 8; and 9-10, respectively.

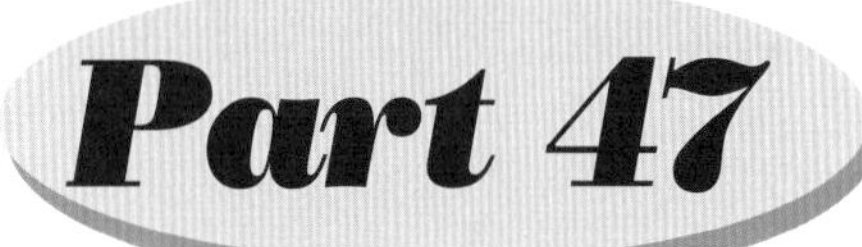

Part 47

Other Diseases and Disorders of Genitourinary Tract

Chapter 1

Nephroptosis

Nephroptosis has been one of the most controversial and often debated urological diagnoses for more than a century. Anatomically, it is defined as a significant descent(>5 cm or two vertebral bodies on IVU) of the kidney as the patient moves from supine to erect. The kidney might move into an abnormal position but is capable of moving back into a normal anatomical site, which differentiates it from an ectopic kidney, which would constantly remain in an abnormal position.

1.1 Etiology

Each kidney with its fibrous capsule rests in a layer of perinephric fat, encompassed by the thick Gerota's fascia. Gerota's fascia is separated from the muscles of the posterior abdominal wall by another layer of adipose tissue(paranephric fat). Although the etiology of nephroptosis is not completely understood, the excessive mobility of the kidney is probably related to deficient support from these perinephric structures, permitting excessive renal mobility. Therefore malrotation or maldescent of the kidney can result in either stretching or torsion of the hilar vessels and/or kinking of the pelviureteric junction or the proximal ureter. Studies in children suggested that nephroptosis is a constitutional rather than an acquired phenomenon, and it is likely that the condition precedes the onset of symptoms, usually in adult life, by several decades.

1.2 Epidemiology

The exact incidence in the general population is unknown but IVU in thin females(where an upright image is included) will show renal mobility amounting to nephroptosis in up to 20% of cases. The male-to-female ratio of radiologically detected nephroptosis is 3 : 100, occurring most frequently in young, slim women. The right side is affected in 70% of cases, the left kidney in 10% and 20% have bilateral renal descent.

1.3 Clinical Manifestation

Most patients are well, and symptomatic nephroptosis is said to be present in 10% –20% of cases. Symptomatic patients are generally young, thin females, some of whom might have previously had unsuccessful surgery for chronic, intermittent abdominal/flank pain. The most frequently associated symptoms are as follows:

(1) Pain. Pain is the principal complaint(90% of patients), usually described as a "dragging" pain in the flank or abdomen, typically when upright, and relieved by recumbency. Acute episodes might present as renal colic, with no detectable ureteric calculi.

(2) Nausea and vomiting. Nausea and vomiting are frequently present, probably due to visceral autonomic nerve stimulation.

(3) Abdominal mass. An abdominal mass might be noted when upright in thin patients, and manipulation of the kidney "mass" into its anatomical position might result in resolution of the symptoms. Occasionally, slim patients might be able to manipulate their kidney into a lower position by themselves.

(4) Transient hematuria, both frank and microscopic.

(5) A history of repeated UTI, renal calculi, and hypertension.

Dietl's crisis is a syndrome attributed to acute hydronephrosis due to kinking or obstruction of the ureter of a "floating kidney", and in its classical form is characterized by violent paroxysms of colicky flank pain, nausea, chills, tachycardia, oliguria, transient haematuria or proteinuria, and a palpable enlarged tender kidney. The immediate resolution of Dietl's crisis was based on gentle manual reduction of the kidney into the renal fossa while the patient was supine, or the patient adopting a supine knee–chest position.

1.4 Laboratory Examination

Laboratory studies add little in terms of establishing the diagnosis of nephroptosis but are recommended to exclude other possible coexisting conditions. They include a mid–stream specimen of urine for dipstick analysis to assess haematuria and proteinuria and formal microscopy, culture and sensitivity to exclude a UTI; and serum creatinine measurement(estimated GFR).

1.5 Imaging Examination

The satisfactory diagnosis of nephroptosis requires the detection of significant renal descent(5 cm) on standing, and ureteric obstruction or diminished arterial flow. For this reason, all suspected cases, especially where surgical intervention is being considered, should undergo the following radiological investigation while both supine and upright: US with colour doppler imaging; IVU(or CT); and radionuclide scans, either dynamic or static renal scanning.

1.6 Treatment

(1) Conservative treatment

Conservative treatment has a negligible role in the current management of symptomatic nephroptosis. Weight gain, abdominal wall exercises, frequent supine rests and abdominal corsets are impractical and unproven short-term solutions.

(2) Surgical treatment

Surgery must be considered in symptomatic patients, with a symptom duration of >3 months, with no other accounting pathology and in whom radiological investigations when both supine and upright, have shown descent of the symptomatic kidney by two vertebral bodies (and/or 5 cm) and obstruction or diminished flow to the symptomatic side in patients who accept the potential morbidity associated with surgery. Surgical intervention can be divided into open nephropexy, percutaneous nephropexy and laparoscopic nephropexy.

Chapter 2

Varicocele

A varicocele is a varicose dilatation of the veins draining the testis.

2.1 Etiology

The veins draining the testis and the epididymis form the pampiniform plexus. The veins gradually join each other as they traverse the inguinal canal and, at or near the inguinal ring, there are only one or two testicular veins, which pass upward within the retroperitoneum. The left testicular vein empties into the left renal vein, the right into the inferior vena cava below the right renal vein. The testicular veins usually have valves near their terminations, but these are sometimes absent. There is an alternative (collateral) venous return from the testes through the cremasteric veins, which drain mainly into the inferior epigastric.

The usual cause is absence or incompetence of valves in the proximal testicular vein. While most varicoceles are idiopathic, obstruction of the left testicular vein by a renal tumour or nephrectomy is a cause of varicocele in later life; characteristically, in such cases the varicocele does not decompress in the supine position.

2.2 Epidemiology

Varicoceles are common, affecting perhaps 15% – 20% of males. 90% are left-sided, reflecting the proximal venous anatomy. In some cases, the dilated vessels are cremasteric veins and not part of the pampiniform plexus.

2.3 Clinical Manifestation and Examination

While most varicoceles are asymptomatic, those that are symptomatic tend to present in adolescence or early adulthood when there may be an annoying dragging discomfort that is worse on standing at the end of the day. This presumably reflects distension of the testicular veins. When examined in the erect position, the scrotum on the affected side hangs lower than normal, and on palpation, with the patient standing, the varicose plexus feels like a bag of worms. There may be a cough impulse. If the patient lies down the veins empty by gravity and this provides an opportunity to ensure that the underlying testis is normal to palpation. In longstanding cases, the affected testis is smaller and softer than its fellow owing to a minor degree of atrophy.

Ultrasonography can be helpful in the diagnosis of small varicoceles and in older men with an apparently recent onset of varicocele, ultrasonography of the kidneys is important in excluding a left renal tumour.

2.4 Treatment

Varicocele treatment should be offered to the male partner of a couple attempting to conceive, when all of the following are present: a varicocele is palpable; the couple has documented infertility; the female has normal fertility or potentially correctable infertility; and the male partner has one or more abnormal semen parameters or sperm function test results. There are two approaches to varicocele treatment: surgery and percutaneous embolization. Surgical repair of a varicocele may be accomplished by various open surgical methods, including retroperitoneal, inguinal and subinguinal approaches, or by laparoscopy. Percutaneous embolization treatment of a varicocele is accomplished by percutaneous embolization of the refluxing internal spermatic vein(s).

Chapter 3

Hydrocele

A hydrocele is an abnormal collection of serous fluid in a part of the processus vaginalis, usually the tunica vaginalis. Acquired hydroceles are primary or idiopathic, or secondary to epididymal or testicular disease.

3.1 Etiology

Hydrocele can be produced in four different ways:

(1) By excessive production of fluid within the sac, e. g., a secondary hydrocele.

(2) By defective absorption of fluid; this appears to be the explanation for most primary hydroceles, although the reason why the fluid is not absorbed is obscure.

(3) By interference with lymphatic drainage of scrotal structures.

(4) By connection with the peritoneal cavity via a patent processus vaginalis (congenital).

Thy types of hydrocele are shown in Figure 47-3-1.

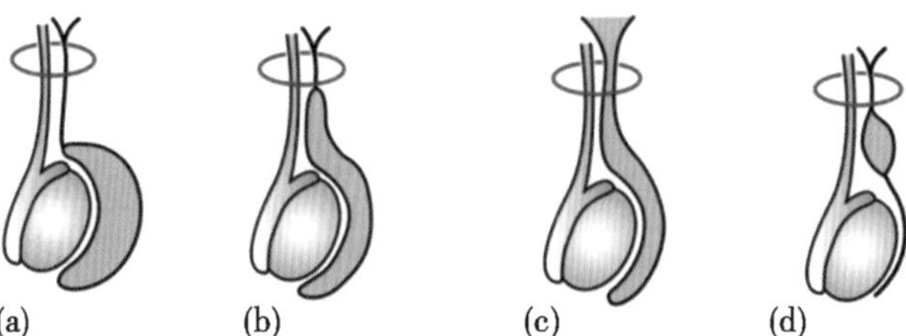

Figure 47-3-1 Different types of hydrocele

(a) Vaginal hydrocele (very common); (b) "infantile" hydrocele; (c) congenital hydrocele; (d) hydrocele of the cord.

Hydrocele fluid contains albumin and fibrinogen. If the contents of a hydrocele are allowed to drain into a collecting vessel, the liquid does not clot; however, the fluid coagulates if mixed with even a trace of blood that has been in contact with damaged tissue.

A secondary hydrocele is most frequently associated with acute or chronic epididymo-orchitis. It is also seen with torsion of the testis and with some testicular tumours. A secondary hydrocele is usually lax and of moderate size; the underlying testis is palpable. If a tumour is suspected, the hydrocele should not be punctured for fear of needle-track implantation of malignant cells. A secondary hydrocele subsides when the primary lesions resolved.

3.2 Clinical Manifestation and Examination

Hydroceles are typically translucent and it is possible to "get above the swelling" on examination of the scrotum. The swelling usually surrounds the testis and epididymis that they may become impossible to be palpated separately.

A primary vaginal hydrocele is seen most commonly in middle and later life but can also occur in older children. Because the swelling is usually painless it may reach a prodigious size before the patient presents for treatment. The testis may be palpable within a lax hydrocele, but an ultrasound scan is necessary to visualise the testis if the hydrocele sac is tense. Be wary of an acute hydrocele in a young man since there may be a testicular tumour.

In congenital hydrocele, the processus vaginalis is patent and connects with the peritoneal cavity. The communication is usually too small to allow herniation of intra-abdominal contents. Pressure on the hydrocele does not always empty it but the hydrocele fluid may drain into the peritoneal cavity when the child is lying down; thus, the hydrocele may be intermittent. Ascites should be considered if the swellings are bilateral.

Encysted hydrocele of the cord is a smooth oval swelling near the spermatic cord which is liable to be mistaken for an inguinal hernia. The swelling moves downwards and becomes less mobile if the testis is pulled gently downwards.

Hydrocele of the canal of Nuck is a similar condition in females. The cyst lies in relation to the round ligament and is always at least partially within the inguinal canal.

3.3 Treatment

Congenital hydroceles are treated by herniotomy if they do not get resolved spontaneously. Small acquired hydroceles do not need treatment. If they are sizeable and bothersome for the patient, then surgical treatment is indicated. Established acquired hydroceles often have thick walls. Lord's operation is suitable when the sac is reasonably thin-walled. Eversion of the sac with placement of the testis in a pouch prepared by dissection in the fascial planes of the scrotum is an alternative (Jaboulay's procedure).

Aspiration of the hydrocele fluid is simple, but the fluid always reaccumulates within a week or so. It may be suitable for men who are unfit for scrotal surgery. Injection of sclerosants such as tetracycline is effective but painful.

Chapter 4

Renovascular Hypertension

Partial or complete occlusion of one or both renal arteries may result in renal ischemia and as a consequence may result in renovascular hypertension(RVH), the most common form of secondary and potentially curable hypertension.

4.1 Etiology and Pathogenesis

The most common forms of RVH are due to atherosclerotic disease and fibromuscular dysplasia, with the former accounting for more than 2/3 of the cases. Atherosclerotic renal artery disease is most frequently seen in those older than 40 years of age, being more often seen in men than women, and generally involves the ostium and/or proximal third of the renal artery. The fibromuscular disease is more often seen in younger Caucasian women, is usually bilateral, and unlike atherosclerotic disease, it involves the more distal segments of the renal arteries.

In the early phases of RVH baroreceptor activation in the ischemic kidney increases renin secretion, causing blood pressure elevation. Thereafter, the renin-angiotensin-aldosterone system(RAAS) activation is progressively attenuated and plasma renin levels may return within the normal range but still remaining inappropriately high for blood pressure levels. It is likely that in RVH the cardiotoxic effects elicited by the activation of the RAAS and of additional humoral factors(cathecholamines, endothelin, cytokynes) contribute to the adverse consequences of blood pressure increase, exposing patients to a global cardiovascular risk particularly high.

4.2 Pathology

Atherosclerotic renal artery disease predominantly affects men and women aged from 40-70 years. The proximal third of the renal artery is usually involved, and in 70% to 80% of the patients there is an aortic plaque that impinges on the renal ostium, whereas the remaining 30% exhibit nonostial narrowing usually 1-3 cm distal to the renal artery ostium. It has been observed that renal arteries with greater degrees of stenosis will more likely and more quickly progress to complete occlusion.

Fibromuscular dysplasia involved various arteries were, with the renal artery being the most common (66%); next was the extracranial carotids(56%); and least common was the vertebral arteries in(18%). There are four types of fibrous dysplasia: medial fibroplasia, perimedial fibroplasia, intimal fibroplasia, and medial hyperplasia. Medial, perimedial, and intimal fibroplastic lesions may affect the renal artery with an incidence of 30%, 5%, and 5%, respectively, and they represent 70%–85%, 10%–25%, and 10%, respectively, of all fibrous renal artery diseases. Medial hyperplasia, the fourth type of fibrous dysplasia, constitutes only 2% to 3% of all fibrous dysplastic lesions.

4.3 Clinical Manifestation

Various clinical signs can suggest RVH but none has sensitivity and specificity high enough to make the diagnosis certain. For example, resistant hypertension was present but this condition is also frequent in patients with essential hypertension. Other signs like renal asymmetry and hypokalemia are characterized-with good specificity but poor sensitivity. However, the predictive value of clinical signs increases by 2–3 folds when two or more of them coexist.

4.4 Laboratory Examination

Renin determination in peripheral blood is still a useful tool to evaluate the hemodynamical relevance of the RAS. However, the diffusion of this test has been hampered both by methodological problems related to the poor reproducibility of plasma renin activity(PRA) determination among laboratories and to the difficulties in interpreting these results related to the pharmacological interference of most antihypertensive drugs on RAAS activity. Recently new methods of the direct determination of plasma renin concentration(PRC) with monoclonal antibodies have been developed. This technique, being faster and simpler than PRA, may allow a wider application of renin determination for the diagnosis of RVH. Various alternative parameters have been proposed for the evaluation of the hemodynamic relevance of RAS(BNP, calculation of trans-stenotic gradient, ultrasound resistive indices), but none of them has reached enough consensus to be exploited for clinical use.

4.5 Imaging Examination

Renal artery stenosis(RAS) is the anatomical substrate of RVH. US, CT, MRI, scintigraphy, and angiography all may be utilized in the diagnosis of RAS. Given the limited scenarios in which testing for RAS is considered appropriate, the decision to perform diagnostic imaging to identify RAS should ideally be based on a multidisciplinary assessment of an individual patient's clinical presentation, comorbidities, and likelihood of response to intervention.

For patients with normal renal function, contrast enhanced CTA and MRA are preferred modalities. US is also an effective modality.

For patients with decreased renal function with eGFR < 30 mL/min/1.73 m^2, US is a preferred screening examination. Unenhanced MRA techniques are available as an alternative to contrast enhanced

MRA to avoid the risk of nephrogenic systemic fibrosis in these patients.

4.6 Treatment

4.6.1 Medical treatment

Due to the uncertainty about the benefits of RA, medical therapy is advisable in patients with RAS < 50% -60% or when blood pressure is under control with a moderate pharmacological burden. RAAS antagonists are particularly effective in reducing blood pressure but they can reduce GFR in the stenotic kidney. This can have little effect on indices of overall renal function because of the compensatory role of the contralateral kidney, but it can cause a progressive deterioration of renal function in the stenotic kidney leading to atrophy. When using a RAAS antagonist in patients with RAS it is advisable to withdraw this therapy in case of increments in serum creatinine values of more than 30% or for potassium above 5.5 mEq/l. Modifications of this magnitude, if confirmed, should always bring about the suspicion of a critical RAS. Also beta blockers can achieve an adequate blood pressure control, inhibiting sympatho-mediated renin secretion without significantly influencing RPF. Calcium antagonists are advisable for their known anti-hypertensive and antiatherogenetic efficacy. Diuretic shouldn't be considered as the first line drugs because they further stimulate the activity of RAAS, unless a severe renal insufficiency coexist. On the basis of the elevated cardiovascular risk profile of RVH patients, the association of antiplatelet agents and statins to antihypertensive treatment is generally recommended.

4.6.2 Surgical treatment

Patients would benefit from surgical intervention, including those with concomitant aneurysmal or occlusive aortic disease, those with macroaneurysms of the renal artery associated with stenosis, those with malignant or accelerated hypertension (with or without acute renal failure) who did not respond or can not tolerate medical therapy, and those in whom transluminal angioplasty is technically impossible to accomplish. Gold standard is represented by renal angioplasty (RA) combined with stent placement.

Part 48

General Principles of Fracture Treatment

48.1 Introduction

Fracture is a break in the structural continuity of bone. If the overlying skin remains intact; it is called closed (Simple) fracture. If the overlying skin or one of the body cavities is breached; it is called open (Compound) fracture.

Mechanism of fracture:

Fracture results from injury; repeatitive stress; abnormal weakening of bone (pathological fracture).

The basic forces-compression, tension, torsion and bending cause the bone to behave in predictable ways. Compression force causes shortening the length of the bone. Tension force can lead to a transverse fracture. Torsion force causes twisting of bones along its long axis. Bending force causes it to bow at the center.

48.2 Characteristic of Fracture

Fractures are described in terms of a number of characteristics:

48.2.1 Etiology: according to the causes of fracture

(1) Traumatic fracture: most fractures are caused by sudden and excessive force, which may be direct or indirect.

With direct force the bone breaks at the point of impact, soft tissues are also damaged. Direct blow usually splits the bone transversely or may bend it over a fulcrum so as to create a break with a "Butterfly" fragment, If crush injury occurs the fracture pattern will be comminuted with excessive soft tissue damage.

The bone breaks at a distance from where the force is applied, soft tissue damage at the fracture site is not inevitable.

Spiral and oblique fracture pattern are usually due to low-energy indirect injuries; bending and transverse patterns are caused by high-energy direct trauma.

(2) Pathological fracture: Pathological fractures occur within diseased bone and often caused by relatively little violence or energy; they are the effect of a normal force on an abnormal bone. The pathology may be localized to one part of bone or generalized.

(3) Fatigue (stress) fracture: These fractures occur in normal bone subject of repeated heavy loading, e.g., in athletes, dancers or military personal. Stress fracture are increasingly seen in patients with chronic inflammatory disease who are on treatment with steroids or methotrexate.

48.2.2 Morphology: the fracture pattern

(1) Transverse and oblique fracture: These fractures are caused by a bending force resulting from a direct blow by a moving object or by a bone striking a resistant object (such as the ground).

(2) Spiral fracture: These are caused by indirect rotational forces. The mechanism of injury is often a simple twist and fall, or a sporting accident.

(3) Avulsion fracture: These fractures are caused by traction from a ligament, tendon or capsular insertion, e.g., anterior inferior iliac spine avulsion caused by rectus femoris whilst kicking, avulsion of the base

of the fifth metatarsal at the peroneus brevis insertion during ankle inversion.

48.2.3 AO Comprehensive Classification System

This alphanumeric system is structured and formulaic. It provides a common description of the principal patterns of diaphyseal and metaphyseal fracture. The classification follows a common pattern.

The bone is first given a number:①Humerus;②Radius and ulna;③Femur;④Tibia and fibula.

· The region of the bone is also numbered:①Proximal metaphysic;②Diaphysis;③Distal metaphysic. The ankle is a special case and is coded 44.

· The fracture type is then denoted by a letter:A,B or C. In general,there is a hierarchy of severity and complexit,with A being the simplest fracture that has the best prognosis,and C being the most complex and difficult to manage. The classification of the fracture type is different for the metaphysic and the diaphysis.

· There are then three groups within each fracture type:1,2 and 3,again numbered in a hierarchy of increasing complexity.

· There are then three subgroups within each group:these are denoted by a decimal point and then three numbers,1,2 and 3.

The type and group codes are common to most fractures,are easy to commit to memory and are helpful descriptors to use in routine clinical practice. The subgroups have poor inter– and intra–observer reliability.

48.2.3.1 AO classification of shaft fractures

The three fracture types are as follow:

(1)A:simple,two–part fractures.

(2)B:wedge fractures with some contact between the two principal fragments(B= butterfly).

(3)C:multifragmentary fractures with no contact between the principal fragments(C=comminuted).

Within each fracture type,the groups indicate increasing complexity,with 1 indicating a spiral pattern, and 2 and 3 increasing comminution. Spiral types are often unstable,are graded lowest,with their large surface area,they often heal most rapidly.

48.2.3.2 AO classification of metaphyseal fractures

The three fracture types are:extra–articular;partial articular;complete articular.

This represents increasing difficulty in reduction and fixation. Within each type are groups indicating increasing complexity. Within type B,these usually represent various saggital and coronal fracture planes, although at either end of the tibia,the B types represent differing degrees of impaction. Within type C,the groups describe increasing comminution of the metaphyseal and articular components of the fracture :

C1 is simple metaphyseal,simple articular.

C2 is complex metaphyseal and simple articular.

C3 is complex metaphyseal,complex articular.

48.4 Clinical Features of Fractures

(1)History

There is usually a history of injury,followed by inability to use the injured limb,but fractures is not always at the site of injury;a blow to the knee may fracture the patella,femoral condyles,shaft of the femur or even acetabulum. The patient's age and mechanism of injury are important. If a fracture occurs with trivial trauma, suspect a pathological lesion. Pain, bruising and swelling are common symptoms. Deformity is more suggestive.

(2) Signs

To elicit crepitus or abnormal movement is unnecessarily painful; X-ray diagnosis is more reliable. Nevertheless the familiar headings of clinical examinations should always be considered, or damage to arteries, nerves and ligaments may be overlooked. A systemic approach is always helpful:

- Examine the most obvious injured part.
- Test for artery and nerve damage.
- Look for associated injuries in the region.
- Look for associated injuries in distant parts.

Look: Swelling and deformity may be obvious, but important point is whether skin is intact; if the skin is broken and wound communicates with the fractures, the injury is called "open". Also note the posture of distal extremity and color of the skin.

Feel: Injured part is palpated for tenderness. Some factures need specifically looked for, e. g. , the classical sign of a fractured scaphoid is tenderness on pressure precisely in the anatomical snuff-box. The common and characteristic associated injuries should also be felt. For example, an isolated fracture of the proximal fibula should always look for the likelihood of an associated fracture or ligament injury of the ankle, and in high energy injuries always examine spine and pelvis.

Move: Crepitus and abnormal movement may be present, but shouldn't inflict pain when X-rays are available. It is more important to ask the patient can move the joints distal to the injury.

(3) X-ray

X-ray examination is mandatory. The rule of twos is important to remember:

Two views: A fracture or a dislocation may not be seen on a single X-ray film, and at least two views (anteroposterior and lateral) must be taken.

Two joints: In the forearm or leg, one bone may be fractured and angulated. The joints above and below the fracture must both be included on the X-ray films.

Two limbs: In children, the appearance of immature epiphyses may confuse the diagnosis of a fracture; X-rays of the uninjured limb are needed for comparison.

Two injuries: Severe force often causes injuries at more than one level. Thus, with fractures of the calcaneum or femur it is important to also X-ray the pelvis and spine.

Two occasions: Some fractures are notoriously difficult to detect soon after injury, but another X-ray examination a week or two later may show the lesion.

(4) Special imaging

Sometimes the fracture or the full extent of the fracture is not appearent on the plain X-ray. Computed tomography may be helpful in lesions of the spine or for complex joint fractures. Magnetic resonance imaging may be the only way of showing whether a fractured vertebra is threatening to compress the spinal cord. Radioisotope scanning is helpful in diagnosing a suspected stress fractures or other undisplaced fractures.

48.5 Secondary Injuries

Certain fractures cause secondary injuries and these should always be assumed to have occurred until proved otherwise. Such as thoracic injuries, spinal cord injuries, pelvic and abdominal injuries.

48.6 Fracture Healing

The way a fracture heals depends on the amount of movement occurring between fragments, described in Perren's strain theory. Where there is some movement at the fracture, secondary bone healing occurs, with a gradual transition of tissue types from flexible to rigid as healing progresses. Where there is no movement bone heals directly with bone.

48.6.1 Secondary bone healing (healing with callus)

Under most circumstances, there is movement at the fracture site and bone heals with callus in four phases:

· Inflammation (week 1): The injury causes a hematoma and local inflammation. There is an influx of neutrophils, macrophages and fibroblasts from surrounding soft tissues, and granulation tissue is formed. There is erythema, heat, swelling, and pain (rubor, calor, tumor and dolor).

· Soft callus (weeks 2-3): the fracture ends become more evident on radiography. The granulation tissue is gradually replaced by fibroblasts and chondroblasts. The fracture ends movement is reduced.

· Hard callus (weeks 4-12): Bone formation (by osteoclasts) begins within the soft callus where the strain is lowest. Bone can be formed in two ways: by intramembranous and by endochondral ossification. Calcium is laid down in the matrix and the callus then becomes visible on radiography. The fracture has consolidated once it has completely healed with bridging bone.

· Remodeling (months to years): Creeping substitution replaces the woven bone with lamellar bone. Bone is laid down according to Wolff's law: the highest density of lamellar bone (and strength) is restored where the load is greatest. In children, the prominent callus bump shrinks and radiographs can return to normal. In adults, this process is rarely complete.

48.6.2 Primary bone healing

If the fracture is reduced and held absolutely rigid then the bone heals directly with bone by the same mechanism as intact or woven bone remodels itself. Osteoclasts form a specialized membrane, which adheres to the woven bone, creating Howship's lacunae. Osteolytic enzymes are discharged into the lacunae and bone is resorbed. A "cutting cone" is formed as the line of osteoclastic resorption is followed by a trail of osteoblasts, which lay down organized lamellar bone to create a brand new Haversian system.

48.6.3 Assessment of healing

A fracture is said to have united when the signs of a fractures have resolved such that the following:

· there is no local tenderness or heat.

· there is no abnormal movement or crepitus.

· there is no pain or normal loading.

· the radiographs demonstrate that the fracture has healed.

48.7 Treatment of Closed Fractures

Treatment consists of manipulation to improve the position of the fragments, followed by splintage to hold them together. The objectives are covered by three simple injunctions: reduction, hold and exercise.

48.7.1 Reduction

Reduction should aim for adequate apposition and normal alignment of the bone fragments. A gap between fragment ends is a common cause of delayed union or non-union. There are two methods of reduction: closed and open.

(1) Closed reduction

Under appropriate anaesthesia and muscle relaxation, the fracture is reduced. This is most effective when periosteum and muscles on one side of the fracture remain intact; the soft tissue strap prevents over-reduction and stabilizes the fracture. Skeletal or skin traction for several days allows better alignment to be obtained. In general, closed reduction is used for all minimally displaced fractures, for most fractures in children and for fractures that are not unstable after reduction and can be held in some form of splint or cast.

(2) Open reduction

Operative reduction of the fracture under direct vision is indicated the following: ①When closed reduction fails. ②When there is a large articular fragment that needs accurate positioning. ③For traction (avulsion) fractures in which the fragments are held apart. As a rule, however, open reduction is merely the first step to internal fixation.

48.7.2 Hold

The objective of holding is prevention of displacement. The restriction of movement is needed to promote soft tissue healing and to allow free movement of the unaffected parts. The available methods of holding reduction are as follows:

- continuous traction.
- cast splintage.
- functional bracing.
- internal fixation.
- external fixation.

(1) Continuous traction

Traction is applied to the limb distal to the fracture, to exert a continuous pulling the long axis of the bone, with a counterforce in the opposite direction. Traction can hold a fracture still; it can pull a long bone straight and hold it out to length but to maintain accurate reduction is sometimes difficult. Meanwhile the patient can move the joints and exercise the muscles.

1) Traction by gravity: This applies only to upper limb injuries. Thus, with a wrist sling the weight of the arm provides continuous traction to the humerus. For comfort and stability, especially with a transverse fracture, a U-slab of plaster may be bandaged on from the axilla to just above the elbow is held on with Velcro.

2) Skin traction: Skin traction will sustain a pull of no more than 4 or 5 kg. Holland strapping or one-way-stretch Elastoplast is stuck to the skin and held on with a bandage. The malleoli are protected by Gam-

gee tissue, and cords or tapes are used for traction.

3) Skeletal traction: A stiff wire or pin is inserted usually behind the tibial tubercle for hip, thigh and knee injuries, or through the calcaneum for tibial fractures and cords tied to them for applying traction. Whether by skin or skeletal traction, the fracture is reduced and held in one of three ways: fixed traction, balanced traction or a combination of the two.

Complications of traction

· Circulatory embarrassment: In children especially, traction tapes and circular bandages may constrict the circulation; for this reason "gallows traction", in which the baby's legs are suspended from an overhead beam, should never be used for children over 12 kg in weight.

· Nerve injury: In older people, leg traction may predispose to peroneal nerve injury and cause a drop foot; the limb should be checked repeatedly to see that it does not roll into external rotation during traction.

· Pin site infection: Pin sites must be kept clean and should be checked daily.

(2) Cast splintage

Plaster of Paris is widely used as a splint. It is safe enough, so long as the practitioner is alert to the danger of a tight cast and provided pressure sores are prevented. Holding reduction is usually no problem and patients with tibial fractures can bear weight on the cast.

(3) Functional bracing

Functional bracing, using either plaster of Paris or one of the lighter thermoplastic materials, is one way of preventing joint stiffness while still permitting fracture splintage and loading. The splints are "functional" in that joint movements are much less restricted that with conventional casts.

(4) Internal fixation

Bone fragments may be fixed with screws, a metal plate held by screws, a long intramedullary rod or nail (with or without locking screws), circumferential bands or a combination of these methods. Properly applied, internal fixation holds a fracture securely so that movement can begin at once; with early movement the "fracture disease" (stiffness and edema) is abolished. As far as speed is concerned, the patient can leave hospital as soon as the wound is healed. Even though the bone moves in one piece, the fracture is not united, it is merely held by a metal bridge and unprotected weight bearing is, for some time, unsafe.

Indication:

· Fractures that can not be reduced except by operation.

· Fractures that are inherently unstable and prone to re-displace after reduction. Also included are those fractures liable to be pulled apart by muscle action.

· Fractures that unite poorly and slowly, principally fractures of the femoral neck.

· Pathological fractures in which bone disease may prevent healing.

· Multiple fractures where early fixation reduces the risk of general complications and late multisystem organ failure.

· Fractures in patients who present nursing difficulties.

Complications: Most of the complications of internal fixations are due to poor technique, poor equipment or poor operating conditions. These are iatrogenic infection, non-union, implant failure and refracture.

(5) External fixation

A fracture may be held by transfixing screws or tensioned wires that pass through the bone above and below the fracture and are attached to an external frame. This is especially applicable to the tibia and pelvis, but the method is also used for fractures of the femur, humerus, lower radius and even bones of hand.

Indication:

· Fractures associated with severe soft-tissue damage (including open fracture) where internal fixation is risky and repeated access is needed for wound inspection, dressing or plastic surgery.

· Fractures around joints that are potentially suitable for internal fixation but the soft tissues are too swollen to allow safe surgery.

· Patients with severe multiple injuries, especially if there are bilateral femoral fractures, fractures with severe bleeding, and those with limb and associated chest or head injuries.

· Ununited fractures, which can be excised and compressed; sometimes this is combined with bone lengthening to replace the excised segment.

· Infected fractures, for which internal fixation might not be suitable.

Complications of external fixation:

The damage to soft tissues, over distraction or pin-track infection are due to injury by transfixing pins or wire, no contact between fracture fragments or because of poor operative techniques.

48.8 Conservative Management

Prevention edema: swelling is almost evitable after fracture and may cause skin stretching and blisters. Persistent edema is an important cause of joint stiffness, should be prevented and treated by a combination of elevation and exercise.

48.9 Treatment of Open Fractures

48.9.1 Initial management

Patient with open fractures may have multiple injuries; a rapid general assessment and any life threatening conditions are addressed. Wound is carefully inspected; any gross contaminated is removed, and the area is covered with a saline-soaked dressing under impervious seal to prevent dessication. This is left undisturbed until the patient is in operating room. The patient is given antibiotics, usually co-amoxiclav or cefuroxime, but clindamycin if the patient is allergic to penicillin. Tetanus prophylaxis is administered: toxoid for those previously immunized, human antiserum if not.

The limb circulation and distal neurological status will need checking repeatedly, particularly after any reduction manoeuvres.

48.9.2 Classifying the injury

Treatment is determined by the type of fracture, the nature of soft tissue injury (including wound size) and the degree of contamination. Gustilo's classification of open fractures is widely used:

Type 1: Wound is small, clean puncture through which a bone spike has protruded. There is little soft tissue damage with no crushing and the fracture is not comminuted.

Type 2: The wound is more than 1 cm long but absence of skin flap. Soft tissue damage is not extensive.

Type 3: There is a large laceration, extensive damage to skin and underlying soft tissue and in most severe examples, vascular compromise. The injury is caused by high energy transfer to the bone and soft tissues. Contamination can be significant.

There are three grades of severity. In type 3A the fractured bone can be adequately covered by soft tissue despite laceration. In type 3B there is extensive periosteal stripping and fracture cover is not possible without use of local or distant flaps. The fracture is classified as type 3C if there is an arterial injury that needs to be repaired, regardless of the amount of other soft-tissue damage.

48.9.3 Principles of treatment

All open fractures must be assumed to be contaminated; it is important to try to prevent them from becoming infected. The four essentials are as follows:

- Antibiotic prophylaxis.
- Urgent wound and fracture debridement.
- Stabilization of the fracture.
- Early definitive wound cover.

Sterility and antibiotic cover: The wound should be kept covered until the patients reaches the operation room. In most cases co-amoxiclav or cefuroxime (or clindamycin in penicillin allergy) is given as soon as possible. At the time of debridement, gentamicin is added. Only cefuroxime or co-amoxiclav is continued thereafter. In case of infections of open fractures are caused by hospital-acquired bacteria, gentamicin and vancomycin are given at the time of definitive wound cover. The total period of antibiotic use for these fractures should not be greater than 72 hours.

Debridement: Under appropriate anaesthesia the dressing previously applied to the wound is replaced by a sterile pad and the surrounding skin is cleaned. The pad is then taken off and the wound is irrigated thoroughly with copious amount of physiological saline. The wound is covered again and the patient's limb then prepared and draped for surgery.

Wound closure: A small, uncontaminated wound in a grade1 or 2 fracture may be sutured without tension. In more severe grades of injury, immediate fracture stabilization and wound cover using split-skin grafts, local or distant flaps is ideal. Adding gentamicin leads under the dressing has been shown to help, as has the use of vacuum dressings. Return to surgery for a "second look" should have definitive fracture cover as an objective. It should be done by 48-72 hours, and not later than 5 days.

48.10 Complications of Fractures

48.10.1 Early complications

Early complications may present as part of the primary injury or may appear only after a few days or weeks. These are visceral injury, vascular injury, compartment syndrome, Haemarthrosis, gas gangrene, infection, plaster and pressure sores, fracture blisters.

Compartment syndrome: Compartment syndrome is the development of muscle swelling within an indestensible fascial compartment, resulting in increased intracompartmental pressure and tissue hypoperfusion. If left untreated, the tissues within the compartment become ischaemic, dysfunctional and then necrotic. Compartment syndrome is therefore a surgical emergency. Some of the causes of compartment syndrome are fractures, blunt contusion, extravasation and reperfusion injury.

Clinical features of compartment syndrome: High-risk injuries are fractures of the elbow, forearm bones, proximal third of the tibia, and also multiple fractures of the hand or foot, crush injuries and circumferential burns. Other precipitating factors are operation (usually internal fixation) or infection. The classic features of ischemia are the five Ps:

- Pain.
- Paraesthesia.
- Pallor.
- Paralysis.
- Pulselessness.

In compartment syndrome the ischemia occurs at the capillary level, so pulses may still be felt and the skin may not be pale. The earliest of the classic features are pain, altered sensibility and paresis (weakness in active muscle contraction).

Treatment of compartment syndrome: The threatened compartment must be promptly decompressed. Casts, bandages and dressings must be completely removed–merely splitting the plaster is useless and the limb should be nursed flat. The *P* should be carefully monitored, if it falls below 30 mmHg, immediate open fasciotomy is performed. The wound should be left open and inspected 2 days later; if there is muscle necrosis, debridement can be carried out, if the tissues are healthy, the wounds can be sutured (without tension) or skin-grafted.

48.10.2 Late complications

Delayed complications of fractures may occur after treatment such as delayed union, non-union, malunion, avascular necrosis, growth disturbance, bed sores, myositis ossificans, nerve compression, muscle contracture, joint stiffness, osteoarthritis, complex regional pain syndrome.

Part 49

Fractures of Upper Limb

Chapter 1

Introduction

Low back pain is common. It occurs in both developed and developed and developing countries and all age groups from children to the elderly population. Globally, people lived with disability caused by low back pain increased population and aging. Low back pain is now the leading cause of disability worldwide, For nearly all people with low back pain, it is not possible to identify a specific nociceptive cause. Only a small proportion of people have a well understood. pathdogical cause, such as a vertebral fracture, malignancy, or infection. People with physically demanding jobs, physical and mental comorbidtities, smokers, and obese individuals are at grecstest risk.

Chapter 2

Disorders of the Scapula and Clavicle

2.1 Clinical Features

Two similar, and possibly related, conditions are encountered: Sprengel's deformity and Klippel-Feil syndrome. Sprengel's deformity is the cardinal symptom and it may be noticed at birth. The shoulder on the affected side is elevated; the scapula looks and feels abnormally high, smaller than usual and somewhat prominent; occasionally both scapulae are affected. The neck appears shorter than usual and there may be kyphosis or scoliosis of the upper thoracic spine. Shoulder movements are painless but abduction and elevation may be limited by the fixation of the scapula. X-rays will show the elevated scapula and any associated vertebral anomalies; sometimes there is also a bony bridge between the scapula and the cervical spine (the omovertebral bar). Klippel-Feil syndrome: This is usually a more widespread disorder. There is bilateral failure of scapular descent associated with marked anomalies of the cervical spine and failure of fusion of the occipital bones. Patients look as if they have no neck; there is a low

2.2 Treatment

Mild cases are best left untreated. Surgical treatment aims to decrease deformity and improve shoulder function. In children under 6 years of age, the scapula can be repositioned by releasing the muscles along the vertebral and superior borders of thescapula, excising the supraspinous portion of the scapula and the omovertebral bar, pulling the scapula down, then reattaching the muscles to hold it firmly in its new position. In older children, this carries a risk of brachial nerve compression or traction between the clavicle and first rib; here it is safer merely to excise the supraspinous portion of the scapula in order to improve the appearance but without improving movement. Before undertaking any operation the cervical spine should be carefully imaged in order to identify any abnormalities of the odontoid process or base of skull.

Chapter 3

Injuries of the Shoudler and Upper Arm

3.1 Fractures of the Clavicle

3.1.1 Mechanism of injury

A fall on the shoulder or the outstretched hand may break the clavicle. In the common midshaft fracture, the lateral fragment is pulled down by the weight of the arm and the inner, medial half is held up by the sternomastoid muscle. In fractures of the lateral end, if the ligaments are intact, there is little displacement; but if the coracoclavicular ligaments are torn, or if the fracture is just medial to these ligaments, displacement may be more severe and closed reduction impossible. The clavicle is also a reasonably common site for pathological fractures.

3.1.2 Clinical features

The arm is clasped to the chest to prevent movement. A subcutaneous lump may be obvious and occasionally a sharp fragment threatens the skin. Although vascular complications are rare, it is prudent to feel the pulse and gently to palpate the root of the neck. Outer third fractures are easily missed or mistaken for acromioclavicular joint injuries.

3.1.3 Imaging

Radiographic analysis requires at least an anteroposterior view and another taken with a 30 degree cephalic tilt. The fracture is usually in the middle third of the bone, and the outer fragment usually lies below the inner. Fractures of the outer third may be missed, or the degree of displacement underestimated, unless additional views of the shoulder are obtained. With medial-third fractures it is also wise to obtain X-rays of the sternoclavicular joint. In assessing clinical progress, remember that "clinical" union usually precedes "radiological" union by several weeks.

CT scanning with three-dimensional reconstructions may be needed to determine accurately the degree of shortening or for diagnosing asternoclavicular fracture-dislocation, and also to establish whether a fracture has united.

3.1.4 Classification

Clavicle fractures are usually classified on the basis of their location:

- Group Ⅰ: middle-third fractures.
- Group Ⅱ: lateral-third fractures.
- Group Ⅲ: medial-third fractures.

3.1.5 Treatment

3.1.5.1 Middle-third fractures

There is general agreement that undisplaced fractures should be treated non-operatively. Most will go on to unite uneventfully with a non-union rate below 5% and a return to normal function. Non-operative management consists of applying a simple sling for comfort. It is discarded once the pain subsides (after 1-3 weeks) and the patient is then encouraged to mobilize the limb as pain allows. There is no evidence that the traditional figure-of-eight bandage confers any advantage and it carries the risk of increasing the incidence of pressures sores over the fracture site and causing harm to neurological structures; it may even increase the risk of non-union. There is less agreement about the management of displaced middle-third fractures. Treating those with shortening of more than 2 cm by simple splintage is now believed to incur a considerable risk of symptomatic malunion—mainly pain and lack of power during shoulder movements-and an increased incidence of non-union. There is, therefore, a growing trend towards internal fixation of acute clavicular fractures associated with severe displacement, fragmentation or shortening. Methods include plating (specific contoured locking plates are available) and intramedullary fixation.

3.1.5.2 Lateral-third fractures

Most lateral clavicle fractures are minimally displaced and extra-articular. The fact that the coracoclavicular ligaments are intact prevents further displacement and non-operative management is usually appropriate. Treatment consists of a sling for 2-3 weeks until the pain subsides, followed by mobilization within the limits of pain. Displaced lateral-third fractures are associated with disruption of the coracoclavicular ligaments and are therefore unstable injuries. A number of studies have shown that these particular fractures have a higher than usual rate of non-union if treated non-operatively. Surgery to stabilize the fracture is often recommended. However, the converse argument is that many of the fractures that develop non-union do not cause any symptoms and surgery can therefore be reserved for patients with symptomatic non-union. Operations for these fractures have higher complication rates and no single procedure has been shown to be better than the others. Techniques include the use of a coracoclavicular screw and plate, hook plate fixation, suture and sling techniques with Dacron graft ligaments and the more recent lateral clavicle locking plates.

3.1.5.3 Medial-third fractures

Most of these rare fractures are extra-articular. They are mainly managed non-operatively unless the fracture displacement threatens the mediastinal structures. Initial fixation is associated with significant complications, including migration of the implants into the mediastinum, particularly when K-wires are used. Other methods of stabilization include suture and graft techniques and the newer locking plates.

3.2 Acromioclavicular Joint Injuries

3.2.1 Mechanism of injury

A fall on the shoulder with the arm adducted may strain or tear the acromioclavicular ligaments and upward subluxation of the clavicle may occur; if the force is severe enough, the coracoclavicular ligaments will also be torn, resulting in complete dislocation of the joint.

Pathological anatomy and classification: The injury is graded according to the type of ligament injury and the amount ofdisplacement of the joint.

- Type Ⅰ: This is an acute sprain of the acromioclavicular ligaments; the joint is undisplaced.
- Type Ⅱ: The acromioclavicular ligaments are torn and the joint is subluxated with slight elevation of the clavicle.
- Type Ⅲ: The acromioclavicular and coracoclavicular ligaments are torn and the joint is dislocated; the clavicle is elevated (or the acromion depressed) creating a visible and palpable "step". Other types of displacement are less common, but occasionally the clavicle is displaced posteriorly (type Ⅳ), very markedly upwards (type Ⅴ) or inferiorly beneath the coracoid process (type Ⅵ).

3.2.2 Clinical features

The patient can usually point to the site of injury and the area may be bruised. If there is tenderness but no deformity, the injury is probably a sprain or a subluxation. With dislocation the patient may be in severe pain and a prominent "step" can be seen and felt. Shoulder movements may also be limited.

3.2.3 X-rays

The acromioclavicular joint is not always easily visualized; anteroposterior, cephalic tilt and axillary views are advisable. In addition, a stress view is sometimes helpful in distinguishing between a type Ⅱ and type Ⅲ injury: this is an anteroposterior X-ray including both shoulders with the patient standing upright, arms by the side and holding a 5 kg weight in each hand. The distance between the coracoid process and the inferior border of the clavicle is measured on each side; a difference of more than 50% is diagnostic of acromioclavicular dislocation.

3.2.4 Treatment

Sprains and subluxations often do not affect function and do not require any special treatment; the arm is rested in a sling until pain subsides (usually no more than a week) and shoulder exercises are then begun. Dislocations are poorly controlled by padding and bandaging, yet the role of surgery in type III injuries remains controversial. The large number of operations described suggests that none is ideal. There is no convincing evidence that surgery provides a better functional result than conservative treatment for a straightforward type III injury. Operative repair should be considered only for patients with extreme prominence of the clavicle, those with posterior or inferior dislocation of the clavicle and those who aim to resume strenuous overarm or overhead activities. While there is no consensus regarding the best surgical solution, there are a number of underlying principles to consider if surgery is contemplated. Accurate reduction should be the goal. The ligamentous stability can be recreated either by transferring existing ligaments (the coracoacromial or conjoined tendons),or by using a free graft(e. g. ,autogenous semitendinosis or a synthetic ligament). This reconstruction must have sufficient stability to prevent re-dislocation during recovery. Any rigid implants which cross the joint will need to be removed at a later date to prevent loosening or fracture. In the modified Weaver-Dunn procedure the lateral end of the clavicle is excised and the coracoacromial ligament is transferred to the outer end of the clavicle and attached by transosseous sutures. Tension on the repair can be reduced either by anchoring the clavicle to the coracoid with various techniques such as anchors or slings around the coracoid and clavicle. Great care is needed to avoid entrapment or damage to a nerve or vessel. Elbow and forearm exercises are begun on the day after operation and active-assisted shoulder movements 2 weeks later,increasing gradually to active movements at 4-6 weeks. Strenuous lifting movementsare avoided for 4-6 months. An alternative procedure is to use a synthetic graft which wraps around the coracoid and is secured around the clavicle by various techniques. Recent advances in instrumentation have made it feasible to perform this type of reconstructive surgery arthroscopically.

Chapter 4

Dislocation of the Shoulder

4.1 Anterior Dislocation of the Shoulder

4.1.1 Mechanism of injury

Dislocation is usually caused by a fall on the hand. The head of the humerus is driven forward, tearing the capsule and producing avulsion of the glenoid labrum (the Bankart lesion). Occasionally the posterolateral part of the head is crushed, giving rise to a Hill–Sachs lesion. Rarely, the acromion process levers the head downwards and the joint dislocates with the arm pointing upwards (luxation erecta); nearly always the arm then drops, bringing the head to its subcoracoid position. In patients with constitutionally lax shoulders, minimal trauma may be involved.

4.1.2 Clinical features

Pain is often severe. The patient supports the arm with the opposite hand and is loathe to permit any kind of examination. The lateral outline of the shoulder may be flattened and, if the patient is not too muscular, a bulge may be felt just below the clavicle. The arm must always be examined for nerve and vessel injury before reduction is attempted.

4.1.3 X–rays

The anteroposterior X–rays will show the overlapping shadows of the humeral head and glenoid fossa, with the head usually lying below and medial to the socket. A lateral view aimed along the blade of the scapula will show the humeral head out of line with the socket. If the joint has dislocated before, special views may show flattening or an excavation of the posterolateral contour of the humeral head, where it has been indented by the anterior edge of the glenoid socket, the Hill–Sachs lesion.

4.1.4 Treatment

Various methods of reduction have been described, some of them now of no more than historical interest. In a patient who has had previous dislocations, simple traction on the arm may be successful. Usually, sedation and occasionally general anaesthesia is required.

· Stimson's technique: The patient is left prone with the arm hanging over the side of the bed. After 15 or 20 minutes the shoulder may reduce.

· Hippocratic method: Gently increasing traction is applied to the arm with the shoulder in slight abduction, while an assistant applies firm countertraction to the body (a towel slung around the patient's chest, under the axilla, is helpful).

· Kocher's method: The elbow is bent to 90 degrees and held close to the body; no traction should be applied. The arm is slowly rotated 75 degrees laterally, then the point of the elbow is lifted forwards, and finally the arm is rotated medially. This technique carries the risk of nerve, vessel and bone injury and is not recommended. Another technique has the patient sitting on a reduction chair and with gentle traction of the arm over the back of the padded chair the dislocation is reduced. An X-ray is taken to confirm reduction and exclude a fracture. When the patient is fully awake, active abduction is gently tested to exclude an axillary nerve injury and rotator cuff tear. The median, radial, ulnar and musculocutaneous nerves are also tested and the pulse is felt. The arm is rested in a sling for about 3 weeks in those under 30 years of age (who are most prone to recurrence) and for only 1 week in those over 30 (who are most prone to stiffness). Then movements are begun, but combined abduction and lateral rotation must be avoided for at least 3 weeks. Throughout this period, elbow and finger movements are practised every day. There has been some interest in the use of external rotation splints, based on the theory that this would reduce the Bankart lesion into a better position for healing. However, a recent Cochrane review has concluded that there is insufficient evidence to inform on the choices for conservative treatment and that further trials are needed to compare different types and duration of immobilization. Young athletes who dislocate their shoulder traumatically and who continue to pursue their sports (particularly contact sports) are at a much higher risk of re-dislocation in the future. The rates of recurrent instability depend on the size of the Hill-Sachs lesion, the presence of other bony injuries such as glenoid rim fractures and thestate of the soft tissues. The rates of recurrent instability vary in particular with the age of the patient. After traumatic dislocation these rates can vary from 17% to 96% with increased rates in younger patients. This knowledge, combined with better arthroscopic instrumentation, has led to a recent increase in surgical stabilization after a single anterior dislocation in young sporting patients.

4.2 Posterior Dislocation of the Shoulder

4.2.1 Mechanism of injury

Indirect force producing marked internal rotation and adduction needs be very severe to cause a dislocation. This happens most commonly during a fit or convulsion, or with an electric shock. Posterior dislocation can also follow a fall on the flexed, adducted arm, a direct blow to the front of the shoulder or a fall on the outstretched hand.

4.2.2 Imaging

On AP X-rays the humeral head, because it is medially rotated, looks abnormal in shape (like an electric light bulb) and it stands away somewhat from the glenoid fossa (the "empty glenoid" sign). A lateral film and axillary view is essential; it shows posterior subluxation or dislocation and sometimes a deep indentation on the anterior aspect of the humeral head. Posterior dislocation is sometimes complicated by fractures of the humeral neck, posterior glenoid rim or lesser tuberosity. Sometimes the patient is too uncomfortable to permit adequate imaging and in these difficult cases CT is essential to rule out posterior dislocation of the shoulder.

4.2.3 Treatment

The acute dislocation is reduced (usually under general anaesthesia) by pulling on the arm with the shoulder in adduction; a few minutes are allowed for the head of the humerus to disengage and the arm is then gently rotated laterally while the humeral head is pushed forwards. If reduction feels stable, the arm is immobilized in a sling; otherwise the shoulder is held widely abducted and laterally rotated in an airplane-type splint for 3-6 weeks to allow the posterior capsule to heal in the shortest position. Shoulder movement is regained by active exercises.

4.3 Inferior Dislocation of the Shoulder

4.3.1 Mechanism of injury and pathology

The injury is caused by a severe hyperabduction force. With the humerus as the lever and the acromion as the fulcrum, the humeral head is lifted across the inferior rim of the glenoid socket; it remains in the sub-glenoid position, with the humeral shaft pointing upwards. Soft-tissue injury may be severe and includes avulsion of the capsule and surrounding tendons, rupture of muscles, fractures of the glenoid or proximal humerus and damage to the brachial plexus and axillary artery.

4.3.2 X-rays

The humeral shaft is shown in the abducted position with the head sitting below the glenoid. It is important to search for associated fractures of the glenoid or proximal humerus.

4.3.3 Treatment

Inferior dislocation can usually be reduced by pulling upwards in the line of the abducted arm, with countertraction downwards over the top of the shoulder. If the humeral head is stuck in the soft tissues, open reduction is needed. It is important to examine again, after reduction, for evidence of neurovascular injury. The arm is rested in a sling until pain subsides and movement is then allowed, but avoiding abduction for 3 weeks to allow the soft tissues to heal.

Chapter 5

Fractures of the Proximal Humerus

5.1 Classification and Pathological Anatomy

The most widely accepted classification is that proposed by Neer in 1970 who drew attention to the four major segments involved in these injuries: the head of the humerus, the lesser tuberosity, the greater tuberosity and the shaft. Neer's classification distinguishes between the number of displaced fragments, with displacement defined as greater than 45 degrees of angulation or 1 cm of separation. Thus, however many fracture lines there are, if the fragments are undisplaced, it is regarded as a one-part fracture; if one segment is separated from the others, it is a two-part fracture; if two fragments are displaced, that is a three-part fracture; if all the major parts are displaced, it is a four-part fracture. Furthermore, a fracture-dislocation exists when the head is dislocated and there are two, three or four parts. This grading is based on X-ray appearances, although observers do not always agree with each other on which class a particular fracture falls into.

5.2 Clinical Features

Because the fracture is often firmly impacted, pain may not be severe. However, the appearance of a large bruise on the upper part of the arm is suspicious. Signs of axillary nerve or brachial plexus injury should be sought.

5.3 Imaging

In elderly patients there often appears to be a single, impacted fracture extending across the surgical neck. However, with good X-rays, several undisplaced fragments may be seen. In younger patients, the fragments are usually more clearly separated. Axillary and scapular-lateral views should always be obtained, to exclude dislocation of the shoulder. It has always been difficult to apply Neer's classification when based on plain X-rays, and not surprisingly there is a relatively high level of both inter- and intraobserver disagreement. Neer himself later noted that, when this classification was developed, the criteria for displacement (distance >1 cm, angulation >45 degrees) were set arbitrarily. The classification was not intended to dictate treatment, but simply to help clarify the pathoanatomy of the different fracture patterns. The advent of 3D CT reconstruction has helped to reduce the degree of inter– and intraobserver error, enabling better planning of treatment than in the past. As the fracture heals, the humeral head is sometimes seen to be subluxated downwards (inferiorly); this is due to muscle atony and it usually recovers once exercises are begun.

5.4 Treatment

5.4.1 Minimally displaced fractures

These comprise the vast majority. They need no treatment apart from period of a week or two of rest with the arm in a sling until the pain subsides, and then gentle passive movements of the shoulder. Once the fracture has united (usually after 6 weeks), active exercises are encouraged; the elbow and hand are, of course, actively exercised from the start

5.4.2 Two–part fractures

Surgical neck fractures The fragments are gently manipulated into alignment and the arm is immobilized in a sling for about 4 weeks or until the fracture feels stable and the X–rays show some signs of healing. Elbow and hand exercises are encouraged throughout this period; shoulder exercises are commenced at about 4 weeks. The results of conservative treatment are generally satisfactory, considering that most of these patients are over 65 and do not demand perfect function. If the fracture can not be reduced closed or if the fracture is very unstable after closed reduction, then fixation is required. Options include percutaneous pins, bone sutures, intramedullary pins with tension band wiring or a locked intramedullary nail. Plate fixation requires a wider exposure and the newer locking plates offer a stable fixation without the need for extensive periosteal stripping. Fracture of the greater tuberosity is often associated with anterior dislocation and it reduces to a good position when the shoulder is relocated. If it does not reduce, the fragment can be reattached through a small incision with interosseous sutures or, in young hard bone, cancellous screws. Anatomical neck fractures are very rare. In young patients the fracture should be fixed. In older patients prosthetic replacement (hemiarthroplasty) is preferable because of the high risk of avascular necrosis of the humeral head.

5.4.3 Three–part fractures

These usually involve displacement of the surgical neck and the greater tuberosity; they are extremely difficult to reduce closed. In active individuals this injury is best managed by open reduction and internal fixation. There is little evidence that one technique is better than another although the newer implants with locked plating and nailing are biomechanically superior in osteoporotic bone.

5.4.4 Four–part fractures

The surgical neck and both tuberosities are displaced. These are severe injuries with a high risk of complications such as vascular injury, brachial plexus damage, injuries of the chest wall and (later) avascular necrosis of the humeral head. The X–ray diagnosis is difficult (how many fragments are there, and are they displaced?). Often the most one can say is that there are "multiple displaced fragments", sometimes together with glenohumeral dislocation. In young patients an attempt should be made at reconstruction (Figure 24.18c,d). In older patients, closed treatment and attempts at open reduction and fixation can result in continuing pain and stiffness and additional surgical treatment can compromise the blood supply still further. If the fracture pattern is such that the blood supply is likely to be compromised, or that reconstruction and internal fixation will be extremely difficult, then the treatment of choice is prosthetic replacement of the proximal humerus. The results of hemiarthroplasty are somewhat unpredictable. Anatomical reduction, fixation and healing of the tuberosities are prerequisites for a satisfactory outcome; even then, secondary displacement of the tuberosities may result in a poor functional outcome. In addition the prosthetic implant should be perfectly positioned. Be warned—these are operations for the expert. More recently the reverse shoulder replacements have been used in these fractures although the longterm outcomes are not yet known. Decision making in all of these fractures remains difficult and current evidence remains unclear whether surgical management actually improves the overall outcome in these serious fractures.

5.4.5 Fracture-dislocations

Two-part fracture-dislocations (greater tuberosity with anterior dislocation and lesser tuberosity with posterior) can usually be reduced by closed means. Three-part fracture-dislocations, when the surgical neck is also broken, usually require open reduction and fixation; the brachial plexus is at particular risk during this operation. Four-part fracture-dislocations have a poor prognosis; prosthetic replacement is recommended in all but young and very active patients.

Chapter 6

Fractured Shaft of Humerus

6.1 Mechanism of Injury

A fall on the hand may twist the humerus, causing a spiral fracture. A fall on the elbow with the arm abducted exerts a bending force, resulting in an oblique or transverse fracture. A direct blow to the arm causes a fracture which is either transverse or comminuted. Fracture of the shaft in an elderly patient may be due to a metastas.

6.2 Clinical Features

The arm is painful, bruised and swollen. It is important to test for radial nerve function before and after treatment. This is best done by assessing active extension of the metacarpophalangeal joints; active extension of the wrist can be misleading because extensor carpi radialis longus is sometimes supplied by a branch arising proximal to the injury.

6.3 Treatment

6.3.1 Non-operative treatment

Fractures of the humerus heal readily. They require neither perfect reduction nor immobilization; the weight of the arm with an external cast is usually enough to pull the fragments into alignment. A "hanging cast" is applied from shoulder to wrist with the elbow flexed 90 degrees, and the forearm section is suspended by a sling around the patient's neck. This cast may be replaced after 2–3 weeks by a short (shoulder to elbow) cast or a functional. The wrist and fingers are exercised from the start. Pendulum exercises of the shoulder are begun within a week, but active abduction is postponed until the fracture has united (about 6 weeks for spiral fractures but often twice as long for other types); once united, only a sling is needed until the fracture is consolidated polypropylene brace which is worn for a further 6 weeks.

6.3.2 Operative treatment

Patients often find the hanging cast uncomfortable, tedious and frustrating; they can feel the fragments moving and that is sometimes quite distressing. The temptation is to "do something", and the "something" usually means an operation. It is as well to remember that the complication rate after internal fixation of the humerus is high; that the great majority of humeral fractures unite with non-operative treatment; there is no good evidence that the union rate is higher with fixation (and the rate may be lower if there is distraction with nailing or periosteal strippingwith plating). There are, nevertheless, some well-de fined indications for surgery:

· Severe multiple injuries.

· An open fracture.

· Segmental fractures.

· Displaced intra-articular extension of the fracture.

· A pathological fracture.

· A "floating elbow" (simultaneous unstable humeral and forearm fractures).

· Radial nerve palsy after manipulation.

· Non-union.

· Problems with nursing care in a dependent person. Fixation can be achieved with the following: ①a compression plate and screws; ②an interlocking intramedullary nail or semi-flexible pins; ③an external fixator (Figures 24.21 and 24.22). Plating permits excellent reduction and fixation, and it has the added advantage that it does not interfere with shoulder or elbow function. However, it requires wide dissection and the radial nerve must be protected. Too much periosteal stripping or inadequate fixation will probably increase the risk of non-union. Antegrade nailing is performed with a rigid interlocking nail inserted through the rotator cuff under fluoroscopic control. It requires minimal dissection but has the disadvantage that it causes rotator cuff problems in a significant proportion of cases (the reported incidence is 5%-40%). The nail can also distract the fracture which will inhibit union; if this happens, exchange nailing and bone grafting of the fracture may be needed. Retrograde nailing with multiple flexible rods is not entirely stable. Retrograde nailing with an interlocking nail is suitable for some fractures of the middle third. External fixation can be an option for high-energy segmental fractures and open fractures, but great care must be taken in placing the pins as the radial nerve is vulnerable.

Chapter 7

Injuries of the Elbow and the Forearm

7.1 Type a Supracondylar Fractures

These extra-articular fractures are rare in adults. When they do occur, they are usually displaced and unstable-probably because there is no tough periosteum to tether the fragments. In high-energy injuries there may be comminution of the distal humerus

Treatment: Closed reduction is unlikely to be stable and K-wire fixation is not strong enough to permit early mobilization. Open reduction and internal fixation is therefore the treatment of choice. The distal humerus is approached through a posterior exposure. It is sometimes possible to fix the fracture without recourse to an olecranon osteotomy using a triceps elevating approach. A simple transverse or oblique fracture can usually be reduced and fixed with a medial and lateral contoured plate and screws.

7.2 Types B and C intra-articular Fractures

Except in osteoporotic individuals, intra-articular condylar fractures should be regarded as high-energy injuries with soft-tissue damage. A severe blow on the point of the elbow drives the olecranon process upwards, splitting the condyles apart. Swelling is considerable but, if the bony landmarks can be felt, the elbow is found to be distorted. The patient should be carefully examined for evidence of vascular or nerve injury; if there are signs of vascular insufficiency, this must be addressed as a matter of urgency.

Imaging: X-rays show that the fracture extends from the lower humerus into the elbow joint; it may be difficult to tell whether one or both condyles are involved, especially with an undisplaced condylar fracture. There is also often comminution of the bone between the condyles, the extent of which is usually underestimated. Sometimes the fracture extends into the metaphysis as a T- or Y-shaped break, or else there may be multiple fragments (comminution). CT scans can be helpful in planning the surgical approach but the surgeon should be prepared for the worst case.

Treatment: These are severe injuries associated with joint damage; prolonged immobilization will certainly result in a stiff elbow. Early movement is therefore aprime objective. Undisplaced fractures These can be treated by applying a posterior slab with the elbow flexed almost 90 degrees; movements are commenced after 2 weeks. However, great care should be taken to avoid the dual pitfalls of underdiagnosis (displacement and comminution are not always obvious on the initial X-rays) and late displacement (always obtain check X-rays a week after injury). Displaced type B and C fractures if the appropriate expertise and facilities are available, open reduction and internal fixation is the treatment of choice for displaced fractures and for most undisplaced fractures in adults. Minor displacement and comminution may be underappreciated and can lead to displacement. The danger with conservative treatment is the strong tendency to stiffening of the elbow and persistent pain. Bridging external fixation can be used for the initial management of open fractures with soft-tissue contamination. This allows for eradication of contaminants prior to staged early definitive treatment. If there is substantial soft-tissue loss that is likely to require involvement of a plastic surgeon, they should be consulted prior to application of the external fixator as this may substantially reduce the reconstructive options. If the articular involvement is minimal, a triceps-preserving approach can be used to access the humerus. For more comminuted fractures a good exposure of the joint is needed. This may require an olecranon osteotomy that can be intra- or extra-articular. The ulnar nerve should be identified, decompressed and protected throughout; some favour transposition in all cases. The fragments are reduced and held temporarily with K-wires. In adults the use of plates and screws is preferred over lag screws or cannulated screws, even for unicondylar fractures. Parallel or orthogonal plates are used depending on the fracture configuration of the lateral column. Pre-contoured locking plates are available that help maintain position in osteoporotic bone. Independent lag screws or headless compression screws may be required for coronal plane fractures but otherwise it is preferable for transverse screws to pass through a plate to engage fragments on the opposite side. Postoperatively the patient is provided with a sling for comfort but immediate active mobilization is initiated with the patient lying supine and the shoulder flexed to 90 degrees. The use of a splint or cast is not recommended and passive stretch should be avoided. Fracture healing usually occurs by 12 weeks. Despite these measures the patient often does not regain full extension and they should be counselled accordingly before surgery. In some cases movement may be severely restricted. A description of this sort fails to convey the real difficulty of these operations, which can provide a real challenge even in the most skilled hands.

Chapter 8

Simple Dislocation of the Elbow

8.1 Mechanism of Injury and Pathology

The majority of dislocations occur as a result of a fall on an outstretched hand with the elbow in extension often with a valgus force. In sports other mechanisms may occur. The medial ligament will be found to be torn on MRI scan in all cases, but in up to 20% the lateral ligament will be either intact or have only alow-grade partial tear. Approximately 8% of elbows will go on to have problems of recurrent instability. It is not known what the risk factors are but they are likely to be related to associated avulsion of the humeral attachments of the secondary stabilizers of the elbow, i. e. , the common flexor and extensor muscles. Simple dislocations may be associated with damage to surrounding nerves and blood vessels, especially if the injury is open-suggesting a more high-energy injury.

8.2 X-rays

X-ray examination is essential to confirm the presence of a dislocation and to identify any associated fractures (see "Fracture-dislocations" above).

8.3 Treatment

The patient should be fully relaxed with sedation or anaesthesia. Reduction can usually be achieved with gentle traction applied to the supinated forearm as the thumb of the surgeon's other hand is applied to the olecranon process to push it anteriorly and the elbow is taken from an extended to a flexed position. After the reduction, the elbow should be put through a full range of motion to see whether it is stable. The distal nerves and circulation are checked again and an X-ray is obtained to confirm that the joint is reduced. The arm is held in a collar and cuff with the elbow flexed above 90 degrees. After 1 week the patient gently moves the elbow while lying supine with the shoulder flexed to 90 degrees and the forearm in neutral rotation. The collar and cuff are discarded when the patient is comfortable. Passive "stretching" of the elbow is to be avoided. The long-term results are usually good. Often the clinician deciding on definitive treatment is not the one who performed the reduction and scant information is likely to be available about the elbow stability. MRI will define the extent of the soft-tissue injury. If the soft-tissue injury extends into the lateral structures, there may be a role for examination under anaesthesia and open stabilization of the elbow.

Chapter 9

Fractures of the Shafts of the Radius and Ulna

9.1 Mechanism of Injury and Pathology

Fractures of the shafts of both forearm bones occur quite commonly. A twisting force(usually a fall on the hand) produces a spiral fracture with the bones broken at different levels. An angulating force causes a transverse fracture of both bones at the same level. A direct blow causes a transverse fracture of just one bone, usually the ulna. Additional rotation deformity may be produced by the pull of muscles attached to the radius: they are the biceps and supinator muscles to the upper third, the pronator teres to the middle third, and the pronator quadratus to the lower third. Bleeding and swelling of the muscle compartments of the forearm may cause circulatory impairment and compartment syndrome. Injuries to the bones of the forearm should be considered intra-articular fractures, because the forearm is a quadrilateral joint—with the proximal distal radioulnar joint at one end and the distal radioulnar joint at the other. Disruption of any one part—the radioulnar joints or the shafts of the long bones—will usually disrupt another part of the quadrilateral ring. Malalignment is likely to affect forearm rotation especially in the skeletally mature

9.2 Clinical Features

Pain and deformity are the most obvious clinical signs; the pulse must be felt and the hand examined for circulatory or neural deficit. Repeated examination is necessary in order to detect an impending compartment syndrome. Pain out of proportion to the injury is the cardinal sign.

9.3 Treatment

9.3.1 Children

In children, closed treatment is often successful because the tough periosteum tends to guide and then control the reduction. The fragments are held in a well-moulded full-length cast, from just distal to the axilla to the metacarpal shafts (to control rotation). The cast is applied with the elbow at 90 degrees and moulded with three-point fixation with an oval shape over the forearm and moulded in the AP direction over the upper arm. If the fracture is proximal to pronator teres, the forearm is supinated; if it is distal to pronator teres, the forearm is held in neutral. The position is checked by X-ray after a week and, if it is satisfactory, splintage is retained until both fractures are united (usually 6-8 weeks). Throughout this period hand and shoulder exercises are encouraged. The child should avoid contact sports for a few weeks to prevent refracture. Occasionally an operation is required, either if the fracture can not be reduced or if the fragments are unstable. Fractures that are initially displaced 100% or more should be held with percutaneous or intramedullary rods even if they can be reduced closed as there is a high risk of redisplacement. Fixation with flexible intramedullary nails is preferred, but they should be inserted with great care to avoid injury to the growth plates. Alternatively, a plate or K-wire fixation can be used. Childhood fractures usually remodel well. One can accept 20 degrees of angulation in the distal third of the radius, 15 degrees in the middle third and 10 degrees in the proximal third, as long as there is at least 2 years or more of growth left. One can accept 100% translation as long as there is no more than 1 cm of shortening.

9.3.2 Adults

Unless the fragments are in close apposition, reduction is difficult and redisplacement in the cast is almost invariable. So predictable is this outcome that most surgeons opt for open reduction and internal fixation from the outset. The fragments are held by interfragmentary compression with plates and screws. Bone grafting is advisable if there is comminution or a loss of continuity in two-thirds of the circumference of the bone. The deep fascia is left open to prevent a build-up of pressure in the muscle compartments, and only the skin is sutured. After the operation the arm is kept elevated until the swelling subsides, and during this period active exercises of the hand are encouraged. If the fracture is not comminuted and the patient is reliable, early range of movement exercises are commenced but lifting and sports are avoided. It takes 8-12 weeks for the bones to unite. With comminuted fractures or unreliable patients, immobilization in plaster is safer.

Chapter 10

Injuries of the Wrist

10.1 Low-energy Dorsally Displaced Fractures ("Colles' fracture")

10.1.1 Mechanism of injury and pathological anatomy

Force is applied in the length of the forearm with the wrist in extension. The bone fractures at the corticocancellous junction and the distal fragment collapses into extension, dorsal displacement, radial tilt and shortening. Normal angles are shown in Figure 26.1.

10.1.2 Clinical features

We can recognize the most common fracture pattern (as Colles did long before radiography was invented) by the "dinner-fork" deformity, with prominence on the back of the wrist and a depression in front. In patients with less deformity there may only be local tenderness and pain on wrist movements.

10.1.3 Imaging

X-rays show there is a transverse fracture of the radius at the corticocancellous junction, and often the ulnar styloid process is broken off. The radial fragment is impacted into radial and backward tilt. Sometimes there is an intra-articular fracture; sometimes it is severely fragmented. If the configuration is not clear, a CT scan is very helpful inplanning treatment.

10.1.4 Treatment

(1) Undisplaced fractures

If the fracture is undisplaced (or only very slightly displaced), a dorsal splint is applied for a day or two until the swelling has resolved, then the cast is completed. An X-ray is taken at 10-14 days to ensure that the fracture has not slipped; if it has, surgery may be required; if not, the cast can usually be removed after 5 weeks to allow mobilization.

(2) Displaced fractures

Displaced fractures must be reduced under anaesthesia (haematoma block, Bier's block, axillary block or general anaesthesia). The hand is grasped and longitudinal traction is applied (sometimes with extension of the wrist to disimpact the fragments); the distal fragment is then pushed into place by pressing on the dorsum while manipulating the wrist into flexion, ulnar deviation and pronation. If it is satisfactory, a dorsal plaster slab is applied, extending from just below the elbow to the metacarpal necks and two-thirds of the way round the circumference of the wrist. The position is then checked by X-ray. It is held in position by a crepe bandage. Extreme positions of flexion and ulnar deviation must be avoided; 20 degrees in each direction is adequate. The arm is kept elevated for the next day or two; shoulder, elbow and finger exercises are started as soon as possible. If the fingers become swollen, cyanosed or painful, there should be no hesitation in splitting the bandage. At approximately 7 days, and if satisfactory then again at about 14 days, fresh X-rays are taken. This is because redisplacement is not uncommon, especially in the elderly after an initial manipulation. If the pattern is particularly unstable, or if there has been substantial slip since the first reduction X-rays but the position is only just acceptable at 14 days, another X-ray at 18-20 days, just prior to the fracture being too "sticky" to manipulate again, is considered. If the position is probably not compatible with a good outcome and if the risks inherent in surgery are understood, manipulation and fixation with either percutaneous wires or a volar locking plate is undertaken. However, in older patients with low functional demands, modest degrees of displacement should be accepted because outcome in these patients is not so dependent upon anatomical perfection; and fixation of the fragile bone can be very difficult and is not without complications. The fracture unites in about 6 weeks and, even in the absence of radiological proof of union, wrist exercises can be commenced. Occasionally the fracture line exits transversely in the central part of the distal radius joint surface; the anterior cortex is intact and the dorsal fragment slips dorsally. These dorsal partial articular shear fractures tend to be more stable in cast but may require surgical stabilization.

(3) Impacted or fragmented low-energy distal radius fractures

With substantial impaction or fragmentation in osteoporotic bone, manipulation and plaster immobilization alone may be insufficient. The fracture can sometimes be reduced and held with percutaneous wires or a volar locking plate but, if impaction is severe, even this may not be enough to hold all the fragments or maintain length; in that case, other techniques, such as dorsal plating, locked intramedullary nails, external fixators, internal plate bridging the radius to the third metacarpal and bone grafts (synthetic or autogenous) are considered.

(4) Volar locking plate or K-wires

· Volar locking plates: There are several volar locking plates available. These are expensive and require surgical skill to apply properly and safely. They are applied to the anterior distal shaft-metaphysis of the radius, approaching the bone beneath pronator quadratus in the safe interval between the flexor carpi radialis and the radial artery, well away from the median nerve and its palmar cutaneous branch. The plate is applied sufficiently distal to support the fracture but proximal enough to avoid abrading the overlying thumb and finger flexors. The screws are fixed to the plate itself and are passed into the relatively stronger subchondral bone distally. These devices, allow stable fixation and thus early mobilization of the forearm.

· K-wires: K-wires are cheaper and more readily available. They must be passed with meticulous care to avoid impinging the vulnerable skin nerves and tendons. Two stout wires are the minimum; with softer or more comminuted bone three or four are preferred. They can be passed through the fragments into the radius shaft or through the fracture line as levers "Kapandji wires". Wires are not strong enough to allow early mobilization and a supplementary plaster, which will need changing once or twice, is needed. The final outcomes and complication rates for the two methods appear the same. Early mobilization and thus earlier return to function might tempt certain patients towards a plate if the device is available and affordable.

(5) Outcome

As Colles himself recognized, the outcome of these fractures in an older age group with lower functional demands is usually good, regardless of the cosmetic or the radiographic appearance. Poor outcomes can usually be improved by performing acorrective osteotomy if undertaken before secondary arthritis intervenes. The amount of displacement that can be accepted depends on patient factors such as age, comorbidity, functional demands, handedness and quality of bone, and treatment factors such as surgical skill and implants available. As a rule, poor outcome is associated with the following:

- Loss of radial length by more than 3 mm.
- Dorsal tilt more than 15 degrees from neutral depending on age and function.
- Palmar tilt more than 20 degrees from neutral.

Early correction should be considered. The tolerances might be less in a younger, higher demand patient.

10.2 Volar Displaced Fracture

10.2.1 Clinical features

The patient presents with a wrist injury, but there is no dinner-fork deformity. Instead, there is a "garden-spade" deformity.

10.2.2 X-rays

There is a fracture through the distal radial metaphysis; a lateral view shows that the distal fragment is displaced or tilted anteriorly. The entire metaphysis can be fractured, or there can be an oblique fracture exiting at the dorsal or volar rim of the radius.

10.2.3 Treatment

These fractures can be reduced by traction, supination and extension of the wrist, and the forearm immobilized in a cast for 6 weeks, but the risk of redisplacement is high and most advocate early surgical intervention with a volar plate to buttress the distal fragment. X-rays should be taken at 7-10 days to ensure that the fracture has not slipped, even when a plate is used. Particular attention should be paid to fragmentation of the volar-ulnar lip of the distal radius as this can readily displace if not adequately supported.

10.3 Fractured Scaphoid

10.3.1 Mechanism of injury and pathological anatomy

The scaphoid lies obliquely across the two rows of carpal bones and is also in the line of loading between the thumb and forearm. The combination of forced carpal movement and compression, as in a fall on the dorsiflexed hand, exerts severe stress on the bone and it is liable to fracture. Fractures occur in three anatomical locations: distal tubercle, waist and proximal pole. Some fractures, especially distal oblique and waist fractures, are unstable, which predisposes to non-union or malunion. The blood supply of the scaphoid arises from the dorsal distal pole. This means that the proximal pole has a poor blood supply and is less likely to heal than the distal pole.

10.3.2 Treatment

(1) Fracture of the scaphoid tubercle

These are treated in a cast for 4-6 weeks. Usually there are no complications but occasionally there is a non-union needing excision of a small fragment or grafting of a larger fragment.

(2) Undisplaced waist fractures

These can be treated in two ways: plaster or percutaneous fixation.

(3) Plaster

Around 90% of waist fractures should heal in plaster (a neutral forearm cast from the upper forearm to just short of the metacarpophalangeal joints of the fingers; the thumb is not incorporated). It is retained (and if necessary repaired or renewed) for 6-8 weeks. The plaster is removed and the wrist examined clinically and radiologically. If there is no tenderness and the X-ray shows full healing, the wrist is left free; a CT scan is the most reliable means of confirming union if in doubt. If the scaphoid is tender, or the fracture is still visible on X-ray, the cast is reapplied for a further 4 weeks. At that stage, one of two pictures may emerge: ①the wrist is painless and the fracture has healed—the cast can be discarded; ② the X-ray shows signs of delayed healing (bone resorption and cavitation around the fracture)—union can be hastened by bone grafting and internal fixation.

(4) Percutaneous fixation

This should be considered for those patients who do not want to endure prolonged plaster immobilization and who want to get back to work or sport earlier (but they must still avoid impact or heavy load on the wrist until the fracture is healed). A screw is passed through a small incision in the front of the scaphoid tubercle. Special cannulated screws and technical perfection are essential.

(5) Displaced fractures

These can also be treated in plaster, but the outcome is less predictable; it may not heal or may heal in a poor position. It is better toreduce the fracture (closed if possible, otherwise open) and to fix it with a compression screw. This should increase the likelihood of union and reduce the time of immobilization.

(6) Proximal pole fractures

These may heal in plaster, and probably will if left long enough. However, the risk of non-union and the disadvantages of prolonged immobilization are such that early surgical fixation (through a small dorsal incision) should be considered.

Chapter 11

Injuries of the Hand

The metacarpal bones are vulnerable to blows and falls upon the hand, or the longitudinal force of the boxer's punch. Injuries are common and the bones may fracture at their base, in the shaft, through the neck or at their head.

(1) Oblique or transverse fractures with slight displacement

These fractures require no reduction. Splintage also is unnecessary, but a firm crepe bandage may be comforting; this should not be allowed to discourage the patient from active movements of the fingers, which should be practised assiduously. As the patient moves the fingers, the fracture may shorten until the intercarpal ligaments between the metacarpal necks tighten, thus limiting further shortening and rotational deformity. After 4–5 weeks callus forms and the fracture becomes stable.

(2) Transverse fractures with considerable displacement

Fractures of this type can be reduced by traction and pressure then held with a plaster cast, but they are usually unstable and should be fixed surgically with compression plates to allow immediate mobilization. If plates are not available, percutaneous K–wires are placed transversely through the neighbouring undamaged metacarpals or up through the medulla, supported by a cast for 4–5 weeks.

(3) Spiral fracturess

piral fractures are liable to rotate. They can be managed non–operatively if there is no rotational displacement and the patient accepts a shorter knuckle profile but, otherwise, they should be perfectly reduced and fixed withlag screws and a plate to allow immediate mobilization. If rigid fixation is not available, percutaneous wires protected by a plaster for 4–5 weeks is an alternative.

Part 50

Fracture of Lower Limb

Chapter 1

Fracture of Femoral Neck

Femoral neck fracture primarily occurs in elderly patients with poor bone quality after low energy falls, it occurs more frequently in women than in men, because of the relatively greater osteoporosis in women. And it also occurs in younger patients after high-energy events such as car accidents, falling from heights, or sports injuries.

1.1 Anatomy

The femoral aspect of the hip is made up of the femoral head with its articular cartilage and the femoral neck, which connects the head to the shaft in the region of the lesser and greater trochanters.

Femoral neck fractures regularly disrupt the blood supply to the femoral head. A large branch of the medial femoral circumflex artery is consist of the extracapsular arterial ring posteriorly and anteriorly by a branch from the lateral femoral circumflex artery. The primary source for the blood supply of the head of the femur depends the deep branch of the medial femoral circumflex artery. The lateral vessels are the most vulnerable to damage in femoral neck fractures. The superior retinacular and lateral epiphyseal vessels are the most important origins of this blood supply. Broadly displaced intracapsular hip fractures tear the synovium and the surrounding vessels. The progressive split of the blood supply can lead to serious clinical conditions and complications, including osteonecrosis and nonunion.

1.2 Classification

1.2.1 Garden classification

In this classification, femoral neck fractures are divided into the following four grades based on the degree of displacement of the fracture fragment. This classification is based on anteroposterior radiographs and does not consider lateral or sagittal plane alignment.

· Grade Ⅰ is an incomplete or valgus impacted fracture.

· Grade Ⅱ is a complete fracture without bone displacement.

· Grade Ⅲ is a complete fracture with partial displacement of the fracture fragments.

· Grade Ⅳ is a complete fracture with total displacement of the fracture fragments.

1.2.2 According to position of the fracture line

The classification of fracture of femoral neck according to position of the fracture line. The fractures are considered intracapsular fractures, include the following:

· Subcapital: femoral head/neck junction.

· Transcervical: midportion of femoral neck.

· Basicervical: base of femoral neck.

1.2.3 Pauwel's classification

The biomechanical understanding of the proximal femur has historically been formed by Pauwels. This classification calculates the angle (Pauwel's angle) between the fracture line of the distal fragment and the horizontal line to determine shearing stress and compressive force. The classification is described as follows:

· Type Ⅰ (Adduction): Pauwel's angle is up to 30°. Compressive forces are dominant.

· Type Ⅱ: Pauwel's angle is 30°–50°. Shearing force occurs and may have a negative effect on bone healing.

· Type Ⅲ (Abduction): Pauwel's angle is 50° and more. Under these circumstances, shearing force is predominant and is associated with a significant amount of varus force which will more likely result in fracture displacement and varus collapse.

1.3 Clinical Manifestation

(1) The patient has a history of trauma, including slight trauma.

(2) The patient reports a gradually worsening deep, achy pain in the hip, groin, or thigh. Usually, pain initially occurs after an activity. As the stress of training continues, pain occurs during training and becomes more intense.

(3) The patient has an externally rotated shortened leg in a supine position.

(4) The patient is unable to lift the extended leg or bear weight on the leg.

(5) An X-ray usually will confirm that you have a fracture and show exactly this fracture, occasionally if X-ray doesn't show a fracture but patient still have hip pain, an MRI, CT or bone scan are used to look for a small hairline fracture.

1.4 Treatment

The treatment of femoral neck fracture depends primarily on the activity of the patient, the severity of fracture displacement, the age of the fracture, and the degree of osteoporosis present. Significant complications such as avascular necrosis and non-union are very common without surgical intervention. The treatment options include non-operative management, internal fixation or prosthetic replacement (Figure 50-1-1).

· Non-operative management may be considered in some patients who are non-ambulators, have minimal pain, and who are at high risk for surgical intervention.

· Internal fixation can be performed with multiple pins, intramedullary hip screw (IHMS), crossed screw-nails or compression with a dynamic screw and plate.

· Replacing the femoral head is achieved with either hemiarthroplasty or total hip arthroplasty.

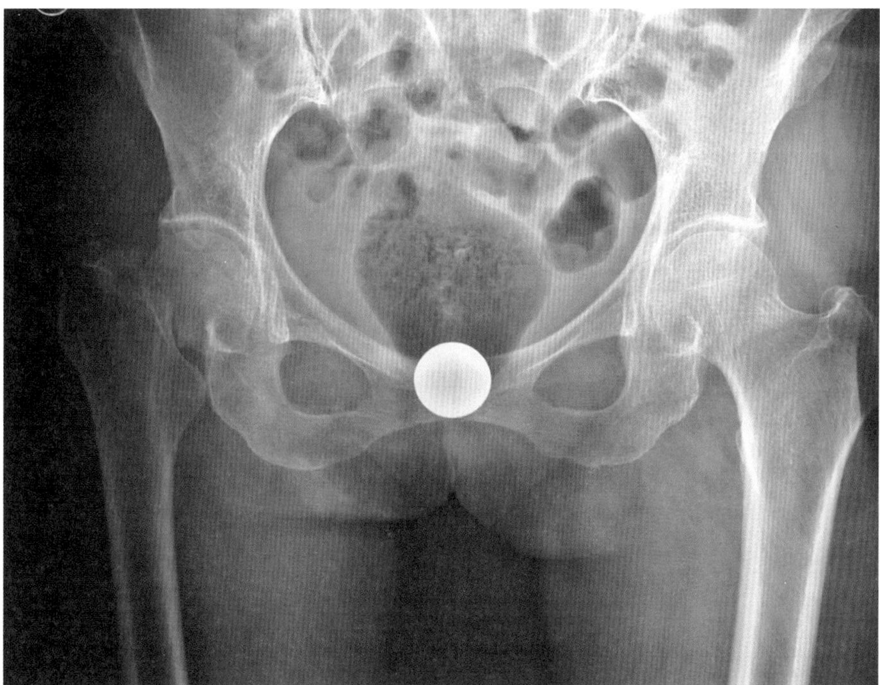

Figure 50-1-1 Femoral neck fracture

Chapter 2

Trochanteric Fracture

Trochanteric fracture is an extracapsular fracture of the proximal femur between the greater and lesser trochanters. Trochanteric fracture frequently occurs in elderly patients with osteoporosis after low energy trauma, and also takes place in younger patients after high-energy events, roughly the same as the femoral neck fracture.

2.1 Anatomy

The anatomy of the pertrochanteric region of the femur is perfectly variable in its combination of cortical and cancellous bone structure. The well-vascularized pertrochanteric region is dependent on the structural integrity of a laminated cancellous bone arcade from the femoral head and epiphyseal scar, around Ward's triangle, to the lesser trochanter, where the solid nature of the structure changes to a tubular construct with the origin of the femoral medullary canal. The femoral aspect of the hip is made up of the femoral head with its articular cartilage and the femoral neck, which connects the head to the shaft in the region of the lesser and greater trochanters.

2.2 Classification

Trochanteric fractures are commonly subdivided into either intertrochanteric (between the greater and lesser trochanter) or pertrochanteric (through the trochanters)

2.2.1 Fractures in these regions can be classified as follows

- Intertrochanteric.
- Pertrochanteric; intertrochanteric, involving both trochanters.
- Subtrochanteric.
- Greater trochanteric avulsion fracture.
- Lesser trochanteric avulsion fracture.

2.2.2 They are subdivided according to the number of fragments, as follows

- Two-part linear intertrochanteric fracture stable.
- Three-part with comminution of lesser trochanter or greater trochanter.
- Four-part with comminution of both trochanters.
- Multi-part with comminution of both trochanters and intertrochanteric region.

2.2.3 The Boyd and Griffin classification is based on the involvement of subtrochanteric region

- Type Ⅰ linear intertrochanteric.
- Type Ⅱ with comminution of trochanteric region.
- Type Ⅲ with comminution associated with the subtrochanteric component.
- Type Ⅳ oblique fracture of the shaft with extension into the subtrochanteric region.

2.3 Clinical Manifestation

(1) Elderly patients frequently have a history of fall or slip.

(2) A younger patient with a high-energy fracture has usually been in a significant accident and has the potential for multiple other injuries.

(3) The patient would complaint of pain in the affected hip.

(4) The patient has a shortened, externally rotated lower extremity.

(5) The patient should undergo complete musculoskeletal examination.

(6) An X-ray usually will confirm that you have a fracture and show exactly this fracture.

2.4 Treatment

Elderly patients may have coexisting conditions that might affect the treatment of the fracture. Hypertension, cardiac problems, diabetes are common issue encountered in elderly. Complete medical evaluation should be done pulmonary insufficiency.

Non-operative treatment has very limited role in management of intertrochanteric fractures. Non-operative management may be considered in some patients who are non-ambulators, declines surgery, and who are at high risk for surgical intervention including unfitness for any kind of anesthesia.

Closed/open reduction and internal fixation is indicated for all intertrochanteric fractures (Figure 50-2-1).

- The intertrochanteric fractures are reduced closely or after opening and fixed with a fixation device.
- Internal fixation can be performed with sliding hip screw, intramedullary hip screw (IHMS), crossed screw-nails or compression with a dynamic screw and plate.
- Total hip arthroplasty has a limited role in treatment and is still evolving. It could be used in very osteoporotic skeleton or as salvage of failed surgery.
- Preventive DT protocol is followed after surgery. Physical therapy includes muscle strengthening and ambulation training. Depending on the patient profile walkers, crutches, four-post canes, and other canes

may be used.

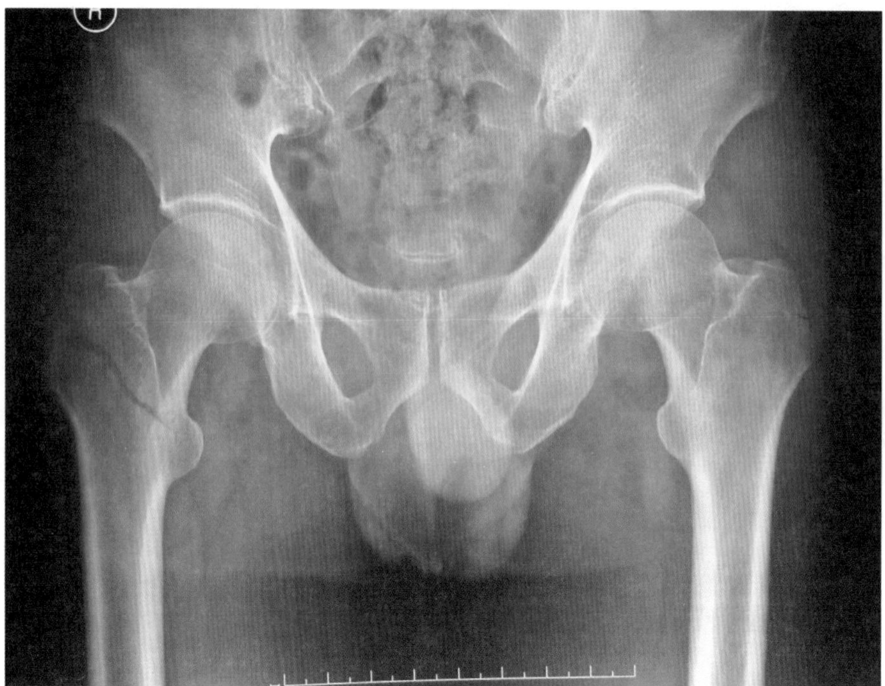

Figure 50-2-1 Trochanteric fracture

Chapter 3

Fracture of the Femoral Shaft

Fractures of the diaphysis (shaft) of the femur are nearly always the result of relatively high-energy trauma. Motor vehicle accidents are the most common cause of femoral shaft fractures. Secondary causes are pedestrians injured by falls from heights and gunshot wounds. Femoral shaft fractures occur in a bimodal age distribution and typically are either high-energy injuries in young men or low-energy injuries in elderly women.

3.1 Anatomy

The femur is the longest and strongest bone in the body. The femur has an anterior bow. The femoral shaft is almost cylindrical in form, is a little broader superiorly and is slightly arched such that it is convex anteriorly and concave posteriorly where it is strengthened by a prominent longitudinal ridge of bone, the linea aspera. A variety of muscles have their origins at and insert into the femoral shaft.

3.2 Classification

The two most commonly used classification systems are those of Winquist and Hansen and the Arbeitsgemunshaft for Osteosynthesefragen/Orthopaedic Trauma Association (AO/OTA).

3.2.1 Winquist and Hansen classification

Based on their degree of diaphyseal comminution.

- Type 0: No comminution.
- Type Ⅰ: Insignificant amount of comminution.
- Type Ⅱ: Greater than 50% cortical contact.
- Type Ⅲ: Less than 50% cortical contact.
- Type Ⅳ: Segmental fracture with no contact between proximal and distal fragment.

3.2.2 OTA classification

The OTA classification is shown in Table 50-3-1.

Table 50-3-1 OTA classification

32A-Simple	· A1—Spiral · A2—Oblique, angle > 30 degrees · A3—Transverse, angle < 30 degrees
32B-Wedge	· B1—Spiral wedge · B2—Bending wedge · B3—Fragmented wedge
32C-Complex	· C1—Spiral · C2—Segmental · C3—Irregular

3.3 Clinical Manifestation

(1) The patient would complaint of severe pain in the thigh.

(2) There would be a tense, swollen thigh.

(3) Blood loss in open fractures may be double that of closed fractures.

(4) Advanced Trauma Life Support (ATLS) should be initiated.

(5) An X-ray usually will confirm that you have a fracture and show exactly this fracture (Figure 50-3-1).

3.4 Treatment

(1) Nonoperative treatment of an adult femoral shaft fracture in the era of modern medicine is essentially nonexistent. Non-operative management may be considered in some patients who are non-ambulators, declines surgery, and who are at high risk for surgical intervention.

(2) A fracture of the femoral shaft in an adult is an indication for surgical management.

(3) Antegrade intramedullary nail with reamed technique is gold standard for treatment of diaphyseal femur fractures.

(4) Retrograde intramedullary nail with reamed technique is used in floating knee (ipsilateral tibial shaft fracture).

(5) External fixation of a femoral shaft fracture is a damage-control procedure typically performed when a polytrauma patient is under-resuscitated or has a significant head injury, a very contaminated open soft tissue envelope, an associated ischemic vascular injury, or other surgical injuries requiring concurrent operating room teams.

(6) ORIF with plate is used at distal metaphyseal-diaphyseal junction.

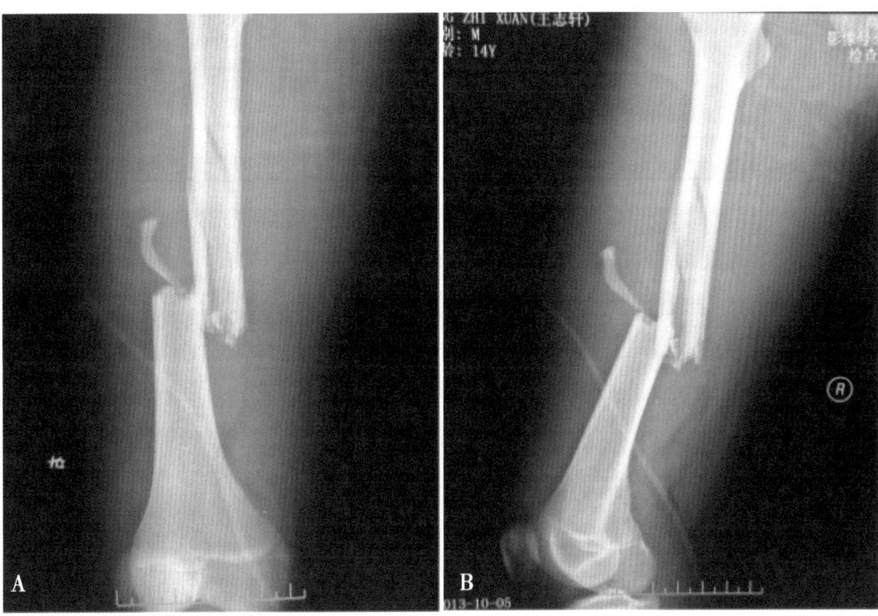

Figure 50-3-1 Femoral shaft fracture

A. AP view of X-ray in right femoral shaft fracture; B. Lateral view of X-ray in right femoral shaft fracture.

Chapter 4

Fracture of the patella

Patella fracture is one of the common knee injuries usually post direct trauma to the patella or sudden forceful contraction of the quadriceps muscles in a context of sports injury.

4.1 Anatomy

The patella is triangular in shape with a superior base and inferior apex. The posterior surface is smooth, composed of articular cartilage, and is divided into medial and lateral facets articulate with the medial and lateral condyles of the femur. The anterior surface is rough, for attachment of tendons and ligaments.

4.2 Classification

Patella fractures are typically classified very simply by the orientation of the fracture line(s) as seen on plain radiographs.

- nondisplaced.
- transverse.
- pole or sleeve(upper or lower).
- vertical.
- marginal.
- osteochondral.
- comminuted(stellate).

4.3 Clincal Manifestation

Patients present with marked swelling and pain over the patella with point tenderness and marked reduction in extension strength. Usually, there is a large joint effusion or hemarthrosis. An X-ray usually will confirm that you have a fracture and show exactly this fracture(Figure 50-4-1).

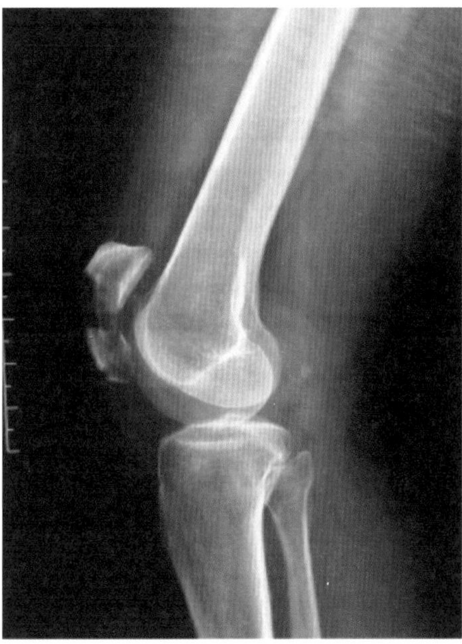

Figure 50-4-1 Patella fracture

4.4 Treatment

Treatment may be with or without surgery, depending on the type of patella fracture. Undisplaced fracture can usually be treated by casting. Even some displaced fractures can be treated with casting as long as a person can straighten their leg without help. Typically the leg is immobilized in a straight position for the first 3 weeks and then increasing degrees of bending are allowed. Other types of fractures generally require surgery, including open patella fractures. Aim of every surgical intervention is to allow a high stability for early active range-of-motion exercises.

Chapter 5

Fracture of the Shafts of the Tibia and Fibula

Tibial and fibula shaft fractures are often the result of high–energy injury. Sometimes they can also be insidious in onset, such as stress fractures. Motor vehicles, snowmobiles, and motorcycles, as well as the growing popularity of extreme sports, contribute to the increasing occurrence of tibial and fibula shaft fractures.

5.1 Anatomy

The tibia is a unique anatomical structure. Its anteromedial surface is entirely subcutaneous prone to injury. The location, morphology, and degree of displacement of the fracture has a marked influence on the outcome of the fracture. Fracture of the upper 1/3 of the tibia may involve the injury of posterior tibial artery. Fracture of the middle 1/3 of the tibia commonly need to pay close attention to the osteofascial compartment syndrome(OCS). Fracture of the lower 1/3 of the tibia frequently happens the delay union and nonunion. Fracture of the neck of fibula may be careful the injury of the peroneal nerve.

5.2 Classification

5.2.1 Oestern and Tscherne classification of closed fracture soft tissue injury

See Table 50–5–1。

Table 50–5–1 Oestern and Tscherne classification of closed fractuer soft tissue injury

Classification	Performance
Grade 0	Injuries from indirect forces with negligible soft–tissue damage
Grade Ⅰ	Superficial contusion/abrasion, simple fractures
Grade Ⅱ	Deep abrasions, muscle/skin contusion, direct trauma, impending compartment syndrome
Grade Ⅲ	Excessive skin contusion, crushed skin or destruction of muscle, subcutaneous degloving, acute compartment syndrome, and rupture of major blood vessel or nerve

5.2.2 Gustilo-Anderson classification of open tibia fractures

See Table 50-5-2。

Table 50-5-2 Gustilo-Anderson classification of open tibia fractures

Classification	Performance
Type Ⅰ	Open fracture, clean wound, wound <1 cm in length
Type Ⅱ	Open fracture, wound > 1 cm but < 10 cm in length; without extensive soft-tissue damage, flaps, avulsions
Type Ⅲ A	Open fracture with adequate soft tissue coverage of a fractured bone despite extensive soft tissue laceration or flaps, or high-energy trauma (gunshot and farm injuries) regardless of the size of the wound
Type Ⅲ B	Open fracture with extensive soft-tissue loss and periosteal stripping and bone damage. Usually associated with massive contamination. Will often need further soft-tissue coverage procedure(i. e. , free or rotational flap)
Type Ⅲ C	Open fracture associated with an arterial injury requiring repair, irrespective of degree of soft-tissue injury
Gustilo and Anderson(JBJS 1976)	

5.3 Clinical Manifestation

Tibial shaft fractures would be visible swelling and deformity in the leg. Often the pain is severe. Undisplaced or partial fractures may be less characteristic in presentation. Tibial shaft fractures without fibula fractures present with lesser deformities than those with fibula fractured.

A patient stress fracture presents with pain on weight bearing, often with an antecedent change in lifestyle or an increase in physical activity. The pain is classically worse with weight bearing exercise and improves with rest. The injured should be examined completely to look for concomitant injuries. The leg should be examined for extent of injury. Ipsilateral knee and ankle joint should be assessed for injury. Deformity, angulation and malrotation should be noted. Contusions, blisters and open wounds must be accounted.

Compartment syndrome evaluation may be done if required.

Particular care taken to assess any open wounds or color changes that may indicate a more serious injury. Distal neuro-vascular examination should be done and compared to opposite side.

5.4 Treatment

Most closed tibial fractures can be treated nonoperatively(Figure 50-5-1).

Operative fixation is required when fractures are unstable.

Instability is defined as any of the following values when leg is in cast.

(1) Shortening> 1.5 cm of shortening.

(2) Valgus/varus angulation>5 degrees.

(3) Anterior or posterior angulation> 20 degrees.

(4) Open fractures and fractures with vascular injuries are surgical emergencies.

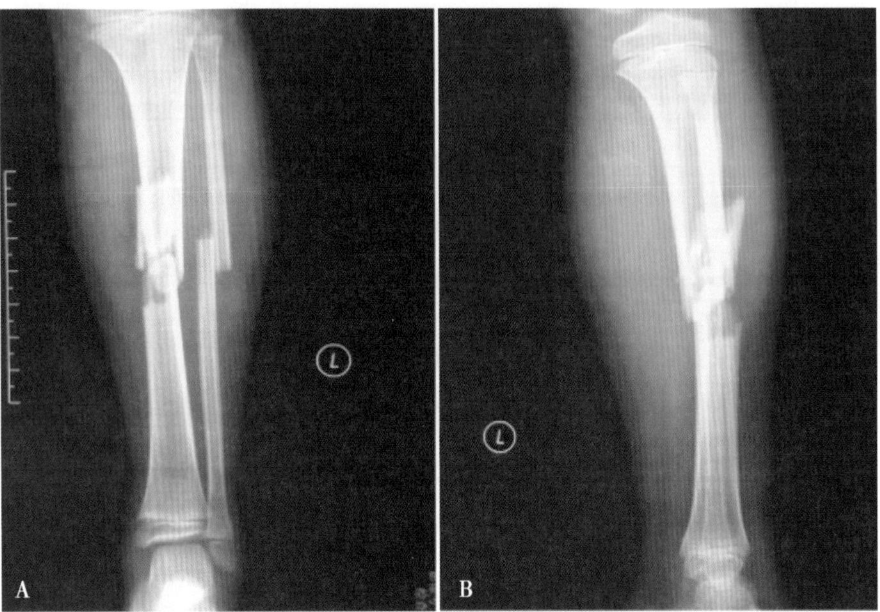

Figure 50-5-1 Tibial and fibula shaft fracture

A. AP view of X-ray in left tibial and fibula shaft fracture; B. Lateral view of X-ray in left tibial and fibula shaft fracture.

Part 51

Fracture and Dislocations of the pelvis

Chapter 1

Fractures and Dislocations of the Pelvis

1.1 Introduction

Pelvic fracture are relatively uncommon with a reported incidence of only 2% –8% of all fractures, but in multiple trauma patients, the frequency can rise up to more than 25%. The literature shows that pelvic fracture results in substantial mortality that ranges from 5% to 50% and is dependent not only on the type of pelvic–ring fracture but also on the severity of associated injuries involving the abdomen, chest, and central nervous system. Although the mortality rate of pelvic fracture has declined so far, the mortality rate of "complex pelvic traumas" remains approximately 18%. Clinically, for the pelvic fracture, surgeons are still confronted with great challenges.

1.2 Anatomy

The pelvis is the key link between the axial skeleton and the major weight–bearing locomotive structures, the lower extremities. The pelvis is a ring structure made up of three bones: the sacrum and the two innominate bones. The innominate bone is formed from the fusion of three ossification centers: the ilium, the ischium, and the pubis. They meet at the triradiate cartilage, which fuses at puberty. Anteriorly, two innominate bones meet at the pubic symphysis. The sacrum meets innominate bones posteriorly at the two sacroiliac joints. The three bones and three joints composing the pelvic ring have no inherent stability without vital ligamentous complexes. The ligamentous complexes include posterior sacroiliac ligaments, anterior sacroiliac ligaments and interosseous ligaments. The most important ligamentous structures is the posterior sacroiliac ligaments around the pelvis. Because the major weight–bearing forces are transmitted across the sacroiliac joints from the lower extremities to the spine (Figure 51–1–1).

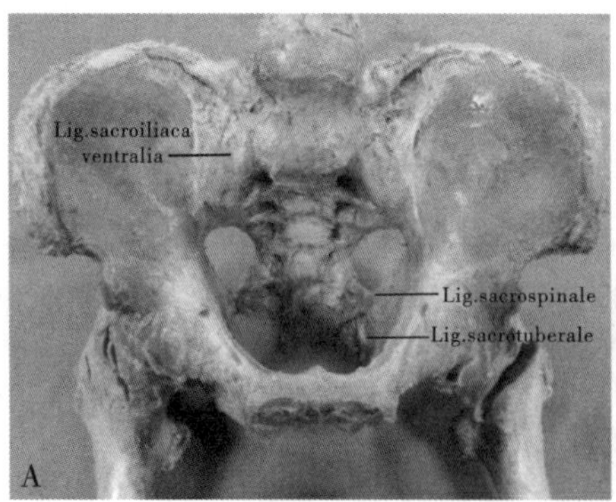

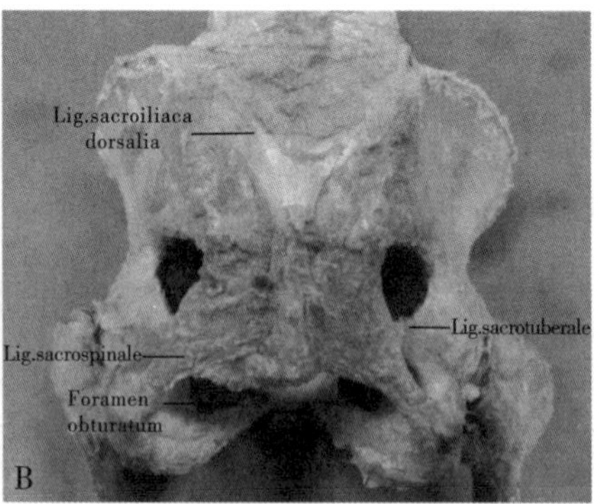

Figure 51-1-1 **Osteoligamentous structures of pelvic**

A. The front view of pelvis includes bony structure and main ligaments; B. Posterior view of pelvis, including bony structure and main ligaments.

The intact pelvis includes the false pelvis(greater pelvis)and the true pelvis(lesser pelvis). No major muscular structures cross the pelvic brim which dividing the false pelvis and the true pelvis. The false pelvis is lined laterally by the iliopsoas muscle. The lateral wall of the true pelvis consists of portions of the pubis, ischium and a small triangular portion of the ilium. The obturator foramen which opens superiorly and laterally for passage of the obturator nerve and vessels also defines the boundary of the true pelvis. The sciatic nerve leaves the pelvis anterior to the piriformis which originates from the lateral aspect of the sacrum and enters the greater sciatic notch.

The lumbosacral coccygeal plexus is made up of the anterior rami of T_{12} through S_4. The lumbar roots L_4 and L_5 enter the true pelvis from the false pelvis. The L_4 root merges with L_5 to form the lumbosacral trunk at the sacral promontory. The sacral roots pass through the sacral foramen and join the plexus. Numerous branches extend to the major muscles within the pelvis. The superior gluteal and inferior gluteal nerves leave ventral to the piriformis and exit the pelvis through the greater sciatic notch.

Major blood vessels lie on the inner wall of the pelvis. The important arteries include the median sacral artery, the superior rectal artery, the internal iliac and the external iliac artery. These branch of arteries and associated veins can all be injured and represent a potential source for significant hemorrhage during pelvic disruption.

Gastrointestinal and genitourinary systems injuries are very common in pelvis. The female perineum consists of the pelvic diaphragm with the urethra, vagina, and rectum. These structures are relatively pliable and are not commonly injured. However, the vagina may be perforated by bone spicules from pubic rami fractures in particular when the injury is due to a lateral compression force. In males, the prostate lies between the bladder and pelvic floor and is invested by a dense fascial membrane. The urethra passes through the prostate and before it exits below the pelvic floor. The junction between the prostate and the pelvic floor is strong, as is the membranous urethra. The weak link in this area is the urethra below the pelvic diaphragm in its bulbous portion.

1.3 Pelvic Stability

The pelvic ring is often considered a single anatomical structure including three bones and ligaments holding these bones anteriorly and posteriorly. Any type of traumatic disruption of the pelvic ring results in-

instability. In general, pelvic instability includes physiological instability (pregnancy), iatrogenic instability (posterior bone graft), division of specific ligaments and division of the pelvic ring structure. The instability we are discussing is the instability caused by damage of ligaments and pelvic ring.

The degree of pelvic instability correlates with the energy of the trauma and the overall physiological status of the patient. A low-energy fall injury in a patient with osteoporosis that results in a minimally displaced pubic ramus fracture is considered completely stable. On the other side, a young healthy man who sustains a complete disruption of the pubic symphysis and a sacroiliac joint in a 50-foot fall has a completely unstable pelvis.

Specific ligaments injury is considered to be the important factors for the pelvic instability. For instance, transection of the pubic symphysis alone allowed motion between the pubic bodies, but the intact posterior structures prevented symphyseal diastasis of more than 2.5 cm. However, when the anterior sacroiliac ligaments were sectioned, the pelvis opened like a book with the intact posterior sacroiliac ligaments simulating the binding of the book. In addition, the method of loading and the order in which ligaments are sacrificed influence the way the pelvis responds to force. If the anterior pelvic ligaments are cut, the degree of stability of the pelvis varies according to the different way of standing. Although the posterior ligamentous structures are more important in maintaining pelvic stability, the anterior structures also play a critical role in maintaining pelvic stability. For example, in double-leg stance, approximately 60% of stability comes from the posterior structures and 40% comes from the anterior structures. Fixation of the posterior injury alone does not address the entire problem of instability; excessive motion will occur resulting in pain, potential disruption of healing, and a greater chance of malunion.

1.4 Clinical Evalution

A pelvic fracture should be considered in all patients that have experienced any significant amount of blunt trauma or fall. A fracture to the pelvis is almost always painful and aggravated by movement of the hip or attempting to walk. Patients will usually try to keep their hips or knees flexed to avoid such aggravation. There may also be swelling or bruising noted in the injured area. Manual palpation may reveal crepitus while compression along the iliac crest can help determine the level of pelvic stability and instability.

As most pelvic fractures occur in the setting of trauma, all patients should undergo routine assessment which includes evaluation for any potentially life-threatening injuries (whether related to the hip or not). Assessment of soft-tissue injuries may provide further insight to the degree of impact sustained by the patient. It is particularly important to assess for any lacerations of the perineum (e.g., rectum or vagina) as this would indicate a severe injury and fractures potentially contaminated by urine, stool, or other environmental contaminants.

Pelvic ring fractures are also commonly associated with injuries to the axial or appendicular spine. Therefore, the spine and extremities should also be examined (e.g., limb length discrepancies, internal/external rotational deformities).

Vascular structures crossing the pelvis may also be involved with injuries to the pelvis. The usual cause of retroperitoneal hemorrhage secondary to pelvic fracture is a disruption of the venous plexus in the posterior pelvis. It may also be caused by a large-vessel injury, such as external or internal iliac disruption. Large-vessel injury causes rapid, massive hemorrhage with frequent loss of the distal pulse and marked hemodynamic instability.

Neurologic injuries associated with pelvic fractures typically involve the L_5 or S_1 nerve roots. If there is a sacral fracture involved, this may also include an S_2–S_5 sacral nerve root injury which could result in bowel or bladder incontinence and sexual dysfunction.

Although most trauma patients undergo routine CT scans to the abdomen and pelvis, an anteroposterior pelvic radiograph should be considered (as a rapid diagnostic tool) for hemodynamically unstable patients, to allow for earlier intervention. Sonography may help identify intraperitoneal bleeding (potentially pinpointing a source of shock) if it is present. Individuals presenting with hematuria in the setting of an intact urethra should undergo a cystography. Pelvic angiography may help to detect occult or obvious arteries injuries after pelvic fracture.

1.5 Classification

There are several main classification systems used to describe pelvic fractures. The tile classification system is developed by Pennal and Tile, divides injuries into lateral compression (LC), anteroposterior compression (APC) or vertical shear (VS) injuries. This classification system also takes into consideration radiographic signs of pelvic stability or instability. The Young–Burgess classification system is commonly used in traumatology, expanded on Tile's classification by including combined fractures. The most common combination fracture is LC/VS.

Another popular fracture classification system is AO classification system. Stable pelvis fractures (type A) do not displace significantly with physiological loading. Patients with these injuries often require protective weight bearing and limited activity until significant fracture healing has occurred. Partially unstable injuries (type B) are characterized by significant rotational instability of the pelvic ring, with sufficient residual ligamentous stability to prevent vertical displacement of the posterior pelvis. If satisfactory reduction and stabilization of the anterior pelvic ring is achieved, both the anterior and posterior pelvic injuries will remain reduced until the injury has healed. Vertically unstable (type C) pelvic injuries are characterized by disruption of both the anterior and the posterior pelvic ring and require more complex fixation to maintain reduction. Stabilization of the anterior pelvis can be achieved with internal or external fixation, but stabilization of the posterior pelvis requires internal fixation.

1.6 Treatment

The primary goal in the acute setting is to provide early stable fixation as it has been associated with decreased blood transfusion, systemic complications, hospital stay and overall improved survival. Excessive movement of the pelvis should also be avoided. Large–bore intravenous access for administration of analgesics and fluids should be obtained as soon as possible, and vital signs should be monitored closely. Therefore resuscitation of the polytrauma patient with an unstable pelvis often requires use of techniques to quickly stabilize the pelvic injury, with the goal of controlling hemorrhage. Spica casts, traction, external fixation and pelvic clamps are often chosen as a temporary method.

For stable fractures in which the bones are nondisplaced or minimally displaced, nonsurgical treatments may be selected. Unstable injuries, which in the early course of resuscitation are provisionally stabilized with one or more of the aforementioned techniques, should be evaluated for definitive stabilization using internal and/or external fixation.

Indications for anterior external fixation include emergency stabilization of an unstable fracture in a patient with hemodynamic instability, definitive stabilization of the rotationally unstable (type B) injury, and definitive stabilization of completely unstable shear injury with concomitant internal fixation posteriorly. The external fixation provides adequate stability for mobilization but does not provide adequate strength for unrestricted weight in the early postoperative period. Satisfactory reduction of the markedly displaced lateral compression pelvic injuries usually can be achieved with external rotation. If not, surgical reduction and internal fixation may be necessary (Figure 51-1-2).

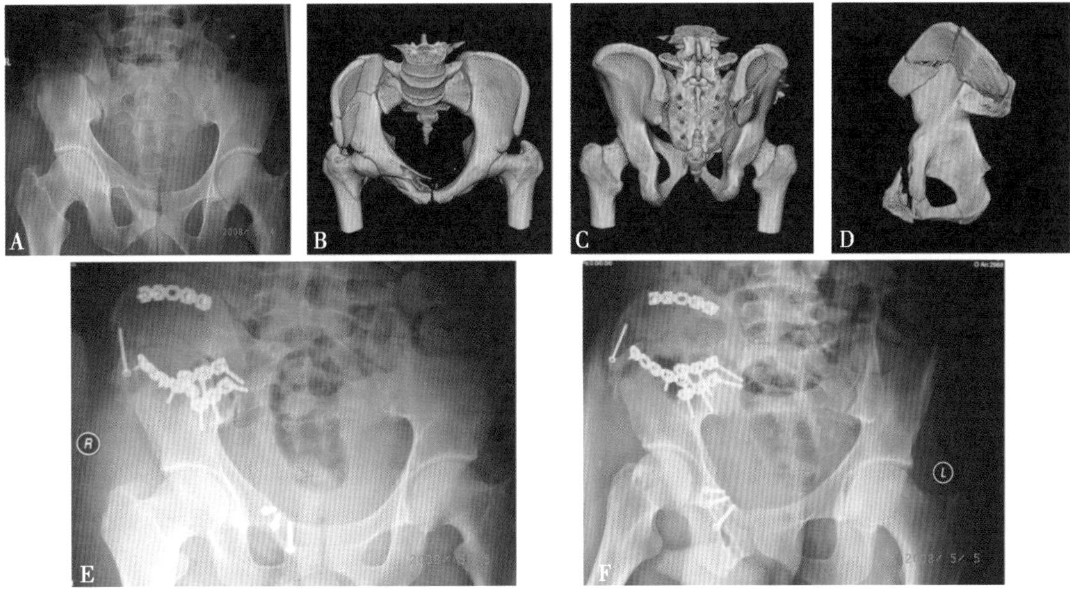

Figure 51-1-2 AO type B pelvic fracture

A-D are pre-operation images and E-F are post-operation images with internal fixation.

Numerous methods including plate, cerclage wiring and nonbioabsorbable suture fixation across the symphysis have been described for stabilizing the pubic symphysis. An injury model comparing external fixation and internal fixation for anterior ring injuries confirms that one or two plates are biomechanically stiffer and stronger than an external fixator.

An unstable iliac fractures passing from the greater sciatic notch, through the pelvic brim, and out the iliac wing is an excellent indication for open reduction and internal fixation of the posterior pelvis. This kind of fractures are often caused by an unstable vertical shear injury. Fixation of the injury at both the iliac crest and pelvic brim provides optimal stability.

Crescent fracture dislocations are defined as fracture dislocations of the sacroiliac joint with dislocation of the inferior sacroiliac joint and fracture through the posterior iliac crest. Anterior fixation of the sacroiliac joint with plates and screws can be used alone or in conjunction with plating of the crescent fracture to achieve stability. And stabilization of a crescent fracture in the posterior ilium can be achieved with plates and screws inserted through posterior or anterior incisions.

The goal of treatment of sacroiliac dislocation should be anatomical reduction and stable fixation. Posterior fixation methods included two iliosacral lag screws, transiliac bars, and double plating of the anterior aspect of the sacroiliac joint. Anterior fixation methods included superior symphyseal plate fixation, anteroinferiorplate fixation, double symphyseal plate fixation, and anteriorexternal fixation (Figure 51-1-3).

Clinically, sacral fractures which typically pass obliquely through the transforaminal region often are comminuted. These injuries can be treated effectively in several ways. Posterior fixation of the sacral fracture can be achieved with iliosacral screws, sacral plating, transiliac bars, or direct exposure of the fracture and open reduction internal fixation. Anterior internal or external fixation will optimize stability of the pelvic ring construct.

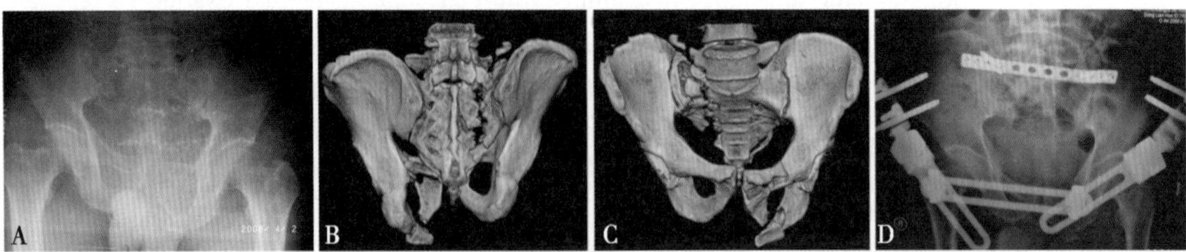

Figure 51-1-3 AO type C pelvic fracture with sacral fracture

A:Care pre-operation images and D is post-operation image withexternal fixation and sacral plating.

Bilateral vertically unstable pelvic (type C3) injuries and sacral fracture with atransverse component (H-shaped) require special consideration. The true nature of these fractures is best appreciated on sagittal-plane reconstructions of the CT scan, which clearly depict the potential for rotational motion in this plane. This type of fracture often requires a variety of approaches and a variety of fixations to treat.

Chapter 2

Fractures of the Acetabulum

2.1 Introduction

Acetabular fractures are usually severe injuries and mostly associated with high-energy trauma. They are challenging orthopedic injuries that require particular attention and expertise for treatment. Traffic accidents reported as the most common cause of injury.

2.2 Anatomy

The acetabulum is a complex geometric structure that can be conceptualized as being built from essentially six principal components. These components are as follows: anterior column, posterior column, anterior wall, posterior wall, acetabular dome or tectum, Medial wall. This structure provides coverage to approximately 170° of the femoral head, less than a hemisphere. The acetabular socket is covered by a cartilaginous surface. This surface has a crescent shape, as cartilage covers the anterior and posterior walls and most of the dome but is absent medially and inferiorly. The arterial network supplying the acetabulum is composed medially of the iliolumbar, obturator, and fourth lumbar arteries, and laterally the superior gluteal, inferior gluteal, and medial femoral circumflex arteries.

2.3 Stability

The posterior wall is the major bony contributor to stability of the hip. Hip stability depends principally on an intact posterior wall and an intact capsule. 100% of hips are stable with as much as 25% of the posterior wall disrupted, but when 33% of the posterior wall isdisrupted only 75% of hips are stable. When 50% of the posterior wall is disrupted, all specimens are found to be unstable. When the posterior capsule is removed, stability is reduced to 89% -14% of hips in the 25% -33% posterior wall disruption groups, respectively.

2.4 Clinical Evaluation

It is necessary to evaluate the airway, breathing, circulation, disability and exposure for acetabular fracture. Patient factors, such as patient age, degree of trauma, presence of associated injuries, and general medical condition are important because they affect treatment decisions as well as prognosis. Careful assessment of neurovascular status is necessary, because sciatic nerve injury may be present in up to 40% of posterior column disruptions. Femoral nerve involvement with anterior column injury is rare, although compromise of the femoral artery by a fractured anterior column has been described. The presence of associated ipsilateral injuries must be ruled out, with particular attention to the ipsilateral knee in which posterior instability and patellar fractures are common. Soft tissue injuries may provide insight into the mechanism of injury.

Radiographic evaluation is needed to process from three different views including an AP view, iliac view, and oblique view. AP view help to show the iliopectineal line, the ilioischial line, the anterior lip, the posterior lip, and the line depicting the superior weight-bearing surface of the acetabulum terminating as the medial teardrop. Iliac oblique radiograph best demonstrates the posterior column (ilioischial line), the iliac wing, and the anterior wall of the acetabulum. Obturator oblique view is best for evaluating the anterior column and posterior wall of the acetabulum. Computed tomography provides additional information regarding size and position of acetabular fractures. Three-dimensional reconstruction allows for digital subtraction of the femoral head, resulting in full delineation of the acetabular surface.

2.5 Classifiation

Letournel-Judet classification divides the acetabular fractures into elementary and associated or complex (Table 51-2-1).

Table 51-2-1 Letournel-Judet classification

Elementary fractures	Posterior wall	Posterior column	Anterior wall	Anterior column	Transverse	
Associated fractures	T-shaped	Posterior wall plus posterior column	Posterior wall with transverse	Anterior column or wall with transverse	Anterior column or wall with posterior hemitransverse	Both columns

AO/OTA classification added additional modifiers on the basis of Letournel-Judet classification. The AO classification is based on the anatomical site, the segment, the type, group and subgroup, and modifiers. The fractures may be divided into type A, type B, and type C (Table 51-2-2).

Table 51-2-2 AO/OTA classification

Type A(62-A) Partial articular fractures, one column involved	Type B(62-B) Partial articular fractures (transverse or T-type fracture, both columns involved)	Type C(62-C) Complete articular fracture (both-column fracture; floating acetabulum)
A1 Posterior wall fracture A2 Posterior column fracture A3 Anterior wall or anterior column fracture	B1 Transverse fracture B2 T-shaped fracture B3 Anterior column plus posterior hemitransverse fracture	C1 Both-column fracture, high variety C2 Both-column fracture, low variety C3 Both-column fracture involving the sacroiliac joint

2.6 Treatment

Although treatment of displaced acetabular fractures has progressed from non-surgical to the surgical approach over the last decade, non-operative treatment is still one of the effective treatment options. Indications for non-operative treatment depend on the assessment of hip joint stability, congruity of the hip joint, and the presence or absence of fracture lines in the weight bearing portion of the hip. Some literatures provide the following indications of non-operative treatment including stable posterior wall fractures, non-both-column and nonposterior wall fractures with intact weight-bearing dome, and both-column fractures with secondary congruence. Nonoperative treatment typically consists of mobilization and progressively weight bearing over 3 months.

Most displaced acetabular fractures should be treated operatively. Emergency surgery is often unnecessary unless for the rare open fractures, irreducible hip dislocation, progressive neurological deficits, and vascular injuries. The choice of the surgical approach depends primarily on various factors, including fracture type, the location of maximal displacement, soft-tissue conditions, and the timing of surgery. The most common approaches are the Kocher-Langenbeck approach, the ilioinguinal approach, the Stoppa approach, and the extended iliofemoral approach. Occasionally, more than one-stage approach is used (Figure 51-2-1).

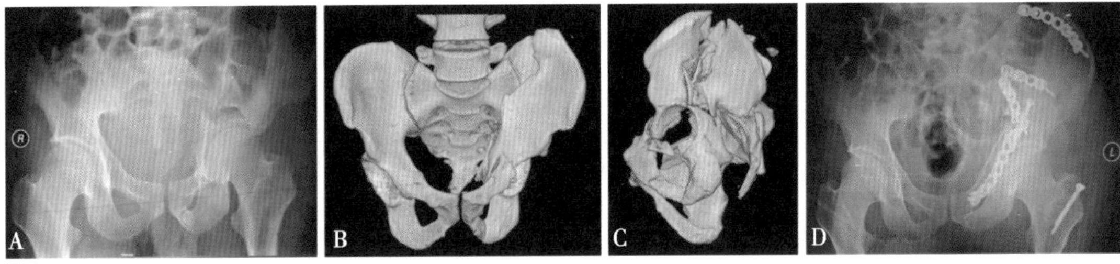

Figure 51-2-1 AO type C acetabular fracture

A-C shows pre-operation images and D shows post-operation image with internal fixation.

Sometimes the fracture itself meets operative indications but the patient does not. Many trauma-related conditions that prevent a patient from being an operative candidate improve or resolve with time. However, the early window for fixation may close in such situations. Other special circumstances include associated fractures, associated soft-tissue injuries, associated bladder injuries, and acetabular dysplasia.

Decision making in the treatment of displaced acetabular fractures is challenging. The current evaluation of a patient with an acetabular fracture should include specific plain X-rays, CT scans, and potentially image intensification-aided stress examinations with the patient under anesthesia. The primary role of the surgery is to obtain a satisfactory anatomical joint reduction.

Part 52

Fracture of the Spine

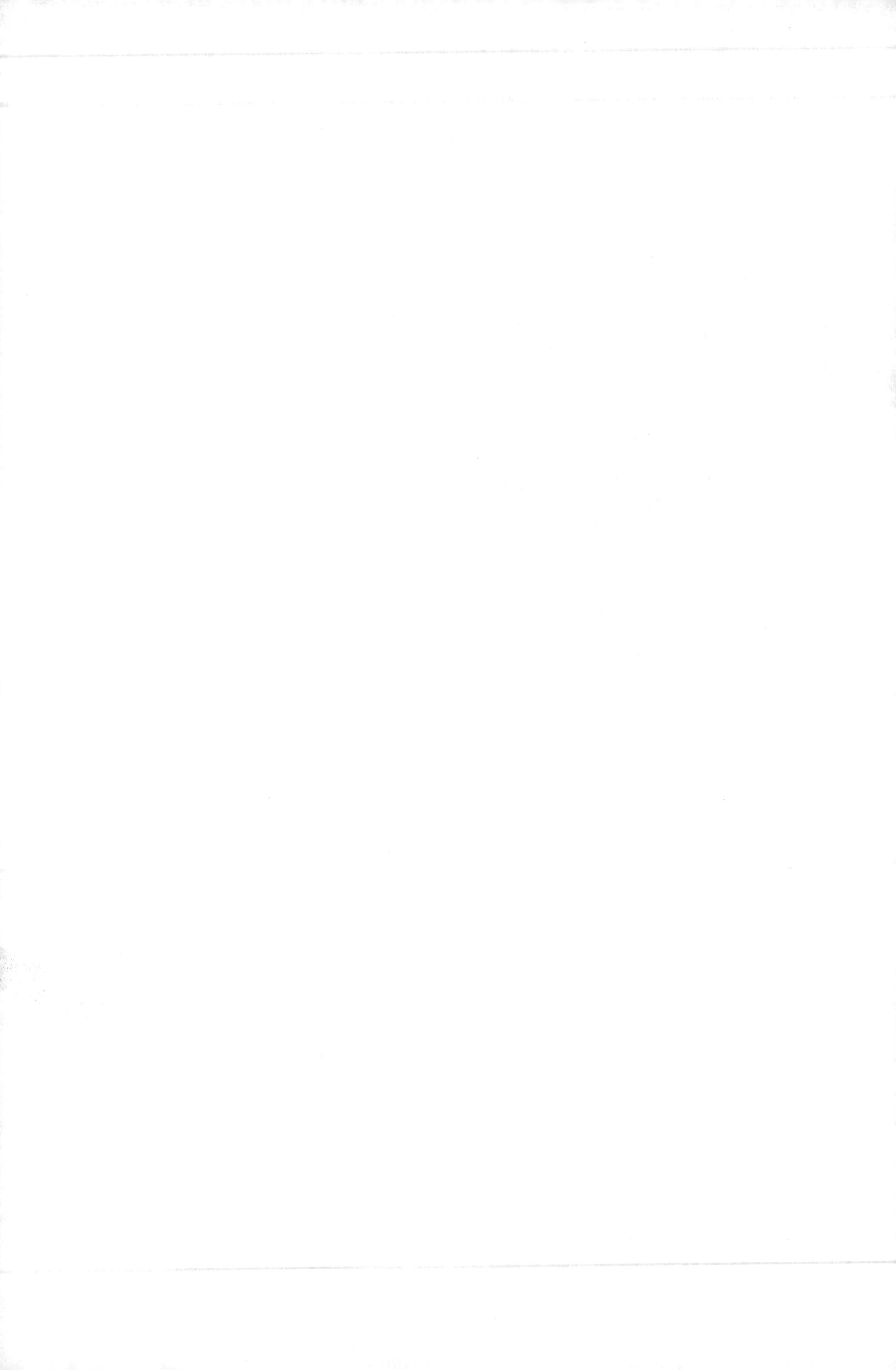

52.1 Introduction

The cervical spine is a dynamic structure tasked with protecting nervous innervation to the entire body while also maintaining range of motion for the head and neck. Fractures of the cervical spine are a leading cause of mobility and mortality in trauma patients, and a bone fracture is associated with 56% of cervical spinal cord injuries. Fractures of the cervical spine can be described based on the level involved and typically divided into three groups: C_1, C_2 and the sub-axial spine(C_3-C_7).

Compression fractures of the spinal column occur due to an axial load and a biomechanical failure of the bone from the added force. This failure is indicated by a decreased vertebral body height at the anterior aspect. Compression fractures do not involve the posterior wall of the vertebral body and do not involve the posterior osseous ligamentous complex. The implications these compression fractures are related to the stability of the resulting structure and potential for deformity progression. Compression fractures are usually considered stable and do not require surgical instrumentation.

52.2 Etiology

Fractures of the cervical spine result from abnormal movement or a combination of movements including hyperflexion, hyperextension, rotation, axial loading, and lateral bending of the spinal column.

While compression fractures to the spine are most frequently due to low-energy mechanisms in osteoporotic individuals(older adults), they can also be caused by higher energies. Due to the ligamentous and anatomical changes noted as one travels from the thoracic to the lumbar level, inherent areas of instability make this a frequent site of injury.

For the spinal column, traditional teaching is that the column can be divided into three sections: ①Anterior column(anterior longitudinal ligament, anterior annulus, the anterior portion of the vertebral body). ②Middle column(posterior vertebral body, posterior annulus, and posterior longitudinal ligament). ③the posterior column(ligamentum flavum, neural arch, facets, posterior ligamentous complex). If two of these three columns are compromised, the injury is considered unstable, and the patient potentially needs surgery.

Compression fractures typically only involve the anterior column and therefore, are considered stable. When they progress to the middle and/or posterior column, they become burst fractures.

52.3 Epidemiology

About 50% of all spine fractures occur at the thoracolumbar junction, and an additional 30% occur at the L_2 to L_5 region. About 50% of spine fractures are due to motor vehicle collisions with another 25% being due to falls. Osteoporosis is another mechanism that can result in vertebral compression fractures. It is estimated that 44 million Americans have osteoporosis and that 50% of Caucasian females will have an osteoporotic compression fracture at some point.

52.4 Pathophysiology

C_1 fractures typically result from axial loading. C_2 fractures typically occur due to a combination of compression, hyperflexion, and hyperextension. Subaxial cervical spine fracture is commonly seen with high impact accidents such as motor vehicle accidents.

During a fall or trauma, the spinal column will rotate around a center of axis for this rotation. There is also an associated axial force applied due to this flexion/extension of the spine. An axial force more than the forces tolerable by the vertebral body leads initially to a compression fracture with more significant forces resulting in a burst fracture. The resulting kyphotic (forward flexion of the spine) deformity of the compression fracture may alter the spine biomechanics, placing additional stresses on other spine levels. The altered biomechanics risk additional fractures and progressive deformity. The occurrence an osteoporotic compression fracture increases the risk of an additional compression fracture.

52.5 History and Physical

Examination of a patient with cervical spine fractures should begin with a thorough trauma examination of ABCs (check of the airway, breathing, and circulation). Injury to the cervical spine has the potential to compromise respiratory and cardiovascular function and even once stabilized these patients must be closely monitored for the ongoing possibility of changes in the respiratory and cardiovascular function. Next, formal strength and sensation testing of the upper and lower extremities, as well as rectal tone and palpation of the cervical spine should be performed. This is most commonly done following the ASIA scoring system. Acute spinal cord injury is important to identify as early decompression within 24 hours can increase the chance of neurological recovery.

Initial evaluation of spine fractures, once the patient has been stabilized, includes evaluation of the neurologic function of the arms, legs, bladder, and bowels. The keys to a thorough exam are organization and patience. Of note, many high-energy compression fractures have associated abdominal, cerebral, and extremity injuries, and these all should be evaluated. One should not only evaluate strength, but also sensation and reflexes. It is also important to inspect the skin along the back and document the presence of tenderness to compression. Documentation is paramount as these initial findings will likely be used as a baseline for all future evaluations.

52.6 Evaluation

Indications for cervical spine imaging includes localized neck pain, deformity, edema, altered mental status, head injury, or neurological deficit. Computed tomography is the preferred imaging in acute spine trauma as it is more sensitive for detection of bony cervical spine injury when compared to plain radiographs (sensitivity of 98% versus 52%). Further evaluation of ligamentous structures of the spinal cord with MRI is important for determining spinal stability and in planning surgical treatment. Scoring systems in dealing with cervical spinal cord injury that includes ligamentous, bony and neurologic injury exist, a common one is called SLICS(Subaxial Cervical Spine Injury Classification System),and this can be used to help with evaluation and guidance of surgical or nonsurgical management. A SLICS score of 1-3 is nonsurgical,a score of 4 is not specified,and a score of 5 or greater is a surgical indication. The scoring system is as follows:

Fracture morphology:

- No abnormality-0.
- Compression endplate disruption or vertebral body fracture-1.
- Burst-2.
- Distraction-3.
- Rotation or translocation-4.

Discoligamentous complex:

- Intact-0.
- Indeterminate-1.
- Disrupted-2.

Neurologic status:

- Intact-0.
- Root injury-1.
- Complete spinal cord injury-2.
- Incomplete spinal cord injury-3.

Continuous cord compression:

- With neuro deficit-1.

Evaluation of patients with suspected back trauma includes anterior-posterior and lateral radiographs of the impacted area. In the trauma setting these initially,should be obtained supine with spine precautions until cleared by the spine team or bracing has been provided. At some point,standing radiographs in the brace are helpful to guide treatment as a supine position may artificially reduce a displaced fracture.

A CT should also be obtained in all trauma settings. If there is a suspected posterior column injury not able to be confirmed on CT,an MRI will indicate disruption of the posterior ligamentous complex. Radiographs showing 30 degrees of traumatic kyphosis (forward flexion of the spine) and 50% vertebral body height loss are historically thought to be unstable fractures,but new evidence is changing this belief. Furthermore,any neurologic deficit necessitates an MRI for additional evaluation. Elderly patients with low energy compression fractures likely will not require an MRI. Serial standing lateral radiographs obtained in the clinic will help track the fracture progression and healing.

52.7 Treatment / Management

Injuries to C_1 and C_2 compose approximately 30% of cervical spine fractures. Fractures of C_1 occur through the lateral mass or arch in single or multiple places(multiple arch fractures,Jefferson fracture). Neurological injury rarely results from an isolated C_1 fracture due to abundant space surrounding the spinal cord. C_1 fractures may be managed in a rigid cervical collar or halo if the transverse alar ligament(TAL) remains intact on MRI. If the TAL is disrupted C_1 to C_2 posterior fusion should be considered.

C_2 fractures can result in fracture through the body,dens,or pars. If the fracture extends bilaterally through the pars interarticularis,a Hangman's fracture is described. Hangman's fracture with less than 3 mm of displacement and no significant angulation may be treated in a hard cervical collar. If the fracture is displaced greater than 3 mm or with greater than 11 degrees of angulation, reduction with halo placement or surgical fixation should be considered. Associated disruption of the C_2 to C_3 disc with a hangman's fracture requires surgical fixation. Fracture through the C_2 dens can be classified as type Ⅰ, Ⅱ, or Ⅲ. Type Ⅰ is avulsion of the dens tip, type Ⅱ is a fracture through the base of the dens, and type Ⅲ is a fracture extending into the C_2 vertebral body. Type Ⅰ and Ⅲ fractures should be treated in a rigid cervical collar or halo. Type Ⅱ fractures without risk of nonunion can be considered for hard cervical collar or halo. Risk factors for nonunion include 5 mm or more of displacement, greater than 10 degrees of angulation, or age older than 50. Type Ⅱ fractures at risk for nonunion should be considered for odontoid screw placement or posterior C_1 to C_2 fusion. All fractures of the C_1 to C_2 complex are considered unstable and should be treated initially with a hard cervical collar, and then evaluated by a spine surgeon.

Subaxial cervical spine fractures follow similar patterns at each level. Compression fractures result in loss of anterior vertebral body height without canal compromise or neural injury. Burst fractures are a variant of compression fractures that result in retropulsion of the vertebral body into the cervical canal. Of note, C_7 burst fractures carry a higher risk of developing kyphotic deformity that other levels of the subaxial cervical spine. Teardrop fractures occur with flexion or flexion-extension of the cervical spine leading to an anterior-inferior fracture of the vertebral body. There are also three column fractures extending through the anterior vertebral body all the way through to the posterior ligaments, and these are highly unstable. Unilateral facet fractures are controversial, but many are highly unstable or can lead to progressive deformity and warrant surgical evaluation. Any fracture extending into the foramina transversarium from C_2 to C_6 should be evaluated for the possibility of co-occurring vertebral artery injury. Surgical fixation of subaxial cervical spine fractures should take into consideration the SLICS scoring system as previously described.

Clay shoveler's fractures describe fractures of the cervical spinous processes.

Each fracture described should warrant cervical collar placement with surgery indicated for restoration of cervical lordosis, decompression of the spinal cord, or fixation as determined by the instability of ligamentous components.

52.8 Pearls and Other Issues

Cervical spine fractures are high-risk injuries with the potential for devastating neurological sequelae. Hence, a trained spine specialist should carry out subsequent evaluation and treatment. All patients with cervical fractures should be closely monitored with a follow-up to ensure continued cervical stability and healing. Any fracture extending into the foramina transversarium from C2 to C6 should be evaluated for the possibility of co-occurring vertebral artery injury. This is most often done with CT angiogram.

Determining the need for surgery is at times controversial. In 2005, a classifications system was introduced to provide more uniformity in management and provide simple treatment recommendations. The Thoracolumbar Injury Classification and Severity (TLICS) scale uses the posterior ligamentous complex, injury morphology, and neurological status to provide a score (1-10) that can guide intervention: less than 4 favoring non-surgical treatment, more than 4 surgical, and 4 being managed by either (Table 52-1-1). Of course, these are general guidelines, predominantly for trauma patients, and each case should be evaluated carefully. Interestingly, newer studies have shown that historical considerations such as loss of vertebral body height, segmental kyphosis, and canal compromise, do not correlate with the need for surgery (in those neurologically intact patients). Of note, currently, there have been no randomized trials evaluating surgery versus brace treatment in "unstable" compression fractures.

Orthosis/bracing modalities accomplish conservative management for a period of 4–12 weeks. Discontinuation of the bracing can be considered when there is radiographic evidence of healing, and the patient no longer is tender over the fracture site. In that bed rest, analgesic medications, and bracing are poorly tolerated in the elderly; many will alternatively consider percutaneous procedures such as kyphoplasties for stabilization of the fracture and faster clinical improvement.

Surgical options are largely dependent on fracture characteristics and neurologic injury. Rarely would compression fractures require instrumented stabilization. For patients with osteoporotic compression fractures, kyphoplasty is a relatively safe and simple procedure relying on the percutaneous insertion of a balloon into the vertebral body to restore the height followed by injection of bone cement to maintain the correction. Recent randomized controlled trials have shown kyphoplasties allowing for significantly more rapid improvement in the quality of life, function, pain, and mobility.

52.9 Pearls and Other Issues

The most important consideration when evaluating fractures of the spine should be the neurologic exam as compression of the spinal canal may alter treatment options. Regarding a kyphoplasty treatment for compression fractures, several contraindications should be remembered. These include current neurologic compromise, burst fractures (fractures of the posterior vertebral body wall), spine infections, current sepsis, or underlying bleeding diatheses. Not addressed above are patients with diffuse idiopathic skeletal hyperostosis (DISH) and ankylosing spondylitis (AS). Both of these result in brittle spinal columns and a fracture of any type should be considered unstable and require CT, MRI, and potentially surgery.

Table 52–1–1 The Thoracolumbar Injury Classification and Severity score

Injury Category	Point Value
Injury morphology	
Compression	1
Burst	2
Translation or rotation	3
Distraction	4
PLC status	
Intact	0
Injury suspected or indeterminate	2
Injured	3
Neurologic status	
Intact	0
Nerve root involvement	2
Spinal cord or conus medullaris injury	
Incomplete	3
Complete	2
Cauda equina syndrome	3

Scores: <4 non–operative, 4 non–operative or operative, >4 operative.

PLC: posterior ligamentous complex.

Toracolumbar injuries usually are the result of high–energy trauma, and often associated visceral injuries are present in patients who have sustained significant injuries in this region. As was discussed for cervical injuries, patients with a suspected thoracolumbar injury need rapid evaluation in the trauma assessment area. This should follow the ATLS protocol with a secondary survey that includes inspection and palpation of the entire spine, ntenderness, step offs mental status, motor and sensory examination in the extremities, and a rectal examination for tone and the presence or absence of spinal reflexes. The ASIA form is used to record the neurologic findings. The radiographic assessment should be completed as expeditiously as possible to allow the spine to be cleared and to remove the patient from the spine board or, if injury is present, to identify the injury so prompt treatment can be undertaken. To this end, CT has become the standard method for evaluation of the thoracic and lumbar regions. CT of the chest, abdomen, and pelvis with contrast enhancement is routinely obtained in the same population at risk for thoracic or lumbar spine fractures to assess for visceral injury. Several authors have shown that CT of the chest, abdomen, and pelvis has superior specificity and sensitivity for detecting injuries compared with plain radiographs. Additionally, CT of the chest, abdomen, and pelvis allows completion of the evaluation more quickly and with fewer transfers of the patient. Hauser et al. found that neither CT of the chest, abdomen, and pelvis nor plain radiographs failed to demonstrate any unstable thoracic or lumbar injuries in the 222 patients studied. Identifcation of additional injuries considered minor by CT of the chest, abdomen, and pelvis compared with plain radiographs was shown to change treatment with respect to pain management and how patients were mobilized. These minor injuries included spinous process and transverse process fractures without displacement.

52.10 Classification

The classifcation of thoracic and lumbar spine injuries is still evolving more than 80 years after the first published report of Böhler. The classification of these injuries remains difficult in part because the goals of classification, anatomic structures to consider, and definitions have not been agreed upon by the community of spine surgeons. Thus, some systems have been developed to direct treatment, whereas others are not intended for this purpose. Terminology, particularly relating to "stability" of the spine, does not have a universally agreed upon definition, which introduces conflicting meanings in different schemes. Nicoll et al. were the first to focus on patient outcomes and found that anatomic reduction was not crucial to good outcomes in a population of miners who were the basis of their studies. They also classifed fractures as stable or unstable based on the probability of increasing deformity and spinal cord injury. Other systems use "instability" as a surrogate term for neurologic injury and consider injuries unstable if a neurologic injury is present without considering the fracture pattern. To classify fractures it is necessary to image the spine, but imaging has changed significantly in the past several years; CT is now the modality of choice in most centers. The use of MRI remains controversial and has a limited role in the thoracic and lumbar regions. There have been some reports indicating MRI can accurately image the ligamentous structures, but to date these have not been corroborated by large multicenter studies. Classification systems have followed treatment options that have become more diverse as instrumentation for posterior segmental fxation, anterior reconstruction and fixation, intraosseous techniques, and minimally invasive systems have been used in the trauma setting. Most of the various classification systems currently in use are either based on a presumed mechanism of injury with specific injury patterns recognized or they are based on fracture morphology. The Denis classification, based on a three column model of the spine, is an example of a mechanistic system that remains in widespread use. The

AO system is based on fracture morphology with more severe injuries progressing from type A to type C with subtypes 1 to 3 within each type of injury. These subtypes are further subdivided into 53 possible patterns. In 2005, a collaborative effort of the Spine Trauma Study Group produced the Toracolumbar Injury Severity Score (TLISS) system. This system incorporates the neurologic examination of the patient in a more direct way than previous systems and uses this information with the fracture morphology and the integrity of the posterior ligamentous complex to derive a numeric score for a given injury. The numeric value is then used to guide treatment options, and these treatment options are based on consensus opinions. This system was subsequently modifed to become the TLICS by the original author in an effort to improve the reliability of classifying injuries. There have been numerous articles evaluating the reliability of various classifcation systems and comparing one system to another or comparing the results of the same surgeons classifying the same cases at different time points. Generally, these studies have not shown one classification system to be superior to another. The TLICS system is appealing because it incorporates the neurologic function of the patient, which is the single most important determinant of functional outcome for a patient with spine injury. Although the reliability of the system has been found to be equivalent to other systems, the validity of the criteria has not been demonstrated, which also is the case for the other classifcations. Also, the treatment recommendations are level IV evidence as consensus opinion.

Wedge compression fractures cause isolated failure of the anterior column and result from forward flexion. They rarely are associated with neurologic defcit except when multiple adjacent vertebral levels are affected. In stable burst fractures, the anterior and middle columns fail because of a compressive load, with no loss of integrity of the posterior elements. In unstable burst fractures, the anterior and middle columns fail in compression and the posterior column is disrupted. The posterior column can fail in compression, lateral flexion, or rotation. There is a tendency for posttraumatic kyphosis and progressive neural symptoms because of instability. If the anterior and middle columns fail in compression, the posterior column can not fail in distraction. Chance fractures are horizontally oriented distraction injuries of the vertebral bodies caused by flexion around an axis anterior to the anterior longitudinal ligament. The entire vertebra is pulled apart by a strong tensile force. In flexion compression injuries, the flexion axis is posterior to the anterior longitudinal ligament. The anterior column fails in compression, whereas the middle and posterior columns fail in tension. This injury is unstable because the ligamentum flavum, interspinous ligaments, and supraspinous ligaments usually are disrupted. Translational injuries are characterized by malalignment of the neural canal, which has been totally disrupted. Usually all three columns have failed in shear. At the affected level, one part of the spinal canal has been displaced in the transverse plane.

The treatment of fractures that involve the thoracic and lumbar spine remains controversial for several reasons. The first is the determination of which injuries are truly best treated operatively and which are best treated non-operatively; the second is the optimal approach for patients who will be treated operatively; and the third is whether operative treatment should include a direct decompression or if indirect decompression is sufcient. The optimal nonoperative treatment likewise is not settled with respect to whether a postural reduction should be performed, whether initial casting or a thoracolumbosacral orthosis (TLSO) should be used for the duration, or whether treatment should include a period of recumbency or if mobilization should be started quickly. To date, there are only two randomized controlled trials comparing operative with non-operative treatment of thoracolumbar fractures. fractures treated nonoperatively. Typically, incomplete injuries (ASIA B-D) will improve one grade with either form of treatment; several studies, including that of Wood et al., showed no benefit to surgery with respect to correcting spinal canal stenosis caused by retropulsion of bony fragments. The type of hospital setting where treatment was rendered was a significant determinant of whether a patient received operative or non-operative care. Patients, with or without neurologic injury, treated at an urban teaching hospital or a high-volume hospital were more likely to have surgery than at a nonteaching hospital.

Patients who have spinal cord, conus medullaris, or cauda equina injuries are most often treated operatively. Short-segment posterior instrumentation is the most common construct used, but specific construct design is dictated by the injury pattern and the neurology of the patient. Anatomic fracture reduction, although desirable, has not been the primary treatment objective. The acceptable limits of residual deformity in the sagittal and coronal planes before functional outcome is compromised have not been determined.

Non-operative treatment consists of a TLSO for most patients with injuries at or caudal to T_7 to help control lateral bending, although Jewett-type braces also are used fairly frequently if lateral bending is less of a concern and if dictated by body habitus. Injuries that are rostral to T_7 are difficult to brace, especially if there are rib fractures at the injured level. Comorbidities, concomitant injuries, and anticipated activity level of the patient are some of the individual factors considered when determining whether brace treatment is a reasonable option for a particular patient. Brace treatment is initiated as soon as possible to begin mobilization, and a postural reduction usually is not done. After the patient has mobilized sufciently, upright radiographs centered at the injury level are reviewed to confirm adequate maintenance of alignment and full-length radiographs are obtained as soon as feasible.

The orthosis is worn at all times when the patient is upright beyond 30 degrees from horizontal for 12 weeks or longer if clinical progress is not as rapid as expected.

52.11 Compression Fractures

Compression fractures are characterized by loss of vertebral height anteriorly, with no loss of posterior vertebral height and no posterior ligamentous or bony injury. MRI is not routinely indicated unless ligamentous injury is suspected because of more than 25 degrees of segmental kyphosis. Compression fracture treatment is with a TLSO for 12 weeks with medical management of pain, which is significant, and graduated return to activity. The most severe pain usually improves after 3-6 weeks. Upright radiographs must be reviewed after mobilization to verify that there is no worsening of deformity. If the patient has a posterior ligamentous injury and an anterior body fracture, operative treatment is an option. Short-segment posterior tension band reconstruction that can be percutaneously placed has shown promise in this setting, but longer-term study is needed. Intraosseous procedures such as kyphoplasty should be reserved for low-energy pathologic fractures. Higher-energy fractures can have fracture lines not visible on CT scan that may extend through the posterior cortex, allowing ingress of bone cement into the spinal canal.

52.12 Burst Fractures

The key features of this injury are posterior vertebral body cortex fracture with retropulsion of bone into the canal and widening of the interpedicular distance relative to the adjacent levels. Multiple studies have shown that there is no reliable correlation between degree of canal compromise and neurologic function, so the percentage of canal compromise is not used as a stand-alone indication for surgery. It is very uncommon for a patient to develop a neurologic deficit with proper immobilization for a burst fracture even in the setting of severe canal compromise. Fractures of the laminae that are nondisplaced and vertic ntrap nerve rootlets, and if neurologic deficits necessitate decompression, then stabilization will be necessary after decompression. If the patient has a neurologic defcit involving more than a single root level, operative decompression and stabilization are recommended. The decompression can be indirect using distraction and ligamentotaxis through the intact posterior longitudinal ligament or a direct decompression that can be done either anteriorly or posteriorly. If there is a horizontally oriented injury posteriorly in the pars interarticularis, laminae, or a facet disruption, this would suggest a distraction force and not an axial load injury, and the posterior longitudinal ligament may be disrupted, so ligamentotaxis should not be employed. For patients without neurologic deficit who are treated operatively, posterior indirect reduction is used. The terms stable burst and unstable burst are ambiguous and in our opinion should be avoided in favor of a structural assessment of each specific portion of vertebrae. This allows an overall assessment of the structural integrity of the spine and forms the most logical basis for treatment. If operative treatment is chosen, it also can help direct the anatomic approach and the extent of stabilization that is needed. If operative stabilization is undertaken, shortsegment constructs to preserve motion segments are desirable, particularly in the mid and lower lumbar levels. The load-bearing fracture classifcation of McCormack et al. is helpful in determining if a short construct is likely to fail based on fracture characteristics. For injuries that can not be stabilized using short constructs, a longer construct can be used in the thoracic spine without sacrificing clinically important motion. In the lumbar spine, anterior decompression and reconstruction usually allow preservation of motion segments and rarely need supplemental posterior stabilization at the same levels. The patient's neurologic status and coexisting injuries must be considered in operative planning. Achieving adequate stability to allow fracture and fusion healing to progress to defnitive stability is the objective. For patients requiring the most complete decompression of the spinal cord, direct anterior decompression is favored.

52.13 Fracture-dislocations

The pathognomonic feature for this type of injury is translational displacement in the axial plane. The displacement may be most evident on either the sagittal or the coronal reconstruction but may not be well demonstrated on the axial images unless two vertebral bodies happen to be imaged on the same axial slice. There also can be a rotational component (either flexion or extension) present; some injuries have distraction as a major component, but the translational displacement identifes the fracture-dislocation. This injury pattern is the most severe and is usually associated with a significant neurologic injury. These injuries are unstable in shear and require long constructs with segmental fxation. Fracture reduction and proper spinal alignment are more important goals in these injuries than decompression because many have complete neurologic injuries that will not be improved by decompression. Achieving final stability is dependent on achieving a solid fusion.

Part 53

Arthrosis Dislocation

Chapter 1

Introduction

If the structure and stability of a joint is imcomplete or injured, dislocation of joint may occur. Almost every joint has a chance of dislocation, but the shoulder joint (glenohumeral joint), elbow joint, and hip joint have much higher chance of arthrosis disclocation.

According to the mechanical or pathological reasons, the arthrosis dislocation usually can be divided into two types, one is traumatic dislocation of joint, the other is pathological dislocation of joint. For example, at normal condition, as the shoulder joint has a motion in any proper direction, ligaments and muscles around the shoulder joint can maintain the proper position of the humeral head in the socket (glenoid fossa). But during forceful motion or injury, these important tissues, especially shoulder cuff ligaments, can be stretched or torn and the humeral head can totally dislocate from the socket. This is a mechanical and complete dislocation the shoulder joint. Sometimes, the term "subluxation" used clinically means that it has only partially dislocated. Therefore, arthrosis dislocation consists of complete and partial (subluxated) types.

On the other hand, many diseases, such as infection, tumor, and deformities of a joint, can pathologically change or destroy the structure and stability of the involved joint. As a result, the pathological dislocation of the joint occurs.

Arthrosis dislocation can not only reduce the motion of involved limb, but also may lead severe neurovascular complications. For example, the traumatically complete shoulder joint dislocation may lead to intractably axillary artery injury. In the lower limb, the posterior dislocation of the hip joint may be a severe challenge of sciatic nerve.

Therefore, in this Part, the details of arthrosis dislocation are systematically taught.

Chapter 2

Dislocation of the Shoulder Joint

2.1 Anatomic Properties and Causes of Shoulder Joint Dislocation

Usually, the shoulder joint dislocation refers to the dislocation of glenohumerl joint. The dislocations are most commonly anterior, meaning that the head of the humerus goes forward out of the joint. An injury where the arm is turned outwards and away from the body, such as a fall sideways on the arm, can cause an anterior dislocation. Occasionally, a dislocation can be posterior, where the humeral head moves backwards out of the joint. This usually occurs from a different type of injury, in which the arm is struck while it is internally rotated.

Importantly, once a shoulder is dislocated, the chances are higher that it will happen again, particularly if you are under age 30. That makes it all the more important that you follow your physician's recommendations and rehabilitation program carefully.

2.2 Symptoms and Diagnosis of the Shoulder Joint Dislocation

The first and foremost symptom is pain. Other symptoms include the following:

· Deformity of the joint.

· Swelling around the joint.

· Bruising of the skin around the joint.

· Displaced bones affecting the surrounding nerves, tendons and blood vessels.

In addition to the pain, patient may experience numbness in his or her upper arm and weakness of the muscles around the shoulder. Patients with glenohumeral instability may also report that their shoulder continually slips out of joint. Dugas sign is positive for these patients. X-rays of the involved shoulder joint may clearly show the complete dislocation and be very useful for the classification of shoulder joint dislocation.

However, X-rays only allow bones and the spaces between them to be visualized. If the shoulder joint is subluxed, some of the signs of dislocation will not be present in the X-rays. Instead, CT scan and MRI can provide much more and detailed information of the dislocated joint including subluxation position, fracture of bone and cartilage, torn ligaments and tendons, broken labrum and compression on important soft tissue.

2.3 Treatment of a Dislocated Shoulder

2.3.1 Reduction

How to treat a dislocated shoulder joint? It's requires a correct manipulation of putting the humeral head back into the socket and keeping the stability of the shoulder as soon as possible. Hippocrates method is an effective way for relatively fresh shoulder joint dislocation. After the successfully close reduction, the patient immediately reports that there is no pain at the involved shoulder. Simultaneously, the deformity of the shoulder joint disappears. At the following situation, surgery must be taken into consideration.

- Close reduction failed.
- Neurovascular injury.
- Severe shoulder cuff and/or labrum injury.
- Displaced fracture affecting the joint reduction.
- Shoulder joint dislocation combined with instable extra-articular fracture.
- Old shoulder joint dislocation.

2.3.2 Stablization and rehabilitation

After a succeed reduction, the corrected shoulder should be kept in a proper position for about 3 weeks. It will be very important to allow the ligaments, labra and muscles to heal. Scarf bandage and plaster can be used for the shoulder joint stability. The elbow joint should be maintained at 90 degrees. Professional rehabilitation training is required for each case. And after a short period of immobilization, structured rehab will start.

Chapter 3

Dislocation of the Elbow

3.1 Anatomic Properties and Causes of Elbow Joint Dislocation

There are three bones of the elbow joint, the humerus, radius and ulna. The elbow is both a hinge joint, and a ball and socket joint. The function of flexion and extension relies on the hinge joint between the humerus and the ulna. The rotation is provided by the ball and socket joint between the humerus and the ulna. On this basis, different functional muscles around the elbow joint contract and relax can provide perfect motions of the elbow. Both bones and ligaments play very important roles in the stability of the elbow joint. Three bones the humerus, radius and ulna at the elbow joint have very distinct shapes and the ligaments connected to the bones can keep these bones in proper alignment. Injuries and dislocations to the elbow can affect either of these motions.

Indirect force such as falling with outstretched forearm is the common reason for elbow joint dislocation. It is known that stability of the elbow joint is determined by the combined stabilizing effects of bones, ligaments and muscles. During a dislocation of the elbow joint, the force can result in bony structure or soft tissue injuries to different degrees. There are two types of elbow joint dislocation. In a complete dislocation, the elbow joint surfaces are completely separated. In a partial dislocation (subluxation), the eblow joint surfaces are only partly separated.

3.2 Symptoms and Diagnosis of the Elbow Joint Dislocation

· Extreme pain and obvious deformity is easily found in a complete elbow dislocation case. As to the elbow subluxation, it is still very painful but the deformity is not obvious.

· Swelling around the joint.

· Bruising of the skin around the joint.

· Displaced bones affecting the surrounding nerves, tendons and blood vessels.

Physical examine of the arm is very essential for diagnosis of the elbow dislocation. The tenderness, swelling, circulation and deformity will be checkcd. If the brachial artery is injured at the elbow due to joint dislocation, the pulse at wrist will be weaker or disappeared and hand will be cool to touch. The elbow joint dislocation may also lead to other complications such as radial or ulnar nerve injury. If radial nerve injured, the dropped wrist deformity can be checked. The numb of medial one and half fingers indicates the ulnar nerve injury.

X-rays are very useful to confirm that the elbow is completely dislocated. If it is difficult to identify on X-rays, a CT scan may be done. If the ligaments are required for an evaluation, a MRI can be used. First, however, the doctor will set the elbow, without waiting for the CT scan or MRI.

3.3 Treatment of a Dislocated Elbow

3.3.1 Conservative management

Usually, a dislocation of the elbow should be treated as an emergency injury, and a reduction maneuver is always required the treatment of an elbow dislocation. Two physicians are usually needed for this maneuver. Just at the beginning, sedatives and pain medications usually will be given. The close reduction is performed gently and skillfully, and after restoration of the elbow joint, the elbow is kept in a splint or sling for 2-3 weeks for stabilization and immobilization. The goal of immediate treatment of a dislocated elbow is to return the elbow to its normal alignment and avoid the neurovascular complications. The long-term goal is to restore function to the arm. Physical therapy from improvement of motion range to muscle strength can be carried out during this period of recovery, and early motion exercise is emphasized. During the recovery, X-rays may be taken periodically to ensure that the bony structure of the elbow joint remains well aligned.

3.3.2 Non-conservative management

Under the following circumstances, surgery should be taken into consideration.

· Close reduction failed.

· Neurovascular injury.

· Important ligament injury.

· Displaced fracture or soft tissue affecting the joint reduction.

· Elbow joint dislocation combined with open injury, instable or intra-articular fracture.

· Joint dislocation with other severe deformities.

For a typical dislocation of the elbow, both bone and ligament are needed to repair. If the neurovascular injury occurs, additional surgery may be required to repair the blood vessels and nerves. As to a relatively old dislocation, surgery will remove soft tissue scar, and extra bone growth or callus to improve the joint movement and avoid the stiffness. After surgery, the elbow may be protected with an external hinge, and correct physiotherapy is encouraged. Improved therapy and rehabilitation techniques, such as continuous motion machines, dynamic splinting (spring-loaded assist devices), and progressive static splinting can improve results.

Chapter 4

Subluxation of Radial Head in Children

4.1 Anatomy and Mechanism of Radial Head Subluxation

The upper ulnar-radial joint consists of proximal ulna, proximal radius (radial head and radial neck) and annular ligament. The annular ligament is a very important ligament for the functional connection, motion and stabilization of the upper ulnar-radial joint. Subluxation of radial head is a special type of elbow joint dislocation in children. This subluxation of radial head is usually caused by indirect force such as pulling with rotation. It typical occurs when a child's arm is suddenly pulled and rotated by his or her parent. Another reason for the subluxation is that the annular ligament of radius is relatively weak in childhood.

4.2 Symptoms and Diagnosis of the Radial Head Subluxation

It is painful although there is no obvious deformity or swelling around the joint. Physical examine of the arm is very essential for the check of subluxed radial head. The pain site is justaround the radial head. Due to the pain, patient is not willing to move his or her involved elbow joint especially in the rotation activity or lifting the arm up. Touch at the pain site is resisted. X-ray is a way to confirm the subluxation. But for young kids, bilateral X-rays may be needed for diagnosis.

4.3 Treatment

Conservative management plays essential roles in the treatment of a radial head subluxation. One skillful physician can easily achieve close reduction of the radial head. During the close treatment, the physician will use one hand to push the radial head, and use the other hand to rotate involved forearm.

After restoration of the upper radial–ulnar joint, the elbow should be kept in a proper position and safe manner is emphasized. Usually the outcome of close reduction is satisfied and sling is used for the stability. As to a recurrent case, plaster should be used to maintain the elbow stability at 90 degrees for 7–10 days.

Chapter 5

Dislocation of the Hip

5.1 Anatomy and Mechanism of Hip Joint Dislocation

The hip joint consists of femoral head and acetabular fossa, and it is a typical ball-and-socket configuration with stability supported by bony and ligamentous restraints. At a normal condition, about 40% of the femoral head is covered by the acetabulum at any position of hip motion. The effect of the acetabular labrum is to deepen the socket and increase the stability of the hip joint. On the other hand, the hip joint capsule and ligaments are very important for the stability of the joint during motion activity. The capsule of the hip is formed by thick longitudinal fibers supplemented by much stronger ligamentous condensations. Exactly, they are the iliofemoral, pubofemoral, and ischiofemoral ligaments.

The dislocation of hip joint almost always results from high-energy trauma, such as a motor vehicle accident or fall from a height. There are two important sources of indirect force transmission to the hip joint. One is the anterior striking on the ipsilateral flexed knee, the other is the force transmission from a sole foot while the ipsilateral leg is extended. There are three types of the hip joint dislocation, anterior, posterior and central dislocations. Direction of dislocation is determined by both the direction of the pathologic force and the position of the lower extremity at the time of injury.

5.2 Anterior Dislocation of the Hip Joint

Alongitudinally stronge force transmitted to the hip with abduction and external rotation can lead to such a dislocation. Besides, according to the degree of hip flexion, there are the following subtypes of anterior dislocation.

Inferior (obturator) dislocation is the result of simultaneous abduction, external rotation, and hip flexion.

Superior (iliac or pubic) dislocation is the result of simultaneous abduction, external rotation, and hip extension.

5.3 Manifestation and Diagnosis of the Anterior Hip Joint dislocation

Usually a high energy trauma and the pain site of hip can be conformed. The deformity of the hip with abduction, external rotation and flexion is obvious. In addition, X-rays or CT scanning are very helpful for the diagnosis of anterior dislocation of the hip joint.

5.4 Treatment

Close reduction should be carried out as early as possible. The Allis's method is always used for close reduction following good anaesthesia. If the close reduction is failure or the dislocation combined with hip fracture or femoral vessels and/or nerve injury, surgery is strongly recommended. As the reduction is achieved, the hip should be kept at a correct position (adduction, internal rotation and extension) for a least of 3 weeks. Professional physiotherapy can be carried out during this period.

5.5 Posterior Dislocation of the Hip Joint

About over 80% of hip dislocation is posterior manner. Alongitudinally strong force transmitted to the hip while the hip and knee flexed and internal rotated. This dislocation is a severe challenge for the sciatic nerve. And according to the hip fracture situation (fractures of acetabular posterior-superior rim or femoral head), there are five subtypes of the posterior dislocation of the hip joint:

Ⅰ: Simple dislocation with or without an insignificant posterior wall fragment.

Ⅱ: Dislocation associated with a single large posterior wall fragment.

Ⅲ: Dislocation with a comminuted posterior wall fragment.

Ⅳ: Dislocation with fracture of the acetabular floor.

Ⅴ: Dislocation with fracture of the femoral head.

5.6 Manifestation and Diagnosis of the Pnterior Hip Joint dislocation

Usually a high energy trauma and the pain site of hip can be conformed. The deformity of short leg and the involved hip with adduction, internal rotation and flexion is obvious. In addition, X-rays or CT scanning are very helpful for the diagnosis of posterior dislocation of the hip joint (Figure 53-5-1 to Figure 53-5-3).

5.7 Treatment

Reduction should be carried out as early as possible. It has been proved that the long-term prognosis worsens if reduction (closed or open) is delayed more than 12 hours. The Allis's method is always used for close reduction following good anaesthesia. This method consists of traction applied in line with the deformity. The patient is placed supine with the surgeon standing above the patient on the stretcher or table. Initially, the surgeon applies in-line traction while the assistant applies countertraction by stabilizing the patient's pelvis. While increasing the traction force, the surgeon should slowly increase the degree of flexion to approximately 70 degrees. Gentle rotational motions of the hip as well as slight adduction will often help the femoral head to clear the lip of the acetabulum. A lateral force to the proximal thigh may assist in reduction. An audible "clunk" is a sign of a successful closed reduction. If the close reduction is failure or the dislocation combined with hip fracture or sciatic nerve injury, surgery is required. As the reduction is achieved, the hip should be kept at a correct position (abduction, external rotation and extension) for a least of 3 weeks. Professional physiotherapy can be carried out during this period.

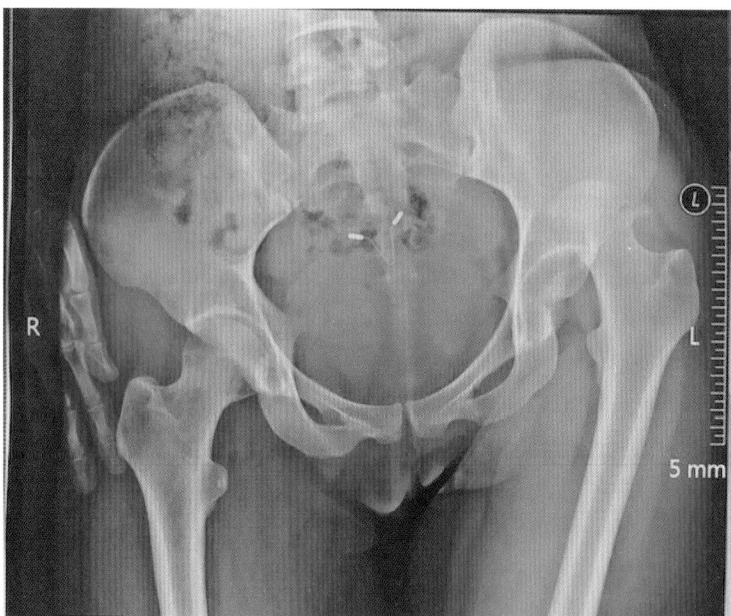

Figure 53-5-1 AP X-ray of pelvis showed the dislocation and fractures of left hip

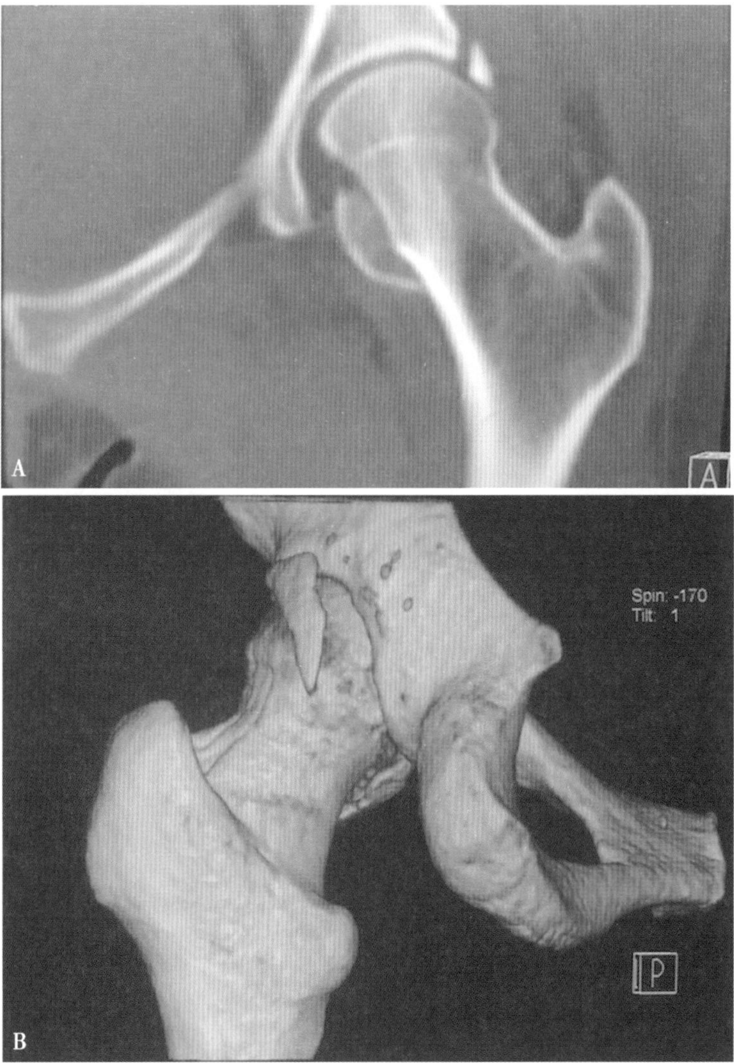

Figure 53-5-2 Hip joint fracture

A. 2D CT view shows acetabular and femoral head fractures; B. 3D CT view shows the posterior aspect of acetabular and femoral head fractures.

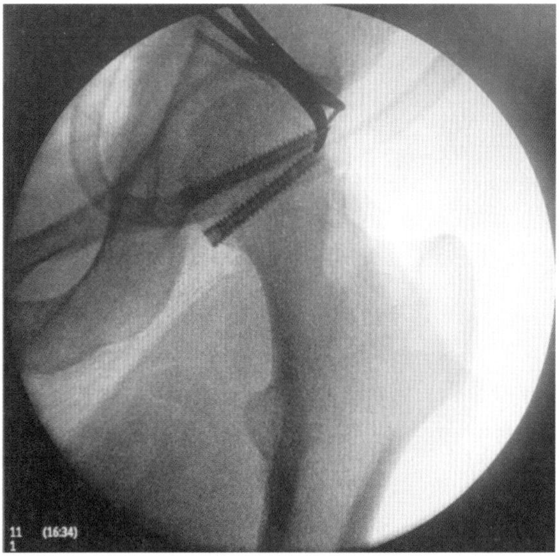

Figure 53-5-3 Post-operative X-ray of the hip

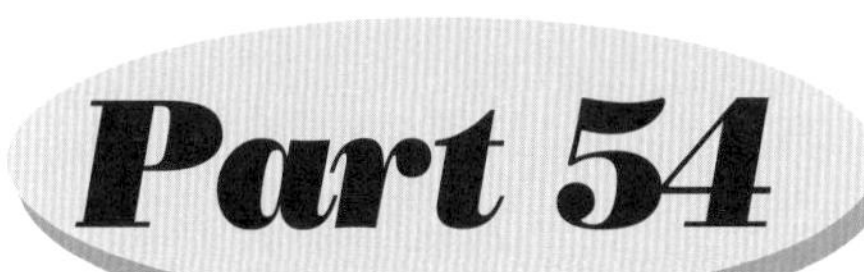

Chronic Lacomotor System Damnification

The diseases of chronic lacomotor system damnification are common in middle aged and elderly people. These conditions are often correlative with chronic and accumulated microdamage, over use, repetitive work, aseptic inflammation of the lacomotor system. These diseases often treated by non-surgical treatment. If the course of disease is long and is not effective after strict non-surgical treatment, surgical treatment may be considered.

Chapter 1

Muscle Ruptures in the Back

1.1 Causes

The back is made up of many muscle groups. Mainly including cowl–muscle, scapular muscle group, latissimus dorsi, erector spinae muscle, psoas and so on. Muscle ruptures in the back is a chronic and accumulated microdamage that occurs in areas where muscle activity is excessive or where muscle tension persists in static postures.

1.2 Clinical Manifestation

The clinical manifestations include muscle weakness, fatigue, pain, tenderness, activity limitation, labor ability, and persistent pain, muscle soreness, induration, dysfunction and so on.

1.2.1 Nature of pain

Local pain which is caused by the lesion or secondary muscle spasm. sometimes there are several localized obvious tenderness points, with anesthetic local blocking treatment, the pain can be relieved immediately.

1.2.2 Tenderness point

In the prone position, it is easy to find accurate tenderness points after relaxing the muscles. The superficial tissue diseases often have special tenderness points. If tenderness occurs in the supraspinous fossa, it is the supraspinatus muscle, in the inferior fossa is the infraspinar muscle, and then in the inferior fossa, it is the teres minor or teres major. If the tenderness is within the inner margin of the scapula, the upper is the levator scapularis muscle, the slightly lower part is the rnomboid minor muscle, and the lower part is the greater muscle, rhomboid muscle. The tenderness points of the lumbar muscle strain often occur at the lateral margin of the spinous muscle of the lumbar spine. Deep muscle lesions are only deep tenderness or percussion pain on the surface of the structure, which is not as clear as superficial muscle lesions.

1.3 Treatment

1.3.1 Non-surgical treatment

A large number of patients of muscle ruptures in the back can be relieved or cured by non-surgical treatment.

(1) Bed rest, reduce back muscle activity, wear branch, avoid all injury factors.

(2) Traction, physiotherapy, massage, short-term, proper traction may relax spasmodic muscles, but violent massage should be prohibited.

(3) Appropriate use of NSAIDs.

1.3.2 Surgical treatment

If the course of disease is long and is not effective after strict non-surgical treatment, surgical treatment may be considered.

Chapter 2

Chronic Trauma of Intervertebral Ligaments and of Supraspinal Ligament

2.1 Anatomy

The intervertebral ligament lies between the adjacent spinous processes, the anterior edge is connected with the ligamentum flavum, and the posterior is transferred to the supraspinal ligament. Because of the lumbar 5 to sacral 1 has no supra-spinal ligament, and between the active lumbar vertebrae and fixed sacral vertebrae, the force is the largest, the opportunity of interspinous ligament injury is also the greatest.

The supraspinous ligament is a strong rope like tissue that connects the tips of the spinous processes from your sacrum up to C_7. Towards the neck, it merges with the ligamente nuchae. The anterior part fused with interspinous ligaments (Figure 54-2-1).

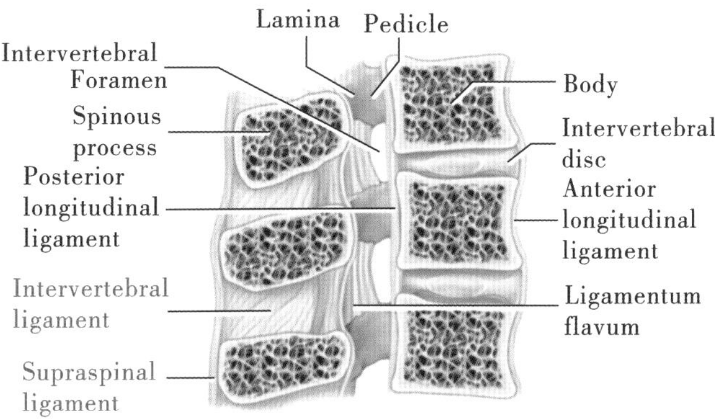

Figure 54-2-1 Anatomy of spine

2.2 Causes

The unprepared sudden movements such as bending over the waist, moving heavy objects, lifting, coughing, sneezing, etc. , cancause sprain or rupture from the tip and forming a small hematoma. The spine bending for a long time and the daily flexion and extension of the waist often cause the ligament deformation, rupture, bleeding.

2.3 Clinical Manifestation

Long-term low back pain, aggravate when bending or extension. Sometimes pain radiates to the sacrum or the buttocks. There is tenderness at the spinous process or interspinous at the injured level.

2.4 Treatment

The vast majority of this condition can be cured by non-surgical treatment. Avoid bending as much as possible, to increase the chance of repair. Physiotherapy is recommended. Local injection of glucocorticoid can significantly relieve pain. Simultaneously using waistline can shorten the course of treatment. Someone perform fascia band repair for long lasting pain, but the effect is still unconfirmed.

Chapter 3

Ganglion of Tendon Sheath

3.1 Cause

The cause of these cysts is unknown although they may form in the presence of joint or tendon irritation or mechanical changes, such as a history of chronic injury and connective tissue mucus degeneration.

3.2 Clinical Manifestation

They occur in patients of all ages, especially among women and teenagers. Ganglion of tendon sheath are very common lumps within the hand and wrist that occur adjacent to joints or tendons. The most common locations are the top of the wrist, the base of the finger on the palm side, the palm side of the wrist, and the top of the end joint of the finger. Ganglions often resembles a water balloon on a stalk, and is filled with clear fluid or slightly yellow gel. These ganglions may change in size or even disappear completely, and they may or may not be painful. The ganglion of tendon sheath is easily diagnosed by ultrasound.

3.3 Treatment

Non-surgical treatment is the first choice. Splints and anti-inflammatory medication can be used to decrease pain associated with activities. Glucocorticoid injection is effective for the treatment of tendon sheath cysts. If non-surgical options fail to provide relief or if the cyst recurs, surgical removal of a generous capsular margin around the cyst is generally successful although cysts may recur.

Chapter 4

Frozen Shoulder

4.1 Causes

The causes of frozen shoulder are not fully understood. Frozen shoulder occurs much more often in people with diabetes, and also associated with hypothyroidism, hyperthyroidism, Parkinson's disease, and cardiac disease. Frozen shoulder can develop after a shoulder has been immobilized for a long period, such as after surgery or an arm fracture(Figure 54-4-1).

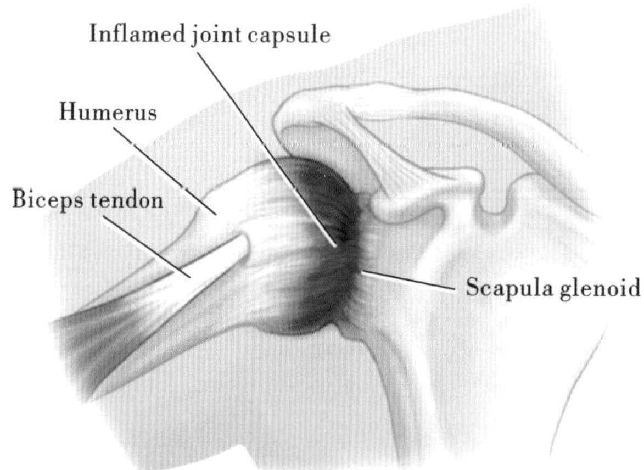

Figure 54-4-1 Frozen shoulder

4.2 Pathology

Frozen shoulder, also known as adhesive capsulitis, The shoulder capsule thickens and becomes stiff and tight. The shoulder becomes very hard to move and difficult to recover.

4.3 Clinical Manifestation

Frozen shoulder most commonly affects people between the ages of 40 and 60, and occurs in women more often than men. The clinical process of primary frozen shoulder consists of three stages. Stage 1: freezing stage. Patients usually develop progressive, diffuse shoulder pain that can last for 6 weeks to 9 months. As the pain worsens, shoulder loses range of motion. Stage 2: frozen stage. Painful symptoms may actually improve during this stage, but the stiffness remains. During the 4-6 months of the "frozen" stage, daily activities may be very difficult. Stage 3: thawing stage. Shoulder motion slowly improves. Complete return to normal or close to normal strength and motion typically takes from 6 months to 2 years. Except osteoporosis of the humeral head, no special findings on X-ray.

4.4 Treatment

Frozen shoulder generally gets better over time, although it may take up to 3 years. However, about 10% of the patients have a long-term problem. The focus of treatment is to control pain and restore motion and strength through physical therapy. The earlier the patient is treated, the faster the patient usually recovers.

Early physical therapy can improve symptoms. Therapy includes NSAIDs, Glucocorticoid can be injected locally or directly into shoulder joint, Hydrodilatation to expand and stretch the shoulder joint capsule, endurable stretching or range of motion exercises for the shoulder. If the symptoms are not relieved by non-surgical treatment, manipulation under anesthesia and shoulder arthroscopy can be offered, especially for stage 2 patients.

Chapter 5

Trigger Finger or Thumb

5.1 Causes

Trigger finger is a painful condition that causes the fingers or thumb to catch or lock when bent. In the thumb its called trigger thumb. when the metacarpal is raised and the hand grasps, the tendon sheath is crushed by the hard flexor tendon and the metacarpal bone, and the friction is increased. The tendon sheath gradually become thicker and the fibrous canals become narrow thus causing difficulty in the patient's flexion and extension and pain(Figrue 54-5-1).

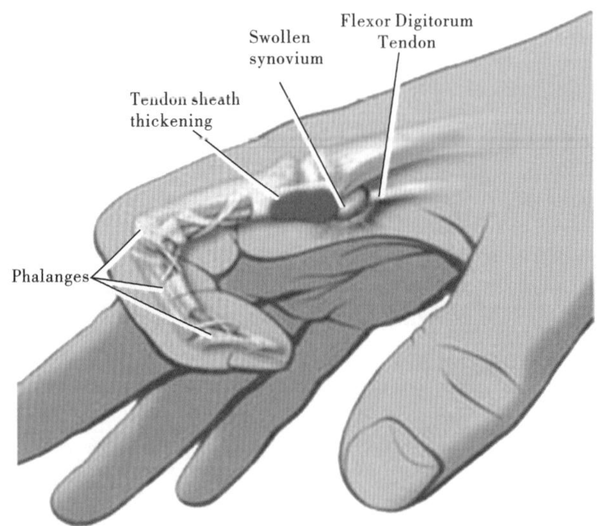

Figure 54-5-1 Tigger finger

5.2 Clinical Manifestation

The triggering is usually more pronounced late at night and into the morning, or while gripping an object firmly. The nodule can be palpated by the examiner's fingertip and moves with the tendon.

5.3 Treatment

In early stages, treatment of trigger digits usually is non-surgical, including stretching, night splinting, corticosteroid injection and combinations of heat and ice. Patients with stable diabetes mellitus may be more refractory to non-surgical management. If non-surgical options is ineffective, surgical release of the thicker tendon sheath are available. Approximately 97% of patients have complete resolution after surgical release.

Chapter 6

The Carpal Tunnel Syndrome

6.1 Anatomy

The carpal tunnel is bounded by the transverse arch of the carpal bones dorsally. The ventral aspect, of the carpal tunnel is formed by the flexor retinaculum, the transverse carpal ligament over the wrist, and the aponeurosis between the thenar and hypothenar muscles distally. The most ventral structure in the carpal tunnel is the median nerve. Lying dorsal to the median nerve in the carpal tunnel are the nine flexor tendons to the fingers and thumb (Figure 54-6-1).

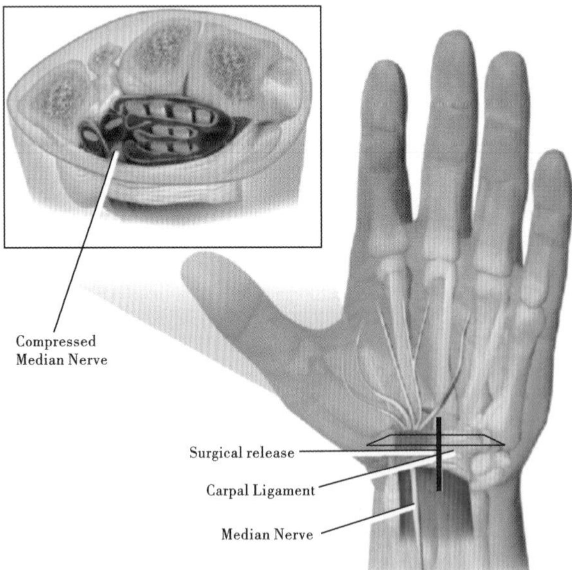

Figure 54-6-1 The Carpal Tunnel Syndrome

6.2 Causes

Carpal tunnel syndrome can be associated with any condition that causes pressure on the median nerve at the wrist, the most common is the incrassated transverse carpal ligament. Repetitive hand motions has been identified as a possible aggravating factor.

6.3 Clinical Manifestation

It occurs most often in patients 30–60 years old and is 2–3 times more common in women than in men. 90% of patients are during the menopause. 30% of them are the bilateral carpal tunnel syndrome.

Carpal tunnel syndrome consists predominantly of tingling and numbness in the typical median nerve distribution in the radial three and a half digits(thumb, index, long, and radial side of ring). Pain, described as deep, aching, or throbbing, occurs diffusely in the hand and radiates up the forearm, is relieved by exercise, especially on the morning and in the evening.

Physical examination: abnormal feeling occurs on the thumb, index, long, and radial side of ring, thenar muscle atrophy usually is seen in the course of the nerve compression. The Tinel nerve percussion (+). Acute flexion of the wrist for 60 seconds(Phalen test) or strenuous use of the hand increases the paresthesia. Electrodiagnostic studies may show signs of nerve damage of the median nerve.

6.4 Treatment

Symptoms can be improved by wearing a wrist splint or with corticosteroid injections. Taking NSAIDs or gabapentin does not appear to be useful. Surgical release the transverse carpal ligament is effective with better results.

Chapter 7

Tennis Elbow

7.1 Causes

Tennis elbow is a type of repetitive strain injury resulting from tendon overuse and failed healing of the tendon(Figure 54-7-1). In addition, the extensor carpi radialis brevis muscle plays a key role. Tennis elbow can occur when these activities that require repetitive supination and pronation of the forearm with the elbow in near full extension, resisted wrist dorsiflexion and forearm supination and when grasping objects be happened frequently. The tennis, table tennis, game of badminton, cook, homework, etc. , may conduces the tennis elbow.

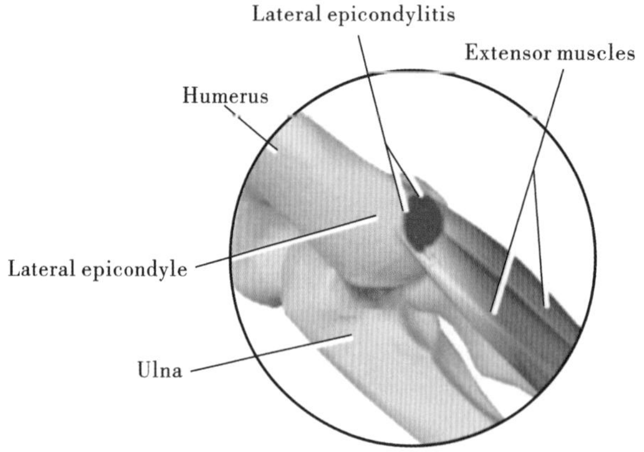

Figure 54-7-1 Tennis elbow

7.2 Clinical Manifestation

The patients often complain pain on the outer part of the elbow, sometimes radiate to the forearm and wrist, weakness of the forearm. When having a physical examination, the tenderness on the place of the radial head, lateral epicondyle or between them can be found. The flexion and extension of the elbow joint is ok. The Mill's test is positive. The clinician palpates the patient's lateral epicondyle with one hand, while pronating the patient's forearm, fully flexing the wrist, the elbow extended. A reproduction of pain in the area of the insertion at the lateral epicondyle indicates a positive Mill's test.

7.3 Treatment

Conservative treatment including physical therapy, orthosis, NSAIDs are useful to most of the tennis elbow. The key of treatment and precaution is avoid the resisted elbow dorsiflexion, wrist flexion, forearm pronation and grasping objects. Local block injection to the area of maximal tenderness are helpful in the near-term. Patients who fail to respond to a non-operative regimen should be operated, incuding release of the entire extensor origin, resection of nerve vessel bundles impingement under the open operation so far as to arthroscopy.

Part 55

Purulent Infection of Bone and Joint

Chapter 1

Acute Haematogenous Osteomyelitis

1.1 Pathology

Suppurative osteomyelitis refers to acute haematogenous osteomyelitis in the arm or leg. The acute haematogenous osteomyelitis is mainly a disease of children. When the resistance of adults is lower, they may also have the chance of such disease. Trauma may determine the site of infection, possibly by causing a small haematoma or fluid collection in a bone, in patients with concurrent bacteraemia.

The causal organism in both adults and children is usually Staphylococcus aureus(found in over 70% of cases), and less often one of the other Gram-positive cocci, such as the Group A beta-haemolytic streptococcus(Streptococcus pyogenes) which is found in chronic skin infections, as well as Group B streptococcus(especially in newborn babies) or the alphahaemolytic diplococcus S. pneumoniae.

The blood stream is invaded, perhaps from a minor skin abrasion, treading on a sharp object, an injection point, a boil, a septic tooth or—in the newborn—from an infected umbilical cord. In adults the source of infection may be a urethral catheter, an indwelling arterial line or a dirty needle and syringe.

In children the infection usually starts in the vascular metaphysis of a long bone, most often in the proximal tibia or in the distal or proximal ends of the femur. Predilection for this site has traditionally been attributed to the peculiar arrangement of the blood vessels in that area. The non-anastomosing terminal branches of the nutrient artery twist back in hairpin loops before entering the large network of sinusoidal veins; the relative vascular stasis and consequent lowered oxygen tension are believed to favour bacterial colonization. It has also been suggested that the structure of the fine vessels in the hypertrophic zone of the physis allows bacteria more easily to pass through and adhere to type 1 collagen in that area.

In adults, haematogenous infection accounts for only about 20% of cases of osteomyelitis, mostly affecting the vertebrae. Staphylococcus aureus is the commonest organism but Pseudomonas aeruginosa often appears in patients using intravenous drugs. Adults with diabetes or immune deficiency may develop contiguous bone infectious disease from soft-tissue infections involving a variety of organisms.

1.2 Clinical Manifestation and Diagnosis

The patients usually suffer from severe pain, malaise and a fever. Physician will notice that the patients refuse to use one limb or to allow it to be handled or even touched. There may be a recent history of infection: a septic teeth or toe, a boil, a sore throat or a discharge from the ear.

During the physical examine, high pulse rate (>100) and temperature (38. 5 ℃) are usual. The involved limb is very painful and can not be touched. It's restricted to any motion. Both the systematic toxaemia and local redness, swelling, warmth and oedema and are noticable.

1.3 Diagnostic Imaging

1.3.1 X-ray and CT

There is no abnormality of the bone from the X-rays taken in the first week after the onset of symptoms. The image of soft-tissue swelling is not specific. By the second week there may be a faint extra-cortical outline due to periosteal new bone formation; this is the classic X-ray sign of early pyogenic osteomyelitis, but treatment should not be delayed while waiting for it to appear. Later the periosteal thickening becomes more obvious in X-rays and CT images. An important late sign of X-ray and CT is the combination of regional osteoporosis with a localized segment of apparently increased density. Osteoporosis is a feature of metabolically active, and thus the bone is living. On the contrary, the segment that fails to become osteoporotic is metabolically inactive and possibly dead.

1.3.2 Ultrasound

Ultrasound may be used for detection of a subperiosteal collection of fluid in the early stages of osteomyelitis, but it can not distinguish between a haematoma and pus.

1.3.3 Magnetic resonance imaging

Magnetic resonance imaging can be helpful in cases of doubtful diagnosis, and particularly in suspected infection of the axial skeleton. It is also the best method of demonstrating bone marrow inflammation. It is extremely sensitive, even in the early phase of bone infection, and can therefore assist in differentiating between soft-tissue infection and osteomyelitis. However, specificity is too low to exclude other local inflammatory lesions.

1.3.4 Laboratory investigations

If osteomyelitis is suspected, blood and fluid samples should be taken for laboratory investigation. The most certain way to confirm the clinical diagnosis is to aspirate pus or fluid from the metaphyseal subperiosteal abscess, the extraosseous soft tissues or an adjacent joint. This is done using a 16- or 18-gauge trocar needle. The sample is sent for detailed microbiological examination and tests for sensitivity to antibiotics. Tissue aspiration will give a positive result in over 60% of cases; blood cultures are positive in less than half the cases of proven infection.

The blood test plays important roles in diagnosis. The white blood cell(WBC) count rises and the haemoglobin concentration may be diminished. C-reactive protein(CRP) values are usually elevated within 12–24 hours and the erythrocyte sedimentation rate(ESR) within 24–48 hours after the onset of symptoms.

1.4 Differential Diagnosis

1.4.1 Acute suppurative arthritis

Tenderness is diffuse, and movement at the joint is completely abolished by muscle spasm. In many cases of young kids, it is very difficult for the distinction between metaphyseal osteomyelitis and septic arthritis of the adjacent joint, as both often coexist. MRI is recommended for the differential diagnosis.

1.4.2 Ewing's tumor

Patients with Ewing's sarcoma always suffer from pain and fever. The temperature, ESR and the white cell count are higher. MRI and biopsy can be used for the differential diagnosis.

1.5 Treatment

Treatment will start immediately. There are four important aspects to the management of the patient.

1.5.1 Supportive treatment

The distressed patient needs to be comforted and treated for pain. Analgesics should be given at repeated intervals. Septicaemia and fever can cause severe dehydration and it may be necessary to give fluid intravenously.

1.5.2 Stability of the affected part

Stability can reduce the pain. Splint and plaster are is desirable for prevention of joint contractures. Simple skin traction may suffice and, if the hip is involved, this also helps to prevent dislocation.

1.5.3 Antibiotics

Blood and aspiration material are sent immediately for examination and culture, but the prompt intravenous administration of antibiotics is so vital that treatment should not await the result.

Initially the choice of antibiotics is based on the findings from direct examination of the pus smear and the clinician's experience of local conditions—in other words, a "best guess" at the most likely pathogen. Staphylococcus aureus is the most common at all ages, but treatment should provide cover also for other bacteria that are likely to be encountered in each age group. Factors such as the patient's age, general state of resistance, renal function, degree of toxaemia and previous history of allergy must be taken into account.

The usual programme is to administer the sensitive antibiotics intravenously until the patient's condition begins to improve and the CRP values return to normal levels. Usually, it will take about 3 weeks. CRP, ESR and WBC values are required for check at regular intervals and treatment can be discontinued when these are seen to remain normal.

1.5.4 Surgery

It has been estimated that more than 30% of the patients with osteomyelitis are likely to need an operation. If there is confirmed deep pus or extensive intramedullary abscess, the surgical drainage should be carried out under anaesthesia. After surgery, the sensitive antibiotics must be used for 3-4 weeks. Simultaneously, splint or traction for affected extremity or brace for affected spine should be used. Once the signs of infection subside, movements are encouraged and the child is allowed to walk with the aid of crutches. Full weight bearing is usually possible after 3-4 weeks.

1.6 Chronic Osteomyelitis

Chronic osteomyelitis is, to a certain extent, from the acute haematogenous osteomyelitis. As the patients have a poor condition or low resistance, the less virulent organism in the bone can lead to chronic osteomyelitis.

1.7 Clinical Features

Patients usually have pain near one of the larger joints for several weeks or even months. He or she may have a limp and often there is slight swelling, muscle wasting and local tenderness. The temperature is usually normal and there is little to suggest an infection. If there is a sinus and necrotic tissue comes out, chronic osteomyelitis can be easily identified. The WBC count and blood cultures usually show no abnormality, but the ESR and/or CRP can be sometimes elevated.

1.8 Imaging

The typical radiographic lesion is a round or oval radiolucent cavity with 1-2 cm in diameter. Most often it is seen in the long bone metaphysis, but it may occur in the epiphysis or in one of the cuboidal bones (e. g., the calcaneum). Sometimes the cavity is surrounded by a halo of sclerosis; occasionally it is less well defined, extending into the diaphysis.

Metaphyseal lesions cause little or no periosteal reaction; diaphyseal lesions may be associated with periosteal new bone formation and marked cortical thickening. If the cortex is eroded the lesion may be mistaken for a malignant tumor. X-rays, CT and MRI are always needed.

1.9 Diagnosis

History, clinical manifestation, etiological and radiological examinations are essential for correct diagnosis of chronic osteomyelitis. At present, bacteriological culture is still an effective way, and Staphylococcus aureus is still the most important organism in this disease.

1.10 Treatment

Conservative treatment may be used in many chronic cases. General support, immobilization and intravenous antibiotics are initially recommended. Then the oral antibiotics could be used for another 6 weeks. Usually, as a result, the healing can be achieved. If the diagnosis is in doubt, an open biopsy is needed and the lesion may be curetted at the same time. Curettage is also indicated if the X-ray shows that there is no healing after conservative treatment; this is always followed by a further course of antibiotics. During the operation, the dead bone and abnormal area must be excised and the exposed surface thoroughly curetted. Bone grafts, bone transport or free bone transfer may be needed for the bone healing.

Chapter 2

Pyogenic Arthritis

2.1 Etiology

A joint can become infected by the following: ①direct invasion through a penetrating wound, intra-articular injection or arthroscopy; ②direct spread from an adjacent bone abscess; ③ blood spread from a distant site.

The causal organism is usually Staphylococcus aureus. Occasionally other microbes, such as Streptococcus, Escherichia coli and Proteus, are encountered. Compared with normal individuals, patients with diabetes, rheumatoid arthritis, intravenous drug abuse and immunosuppressive conditions are easily for this infection.

2.2 Pathology

The usual trigger is a haematogenous infection which settles in the synovial membrane; there is an acute inflammatory reaction with a serous or seropurulent exudate and an increase in synovial fluid. As pus appears in the joint, articular cartilage is eroded and destroyed, partly by bacterial enzymes and partly by proteolytic enzymes released from synovial cells, inflammatory cells and pus. If the infection goes untreated, it will spread to the underlying bone or burst out of the joint to form abscesses and sinuses.

2.3 Clinical Features

The patients usually suffer from severe pain and a fever. Physician will notice that the patients refuse to use one limb or to allow the affected joint to be handled or even touched. The affected joint may be swelling and local temperature is higher. At the acute phase, the systematic toxaemia, high body temperature and increased pulse rate are noticable. The infectious joint is painful and contractured.

2.4 Imaging

(1) Ultrasound

Ultrasound is the most reliable method for revealing a joint effusion in early cases. Widening of the space between capsule and bone of more than 2 mm is indicative of an effusion.

(2) X-ray

X-ray examination is usually normal at early stage. With E. coli infections there is sometimes gas in the joint. Narrowing and irregularity of the joint space are late features.

(3) MRI

MRI is helpful in diagnosing arthritis and can make a good differential diagnosis.

2.5 Treatment

The first step is to aspirate the joint and examine the fluid. Treatment is then started without further delay and follows the same lines as for acute osteomyelitis. Once the blood and tissue samples have been obtained, there is no need to wait for detailed results before giving antibiotics. If the aspirate looks purulent, the joint should be drained without waiting for laboratory results.

General supportive care and analgesics must be given immediately. The joint should be rested and immobilized by using splint, plaster cast or traction. Antibiotic treatment follows the same guidelines as presented for acute haematogenous osteomyelitis. The initial choice of antibiotics is based on judgement of the most likely pathogens. Simultaneously, the safety of medicine must be taken in account. Usually, antibiotics should be given intravenously for 4-7 days and then orally for another 3 weeks.

2.6 Surgery

Under anaesthesia the joint is opened through a small incision, drained and washed out with physiological saline. At present, more and more operations are performed by arthroscopy. It is a much more minimally invasive surgery, but the surgical outcome is not obviously superior to open surgery. After the surgery, a small catheter is left in place and the wound is closed, and suction-irrigation is continued for another 2 or 3 days. After surgery, the use of sensitive antibiotics and immobilization is 2-3 weeks. Once the signs of infection subside, movements are encouraged.

Part 56

Pain Syndrome of Low Back and Leg

Chapter 1

Introduction

Low back pain is a very common symptom. It occurs in high-income, middle-income, and low-income countries and all age groups from children to the elderly population. Globally, years lived with disability caused by low back pain increased by 54% between 1990 and 2015, mainly because of population increase and ageing, with the biggest increase seen in low-income and middle-income countries. Low back pain is now the leading cause of disability worldwide. For nearly all people with low back pain, it is not possible to identify a specific nociceptive cause. Only a small proportion of people have a well understood pathological cause, such as a vertebral fracture, malignancy, or infection. People with physically demanding jobs, physical and mental comorbidities, smokers, and obese individuals are at greatest risk of reporting low back pain.

Chapter 2

Lumbar Intervertebral Disc Herniation

Lumbar disc herniations are a common manifestation of degenerative disease. They tend to occur early within the degenerative cascade, representing the tensile failure of the anulus to contain the gel-like nuclear portion of the disc. With improvements in advanced imaging techniques, lumbar disc herniations have been increasingly recognized in symptomatic and asymptomatic individuals.

2.1 Pathophysiology

Disc herniation is one stage of the lumbar degenerative cascade. It is considered one of the earlier stages, following internal disc disruption. Herniation occurs through a tear in the anulus fibrosus. The anulus is the thick outer layer that normally withstands tensile forces transferred from the compressed nucleus pulposus. Force transfer works only if the nucleus-anulus-endplate complex acts as a closed volume system. Normally, compression across the disc space leads to increased pressure within the nucleus. The soft nucleus deforms and flattens, pushing against the annular fibers, which then generates tensile hoop stresses. The circumferential fibers are placed under tension, dissipating stresses and containing the anulus. With disruption of the anulus, the soft nucleus can be pushed through if placed under sufficient pressure. The nucleus must be fluid enough to permit herniation to occur. Acute sciatica from a disc herniation is often associated with a prodromal history of back pain. Postural variations can influence intradiscal pressures.

The most classic symptom of a herniated disc is radicular pain in the lower extremity following a dermatomal distribution. Focal neurologic deficits attributable to the same nerve root are sometimes present and lend further diagnostic accuracy. The relationship between disc herniation and sciatica is incompletely understood. Inflammation may be produced by prolonged neuroischemia of the microvasculature of the nerve root from mechanical compression or by nonmechanical, possibly biochemical factors. Neurochemical factors also have a role in the production of sciatic pain.

2.2 Clinical Findings

2.2.1 Symptoms

Patients do not have this complaint. Radicular pain is more typical and often the more "treatable" of the complaints. S_1 radicular pain may radiate to the back of the calf or the lateral aspect or sole of the foot. L_5 radicular pain can lead to symptoms on the dorsum of the foot. Radiculopathy from involvement of the upper lumbar roots can lead to more proximal symptoms. L_2 and L_3 radiculopathy can produce anterior or medial thigh and groin pain. Groin pain may also be indicative of L_1 pathology. The character of radicular pain can be sharp, dull, burning, or dysesthetic. It can be exacerbated by coughing, bending, or lifting. A relieving maneuver may be lying supine with the knees and hips flexed, particularly with lower lumbar herniations. In contrast to patients with lumbar stenosis, patients with disc herniations more typically complain of constant pain that is not exacerbated by ambulation. Buttock pain is also common and can be referred or radicular in nature. Patients may interpret this as back pain, but the pathoanatomic significance of pain in this area is different than true axial pain. Pain is one component of radiculopathic complaints. Nerve compression can lead to motor and sensory deficits. Acute bowel or bladder symptoms can be the sign of a cauda equina syndrome, which should mandate urgent surgical decompression.

2.2.2 Signs

Compression of nerve roots often produces objective sensory changes early, with paresthesia and loss of sensation detectable in the affected dermatome. With continued root compression, motor weakness corresponds to the specific myotomes innervated by the compressed nerve root. With involvement of the L_4 root, the patellar tendon reflex may be diminished, and slight quadriceps weakness may be observed. Sensation may be diminished over the medial calf. With involvement of thc L_5 root, weakness is frequently manifested by loss of strength in great toe dorsiflexion. Pain and numbness are present in the anteromedial leg and foot. First sacral root involvement affects the calf muscles, and the Achilles tendon reflex may be lost on the involved side. Sensory findings include pain and numbness in the posterolateral leg and foot. Muscle atrophy may accompany sensory and motor changes.

2.2.3 Diagnostic tests

2.2.3.1 Inspection

There can be loss of normal lumbar lordosis from muscular spasm. Hip flexion can relieve pain, leading some patients to lean forward or be reluctant to place the affected foot flat on the floor. In some cases, a nonstructural "sciatic scoliosis" can be noted on radiographs or examination of the back.

2.2.3.2 Palpation and percussion

Tenderness to palpation of one or two levels is more consistent with bony pathology than tenderness at multiple levels. In some cases, pressure on the spinous processes can reproduce sciatic symptoms. The paraspinal muscles should be palpated. Spasm can be noted in addition to tenderness.

2.2.3.3 Neurologic examination

A neurologic examination is required in all patients with suspected herniated discs. Sensation of light touch is tested along dermatomes from L_1 to S_1. The motor examination should proceed in a routine manner. S_1 motor function is assessed by testing plantar flexion, whereas L_5 is tested by toe dorsiflexion particularly the great toe (extensor hallucis longus), and hip abduction. L_4 involvement most often affects ankle dorsiflexion (anterior tibialis), although quadriceps function can be compromised. Deep tendon reflexes are tested at the patella and Achilles tendons which mainly related to L_4 or S_1 lesion.

2.2.3.4 Specific tests

The straight-leg raise (SLR) test is an extremely useful provocative test in examining patients with a herniated disc. The SLR test is best for eliciting L_4, L_5, or S_1 radiculopathy. It is not useful for upper lumbar roots, for which a femoral stretch test should be used.

2.2.4 Imaging studies

X-ray examination may reveal degenerative changes, such as disc space narrowing and osteophytosis, or the results may be entirely normal. A myelogram, CT scan and MRI will confirm the diagnosis (Figure 56-2-1, Figure 56-2-2).

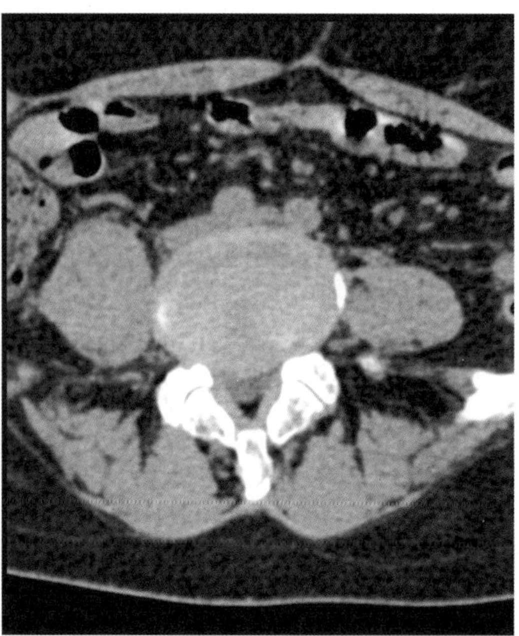

Figure 56-2-1 Transverse CT images of a patient with low back pain radiating down the posterior leg due to $L_{4/5}$ disc herniation

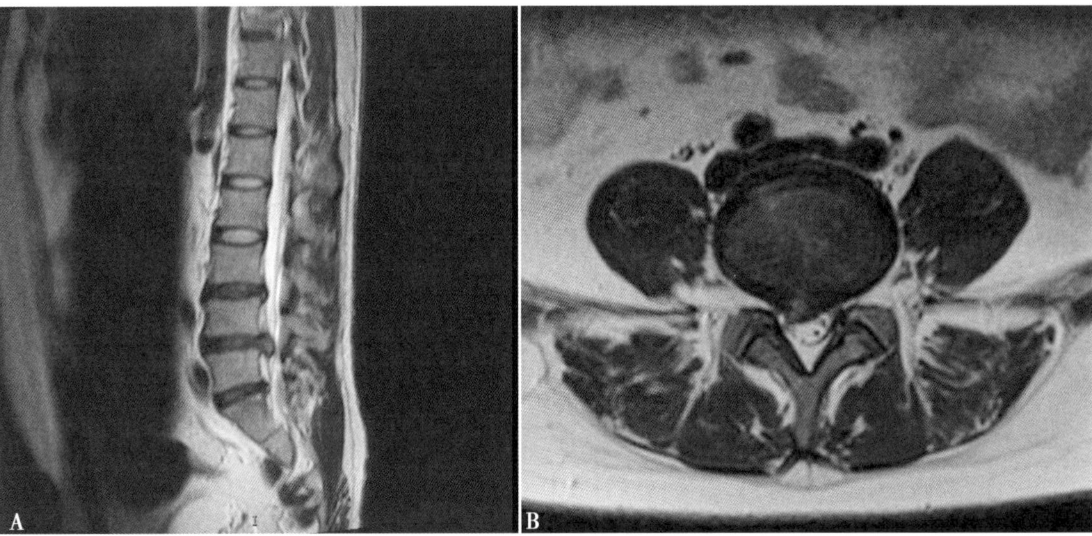

Figure 56-2-2 Sagittal and axial T2-weighted magnetic resonance images

1. Disc herniation at L4/5 level for sagittal view, causing almost complete CSF block; B. Large extrusion compressing dural sac.

2.3 Differential Diagnosis

The differential diagnosis should be narrowed based on history, physical examination, and selected imaging tests. Radicular pain can be caused by numerous compressive disorders, such as spinal stenosis, abscess, tumor, or vascular disease. Intrinsic nerve problems, such as nerve tumors or multiple sclerosis, can produce similar symptoms. Peripheral neuropathies, such as tarsal tunnel syndrome, meralgia paresthetica, and obturator or piriformis syndrome, can also lead to similar sciatic-type pain.

2.4 Treatment

2.4.1 Conservative management

If symptoms are produced by bulging rather than by extrusion of the herniated disc, conservative measures such as bed rest, analgesics, and anti-inflammatory medications often result in complete resolution of symptoms.

2.4.2 Operative treatments

It is still controversial about operative and non-operative treatments. If pain or neurologic symptoms fail to respond to conservative measures (usually longer than 3-6 months), surgery would be recommended.

In the patients with persistent neurogenic claudication that fails to respond to conservative measures, the possible cause is spinal stenosis, thus the decompressive laminectomy is very effective in relieving symptoms and improving function. If spinal instability (degenerative spondylolisthesis) of deformity is also present, the spine should be stabilized and fused over the affected levels.

Chapter 3

Cervical Spondylosis Syndrome

3.1 Pathophysiology

The degenerative changes typically associated with aging are collectively termed spondylosis of the cervical spine. Men and women are affected equally. Among persons over age 50, radiologic signs of degeneration of the cervical spine are extremely common. It is estimated that by the seventh decade, 75% of individuals demonstrate such degeneration. though most are asymptomatic. Disk degeneration is therefore considered a natural aging phenomenon.

Cervical spondylosis is characterized initially by tears in the posterior annulus followed by softening and fragmentation of the disk. The weakest area of the annulus is the posterolateral region, which is the commonest site of bulging of the disk. The hydrostatic support provided by the degenerating disk steadily diminishes, and the adjacent vertebral bodies converge. The longitudinal ligaments become lax and are stripped from their bony attachments by the bulging disks. Degenerative calcification of the ligaments produces the familiar bony spurs. The ligamentum flavum also becomes lax and may bulge into the spinal canal. The posterolateral regions of the vertebral bodies become closely approximated and ultimately form an area of friction. These so-called uncovertebral joints of Luschka become increasingly hypertrophic, creating prominent spurs that may encroach onto the neural foramen and spinal canal.

As the vertebral bodies converge because of loss of disk support, the facet joints become subluxated as the superior facet slides posteriorly. Mechanical dysfunction of the joints results in osteoarthritic degeneration and osteophyte formation. Osteophytes about the facets may project into the intervertebral foramina and impinge upon the exiting nerve roots.

3.2 Clinical Findings

3.2.1 Cervical spondylotic radiculopathy

3.2.1.1 Symptoms

Cervical spondylotic radiculopathy results from pressure on a nerve root as it emerges from the cord to pass peripherally through the intervertebral foramen. A bulging or herniated disk or osteophytes are usually the cause of the compression. The onset of symptoms may be acute or insidious. Patients will usually complain of neck pain with radiation into the infrascapular area. Symptoms of root compression usually are associated with pain radiating into the arm or chest with numbness in the fingers and motor weakness.

3.2.1.2 Signs

Rupture of the C_{4-5} disc with compression of the C_5 nerve root should result in weakness in the deltoid and biceps muscles. Sensory testing should show a patch on the lateral of the proximal arm to be diminished. Rupture of the C_{5-6} disc with compression of the C_6 root can be confused with other root levels because of dual innervation of structures. Weakness may be noted in the biceps and extensor carpi radialis longus and brevis. Sensory testing usually indicates a decreased sensibility over the lateral proximal forearm, thumb, and index finger. Rupture of the C_{6-7} disc with compression of the C_7 root frequently results in weakness of the triceps. Weakness of the wrist flexors, especially the flexor carpi radialis, also is more indicative of C_7 root problems. Sensation is lost in the middle finger. Rupture between C_7 and T_1 with compression of the C8 nerve root results in no reflex changes. Weakness may be noted in the finger flexors and in the interossei of the hand. Sensibility is lost on the ulnar border of the palm, including the ring and little fingers. By evaluating multiple motor groups, multiple levels of deep tendon reflexes, and sensory abnormalities the level of the lesion can be localized as accurately as any other lesion in the nervous system. The multiple innervation of muscles can sometimes lead to confusion in determining the exact root involved. For this reason, myelography or other studies done for roentgenographic confirmation of the clinical impression usually are helpful.

3.2.2 Cervical spondylotic myelopathy

3.2.2.1 Cause and mechanism

Cervical spondylotic myelopathy is the most common form of spinal cord dysfunction in people over the age of 55. Patients over age 60 are more likely to have multisegmental disease. Spinal cord compression is caused by a combination of factors, including anterior and posterior osteophytes, bulging or herniated intervertebral disks, and a buckled ligamentum flavum. Ossification of the posterior longitudinal ligament is a common cause of multisegmental cervical compression.

In addition to the mechanical compression of the spinal cord, vascular insufficiency from compression of the anterior spinal artery and the radicular arteries contributes to the neurologic injury. The severity of the myelopathy is dependent upon three factors: ① the degree of initial compression on the spinal cord; ②the length of time over which the com pression occurs; ③the constancy or intermittency of the compressive force. The average space available for the spinal cord in the subaxial cervical spine is between 17 mm and 18mm. Cervical stenosis is felt to exist if the space available for the spinal cord is less than 13 mm(Figure

45-4). It is important to note that these measurements are taken using the lateral cervical spine radiograph with the neck in neutral position. In the case of multisegmental disease, the actual space available for the cord may be much smaller when the neck is extended.

3.2.2.2 Symptoms and signs

(1) Axial neck pain

Pain along the posterior neck and trapezius muscles without radiation into the upper extremity is an extremely common, but nonspecific presenting symptom.

(2) Cervical radiculopathy

It refers to symptoms in a specific dermatomal distribution in the upper extremity. Patients describe sharp pain, tingling, or burning sensations in the involved area. There may be sensory or motor loss corresponding to the nerve root involved, and reflex activity may be diminished.

(3) Cervical myelopathy

The subtle nature of the clinical findings of early cervical spondylotic myelopathy makes diagnosis a challenge. The physical findings in cervical spondylotic myelopathy can vary significantly depending on the anatomic portion of the cord primarily involved. Sensory symptoms arise from compression at three discrete anatomic locations: ①the spinothalamic tract, affecting contralateral pain and temperature sensation with light touch often preserved. ②posterior columns, affecting ipsilateral position and vibration sense, possibly leading to gait disturbances. ③ dorsal root compression, leading to decreased dermatomal sensation. The motor and reflex examination typically reveals lower motor neuron signs at the levels of the cervical lesions (hyporeflexia and weakness in the upper extremities) and upper motor neuron signs below the lesions (hyperreflexia and spasticity in the lower extremities).

3.2.3 Diagnostic tests

These are very suggestive of cervical disc herniation when present but are frequently absent in the presence of the disease (that is, they are specific but not sensitive). Spurling's sign refers to the reproduction or exacerbation of pain upon pushing down on the head and bending it toward the involved side. The reduction of when axial traction is applied to the head is also suggestive of a disc protrusion. Finally, raising the affected arm above the head (the shoulder abduction test) reduces the pain.

3.2.4 Imaging studies

The roentgenographic changes in cervical spondylosis include narrowing of the disk space, seen most clearly on a lateral projection. Osteophyte formation at the vertebral body margins and in particular at the posterolateral uncovertebral joints is best observed on an anteroposterior projection. Arthritic degeneration of the facet joints with osteophyte formation is best demonstrated in oblique views. The highest incidence of degeneration is observed in segments C_{5-6} because of the concentration of mechanical forces in this region. C_{6-7} is the next most common level. In the lateral projection, the size of the spinal canal can be measured to assess the degree of cervical stenosis. MRI has improved our ability to determine the levels that are affected by the compression. Electromyography may be useful to demonstrate generalized motor impairment resulting from motor neuron involvement.

3.3 Treatments

3.3.1 Cervical spondylotic radiculopathy

Most patients with acute onset of cervical spondylotic radiculopathy have regression of symptoms over 4-6 weeks. Progression to myelopathy is rare, and most patients require only rest, analgesics, and immobilization to relieve pain. Paresthesias and slight sensory changes may persist after neck and arm pain have subsided. Chronic symptoms may involve an element of nerve root inflammation that may require vigorous anti-inflammatory drug therapy. If pain persists longer than expected, MRI of the cervical spine should be performed to accurately localize the site of compression. Only when a discrete herniation is documented is surgical decompression required, either with foraminotomy through a posterior approach or by complete removal of the involved cervical disk and osteophytes through an anterior approach followed by anterior interbody fusion.

3.3.2 Cervical spondylotic myelopathy

Management of cervical spondylotic myelopathy depends upon the course and severity of symptoms:

(1) Medical measures: The management of slowly progressive disease in elderly patients is conservative, and judicious use of a cervical collar for support is generally sufficient. New anti-inflammatory medications (such as celecoxib, rofecoxib) that are cyclooxygenase 2 selective hold great promise for symptom relief while minimizing the chance of gastrointestinal ulceration.

(2) Surgical treatment: When symptoms are more severe or progressive despite use of a collar and when they occur in younger patients, operative treatment may be necessary. The choice of treatment depends upon the nature of the compression, the sagittal alignment of the cervical spine, and the number of levels involved. Compression confined to the intervertebral disks can be relieved by means of single-level or multiple-level anterior discectomies and fusion. When the disease is limited to two vertebral body levels or if there is a preexisting kyphosis greater than 15 degrees, anterior vertebrectomy, foraminotomy, and fusion with a strut graft allows excellent decompression and stabilization of the degenerative segments. When the compression involves more than two vertebral body levels, the morbidity associated with the anterior approach increases significantly. In this case, a posterior decompression via multilevel laminectomy with or without fusion or laminoplasty is preferred.

Part 57

Bone and Joint Tuberculosis

Chapter 1

Introduction

Tuberculosis(TB) can infect any organ of the body. About 14% of the patients have extrapulmonary tuberculosis, and 1% –8% have bone tuberculosis. Of the patients with bone tuberculosis, 30% –50% had spinal tuberculosis. Tuberculosis of the extremities mostly involves the major weight–bearing joints of the lower extremities, such as the hip or the knee, while the ankle, foot, and upper limb joints are rarely affected. There are also reports of soft tissue tuberculosis abscess.

1.1 Causes

Tuberculosis occurs mostly in the lungs, but it can also occur in any organ of the body. About 50% tuberculosis patients first occurred in the lungs, after the lung infection, access to other systems through the circulation of blood, can lead to bone system tuberculosis, urinary tuberculosis, digestive system tuberculosis. In this case, tuberculosis is not a simple lesion, it is the manifestation of systemic disease in the local.

1.2 Pathology

Typical pathological features were caseous necrosis in tuberculous granuloma, osteolysis was the main change of bone tissue, and new bone formation was rare. The pathological process is divided into exudation stage, proliferative stage and caseous denaturation stage.

1.3 Clinical Manifestation

The main pathogens of tuberculosis are Mycobacterium tuberculosis or tuberculous bovine bacteria, which are then disseminated through human lymph nodes, blood or directly around them. Systemic symptoms include fever, shivering, coughing, accompanied by pleural pain, weight loss and fatigue. The patient may present with acute or chronic symptoms.

Spinal column is the most common site of bone tuberculosis, especially in the elderly. But it is also common in developing countries for children and adolescents. Some patients have primary TB lesion in the lungs or urinary system, and some patients can not find the primary lesion. Spinal tuberculosis is divided into central type, marginal type and disc lesion according to the location of lesion, in which marginal type and intervertebral disc tuberculosis are more common in adults. Children often present with central tuberculosis and should be distinguished from spinal tumors.

Joint tuberculosis of extremities mainly involves the weight-bearing joints of the lower extremities. The lesion invades the articular cartilage, and the resulting granuloma will strip the cartilage. The invasion of the trabeculae of the subchondral bone will affect the weight-bearing function of the joint and accelerate the degeneration of the articular surface. Pathological examination revealed necrotic tissue and multinucleated giant cells in the center of the lesion.

Other affected joints include ankle, foot, and upper limb joints. The patient may have a limp, and the joint will appear elevated skin temperature, swelling and decreased range of activity. Joint TB can seriously affect joint function, even after positive and correct treatment, the lesion will recur in an isolated site. Tuberculosis of the surrounding facet joints is sometimes confused with other rheumatic diseases (e. g., gout and rheumatoid arthritis).

1.4 Laboratory Examination

Patients may have normal pigmentation or normal cell anemia, whole blood cytopenia or thrombocytopenia. White blood cell count is normal generally, erythrocyte sedimentation rate may rise or normal. Tuberculin test generally has diagnostic effect. The detection of acid-fast bacillus tuberculosis from tissue or pus is a marker of diagnosis. The positive rate of the bone tissue from the intervertebral disc was 60%-80%. The positive rate of sputum and gastric contents in patients with lung disease was more than 50%.

For patients with lung lesions, the positive rate of bronchial biopsy can reach 70%-80%. The main components of respiratory secretions are white cells or nucleated leukocytes, and the pH value is slightly sour. Molecular spectrogram can be used to determine the form of infection and the sensitivity to drugs.

1.5 Radiological Examination

X-ray films of the diseased joints can guide the treatment. When a joint is involved, the synovium often invades the subarticular bone. Invasive lesions at the edge of the joint are usually shown as osteolytic lesions on X-ray films, which can be similar to infection, non-infectious arthropathy or malignant tumor. Spinal lesions are much more common in the anterior edge of the vertebral body than in the center of the vertebral body. The late stage can result in the collapse of the involved segment, anterior wedge-shaped vertebral body and humpback, which is a typical manifestation of Pott's disease. MRI and CT scans can also provide specific information about the disease and early detection of tuberculosis.

1.6 Surgical Indication

(1) Bone and joint tuberculosis with obvious dead bone and large abscess formation.

(2) Sinus drainage does not heal for a long time.

(3) Excessive pressure of pyogeny in medullary cavity of simple bone tuberculosis.

(4) The drug treatment of simplc joint tuberculosis is not good.

(5) Spinal tuberculosis with spinal cord compression.

1.7 Surgery Contraindication

(1) Those who are too old to bear the operation.

(2) Systemic weakness and generalized multiple tuberculosis.

(3) Patients with heart and kidney diseases.

(4) Osteoarticular tuberculosis not suitable for acute active stage.

Chapter 2

Tuberculosis of the Thoracic or Lumbar Spine

Spinal tuberculosis has the highest incidence of total bone and joint tuberculosis, accounting for about half of the total number of bone and joint tuberculosis, especially in children and adolescents. All the spine can be involved, in the past, lumbar tuberculosis is the most, in recent years, thoracic vertebrae, lumbar vertebrae, followed by the sacrum and cervical vertebrae, and so on.

Vertebral tuberculosis accounts for the majority, and simple adnexal tuberculosis is rare. Thoracic tuberculosis often forms prevertebral and paravertebral abscess, and may also occur in the posterior mediastinal area or develop along the intercostal chest wall. Vertebral lesions due to circulatory disorders and tuberculosis infection, there is bone destruction and necrosis, there are changes in cheese and abscess formation, vertebral body due to lesions and load-bearing collapse, so that the spine bending, lumbar back can appear "hump" deformity. Paraplegia is caused by compression of the spinal cord or blood supply due to the collapse of the vertebral body and the formation of the tissue and abscess of the dead flesh bud (Figure 57-2-1).

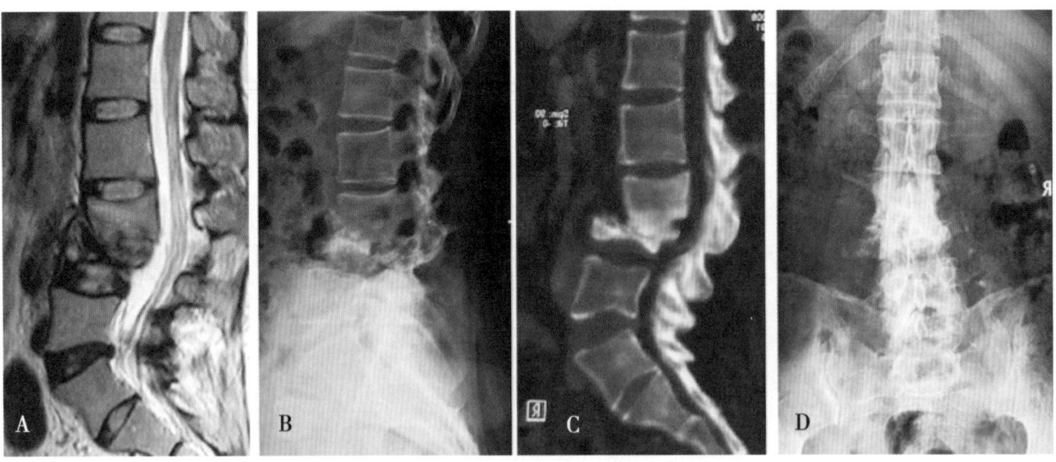

Figure 57-2-1 Lumbar spinal tuberculosis

A. Preoperative MRI showed vertebral signal changes and intervertebral disk compromise at the L3 -L4 level; B-D. X-ray and sagittal CT scans indicated posterior displacement of L3 and severe bony destruction of the L4 vertebra with narrowing of the intervertebral space at the involved segment.

2.1 Causes

The tuberculosis of the thoracic vertebra, like other parts of the tuberculosis, is mostly caused by tuberculosis. The tuberculosis bacteria spread to the bone tissue with the blood. Most of the tuberculosis bacteria are eliminated. The cause of the tuberculosis of the thoracic vertebrae is only a few tuberculous bacteria that escape the anti-tuberculosis drugs and hide in the body. When the body's immunity drops, the colonization infection causes bone destruction to develop into bone tuberculosis.

2.2 Clinical Manifestation

Main performance: Back pain is the most common symptom of thoracic tuberculosis, the nature of pain is mostly blunt pain or pain, accompanied by tenderness and percussion pain, rest can be alleviated or temporarily disappeared, in walking, weight bearing, cough, sleep pain aggravation. The specific manifestations are as follows:

2.2.1 Pain

Initial local pain is much less obvious, the disease develops to stimulate or oppress its neighboring nerve roots, such as the thoracic tuberculosis of the intercostal neuralgia. Lumbar tuberculosis stimulation or compression of lumbar plexus caused leg pain, simple tuberculosis or synovial tuberculosis development of total joint TB pain, often at this time to cause patients attention.

2.2.2 Spinal movement restriction

In order to alleviate the pain, the affected muscles have been in a state of spasm, so as to play a protective role. When the patient's posture changes, especially when nocturnal sleep loses the protection of muscle spasm, the pain is more obvious, children often show night cry and so on.

2.2.3 Swelling

Joint tuberculosis of the extremities is easy to find local swelling, skin color is usually normal, a little local heat. Joint swelling gradually increased, limb muscle atrophy, diseased joints more spindle shape.

2.2.4 Functional disorders

Often, the patient's joint dysfunction occurs earlier than pain in the affected part. In order to alleviate the pain in the affected part, the joints are often forced to be in special positions, such as shoulder droop, elbow semi-flexion, hip flexion, ankle foot droop. Cervical tuberculosis is commonly used to support the mandible, thoracic or lumbar spine tuberculosis muscle protective spasm, resulting in difficult bending and careful squatting pick up special posture.

2.2.5 Deformities

With the development of lesions, bone joint or vertebral mass destruction, the unique posture of the persistent and further development, joint activities further limited and deformity, spinal tuberculosis more than ready-made horn kyphosis.

2.3 Radiographic Examination

2.3.1 X-ray photography

Bone destruction and intervertebral space stenosis were the main manifestations on X-ray films. Bone destruction is concentrated in the upper or lower edge of the vertebral body, quickly invading the intervertebral disc, manifested as the destruction of the end plate of the vertebral body and progressive narrowing of the intervertebral space, and involving the adjacent two vertebrae. Multiple calcification shadows can be seen in chronic cases.

2.3.2 CT

CT can clearly show the location of lesion, cavity and dead bone formation. Even small paravertebral abscesses can be found on CT scans. CT examination has a unique value for psoas major abscess.

2.3.3 MRI

MRI has the value of early diagnosis and can display abnormal signals during inflammatory infiltration, but it is mainly used to observe the compression and degeneration of the spinal cord.

2.4 Diagnosis

According to symptoms, signs and imaging manifestations, typical cases are not difficult to diagnose, but they must be distinguished from the following diseases.

2.4.1 Ankylosing spondylitis

This disease all has sacroiliac arthritis, does not have the whole body poisoning symptom X-ray examination not to see the bone destruction and the dead bone, after the thoracic vertebra will have the chest dilatation limit and other clinical manifestation sufficient differentiation.

2.4.2 Suppurative spondylitis

Acute onset, high fever and obvious pain, rapid progress, early blood culture can detect pathogenic bacteria. The X-ray performance is fast and its characteristic X-ray manifestations can be identified.

2.4.3 Spinal tumors

More commonly seen in the elderly, the pain aggravated day by day. X-ray film can be seen bone destruction involving the pedicle, vertebral space height is normal, there is generally no parenchymal soft tissue shadow.

2.5 Treatment

2.5.1 Supportive therapy

Pay attention to rest, nutrition, daily intake of adequate protein and vitamins. Usually more bed rest, if necessary as required strict bed rest. Anemia can be given blood tonic, severe anemia or repeated fever can be intermittently lost to a small amount of fresh blood. The acute phase of mixed infection can be treated with antibiotics.

2.5.2 Antituberculosis drug therapy

Currently isoniazid rifampicin and ethambutanol are the first line drugs. Isoniazid and rifampicin were the first drug of choice. In order to improve the curative effect and prevent the drug resistance caused by long-term antituberculotic drugs, it is currently advocated that combined use of drugs. The adult dose of isoniazid was 300 mg per day, either orally or once in the morning. Because of the poor blood supply in the focus of bone and joint tuberculosis, the drug infiltration is slow, so the time should not be too short. Generally, it is advocated that isoniazid should be taken orally for 2 years. Rifampicin was administered once in the morning at 450 mg in adults. Rifampicin has toxic effect to liver, should examine liver function immediately after 3 months of medication, depending on the condition of liver function decide whether to continue to use rifampicin. Rifampicin was generally used for 3 months. Ethambutanol has obvious bacteriostatic effect on Mycobacterium tuberculosis. It has a strong ability to penetrate into the lesion and is administered at a dose of 750 mg per dose in adults. Ethambutanol occasionally showed optic nerve damage. Isoniazid + rifampicin or isoniazid + ethambutanol are generally advocated. Severe patients can be treated with three drugs at the same time. The tuberculosis systemic symptom is obvious, the fever does not withdraw the person may use to the aminosalicylate sodium or the amikacin intravenous injection. The dose of sodium aminosalicylate was 12 g per day, which was injected intravenously without light. The dose of amikacin was 1 g per day. Because of toxic reactions, intravenous administration should be controlled within 2 weeks. After antituberculosis drug treatment, systemic symptoms and local symptoms will gradually reduce.

2.5.3 Surgical treatment

There are three types of surgery: ①Incision and discharge of pus: Cold abscess caused secondary infection by extensive drainage, and the symptoms of systemic poisoning were obvious, which could save lives by incision and drainage of pus. ②Debridement: Postoperative antituberculous drug therapy and local immobilization can not be ignored. ③Orthopaedic surgery: Correct kyphosis.

2.6 Prognosis

Generally, antituberculous treatment before and after surgery and surgical focus clearance and internal fixation, the focus of bone healing, the patient symptoms disappeared, clinical recovery.

Chapter 3

Tuberculosis Arthritis of the Hip

Tuberculosis of the hip joint accounts for about 7.20% of the total body and joint tuberculosis, which is the second only second to the tuberculosis of the spine. It is more common in children and young adults than in women. 7% – 10% cases of sacroiliac joint tuberculosis or lower lumbar conical tuberculosis were found.

3.1 Causes

Mycobacterium tuberculosis can pollute the air and cause respiratory tract infections. Gastrointestinal infections are rare. Food can be treated with low temperature sterilization to prevent gastrointestinal tract infection. Tuberculosis does not pass through healthy skin and can cause infection when it is ruptured.

3.2 Clinical Manifcstation

(1) Systemic poisoning symptoms. Patients often have anorexia, wasting, general weakness, bad temper and low fever, night sweats and so on.

(2) Pain and tenderness. Generally, the onset of hidden gradually, the earliest hip pain is relatively mild, aggravated activities, rest relief, often accompanied by the lower extremity of the affected side of the weakness or heavy feeling.

(3) Lameness.

(4) Muscular atrophy. Muscular atrophy of the contralateral limb is another feature of hip tuberculosis. Due to muscular malnutrition and loss of sexual atrophy.

(5) Swelling, abscess, or sinus formation.

(6) Limited hip movement.

(7) Malformations.

3.3 Radiographic Examination

(1) X-ray examination is very important for the diagnosis of hip tuberculosis. It is necessary to take simultaneous radiography of both hip joints for comparison. In the early stage of the disease, only localized osteoporosis can be found, and a good quality X-ray film can show swelling of the joint capsule. Progressive articular space narrowing and marginal bone destruction were early X-ray signs. With the exacerbation of destruction, cavity and dead bone appeared, and the femoral head almost disappeared in severe cases.

(2) CT and MRI can obtain early diagnosis. They can clearly show how much fluid in the hip joint, can reveal the ordinary X-ray film can not show the small bone lesions. MRI can also show the inflammatory infiltration in bone.

3.4 Diagnosis

The diagnosis of hip tuberculosis is generally not difficult to diagnose on the basis of history, symptoms, signs and X-ray manifestations.

3.5 Treatment

3.5.1 Non-surgical therapy

(1) Rest, immobilization and nutrition of the whole body are closely related to the improvement and deterioration of the lesion. Rest and nutrition are essential for the treatment of hip tuberculosis as an important step in improving the overall health of the body.

(2) The use of antituberculosis drugs on the basis of enhancing the body's resistance to choose appropriate drugs to treat various types of tuberculosis, for the treatment of hip tuberculosis is no exception.

3.5.2 Surgical treatment

(1) Focal debridement was performed by surgical procedure. Enter the focus directly, remove abscesses, caseous substances, dead bones, remove hypertrophic synovial tissue, and chisel the sclerosing cavity wall.

(2) Correction of deformities and functional reconstruction of the local focus has been cured, the joint can still be active or have ankylosis, but in non-functional position can be corrected by osteotomy.

Chapter 4

Tuberculosis Arthritis of the Knee

Tuberculosis of the knee joint, like other bone and joint tuberculosis, is a secondary lesion, most of it from tuberculosis. Tuberculosis of the knee joint is more than 10 years old children, no significant differences in gender, children's knee tuberculosis due to long course of disease, easy to involve epiphyseal, it often causes the development and growth of limb deformities. Tuberculosis of the knee joint usually occurs on one side, and it is rare in both sides. It is usually divided into simple synovial tuberculosis, simple bone tuberculosis and total joint tuberculosis.

Treatment:

(1) Support therapy and anti-TB drug therapy

Improve your overall health.

(2) Early bed rest and traction

Can alleviate the symptom quickly, with the skin traction causes the joint to straighten.

(3) Synovial tuberculosis

Early intraarticular injection, if not effective, should be early surgery.

(4) Surgical treatment

1) Bone tuberculosis should be removed as early as possible to avoid the spread to the joint.

2) Synovial tuberculosis, if most of the cartilage is intact, can be done focus clearance, remove the lesion of synovium, superpatellar fat, cartilage on the surface of the granulation; If the meniscus is involved also need to be excised, complete hemostasis after operation, place the affected limb on Thomas's splint, carry on the skin traction, keep the joint straight. After the gradual movement of the joint, but when the rest of the knee to maintain the straight position, antituberculosis drug treatment for more than 6 months, children can retain the full joint of a certain range of motion.

3) When the bone of whole joint tuberculosis is obviously destroyed, the knee joint should be fused in the functional position after thoroughly clearing the focus. Children should be fused at the 180 degree of knee extension, and should not hurt the epiphysis.

Part 58

Tumors of the Bone

Chapter 1

Introduction

1.1 General Properties of Bone Tumors

Bone tumors are important parts of orthopaedics. There are many kinds of bone tumors in human beings including benign, malignant, and bone-tumor like lesions. As to the real bone tumors, they can be divided into primary and secondary bone tumors. The properties of different bone tumors may be quite different. Osteosarcoma, a malignant bone tumor, is relatively easy for individuals between 10-20 years of age or adults over 60 years of age. The incidence of Ewing's tumor, another malignancy, goes up while the ages of patients increase. However, in patients over 65-70 years of age, metastatic bone lesions are more common than all primary tumors together. On the other hand, the location and prognosis of different bone tumors are various. At present, most classifications of bone tumors are based on the recognition of the dominant tissue in the various lesions. Knowing the cell line from which the tumor has sprung may help with both diagnosis and planning of treatment. Among the various classifications, the Enneking's method is widely used clinically. The grade (G0-G2), territory (T0-T2) and situation of metastasis (M0-M1) of a bone tumor can be taken into account. Therefore, the Enneking's strategy, to a certain extent, plays important roles in clinical classification, surgical planning, and prognosis of bone tumors.

1.2 Examination

Lump, swelling, fever and pain are important but less specific. On basis of the manifestation, it can be difficult to distinguish a tumor from infection or a haematoma. Therefore, other essential methods or techniques must be used systematically.

1.3 Imaging

1.3.1 X-rays

Plain X-rays are still the most useful of all imaging techniques. There may be an obvious abnormality in the bone such as abnormal change of a cortical or spongy bone, a lump around the long bone or a mass within a vertebral body. If the boundary of the bony cyst is sharply defined it is probably benign, if it is hazy and diffuse it suggests an invasive tumor. Signs of Codman and light rays may indicate active bone tumors. Stippled calcification inside a cystic area is characteristic of cartilage tumors. For all its informative detail, the X-ray alone can seldom be relied on for a definitive diagnosis. If other forms of imaging are planned (bone scans, CT or MRI), they should be done before undertaking a biopsy, which itself may distort the appearances.

1.3.2 Computed tomography

CT can show more accurately both intraosseous and extraosseous extension of the tumor and the relationship to surrounding structures. It may also reveal suspected lesions in inaccessible sites, like the spine or pelvis; and it is a reliable method of detecting pulmonary metastases.

1.3.3 Magnetic resonance imaging

MRI provides further information. Its greatest value is in the assessment of tumor spread: ①within the bone; ②into a nearby joint; ③into the soft tissues. Besides, blood vessels and the relationship of the tumor to the perivascular space are well defined. MRI is also useful in assessing soft-tissue tumors and cartilaginous lesions.

1.3.4 Laboratory tests

Blood tests are often necessary to exclude other conditions, e. g. , infection or metabolic bone disorders. Anaemia, increased ESR and elevated serum alkaline phosphatase levels are non-specific findings, but if other causes are excluded they may help in differentiating between benign and malignant bone lesions. Serum protein electrophoresis may reveal an abnormal globulin fraction and the urine may contain Bence Jones protein in patients with myeloma. A raised serum acid phosphatase suggests prostatic carcinoma.

1.3.5 Biopsy

Biopsy plays essential roles in bone tumor diagnosis and differential diagnosis. There are two kinds of biopsy, needle biopsy and open biopsy.

1.3.6 Needle biopsy

Needle biopsy should be performed either by the surgeon planning definitive treatment or by an experienced radiologist. Often it is carried out with the help of ultrasound or CT guidance. It is important to ensure that a representative sample of the tumor is taken and that it is adequate to make a histological diagnosis. If infection is suspected then a sample should be sent for microbiology. It is also essential that the biopsy is carried out in the line of any further surgical incision so that the tract can be excised at the time of definitive surgery.

1.3.7 Open biopsy

This is a more reliable way of obtaining a representative sample. The site is selected so that it can be included in any subsequent operation. As little as possible of the tumor is exposed and a block of tissue is removed. It is ideally in the boundary zone, so as to include normal tissue, pseudocapsule and abnormal tissue. Drains should be avoided, so as to minimize the risk of tumor contamination.

1.3.8 Principles of treatment

If it is a benign, but symptomatic or enlarging tumor, or a benign tumor is painful and continue to enlarge after the end of normal bone growth, biopsy is required for confirmation of the diagnosis. Unless they are unusually aggressive, they can generally be removed by local (marginal) excision or by curettage in the case of benign cysts.

If the lesion is thought to be a malignant tumor, the patient is admitted for more detailed examination, blood tests, chest X-ray, further imaging (including pulmonary CT and MRI) and biopsy. This should allow a firm diagnosis and staging to be established. The various treatment options can then be discussed with the patient (or the parents, in the case of a young child). A choice may be excision followed by bone transplantation or prosthesis implantation. Many other surgeries such as amputation and limb-sparing operations and different types of adjuvant therapy are required for various malignant cases.

Chapter 2

Chondroma

2.1 Manifestation

Chondromas are usually asymptomatic and are discovered incidentally on X–ray or after a pathological fracture. This disease is seen at any age(but mostly in young people) and in any bone preformed in cartilage (most commonly the tubular bones of the hands and feet). Islands of cartilage may persist in the metaphyses of bones formed by endochondral ossification. Sometimes they grow and take on the characteristics of a benign tumor. Lesions may be solitary or multiple and part of a generalized dysplasia.

2.2 Radiology

X–ray shows a well–defined, centrally placed radiolucent area at the junction of metaphysis and diaphysis; sometimes the bone is slightly expanded. In mature lesions there are flecks or wisps of calcification within the lucent area; when present, this is a pathognomonic feature.

2.3 Pathology

The lesion consist of pearly–white cartilaginous tissue, often with a central area of degeneration and calcification. Histologically the appearances are those of simple hyaline cartilage.

2.4 Treatment

Treatment is not always necessary, but if the tumor appears to be enlarging, or if it presents as a pathological fracture, it should be removed as thoroughly as possible by curettage. The defect is then filled with bone graft or bone cement. There is a fairly high recurrence rate and the tissue may be seeded in adjacent bone or soft tissues. Chondromas in expendable sites are better removed en bloc.

Chapter 3

Osteochondroma

3.1 Manifestation

Osteochondroma is a developmental lesion which starts as a small overgrowth of cartilage at the edge of the physeal plate and develops by endochondral ossification into a bony protuberance still covered by the cap of cartilage. Any bone that develops in cartilage may be involved; the commonest sites are the fast-growing ends of long bones and the crest of the ilium. In long bones, growth leaves the bump stranded further down the metaphysis. Here it may go on growing but at the end of the normal growth period for that bone it stops enlarging. Any further enlargement after the end of the growth period is suggestive of malignant transformation.

The patient is usually a teenager or young adult when the lump is first discovered. Occasionally there is pain due to an overlying bursa or impingement on soft-tissues, or, rarely, paraesthesia due to stretching of an adjacent nerve.

3.2 Radiology

The X-ray appearance is pathognomonic. There is a well-defined exostosis emerging from the metaphysis, its base co-extensive with the parent bone. It looks smaller than it feels because the cartilage cap is usually invisible on X-ray; however, large lesions undergo cartilage degeneration and calcification and then the X-ray shows the bony exostosis surrounded by clouds of calcified material. MRI may be needed to reveal malignants.

3.3 Pathology

At operation the cartilage cap is seen surmounting a narrow base or pedicle of bone. The cap consists of simple hyaline cartilage; in a growing exostosis the deeper cartilage cells are arranged in columns, giving rise to the formation of endochondral new bone. Large lesions may have a "cauliflower" appearance, with degeneration and calcification in the centre of the cartilage cap.

3.4 Treatment

If the tumour causes symptoms it should be excised; if, in an adult, it has recently become bigger or painful then operation is urgent, for these features suggest malignancy. If there are suspicious features, further imaging and staging should be carried out before doing a biopsy. If the histology is that of benign cartilage but the tumor is known for certain to be enlarging after the end of the growth period, it should be treated as a chondrosarcoma.

Chapter 4

Giant Cell Tumor

4.1 Manifestation

Giant cell tumor, which represents 5% of all primary bone tumors, is a lesion of uncertain origin that appears in mature bone, most commonly in the distal femur, proximal tibia, proximal humerus and distal radius, though other bones also may be affected. It is hardly ever seen before closure of the nearby physis and characteristically it extends right up to the subarticular bone plate. Rarely, there are multiple lesions.

The patient is usually a young adult who complains of pain at the end of a long bone; sometimes there is slight swelling and pathological fracture occurs in 10% –15% of cases. On examination there may be a palpable mass with warmth of the overlying tissues.

4.2 Radiology

X–rays show a radiolucent area situated eccentrically at the end of a long bone and bounded by the subchondral bone plate. The endosteal margin may be quite obvious, but in aggressive lesions it is ill–defined. The centre sometimes has a soap–bubble appearance due to ridging of the surrounding bone. The cortex is thin and sometimes ballooned; aggressive lesions extend into the soft tissue. The appearance of a "cystic" lesion in mature bone, extending right up to the subchondral plate, is so characteristic that the diagnosis is seldom in doubt. However, it is prudent to obtain estimations of blood calcium, phosphate and alkaline phosphatise concentrations so as exclude an unusual "brown tumor" associated with hyperparathyroidism.

Because of the tumor's potential for aggressive behavior, detailed staging procedures are essential. CT scans and MRI will reveal the extent of them tumor, both within the bone and beyond. It is important to establish whether the articular surface has been breached.

4.3 Pathology

Biopsy is essential. This can be done either as a frozen section before proceeding with operative treatment or as a separate procedure. The tumor has a reddish, fleshy appearance. It comes away in pieces quite easily when curetted but is difficult to remove completely from the surrounding bone. Aggressive lesions have a poorly defined edge and extend well into the surrounding bone. Histologically the striking feature is an abundance of multinucleated giant cells scattered on a background of stromal cells with little or no visible intercellular tissue. Aggressive lesions tend to show more cellular atypia and mitotic figures, but histological grading is unreliable as a predictor of tumor behavior. Rarely metastases are discovered in the lungs. The tumor has the potential to transform into an osteosarcoma.

4.4 Treatment

Well-confined, slow-growing lesions with benign histology can safely be treated by thorough curettage and "stripping" of the cavity with burrs and gouges, followed by swabbing with hydrogen peroxide or by the application of liquid nitrogen; the cavity is then packed with bone chips. More aggressive tumors, and recurrent lesions, should be treated by excision followed, if necessary, by bone grafting or prosthetic replacement. Tumors in awkward sites (e. g., the spine) may be difficult to eradicate; supplementary radiotherapy is sometimes recommended, but it carries a significant risk of causing malignant transformation.

Chapter 5

Malignant Tumors of Bone

5.1 Osteosarcoma

5.1.1 Manifestation

In its classic(intramedullary) form, osteosarcoma is a highly malignant tumor arising within the bone and spreading rapidly outwards to the periosteum and surrounding soft-tissues. It is said to occur predominantly in children and adolescents, but epidemiological studies suggest that between 1972 and 1981 the age of presentation rose significantly(Stark et al. , 1990). It may affect any bone but most commonly involves the long-bone metaphyses, especially around the knee and mat the proximal end of the humerus.

Pain is usually the first symptom; it is constant, worse at night and gradually increases in severity. Sometimes the patient presents with a lump. Pathological fracture is rare. On examination there may be little to find except local tenderness. In later cases there is a palpable mass and the overlying tissues may appear swollen and inflamed. The ESR is usually raised and there may be an increase in serum alkaline phosphatase.

5.1.2 X-rays

The X-ray appearances are variable: hazy osteolytic areas may alternate with unusually dense osteoblastic areas. The endosteal margin is poorly defined. Often the cortex is breached and the tumor extends into the adjacent tissues; when this happens, streaks of new bone appear, radiating outwards from the cortex—the so-called "sunburst" effect. Where the tumor emerges from the cortex, reactive new bone forms at the angles of periosteal elevation(Codman's triangle). While both the sunburst appearance and Codman's triangle are typical of osteosarcoma, they may occasionally be seen in other rapidly growing tumors(Figure 58-5-1).

5.1.3 Diagnosis and staging

In most cases the diagnosis can be made with confidence on the X-ray appearances. However, atypical lesions can cause confusion. Conditions to be excluded are post-traumatic swellings, infection, stress fracture and the more aggressive "cystic" lesions.

Other imaging studies are essential for staging purposes. Radioisotope scans may show up skip lesions, but a negative scan does not exclude them. CT and MRI reliably show the extent of the tumor. Chest X-rays are done routinely, but pulmonary CT is a much more sensitive detector of lung metastases. About 10% of patients have pulmonary metastases by the time they are first seen (Figure 58-5-2).

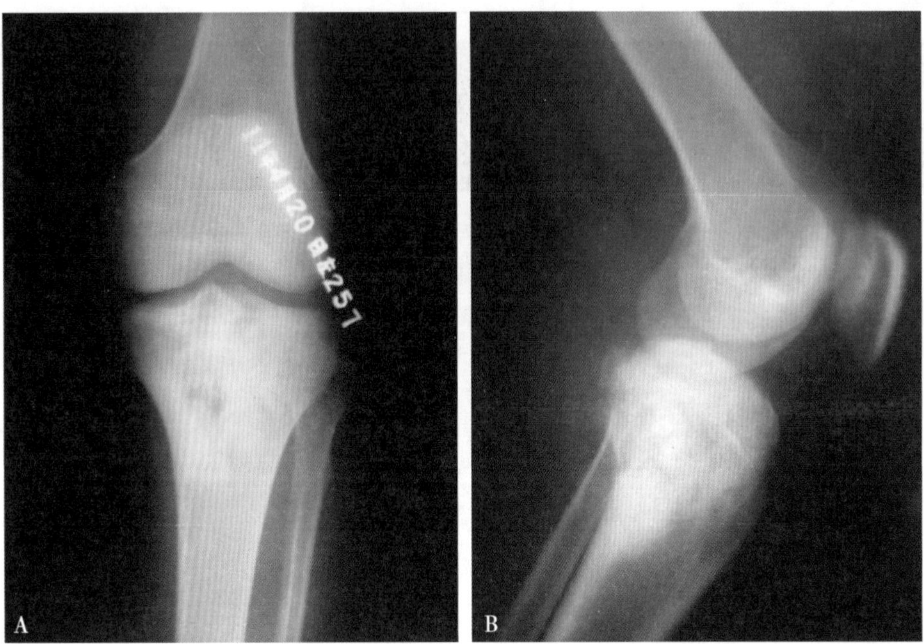

Figure 58-5-1 X-rays images of proximal tibial osteosarcoma

A. AP view, and B. lateral view.

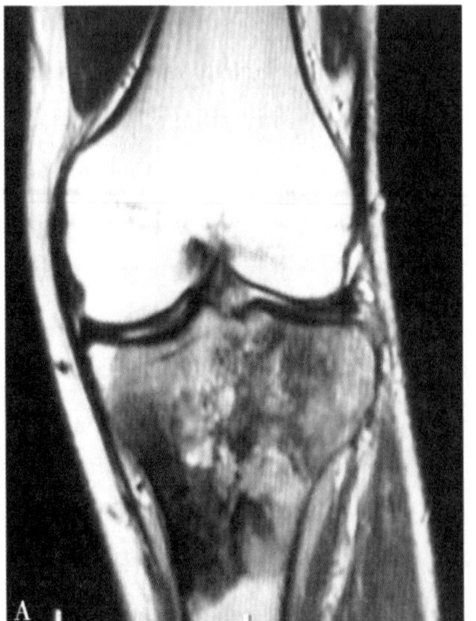

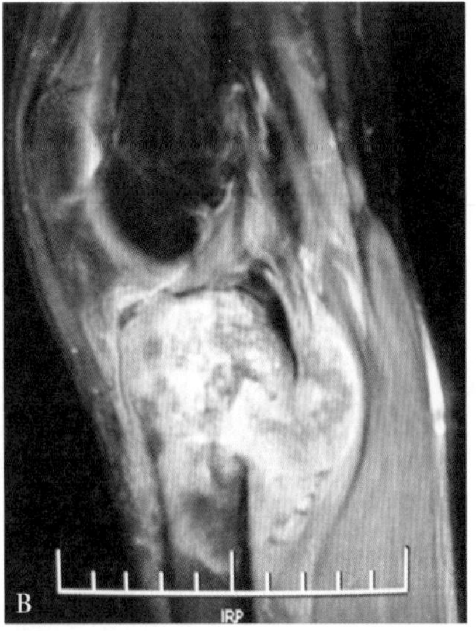

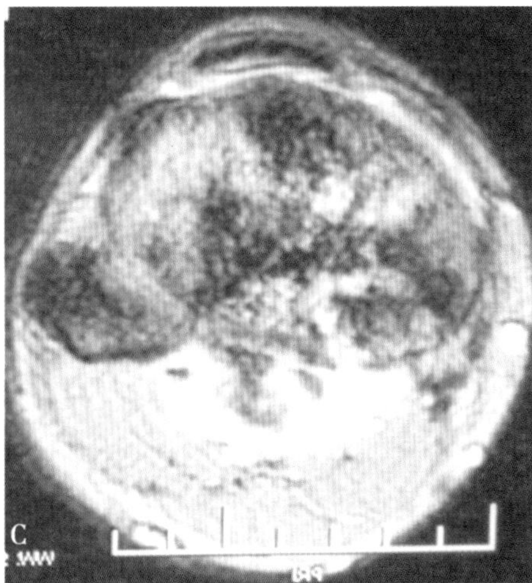

Figure 58-5-2 The coronal(a), sagittal(b), and horizontal(c) MRI images of proximal tibial osteosarcoma

5.1.4 Pathology

A biopsy should always be carried out before commencing treatment; it must be carefully planned to allow for complete removal of the tract when the tumor is excised.

The tumor is usually situated in the metaphysis of a long bone, where it destroys and replaces normal bone. Areas of bone loss and cavitation alternate with dense patches of abnormal new bone. The tumor extends within the medulla and across the physeal plate. There may be obvious spread into the soft-tissues with ossification at the periosteal margins and streaks of new bone extending into the extraosseous mass.

The histological appearances show considerable variation: some areas may have the characteristic spindle cells with a pink-staining osteoid matrix; others may contain cartilage cells or fibroblastic tissue with little or no osteoid. Several samples may have to be examined; pathologists are reluctant to commit themselves to the diagnosis unless they see evidence of osteoid formation (Figure 58-5-3).

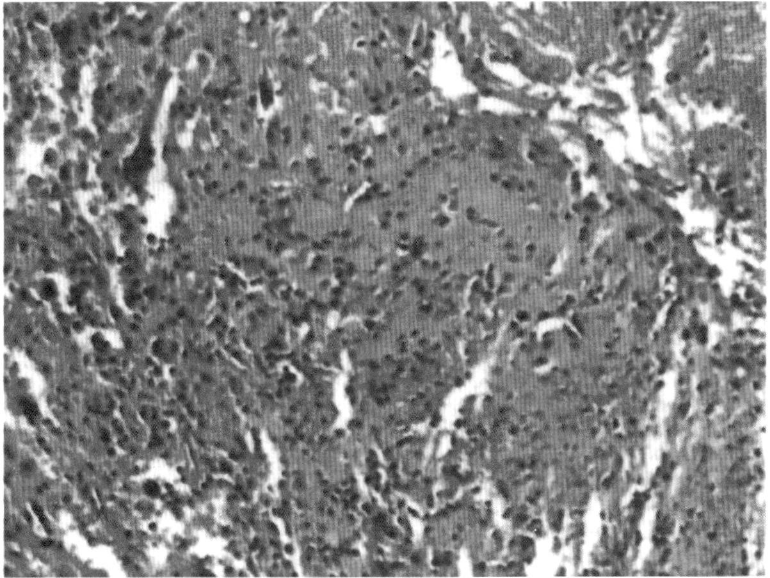

Figure 58-5-3 HE staining of a metaphyseal osteosarcoma (100×)

5.1.5 Treatment

The appalling prognosis that formerly attended this tumor has markedly improved, partly as a result of better diagnostic and staging procedures, and possibly because the average age of the patients has increased, but mainly because of advances in chemotherapy to control metastatic spread. However, it is still important to eradicate the primary lesion completely; the mortality rate after local recurrence is far worse than following effective ablation at the first encounter.

After clinical assessment and advanced imaging, the patient is admitted to a special centre for biopsy. The lesion will probably be graded Ⅱ A or Ⅱ B. Multiagent neoadjuvant chemotherapy is given for 8–12 weeks and then, provided the tumor is resectable and there are no skip lesions, a wide resection is car–preparations would have been made to replace that segment of bone with either a large bone graft or a custom made implant; in some cases an amputation may be more appropriate (Figure 58–5–4).

The pathological specimen is examined to assess the response to preoperative chemotherapy. If tumor necrosis is marked (more than 90%), chemotherapy is continued for another 6–12 months; if the response is poor, a different chemotherapeutic regime is substituted.

Pulmonary metastases, especially if they are small and peripherally situated, may be completely resected with a wedge of lung tissue.

5.1.6 Outcome

Long–term survival after wide resection and chemotherapy has improved from around 50% to over 60% in the past three decades. Tumor–replacement implants usually function well (Figure 58–5–5). There is a fairly high complication rate (mainly wound breakdown and infection) but, in patients who survive, 10–year survival with mechanical failure as the end point is 75% and for failure for any cause is 58%. The limb salvage rate at 20 years is 84%. Aseptic loosening is more prevalent in younger patients.

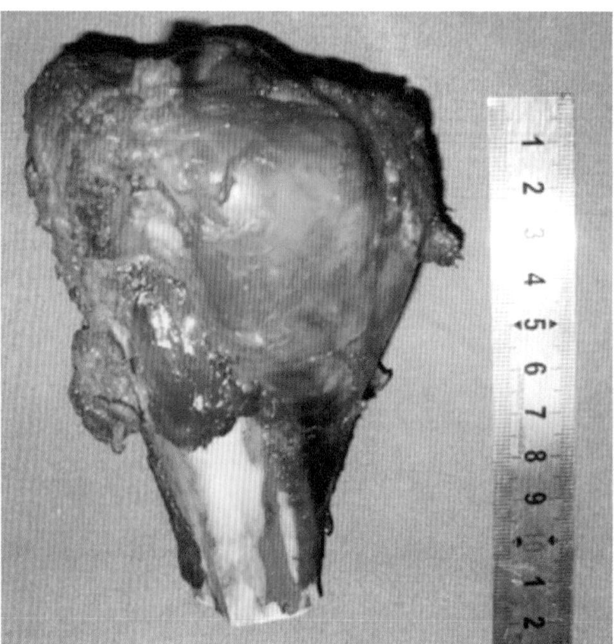

Figure 58–5–4 Completely eradicated proximal tibial osteosarcoma by surgery

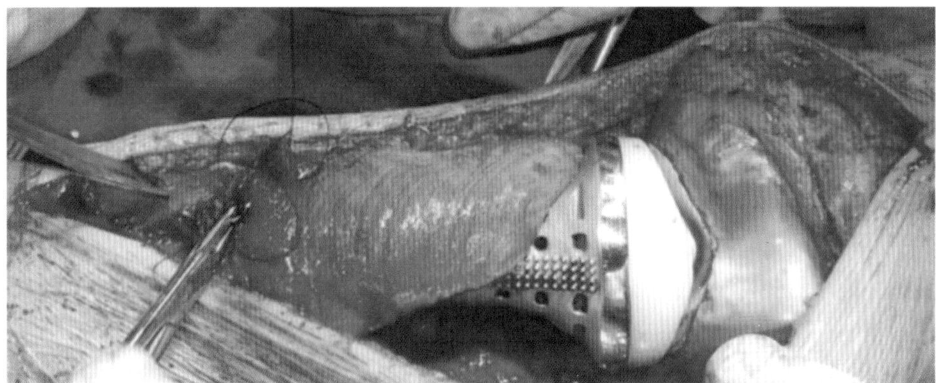

Figure 58-5-5 The use of tumor-replacement implant after surgical resection of osteosarcoma

5.2 Variants of Osteosarcoma

5.2.1 Parosteal osteosarcoma

This is a low-grade sarcoma situated on the surface of one of the tubular bones, usually at the distal femoral or proximal tibial metaphysis. The patient is a young adult who presents with a slowly enlarging mass near the bone end.

(1) Radiology

X-ray shows a dense bony mass on the surface of the bone or encircling it; the cortex is not eroded and usually a thin gap remains between cortex and tumor. The picture is easily mistaken for that of a benign bone lesion and the diagnosis is often missed until the tumor recurs after local excision. CT and MRI will show the boundary between tumor and surrounding soft-tissues. Although the lesion is outside the bone, it does not spread into the adjacent muscle compartment until fairly late. Staging, therefore, often defines it as a low grade intra-compartmental tumor (stage Ⅰ A).

(2) Pathology

At biopsy the tumor appears as a hard mass. On microscopic examination the lesion consists of well-formed bone but without any regular trabecular arrangement. The spaces between trabeculae are filled with cellular fibroblastic tissue. A few atypical cells and mitotic figures can usually be found. Occasionally the tumor has a much more aggressive appearance, and that is dedifferentiated parosteal osteosarcoma.

(3) Treatment

For a low-grade parosteal osteosarcoma, wide excision without adjuvant therapy is sufficient to ensure a recurrence rate below 10%. Dedifferentiated parosteal osteosarcoma should be treated in the same way as intramedullary sarcoma.

5.2.2 Periosteal osteosarcoma

This rare tumor is quite distinct from parosteal osteosarcoma. It is more like an intramedullary osteosarcoma, but situated on the surface of the bone. It occurs in young adults and causes local pain and swelling.

(1) Radiology

X-ray shows a superficial defect of the cortex, but CT and MRI may reveal a larger soft-tissue mass. The appearances sometimes suggest a periosteal chondroma and the diagnosis may not be certain until a biopsy is performed.

(2) Pathology

Histologically this is a true osteosarcoma, but characteristically the sections show a prominent cartilaginous element.

(3) Treatment

Treatment is the same as that of classic osteosarcoma.

5.2.3 Paget's sarcoma

Paget's disease affects about 2% of western Europeans. Although malignant transformation is a rare complication of this disease, most osteosarcomas appearing after the age of 50 years fall into this category. Warning signs are the appearance of pain or swelling in a patient with longstanding Paget's disease. In late cases, pathological fracture may occur.

(1) Radiology

X-ray shows the usual features of Paget's disease, but with areas of bone destruction and soft-tissue invasion.

(2) Histology

This is a high-grade tumor if anything even more malignant than classic osteosarcoma. Staging usually shows that extra-compartmental spread has occurred; most patients have pulmonary metastases by the time the tumor is diagnosed.

(3) Treatment

Even with radical resection or amputation and chemotherapy the 5-year survival rate is low. If the lesion is definitely extra-compartmental, palliative treatment by radiotherapy may be preferable. Chemotherapy is usually difficult because of the patient's age and uncertainty about renal and cardiac function.

5.2.4 Fibrosarcoma of bone

Fibrosarcoma is rare in bone, but it is more likely to arise in previously abnormal tissue (a bone infarct, fibrous dysplasia or after irradiation). The patient—usually an adult—complains of pain or swelling; there may be a pathological fracture.

(1) Radiolgy

X-ray shows an undistinctive area of bone destruction. CT or MRI will reveal the soft-tissue extension.

(2) Pathology

Histologically the lesion consists of masses of fibroblastic tissue with scattered atypical and mitotic cells. Appearances vary from well-differentiated to highly undifferentiated, and the tumors are sometimes graded accordingly.

(3) Treatment

Low-grade, well-confined tumors (stage ⅠA) can be treated by wide excision with prosthetic replacement. High-grade lesions (ⅡA or ⅡB) require radical resection or amputation; if this cannot be achieved, local excision must be combined with radiation therapy. The value of adjuvant chemotherapy is still uncertain.

5.3 Chondrosarcoma

(1) Clinical manifestation and diagnosis

Chondrosarcoma is one of the commonest malignant tumors originating in bone. The highest incidence is in the fourth and fifth decades and men are affected more often than women.

These tumors are slow-growing and are usually present for many months before being discovered. Patients may complain of a dull ache or a gradually enlarging lump. Medullary lesions may present as a pathological fracture. However, despite the fact that it is very slow-growing, it does eventually metastasize.

Although chondrosarcoma may develop in any of the bones that normally develop in cartilage, almost 50% appear in the metaphysis of one of the long tubular bones, mostly in the lower limbs. The next most common sites are the pelvis and the ribs. Despite the relatively frequent occurrence of benign cartilage tumors in the small bones of the hands and feet, malignant lesions are rare at these sites.

By far the majority of chondrosarcomas fall into two well-defined categories: central tumors occupying the medullary cavity of the bone, and so-called "peripheral tumors" growing out from the cortex. Less common varieties are clear-cell chondrosarcoma, interstitial chondrosarcoma and undifferentiated chondrosarcoma. Prognosis of chonrosarcoma is determined by surgical intervention and histological staging. In general, Peripheral and periosteal chondrosarcomas are better than central lesions.

If a chondrosarcoma is suspected, full staging procedures should be employed. CT scans and MRI must be carried out before performing a biopsy. A biopsy is essential to confirm the diagnosis. However, low-grade chondrosarcoma may show histological features no different from those of an aggressive benign cartilaginous lesion. High-grade tumors are more cellular, and there may be obvious abnormal features of the cells, such as plumpness, hyperchromasia and mitoses.

(2) Treatment

Since most chondrosarcomas are slow-growing and metastasize late, they present the ideal case for wide excision and prosthetic replacement, provided it is certain that the lesion can be completely removed without exposing the tumor and without causing an unacceptable loss of function; in that case amputation may be preferable. In some cases isolated pulmonary metastases can be resected. The tumor does not respond to either radiotherapy or chemotherapy. Prognosis is determined largely by the cellular grade and the resection margin. There is a tendency for these tumors to recur late and the patient should therefore be followed up for 10 years or longer.

(3) Central chondrosarcoma

The tumor develops in the medullary cavity of either tubular or flat bones, most commonly at the proximal end of the femur or in the innominate bone of the pelvis. The incidence of this tumor in men and women is (1.5-2) : 1. X-rays show an expanded, somewhat radiolucent area in the bone, with flecks of increased density due to calcification within the tumor. Aggressive lesions may take on a globular appearance with scalloping or destruction of the cortex.

When a benign medullary chondroma (enchondroma) undergoes malignant transformation, it is difficult to be sure that the lesion was not a slowly evolving sarcoma from the outset.

At present, surgery is the effective way for treatment of this tumor. En bloc wide resection is required for this tumor at different stages. The most common malignant transformation occurs still in lungs.

(4) Peripheral chondrosarcoma

This tumor usually arises in the cartilage cap of an osteochondroma that has been present since childhood. Osteochondroma of the pelvis and scapula seem to be more susceptible than others to malignant change, but perhaps this is simply because the site allows a tumor to grow without being detected and removed at an early stage. X-rays show the bony osteochondroma, often surmounted by clouds of patchy calcification in the otherwise unseen lobulated cartilage cap. A tumor that is very large and calcification that is very fluffy and poorly outlined are suspicious features, but the clearest sign of malignant change is a demonstrable progressive enlargement of an osteochondroma after the end of normal bone growth. MRI is the best means of showing the size and internal features of the cartilage cap.

(5) Malignant fibrous histiocytoma

Like fibrosarcoma, this tumor tends to occur in previously abnormal bone (old infarcts or Paget's disease). Patients are usually middle-aged adults and X-rays may reveal a destructive lesion adjacent to an almost invariably show that the tumor has spread beyond the bone.

Histologically it is a fibrous tumor, but the arrangement of the tissue is in interweaving bundles, and the presence of histiocytes and of giant cells distinguishes it from the more uniform fibrosarcoma.

Treatment consists of wide or radical resection and adjuvant chemotherapy. For inaccessible lesions, local radiotherapy may be needed.

(6) Ewing's sarcoma

Ewing's sarcoma is believed to arise from endothelial cells in the bone marrow. It occurs most commonly between the ages of 10 and 20 years, usually in a tubular bone and especially in the tibia, fibula or clavicle.

The patient presents with pain—often throbbing in character—and swelling. Generalized illness and pyrexia, together with a warm, tender swelling and a raised ESR, may suggest a diagnosis of osteomyelitis.

(7) Imaging

X-rays usually show an area of bone destruction which, unlike that in osteosarcoma, is predominantly in the mid-diaphysis. New bone formation may extend along the shaft and sometimes it appears as fusiform layers of bone around the lesion—the so-called "onion-peel" effect. Often the tumor extends into the surrounding soft tissues, with radiating streaks of ossification and reactive periosteal bone at the proximal and distal margins. These features (the "sunray" appearance and Codman's triangles) are usually associated with osteosarcoma, but they are just as common in Ewing's sarcoma.

CT and MRI reveal the large extraosseous component. Radioisotope scans may show multiple areas of activity in the skeleton.

(8) Pathology

Macroscopically the tumor is lobulated and often fairly large. It may look grey (like brain) or red (like redcurrant jelly) if haemorrhage has occurred into it. Microscopically, sheets of small dark polyhedral cells with no regular arrangement and no ground substance are seen.

(9) Diagnosis

The condition which should be excluded as rapidly as possible is bone infection. On biopsy the essential step is to recognize this as a malignant round-cell tumor, distinct from osteosarcoma. Other round-cell tumors that may resemble Ewing's are reticulum-cell sarcoma and metastatic neuroblastoma.

(10) Treatment

The prognosis is always poor and surgery alone does little to improve it. Radiotherapy has a dramatic effect on the tumor but overall survival is not much enhanced. Chemotherapy is much more effective, offering a 5-year survival rate of about 50%. The best results are achieved by a combination of all three methods: a course of preoperative neoadjuvant chemotherapy; then wide excision if the tumor is in a favorable site, or radiotherapy followed by local excision if it is less accessible; and then a further course of chemotherapy for 1 year. Postoperative radiotherapy may be added if the resected specimen is found not to have a sufficiently wide margin of normal tissue. The prognosis for these tumors has improved dramatically since the introduction of multi-agent chemotherapy—from an erstwhile 10% survival rate to the current 70 per cent for patients with nonmetastatic Ewing's sarcoma.

(11) Multiple myeloma

Multiple myeloma is a malignant B-cell lymphoproliferative disorder of the marrow, with plasma cells predominating. The effects on bone are due to marrow cell proliferation and increased osteoclastic activity, resulting in osteoporosis and the appearance of particularly large colony of plasma cells may form what appears to be a solitary tumor (plasmacytoma) in one of the bones, but sooner or later most of these cases turn out to be unusual examples of the same widespread disease.

Associated features of the marrow-cell disorder are plasma protein abnormalities, increased blood viscosity and anaemia. Bone resorption leads to hypercalcaemia in about 1/3 of cases. Late secondary features are due to renal dysfunction and spinal cord or root compression caused by vertebral collapse.

The patient, typically aged 45-65, presents with weakness, backache, bone pain or a pathological fracture. Hypercalcaemia may cause symptoms such as thirst, polyuria and abdominal pain. Clinical signs (apart from a pathological fracture) are often unremarkable. Localized tenderness and restricted hip movements could be due to a plasmacytoma in the proximal femur. In late cases there may be signs of cord or nerve root compression, chronic nephritis and recurrent infection.

(12) Imaging

X-rays often show nothing more than generalized osteoporosis; but remember that myeloma is one of the commonest causes of osteoporosis and vertebral compression fracture in men over the age of 45 years. The "classical" lesions are multiple punched-out defects with "soft" margins (lack of new bone) in the skull, pelvis and proximal femur, a crushed vertebra, or a solitary lytic tumor in a large-bone metaphysis. Investigations mild anaemia is common, and an almost constant feature is a high ESR. Blood chemistry may show a raised creatinine level and hypercalcaemia. Over half the patients have Bence Jones protein in their urine, and serum protein electrophoresis shows a characteristic abnormal band. A sternal marrow puncture may show plasmacytosis, with typical "myeloma" cells.

CT and MRI can not only reveal detirioration within and beyond the bone, but also the compression and invalidation in the surrounding soft tissues. Radioisotope scans may show multiple areas of activity in the skeleton.

(13) Diagnosis

If the only X-ray change is osteoporosis, the differential diagnosis must include all the other causes of bone loss. If there are lytic lesions, the features can be similar to those of metastatic bone disease. Paraproteinaemia is a feature of other (benign) gammopathies, and it is wise to seek the help of a haematologist before reaching a clinical diagnosis.

(14) Pathology

At operation the affected bone is soft and crumbly. The typical microscopic picture is of sheets of plasmacytes with a large eccentric nucleus containing a spoke-like arrangement of chromatin.

(15) Treatment

The immediate need is for pain control and, if necessary, treatment of pathological fractures. General supportive measures include correction of fluid balance and(in some cases)hypercalcaemia.

Limb fractures are best managed by internal fixation and packing of cavities with methylmethacrylate cement(which also helps to staunch the profuse bleeding that sometimes occurs). Perioperative antibiotic prophylaxis is important as there is a higher than usual risk of infection and wound breakdown.

Spinal fractures carry the risk of cord compression and need immediate stabilization, either by effective bracing or by internal fixation. Unrelieved cord pressure may need decompression.

Solitary plasmacytomas can be treated by radiotherapy.

Specific therapy is with alkylating cytotoxic agents(e. g. , melphalan). Corticosteroids are also used—especially if bone pain is marked—but this probably does not alter the course of the disease. Treatment should be carried out in a specialized unit where dosages and response parameters can be properly monitored.

The prognosis in established cases is poor, with a median survival of between 2 and 5 years.

Part 59

Musculoskeletal Malformation

Chapter 1

Introduction

(1) Congenital disorders are defined as those abnormalities of development that are present at the time of birth. It is quite a common problem exceeded in frequency only by those of CNS (central nervous system) and CVS (cardiovascular system).

Congenital disorders can be placed in three groups:

· Those easily noticed by the mother, e. g., club-foot.

· Those not readily noticed, e. g., congenital dislocation of the hip (CDH, DDH developmental dysplasia of hip).

· Those clinically undetected but diagnosed radiologically, e. g., spondylosithesis.

Congenital disorders are more prevalent in diabetic mothers, multiple pregnancies, older mother, etc. Male and female have equal predilection.

(2) Cause: The exact cause is not known. Most congenital disorders begin early in the life of the embryo when cell division is most active. Although a few congenital disorders may be due to uterine malposition, most are believed to be due to genetic defects, environmental influences or a combination of both.

(3) Genetic factors: Defects in the chromosomes of sperm and ovum result in specific disorders which follows Mendel's law.

(4) Embryonic trauma: Congenital disorders can also result from injury to the developing embryo at the time of differentiation of embryonic tissue into specific tissues by extraneous factors.

Chapter 2

Congenital Muscular Torticollis

Congenital muscular torticollis(CMT) is a condition where the sternocleidomastoid muscle of the neck undergoes contractures pulling it to the same side and turning the face to the opposite side.

The exact cause of this condition is unknown; but hypothetically, it may be due to fibromatosis within the sternomastoid muscle.

2.1 Aetiology

Middle part of the sternomastoid is supplied by an end artery, which is a branch of the superior thyroid artery that gets blocked due to trauma, etc.

Birth trauma—Breech delivery, improper application of forceps, etc., may cause injury to the sternomastoid muscle.

The above two reasons can result in sternocleidomastoid muscle ischaemia, necrosis and fibrosis later on.

2.2 Clinical Features

Deformity is the only complaint initially. Later, facial changes and macular problems in the retina may develop.

2.3 Treatment

(1) Principles

During infancy, conservative treatment consists of stretching of the sternomastoid by manipulation and physiotherapy. Excision is unjustified in infancy.

Surgery is delayed till fibroma is well formed. The muscle may be released at one or both ends or the muscle may be excised as a whole.

If muscle is still contracted at the age of 1 year, it should be released.

If CMT is persistent for 1 year, it will not resolve spontaneously and need to be interfered operatively.

(2) Exercise programme is successful

When restriction of motion is less than 30°.

When there is no facial asymmetry.

Nonoperative treatment after 1 year is rarely successful.

Any permanent torticollis becomes worse during growth. Head is inclined towards the affected side, face is turned towards the opposite side, ipsilateral shoulder is elevated and the fronto-occipital diameter is increased.

2.4 Surgical Methods

The most commonly employed surgical methods is subcutaneous tenotomy of the clavicular attachment of the sternomastoid muscle. This procedure is inaccurate and dangerous as there could be an injury to the external jugular vein and phrenic nerve. Hence release from its attachment on the mastoid process is also tried. Open tenotomy if done before the child is 1 year old, tethering of the scar takes place. If the surgery is done between 1 and 4 years of age, tilt of the head and facial asymmetry are corrected less satisfactorily. If done after 5 years of age, the secondary deformities are less corrected.

For older children or after failed operation, bipolar release of the muscle from both sides, Ferkel's modified bipolar release or Z-plasty of the muscle are tried.

Chapter 3

Developmental Dysplasia of Hip

Earlier known as congenital dislocation of the hip.

Definition developmental dysplasia of hip is defined as partial or complete displacement of the femoral head from the acetabular cavity since birth.

This is a spontaneous dislocation of the hip occurring before, during or shortly after birth. In western races, it is one of the commonest congenital disorder. The general term "dysplastic hip" is sometimes used for these congenital malformations of the hip.

The incidence of dislocation is 1 in 1000 infants. Both hips may be involved. DDH is more common in females and in patients with other congenital deformities. It is neither painful nor disabling in children but causes significant symptoms in adults if successful atraumatic closed reduction is not achieved in early childhood. If atraumatic reduction is not possible, surgical release of the obstructing or limiting soft tissues should be performed.

3.1 Aetiology

The aetiology is not well understood, but the following factors appear to be important:

(1) Hereditary predisposition to joint laxity: heredity related lax joints are predisposed to hip dislocation in some positions.

(2) Hormone induced joint laxity: DDH is 3–5 times more common in females. This may be due to the fact that the maternal relaxin (a ligament relaxing hormone in the mother during pregnancy) crosses the placental barrier to enter the foetus. If the hormonal environment of the foetus is a female, relaxin acts on the foetus's joints in the same way as it does on those of the mother. This produces joint laxity, and thus dislocation.

(3) Breech malposition: the incidence of an unstable hip is about 10 times more in newborns with breech presentation than those with vertex presentation the foetal legs are pressed inside the uterus in such a way that if the hip ligaments are lax, dislocation may occur.

3.2 Pathology

The present evidence suggests that there are two distinct types of dysplastic hip—those dislocated at birth(classic DDH)and those dislocatable after birth. The first are primarily due to a hereditary faulty development of the acetabulum,and are difficult to,treat. The second are due to underlying joint laxity,with a precipitating factor causing the dislocation. The following changes are seen in a dislocated joint:

The femoral head is dislocated upwards and laterally;its epiphysis is small and ossifies late.

The femoral neck is excessively anteverted.

The acetabulum is shallow,with a steep sloping roof.

The ligamentum teres is hepertrophied.

The fibrocartilaginous labrum of the acetabulum(limbus)may be folded into the cavity of the acetabulum(inverted limbus).

The capsule of the hip joint is stretched.

The muscle around the hip,especially the adductors,undergo adaptive shortening.

3.3 Diagnosis

Diagnosis is easy in an older child;but may be very difficult in younger children,especially during infancy. This is because of subtle clinical findings and difficulties in interpreting X-rays of these children (Figure 59-3-1).

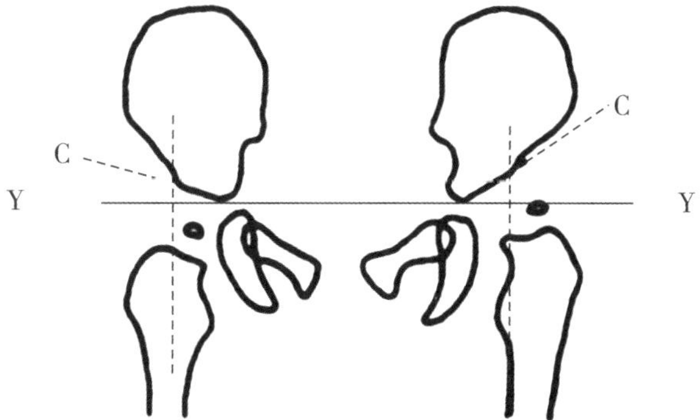

Figure 59-3-1 Developmental dysplasia of left hip demonstrated on Perkin square

Sketch demonstrates the radiological parameters seen in normal and abnormal hip. Y:a straight horizontal line through the triradiate cartilages center of both hips; C:the slope line of the acetabular-sourcil. Acetabular index is defined as the angle between lines of Y and C; P:a vertical line through the outer margin of acetabular (Perkin line) and the hip divided into four quadrants by lines of Y and P and the development of hip evaluated according to the position of femoral head on Perkin square.

3.4 Clinical Features

Girls are affected 6 times more often than boys. In 1/3 of all cases both hips are affected. DDH may be detected at birth or soon after; sometimes not noticed until the child starts walking. The following are the salient clinical features at different ages:

At birth: Routine screening of all newborn children is necessary. The examining paediatrician may notice signs suggestive of a dislocated or a dislocatable hip, as discussed subsequently.

Early childhood: Sometimes, the child is brought because the parents have noticed an asymmetry of creases of the groin, limitation of movements of the affected hip, or a click everytime the hip is moved.

Older child: DDH may become apparent once the child starts walking. The parents notice that the child walks with a "peculiar gait" though there is no pain. On examination a DDH may be found to be the underlying cause.

A meticulous examination is the key to the early diagnosis of DDH. There may be limitation of hip abduction, asymmetry of groin-creases or an audible click. Physical findings in a younger child may be little, and diagnosis may only be possible by special tests designed to elicit instability. These are as follows:

Barlow's test: The test has two parts. In the first part, the surgeon faces the child's perineum. He grasps the upper part of each thigh, with his fingers behind on the greater trochanter and thumb in front. The child's knee is fully flexed and the hips flexed to a right angle. The hip is now gently adducted. As this is being done, gentle pressure is exerted by the examining hand in a proximal direction while the thumb tries to " push out " the hip. As the femoral head rolls over the posterior lip of the acetabulum, it may, if dislocatable (but not, if dislocated) slip out of the acetabulum. One feels an abnormal posterior movement, appreciated by the fingers behind the greater trochanter. There may be a distinct "clunk". If nothing happens, the hip may be normal or may already be dislocated; in the latter, second part of the test would be more relevant.

In the second part of the test, with the hips in 90 degrees flexion and fully adducted, held as described above, thighs are gently abducted. The examiner's hand tries to pull the hip while the fingers on the greater trochanter exert pressure in a forward direction, as if one is trying to put back a dislocated hip. If the hip is dislocated, either because of the first part of the test or if it was dislocated to start with, a "clunk" will be heard and felt indicating reduction of the dislocated hip. If nothing happens, the hip may be normal or it is an irreducible dislocation. In the latter case, there will be limitation of hip abduction. In a normal hip, it is possible to abduct the hips till the knee touches the couch.

Ortolani's test: This test is similar to the second part of Barlow's test. The hip and knees are held in a flexed position and gradually abducted; a "click of entrance" will be felt as the femoral head slips into the acetabulum from the position of dislocation.

In an older child, the following findings may be present:

Limitation of abduction of the hip.

Asymmetrical thigh folds.

Galeazz's sign: The level of the knees are compared in a child lying with hip flexed to 70 degrees and knees flexed. There is a lowering of the knee on the affected side.

Ortolani's test may be positive.

Trendelenburg's test is positive: This test is performed in an older child. The child is asked to stand on the affected side. The opposite ASIS(that of the normal side) dips down.

The limb is short and slightly externally rotated. There is lordosis of the lumbar spine.

Telescopy positive: In a case of a dislocated hip, it will be possible to producc an up and down piston-like movement at the hip. This can be appreciated by feeling the movement of the greater trochanter, under the fingers.

A child with unilateral dislocation exhibits a typical gait in which the body lurches to the affected side as the child bears weight on it(Trendelenburg's gait). In a child with bilateral dislocation, there is alternate lurching on both side.

Radiological features: In a child below the age of 1 year, since the epiphysis of the femoral head is not ossified, it is difficult to diagnose a dislocated hip on plain X-rays. Von Rosen's view may be helpful in diagnosis.

In an older child, the following are the important X-ray findings:

Delayed appearance of the ossific center of the head of the femur.

Retarded development of the ossific center of the head of the femur.

Sloping acetabulum.

Lateral and upward displacement of the ossific center of the femoral head.

A break in Shenton's line.

3.5 Treatment

3.5.1 Principles of treatment

The aim is to achieve reduction of the head into the acetabulum, and maintain it until the hip becomes clinically stable and a "round" acetabulum covers the head. In most cases, it is possible to reduce the hip by closed means; in some an open reduction is required. Once the head is inside the acetabulum, in younger children, under the mould-like effect of the head, it develops into a round acetabulum. If the reduction has been delayed for more than 2 years, acetabular remodeling may not occur even after the head is reduced for a long time. Hence, in such cases, surgical reconstruction of the acetabulum may be required.

3.5.2 Methods of reduction

The following methods of reduction may be used:

(1) Closed manipulation: It is sometimes possible in younger children to reduce the hip by gentle closed manipulation under general anaesthesia.

(2) Traction followed by closed manipulation: In cases where the manipulative reduction requires a great deal of force or if it fails, the hip is kept in traction for some time, and is progressively abducted. As this is done, it may be possible to reduce the femoral head easily under general anaesthesia. An adductor tenotomy is often necessary in some cases to allow the hip to be fully abducted.

(3) Open reduction: This is indicated if closed reduction fails. The reasons of failure of closed reduction could be the presence of fibro-fatty tissue in the acetabulum or a fold of capsule and acetabular labrum (inverted limbus) between the femoral head and the superior part of the acetabulum. In such situations, the hip is exposed, the soft-tissues obstructing the head excised or released, and the head repositioned in the acetabulum.

Maintenance of reduction: Once the hip has been reduced by closed or open methods, the following methods may be used for maintaining the head inside the acetabulum.

Plaster cast: A flog-leg or Batchelor's cast.

Splint: Some form of splint such as Von Rosen's splint.

External splints can be removed once the acetabulum develops to a round shape. The hip is now mobilized, and kept under observation for a period of 2-3 years for any recurrence.

Acetabulum reconstruction procedures: The available procedures are as follows:

(1) Salter's osteotomy: This is an osteotomy of the iliac bone, above the acetabulum. The roof of the acetabulum is rotated with the fulcrum at the pubic symphysis, so that the acetabulum becomes more horizontal, and thus covers the head.

(2) Chiari's pelvic displacement osteotomy: The iliac bone is divided almost transversely immediately above the acetabulum, and the lower fragment (bearing the acetabulum) is displaced medially. The margin of the upper fragment provides additional depth to the acetabulum.

(3) Pemberton's pericapsular osteotomy: The roof of the acetabulum is deflected downwards over the femoral head, with the fulcrum at the triradiate cartilage of the acetabulum.

In some cases, reduction of the hip may be possible only in extreme of abduction or internal rotation of the thigh. In such cases a uarus-derotation osteotomy is done at the subtro-chanteric region. The distal fragment is realigned and the osteotomy fixed with a plate.

3.5.3 Treatment plan

Treatment varies according to the age at which the patient presents. For the convenience of discussion, this has been divided into four groups on the basis of age of the patient:

Birth to 6 months: The femoral head is reduced into the acetabulum by closed manipulation, and maintained with plaster cast or splint.

Months to 6 years: It may be possible up to 2 years to reduce the head into the acetabulum by closed methods. After 2 years, it is difficult and also unwise to attempt closed reduction. This is because, when the head has been out for some time, the soft-tissues around the hip become tight. Such a hip, if reduced forcibly into the acetabulum, develops avascular necrosis of the femoral head. In those cases, reduction is achieved by open methods, and an additional femoral shortening may be required. In older children, an acetabular reconstruction may be performed at the same time or later. Salter's osteotomy is preferred by most surgeons.

6-10 years: The first point to be decided in children at the age is whether or not to treat the dislocation at all. No treatment may be indicated for children with bilateral dislocation because of the following reasons:

The limp is less noticeable.

Although having some posture and gait abnormalities, these patients tend to live normal lives until their 40's or 50's.

The results of treatment are unpredictable and a series of operations may be required.

In unilateral cases, an attempt at open reduction with reconstruction of the acetabulum may be made. A derotation osteotomy is needed in most cases.

11 years onwards: The indication for treatment in these patients is pain. If only one hip is affected, a total replacement may be practicable once adulthood is reached. Sometimes, arthrodesis of the hip may be a reasonable choice.

Chapter 4

Clubfoot

Talipes equinovarus, or clubfoot, is most commonly an idiopathic congenital condition affecting approximately 1 in 1000 children. It occurs twice as often in boys and is bilateral half the time. There is familial tendency, with a 5% chance that a sibling will also be affected.

4.1 Clinical Findings

4.1.1 Symptoms and signs

In congenital clubfoot, there is more or less rigid inversion of the hindfoot, adduction of the forefoot, and limited dorsiflexion—an equinovarus deformity. While the cause is not certain, the deformity involves medial subluxation of the navicular and calcaneus on the talus. The joints principally involved are thus the subtalar and talonavicular joints. The adjacent ankle and midtarsal joints are affected to a lesser degree. The overlying soft-tissues are contracted, and the longer the subluxation remains, the more deformed become the involved bones, which are composed largely of malleable cartilage. Successful treatment requires early reduction of joint subluxations and maintenance of correction throughout growth.

4.1.2 Imaging studies

X-rays are useful primarily for assessing the adequacy of correction rather than for establishing the diagnosis of clubfoot. At birth, only the ossific nuclei of the calcaneus, talus, and metatarsals are present. Navicular ossification does not begin until about age 4. Therefore, radiographs of the newborn foot provide less information than the clinical examination. A good photograph documents the deformity more adequately. By 2-3 months of age, the ossification centers of the talus and calcaneus have elongated sufficiently to indicate their long axes, so that radiographs can provide helpful data about interosseous relationships. An anteroposterior view of a normal foot shows divergence of the talus and calcaneus, the former directed along the first ray and the latter along the fifth ray. In clubfoot, the talus usually points more laterally and may actually appear superimposed upon the calcaneus. On the lateral radiograph of a normal foot in maximal dorsiflexion, the calcaneus is dorsiflexed, so that its axis crosses that of the navicular, and the anterior ends of their shadows overlap. Full calcaneal dorsiflexion is a valuable radiographic indicator of adequate treatment.

4.2 Treatment

4.2.1 Manipulation

Gentle manipulation into a corrected position should be done in order to stretch the contracted soft tissues—specifically, to align the calcaneus and navicular relative to the talus. Gentleness is required to avoid tissue trauma and to prevent overcorrection of the forefoot relative to persisting tarsal deformity.

4.2.2 Casting

After several minutes of manipulation, a plaster cast is applied and molded to maintain the maximally corrected position. Manipulation and cast application should be repeated weekly. Casts are advisable for at least 6 months, followed by a Denis Browne bar with attached out-flare shoes. Similar shoes are worn when the child begins to walk, but the Denis Browne bar splinting should be continued at night and during nap times for several more years. During this time, close follow-up is required, with immediate use of a plaster cast if deformity recurs. Corrections achieved by age 7 years is usually permanent. Carefully and conscientiously pursued, non-operative treatment has been sufficient to correct clubfoot deformity in 35%-90% of cases in large series. If satisfactory correction has not been achieved by age 3 months, operative management should be considered.

4.2.3 Surgical treatment

Operations for clubfoot are many and varied. The present trend is toward a single combined procedure to release all of the posteromedial contracted tissues and permit open realignment of the talonavicular and talocalcaneal joints. Temporary percutaneous wire fixation is advocated by some surgeons. Postoperative care requires persistent follow-up and prolonged support in a plaster cast, splints, and special shoes. Satisfactory results from posteromedial release are reported in 75%-85% of patients. Triple arthrodesis and other surgical procedures provide salvage for symptomatic patients in whom posteromedial release does not provide good results.

Chapter 5

Spinal Deformity

5.1 Scoliosis

A scoliosis is a lateral curvature of the spine but it is usually accompanied by rotational deformity because the spinal column starts to buckle as it collapses. In the thoracic region the rotation throws the ribs into prominence, producing the cosmetically deforming rib hump, whereas in the lumbar region the same degree of curvature may not be so noticeable. A curve is described as structural or fixed when there is loss of mobility in the involved segment. This usually occurs because of alterations in the shape of the vertebrae and adaptive changes in the soft tissues. A curve is described as mobile when normal flexibility is preserved; such curves are often described as postural, although strictly speaking the terms are not interchangeable. A postural curve is secondary to the position of the body, one of the most common causes being leg length inequality. Curves are also described on the basis of their anatomical site and whether they are primary (major) or secondary (compensatory) to the primary curve in an attempt to maintain spinal balance.

5.2 Idiopathic Scoliosis

This is the common form of but the precise cause remains unknown. Three distinct types are recognized depending on the age at onset.

5.2.1 Infantile idiopathic scoliosis

This is usually noted between birth and 3 years old, although most cases are diagnosed under the age of 1 year. These curves are usually convex to the left, occur in males and are associated with other features of intrauterine moulding (moulded baby syndrome), such as plagiocephaly, torticollis, foot deformity and tightness of hip adductors. The majority resolve without treatment, but 10% – 15% may progress to severe deformity if left untreated. Serial examination and radiographs are therefore important to detect progressive cases. Measurement of the rib–vertebral angle difference is helpful in predicting which cases are likely to progress. Treatment is by the application of serial, corrective plaster jackets. If this is unsuccessful there may be a case for surgical anterior spinal release.

5.2.2 Juvenile idiopathic scoliosis

This occurs between the ages of 3 years and puberty. The distinction between juvenile and early adolescent idiopathic scoliosis is ill defined, although juvenile curves frequently progress and early brace treatment is advisable.

5.2.3 Adolescent idiopathic scoliosis

This is the most common form of scoliosis and occurs at puberty. It is slightly more common in girl and usually convex to the right.

A number of different patterns of curves have been described, depending on site and distinguishing between the major and secondary compensatory curves. Appreciation of these patterns is important in assessing the level and extent of spinal fusion. In general, treatment is required for all curves that are progressing. Not all curves progress and not all at the same rate. The following factors are important in determining progression.

Sex—progression is much more common in girls.

Age—curves are more likely to progress when there is still potential for skeletal growth, and those curves presenting before the menarche have more potential for progression. Ossification of the iliac apophysis (Risser's sign) is helpful in estimating skeletal maturity (Figure 59-5-1).

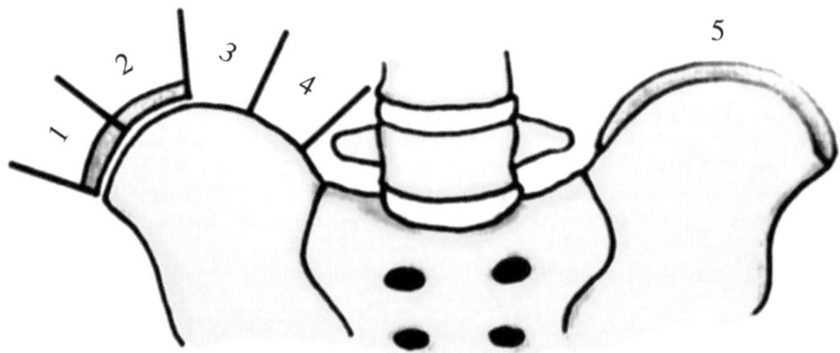

Figure 59-5-1 Skeletal maturityevaluated with Risser grading system in Idiopathic scoliosis

The iliac crest apophysis is divided into four quarters. The fusion of the iliac crest in a lateral to medial manner can be identified radiographically, i. e. stage 0 = none, stage 5 = complete.

Curve pattern—double curves are more likely to progress than single thoracic curves which in turn are more likely to progress than lumbar curves.

Curve magnitude—progression is more likely with curves over 30°.

Miscellaneous—experience suggests that slender patients are more likely to progress.

5.3 Clinical Features

In the history it is important to note those features relevant to curve progression. Also, a history of pain or neurological symptoms should be sought as it is important to exclude other causes of scoliosis, such as spinal tumor. On examination the site, flexibility and appearance of the curve should be noted as well as spinal balance, the head should be centered over the natal cleft. Neurocutaneous stigmata should be sought for example a dimple over the spine or café-au-lait spots. A neurological examination should be carried out and any leg length discrepancy noted. The curve can only be measured accurately by radiography (Figure 59-5-2).

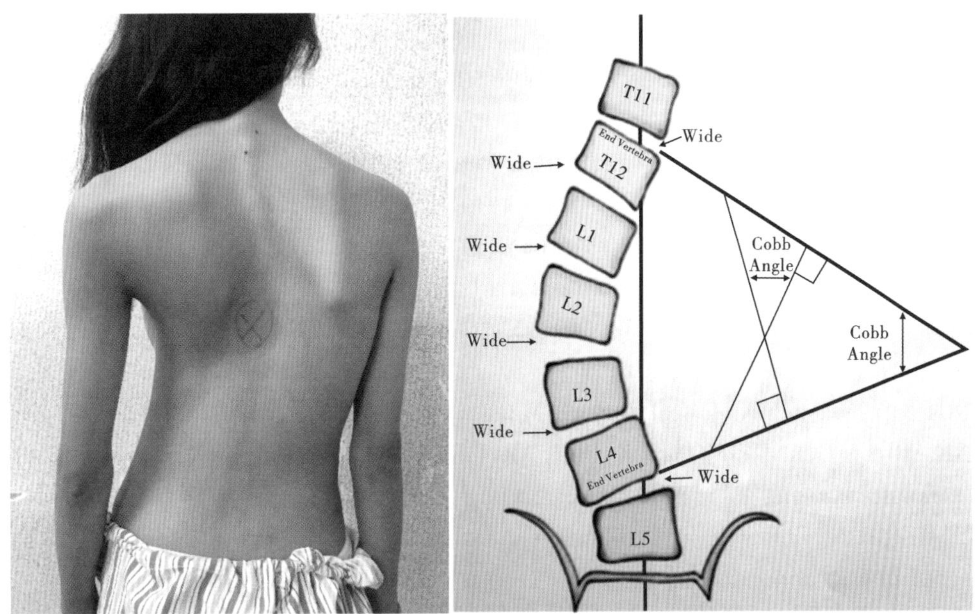

Figure 59-5-2 Idiopathic scoliosis

A. posterior view of patient with idiopathic scoliosis; B. calculation of the Cobb angle. The Cobb angle is formed by the intersection of two lines constructed from the superior and inferior vertebra of the curve.

5.4 Management

Idiopathic scoliosis can only be managed by bracing or surgery. In general, curves that measure less than 30° should be managed conservatively with regular clinical checks and imaging. However, it is important to have an appreciation of which curves are likely to progress, as earlier intervention may be warranted. Once there is clear evidence of progression, bracing is used for curves between 30° and 45°. There are two commonly used types of brace. The Milwaukee incorporates anterior and posterior struts attached to a contoured pelvic support and a neck ring supporting suboccipital pads. The Boston is an underarm brace constructed from a prefabricated pelvic module fitted with individualized pads to correct lumbar and thoraco-lumbar curves. As it can be worn under clothes, it is more acceptable to patients than Milwaukee brace, although it is not suitable for high thoracic curves.

Surgery is generally indicated when:

Bracing is judged likely to be ineffective because:

—the curve is too great, usually over 45°;

—the site of the makes it difficult to brace for example a true double-thoracic curve;

—the curve is fixed.

The basic surgical procedure is a spinal fusion accompanied by instrumentation. The deformity, including the rotational component is corrected keeping the fused segment as short as possible. It is desirable to leave the lumbar mobile, provided the spine is balanced, as this leads to the laest number of long-term complications. An anterior soft-tissue release may be required and instrumentation can be anterior and posterior.

References

[1]TOWNSEND JR C M,BEAUCHAMP R D,EVERS B M,et al. Sabiston Textbook of Surgery[M]. 20th ed. Amsterdam:Elsevier,2016.

[2]GROPPER M A,ERIKSSON L I,FLEISHER L A,et al. Miller's Anesthesia[M]. 9th ed. Amsterdam: Elsevier,2019.

[3]KOUCHOUKOS N T,BLACKSTONE E H,HANLEY F L,et al. Kirklin/Barratt-Boyes Cardiac Surgery [M]. 4th ed. Philadelphia: Saunders,2012.

[4]GROSFELD J L,FONKALSRUD E W,CORAN A G,et al. Pediatric Surgery[M]. 6th ed. Singapore: Elsever,2009.

[5]WINN H R. Youmans Neurological Surgery[M]. 7th ed. Amsterdam:Elsevier,2016.

[6]BRUNICARDI F C,ANDERSON D K,BILLIAR T R,et al. Schwartz's Manual Surgery[M]. 8th ed. New York:McGraw-Hill Education/Medical,2006.

[7]ZOLLINGER R M,ELLISON E C. Zollinger's Atlas of Surgical Operations[M]. 10th ed. New York: McGraw-Hill Education/Medical,2016.

[8]WILLIAMS N S,O'CONNELL P R. Bailey & Love's Short Practice of Surgery[M]. 26th ed. Boca Raton: CRC Press,2013.

[9]YEO C J,MCFADDEN D W,PEMBERTON J H,et al. Shackelford's Surgery of the Alimentary Tract [M]. 7th ed. Philadelphia: Saunders,2012.

[10]JARNAGIN W R. Blumgart's Surgery of the Liver,Biliary Tract and Pancreas[M]. 6th ed. Amsterdam:Elsevier,2016.

[11]SIDAWY A N,PERLER B A. Rutherford Vascular Surgery and Endovascular Therapy[M]. 9th ed. Amsterdam:Elsevier,2018.

[12]WEI A J,KAVOUSSI L R,NOVICK A C,et al. Campbell-Walsh Urology[M]. 10th ed. Philadelphia: Saunders,2011.

[13]AZAR F M,CANALE S T,BEATY J H. Campbell's Operative Orthopaedics[M]. 14th ed. Amsterdam:Elsevier,2020.

[14]GARFIN S R,EISMONT F J,BELL G R,et al. Rothman-Simeone the Spine[M]. 7th ed. Amsterdam: Elsevier,2017.

[15]SALTZMAN C L,ANDERSON R B,COUGHLIN M J. Mann's Surgery of the Foot and Ankle[M]. 9th ed. St. Louis: Mosby,2013.

[16]TJANDRA J J,CLUNIE G J,KAYE A H,et al. Textbook of Surgery[M]. 3rd ed. Hoboken:Wiley-Blackwell,2006.

[17]PHILLIPS F M,LIEBERMAN I H,POLLYJR D W JR. Minimally Invasive Spine Surgery[M]. New York: Springer,2014.

[18]钦伦秀. 外科微创手术基础与临床应用进展[M]. 上海:复旦大学出版社,2017.

[19]赵玉沛,陈孝平. 外科学[M]. 3 版. 北京:人民卫生出版社,2015.

[20]汤锦波. 肌腱外科学[M]. 上海:上海科学技术出版社,2015.

[21]沈周俊. 现代肾上腺外科诊疗学[M]. 上海:上海科学技术出版社,2015.

[22]陈孝平,汪建平. 外科学[M]. 8 版. 北京:人民卫生出版社,2013.

[23]吴孟超,吴在德. 黄家驷外科学 [M]. 7 版. 北京:人民卫生出版社,2008.